Y0-BQW-865

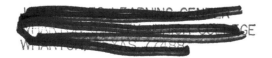

MANUAL OF
LABORATORY IMMUNOLOGY

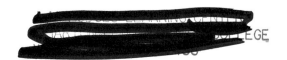

MANUAL OF
LABORATORY IMMUNOLOGY

Linda E. Miller, Ph.D., I(ASCP)SI
Associate Professor, Baccalaureate Program in Medical Technology
Assistant Director, Masters Program in Medical Technology
State University of New York Health Science Center at Syracuse
Syracuse, New York

Harry R. Ludke, B.S., MT(ASCP)
Immunology Supervisor
Division of Clinical Pathology
State University of New York Health Science Center at Syracuse
Syracuse, New York

Julia E. Peacock, M.S., M(ASCP)SI
Department Chairman, Medical Laboratory Technology
Broome Community College
Binghamton, New York

and

Russell H. Tomar, M.D.
Director, Division of Laboratory Medicine
University of Wisconsin Hospital and Clinics
Madison, Wisconsin

74784

SECOND EDITION

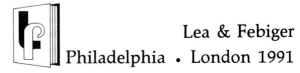
Lea & Febiger
Philadelphia • London 1991

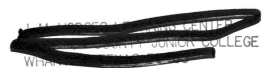

Lea & Febiger
200 Chester Field Parkway
Malvern, PA 19355
U.S.A.
800-444-1785

Lea & Febiger(UK) Ltd.
45a Croydon Road
Beckenham, Kent BR3 3RB
U.K.

Chapter and page reprints may be purchased from
Lea & Febiger in quantities of 100 or more.

Library of Congress Cataloging-in-Publication Data

Manual of laboratory immunology.—2d ed./Linda E. Miller . . . [et
al.]
    p. cm.
   Rev. ed. of: Manual of laboratory immunology/Julia E. Peacock
and Russell H. Tomar. 1980.
   Includes bibliographical references.
   ISBN 0-8121-1319-5
   1. Immunodiagnosis—Laboratory manuals. 2. Immunology—Laboratory
manuals. I. Miller, Linda E. II. Peacock, Julia E. Manual of
laboratory immunology.
   [DNLM: 1. Allergy and Immunology—laboratory manuals.
2. Serology—laboratory manuals. QW 525 M294]
RB46.5.M37 1990
616.07′56—dc20
DNLM/DLC   89-13712
for Library of Congress   CIP

PRINTED IN THE UNITED STATES OF AMERICA

Print number: 5 4 3 2 1

To our colleagues—the medical technologists, students, and residents whose labors are reflected in this publication.

This text is intended to serve as a procedural manual of laboratory assays in humoral and cellular immunology, and has been designed to meet the needs of a wide range of laboratory professionals: Medical Technologists, Educators and Students of Medical Technology, Medical Residents, and Clinical Pathologists. Although cost constraints prevent us from presenting an all inclusive review of clinical immunology procedures, we describe a number of methods that are in widespread use in immunology laboratories. Detailed methods of virtually every procedure performed in the Clinical Immunology Laboratory, Division of Clinical Pathology, SUNY Health Science Center at Syracuse, are presented.

As in the first edition of this manual, for each procedure we have included a brief description of the principle of the test, interpretations of the results in view of procedural limitations, and carefully referenced reviews of background information pertinent to the assay and disease states for which its performance is indicated. References we considered most useful for additional review are indicated on reference lists by an asterisk (*). In the second edition, we have reorganized the topics in the text and have included an index to enable the reader to have easier access to the information in the manual. We have also added an introductory chapter, which we hope will facilitate the roles of educators in instructing students on the basic principles of the immune system.

All the information in this edition has been thoroughly revised and updated, and reflects the dynamic pace at which the field of laboratory immunology has continued to grow. The years since the publication of the first edition have seen the advent and increased usage of new technologies and the discovery of a new disease. Thus, in the second edition, we include new information on double labeling immunofluorescence tests for lymphocyte markers and flow cytometry, AIDS and HIV antibody testing, fluorescence polarization, hepatitis B and EBV panels, immunofixation electrophoresis for detection of paraproteins, tests for autoantibodies, and assays for tumor markers.

We feel that this is both an exciting and challenging time to be involved in immunology, as we continue to watch the field grow exponentially. We hope that this manual will serve as a vehicle in helping professionals to meet some of the challenges of immunology as they affect the clinical laboratory, and welcome any comments on the second edition from our readers.

We would like to take this opportunity to express our gratitude to the individuals who made invaluable contributions to the preparation of this manuscript. First, we wish to extend our appreciation to Joan Benjamin and Judith Kelsey for their diligent labors in typing portions of this manuscript. We thank Charlene Hubbell, Histocompatibility Laboratory Supervisor, Division of Clinical Pathology, SUNY Health Science Center at Syracuse, for consultation on the HLA laboratory procedures. Finally, we thank Brian Harris and Janet Junco for their expert assistance in preparing most of the illustrations for this manual.

Syracuse, New York	Linda E. Miller
Syracuse, New York	Harry R. Ludke
Binghamton, New York	Julia E. Peacock
Madison, Wisconsin	Russell H. Tomar

CONTENTS

INTRODUCTION TO IMMUNOLOGY

The body's ability to defend itself against the myriad of infectious organisms in our environment is caused by the actions of a remarkable organization of interrelated cells and their biologic mediators, collectively known as the immune system.

Responses of the immune system are influenced by a variety of host-related factors (e.g. genetics, age, and general state of health), and environmental factors (e.g. nutrition, living conditions, and rate of exposure to pathogenic agents), as well as the dose and inherent properties of the provoking stimulus.[5,9] These responses may be characterized as (1) nonspecific defenses or (2) specific immune responses.

Nonspecific defenses employ the same biologic machinery against a diverse array of injurious agents, and provide the body's first line of protection. Innate resistance is provided by the skin, mucous membranes, and their secreted products, which serve as both physical and chemical barriers at potential portals of entry into the body.[12,44] In addition, mechanisms such as phagocytosis, natural killer cell activity, and inflammation (see below) may be activated rapidly against the injurious agent, and do not require previous exposure of the host to the stimulus.

A substance that stimulates and subsequently reacts with products of specific immune responses is referred to as an *antigen.* Most antigens are protein molecules, although other types of molecules, including polysaccharides, lipoproteins, and nucleic acids, may also serve as antigens.[9] Various physical and chemical properties of each antigen determine its effectiveness in inducing an immune response.[9]

Specific immune responses are characterized by three fundamental properties:[5,9]

1. *Recognition.* This characteristic refers to the ability of the immune system to recognize the vast numbers of heterogeneous antigens in our environment as foreign, and to distinguish between self and nonself.

2. *Specificity.* This property describes the ability of a single immune response to be directed solely toward the inducing antigen, and not to react with other substances.

3. *Memory.* Memory, or *anamnestic* response, refers to the ability of the immune system to remember an antigen long after the body's initial contact with that antigen. Memory responses are activated rapidly and aggressively upon subsequent exposure to the antigen and provide protection (often lifelong) against the recurrence of a variety of infectious diseases (e.g. measles and mumps); they serve as a basis for immunization.

The specific immune responses are categorized as two major types: (1) *humoral* immune responses, which are mediated by glycoprotein molecules called *antibodies*, which are a product of B lymphocytes and plasma cells (see below); and (2) *cell-mediated* immune responses, which are mediated primarily by T lymphocytes and their secreted products (see below).

CELLS OF THE IMMUNE SYSTEM[33,44,45,53]

The cells of the adult immune system are all derived from undifferentiated stem cells in the bone marrow, and undergo various stages of maturation. Only the mature forms will be discussed below. These cells may be categorized into two major groups based on the morphology of their nuclei (Fig. 1–1):

1. *Mononuclear Cells.* These cells have single, uniformly round or kidney-shaped nuclei, and include the *lymphocytes* and *monocytes.*

2. *Polymorphonuclear Cells* (PMN). These cells have segmented nuclei containing a variable number of connected lobes, and include the *neutrophils, basophils,* and *eosinophils.*

Lymphocytes are the cells central to the specific immune responses. They are round in shape, approximately 6 to 15 μm in diameter, and possess a high nucleus:cytoplasm ratio. With Wright-Giemsa stain, the nucleus stains intensely and has coarse chromatin masses, while the cytoplasm appears pale blue with no granules or a few fine azurophilic granules. Lymphocytes comprise approximately 20 to 50% of the white blood cells in the peripheral blood of a normal adult.[24,45]

There are two major classes of lymphocytes: B lymphocytes (B cells) and T lymphocytes (T cells). B cells constitute approximately 10 to 20% of peripheral blood lymphocytes.[24,44] *B lymphocytes* mature in an organ called the *Bursa of Fabricius* in birds, or its as yet unknown human equivalent. Then they travel to peripheral lymphoid organs (see below), come into contact with antigens, and differentiate further into *plasma cells.* With Wright-Giemsa stain, plasma cells usually appear as oval-shaped cells (7 to 15 μm in diameter), with a round, eccentrically placed nucleus, and intense blue cytoplasm. These are the cells that actually secrete *antibody* molecules into the bloodstream and other body fluids. Plasma cells are rarely seen in the peripheral blood, but are common in the lymph nodes, spleen, and other sites of immune activity.

T cells constitute approximately 60 to 80% of peripheral blood lymphocytes.[24,44] *T lymphocytes* mature in the *thymus,* and circulate to the peripheral lymphoid organs, where they come into contact with antigens, and are transformed into an activated state. Upon activation, these cells produce a number of secretory products, or *lymphokines,* which regulate immune responses or participate in effector functions. T cells have also been divided into subpopulations on

Mononuclear Cells

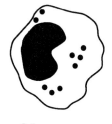

Lymphocyte   Monocyte

Polymorphonuclear Cell

Neutrophil

Fig. 1–1. Cells of the immune system.

the basis of their function and surface phenotype (see also Chap. 4). The major T cell subsets are:

a. *T helper cells (Th).* These cells are responsible for producing lymphokines that positively regulate or "help" B cells in the process of antibody production and aid effector T cells in cell-mediated immune responses. The vast majority of these cells possess the CD4 surface marker.

b. *T suppressor cells (Ts).* These cells are responsible for producing lymphokines that negatively regulate or "suppress" antibody production and cell-mediated immune responses. These cells are positive for the CD8 surface marker. The existence of Ts as a separate lymphocyte population, however, has recently become a subject of controversy.[32]

c. *T inducer cells.* These cells induce the generation of mature T suppressor cells, and are positive for the CD4 surface marker.

d. *T cytotoxic cells (Tcx).* These cells play a role in defense against virus-infected cells and tumor cells, and mediate rejection of foreign graft tissue by secreting lymphokines which have a cytolytic effect on targets of the response. The vast majority of these cells possess the CD8 surface marker.

e. *T delayed type hypersensitivity cells (Td).* These cells secrete lymphokines, which produce an inflammatory response in defense against bacteria, fungi, parasites, and in delayed allergic reactions. They are positive for the CD4 surface marker.

Natural killer (NK) cells are large granular lymphocytes that mediate rapid lysis of virus-infected cells, tumor cells, and foreign graft cells without requiring previous exposure to the targets of this response. They constitute approximately 3% of the peripheral blood lymphocytes.[5] NK cells are sometimes referred to as null cells, since they lack traditional T or B cell surface markers.

Monocytes constitute 3 to 10% of leukocytes in the peripheral blood. These cells are approximately 14 to 21 μm in diameter, with an indented, bilobed nucleus and a dull blue cytoplasm containing occasional dense azurophilic granules and vacuoles. The nucleus:cytoplasm ratio is approximately 1:1. After the cells migrate from the bone marrow to lymphoid and other tissues, they are referred to as *macrophages.* Cells of the macrophage lineage comprise a heterogeneous group, classified on the basis of tissue location, function, and surface phenotype (see Chap. 8). Macrophages (Greek translation, "large eaters")[44] are intimately involved in nonspecific defenses, where they carry out *phagocytosis,* or ingestion of infectious organisms, damaged cells, and debris. This process, and the subsequent destruction of ingested organisms by enzymes contained within the cytoplasmic granules and by metabolic products of the macrophage, are described in detail in Chapter 8. Macrophages also liberate soluble factors (monokines) which perpetuate the inflammatory response. In addition, macrophages play a key role in specific immune responses, where they mediate antigen processing and presentation to T lymphocytes (see below), and liberate monokines which regulate these responses.

Neutrophils comprise 40 to 75% of the leukocytes in the peripheral blood. The mature neutrophil is approximately 10 to 12 μm in diameter, and contains a segmented nucleus with coarse chromatin and 2 to 5 lobes connected by thin nuclear filaments. The cytoplasm stains faint pink with Wright-Giemsa, and has an abundance of fine azurophilic granules. Neutrophils function as the primary effectors of nonspecific defenses, a result of their ability to phagocytize and subsequently kill infectious organisms with enzymes released from their granules. Neutrophils are readily mobilized and are the major cell type present in sites of early acute inflammation (see below).

Eosinophils comprise 1 to 5% of white cells in the peripheral blood. The mature eosinophil is approximately 10 to 12 μm in diameter, and like the neutrophil, contains a segmented nucleus, but usually with only two lobes present. Its most prominent feature with Wright-Giemsa stain is the presence of large orange-red granules scattered abundantly throughout the cytoplasm. Eosinophils play a role in defense against parasites and modulate the inflammatory response. Their numbers are frequently elevated in the blood of patients with parasitic infections or Type I allergic conditions (see below).

Basophils comprise 0 to 2% of peripheral blood leukocytes. The mature basophil is approximately 8 to 10 μm in diameter and contains a segmented nucleus with 2 to 4 lobes. With Wright-Giemsa stain, large bluish black granules are visible in the cytoplasm. Cells bearing similarities to the basophil, called *mast cells,* are present in the tissues. Basophils and mast cells release substances from their granules which promote inflammation and Type I allergic reactions (see below).

TISSUES AND ORGANS OF THE IMMUNE SYSTEM[8,9,44,53]

As mentioned above, all cells of the human immune system derive from undifferentiated stem cells in the bone marrow. In the bone marrow environment, the stem cells become committed to subsequent development into erythrocytes, platelets, monocytes, PMN, or lymphocytes. The lymphocyte-committed stem cells then migrate to one of two *primary lymphoid organs,* where further maturation occurs (Fig. 1–2):

1. The *thymus* is a bilobed capsulated organ located in the upper chest cavity. It reaches its maximum weight at puberty, then atrophies with age. Here, lymphocyte-committed stem cells develop into T lymphocytes under the influence of thymic hormones (e.g. thymosin and thymopoeitin). Immature T cells are located in the cortex, or the layer of the thymus just underneath its outer capsule, while more mature forms are present in the medulla, or inner layer of the thymus.

2. The *Bursa of Fabricius* is a primary lymphoid organ located near the terminal end of the gut in birds. In this organ, lymphocyte-committed progenitors develop into B lymphocytes. An equivalent to this organ has not yet been identified in humans or other mammals, but it has been hypothesized that early B cell development may occur in the liver or yolk sac during fetal life, and the bone marrow or gut-associated lymphoid tissue in the adult.

From the primary lymphoid organs, B and T lymphocytes migrate to the peripheral or *secondary lymphoid organs,* where they encounter antigens, are transformed into an activated state, and become effectors of humoral or cell-mediated immunity (Fig. 1–2). A list of secondary lymphoid organs is found in Table 1–1. Two of these organs are discussed briefly.

The *spleen* is a secondary lymphoid organ located in the left abdominal cavity. In addition to serving as a site of lymphocyte activation, the spleen functions as a filter for the blood by removing effete cells from the circulation, releasing iron back into the blood, and converting hemoglobin to bilirubin. The spleen contains two major areas, the red pulp, which is rich in erythrocytes and macrophages, and the white pulp, or areas of immune activity. Within the white pulp are lymphatic nodules (follicles) that contain B lymphocytes. Follicles containing resting B cells are termed primary follicles, and those containing stimulated B cells are called secondary follicles; the latter contain central clusters of actively dividing B cells called germinal centers. Surrounding the lymphatic nodules are periarterial sheaths containing a predominance of T cells. Usually, the white pulp constitutes about 20% of the total weight of the spleen; however, in highly activated spleens, the white pulp may increase to over 50%, and *splenomegaly,* or enlargement of the spleen, may result.

Lymph nodes (LN) are located in several areas of the body, including the neck and those points where the arms and legs join the trunk of the body. Lymph nodes serve as a filter for the tissue fluid, or lymph, and serve as stations from which lymphocytes can recirculate from blood to lymph and vice versa through vessels of the lymphatic and

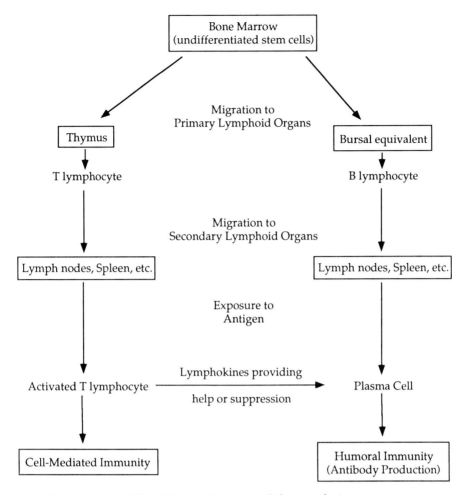

Fig. 1–2. Development of T and B lymphocytes and the specific immune responses.

Table 1–1. Examples of Secondary Lymphoid Organs and Tissues

Spleen
Lymph Nodes
Gut Associated Lymphoid Tissue (GALT)
Tonsils
Peyer's patches
Appendix
Bronchus Associated Lymphoid Tissue (BALT)
Mammary glands
Lacrimal glands
Salivary glands
Blood
Lymph

circulatory systems. The outer region of the LN, just underneath its capsule, is called the cortex, and contains macrophages and B cells which are clustered into primary (resting) and secondary (activated) follicles. T lymphocytes are found in the medulla, or inner region of the LN, and in the paracortical region, just within the cortex. *Lymphadenopathy,* or enlargement of the LN due to cellular infiltration and proliferation, is commonly seen during infection and inflammation.

THE INFLAMMATORY RESPONSE[34,35,44,52]

Inflammation is a nonspecific defense mechanism in which proteins and cells derived from the blood respond to tissue injury. While the cause of injury (e.g. infection, immunopathologic events, exposure to chemicals, radiation, or physical changes) and its bodily location may be varied, the basic manifestations of inflammation are very similar.

The inflammatory response involves a vascular phase and a cellular phase (Fig. 1–3 and discussion below), and is charac-terized by five classical signs—redness, swelling, heat, pain, and loss of function. The *vascular phase* is initiated soon after the injury event, by the release of *immediate phase products* such as histamine from mast cells and basophils, and serotonin from platelets. These chemical mediators are released with-in minutes after the injury, and cause *va-*

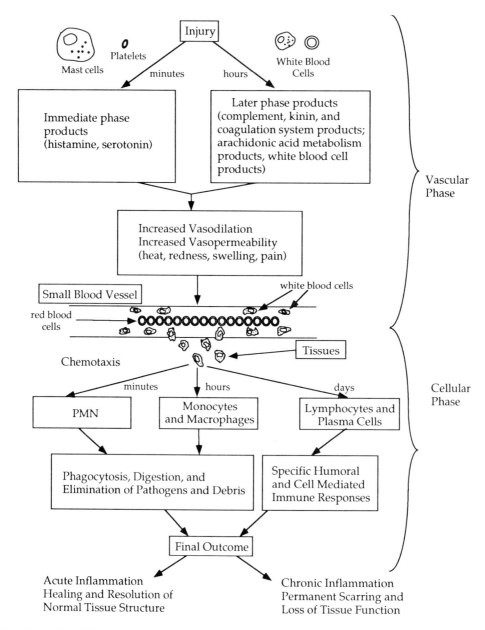

Fig. 1–3. The inflammatory response.

sodilation of small blood vessels in the area, with a resulting increase in blood flow, creating redness and heat, and an increase in *vasopermeability*, with consequent leakage of plasma fluids into the extravascular tissue, and production of edema fluid (i.e. transudates and exudates), creating swelling and pain. These effects may be prolonged by the release of *later phase products* beginning 6 to 12 hours after the injury event, including products of the complement (C3a, C4a, and C5a), kinin (e.g. bradykinin), and coagulation systems (e.g. fibrin split products), products of arachidonic acid metabolism (e.g. prostaglandins, leukotrienes), and products of bacteria, neutrophils, monocytes, and lymphocytes.

The resulting increase in blood flow and loss of vascular fluid leads to the *cellular phase* of inflammation. Red blood cells form stacks (rouleaux) in the center of affected vessels, while the white blood cells are pushed to the periphery (margination). PMN stick to the sides of the vessel (pavementing), move through the endothelial cells of the vessel (diapedesis), and are attracted toward the site of injury (chemotaxis) by products of bacteria, the complement system, damaged tissue, or inflammatory cells. Neutrophils, which begin their mobilization 30 to 60 minutes after the injury, are the major cell type present at the site of *acute inflammation.* There, they phagocytize and digest infectious organisms, cellular debris, and immune complexes, if present. Release of lysosomal enzymes during this process and rapid death of the PMN due to their short lifespan (about 3 days) can result in further tissue damage and the formation of pus. Eosinophils can also participate in phagocytosis and digestion, and furthermore, modulate the inflammatory response through the release of factors which inhibit the action of inflammatory proteins.

Next, migration of macrophages derived from surrounding tissues and from blood monocytes begins under the chemotactic influence of a variety of factors (e.g. bacterial products, the C5a component of complement, and lymphokines). These slower moving cells begin their mobilization about 4 to 5 hours after injury and peak at 12 to 48 hours. Like the neutrophils, macrophages attempt to resolve the process by phagocytosis and killing of infectious organisms, if present, and elimination of necrotic debris. Resolution of the process at this stage marks the end of acute inflammation and results in healing with a return of normal tissue structure. Slightly prolonged inflammation, with greater infiltration of macrophages and eosinophils, and proliferation of fibroblasts, characterize *subacute inflammation.* Failure to resolve the process at this stage results in *chronic inflammation,* which may involve activation of specific immune defenses, as evidenced by infiltration of lymphocytes and plasma cells; complications, including scarring and loss of function, may occur. The final outcome of the inflammatory response depends on the type and dose of injury, and the status of the host's resistance. The involvement of specific immunologic mechanisms can provide a second line of defense which is more directed toward the stimulus and more effective in bringing about resolution of the injury.

HUMORAL IMMUNITY[5,8,9,23,37,39,44,46]

Antibody molecules, a product of B lymphocytes and plasma cells, are central to humoral immune responses. Antibodies circulate throughout the bloodstream and mediate elimination of a variety of infectious organisms and toxins. They are glycoproteins contained primarily in the gamma globulin fraction of serum protein electrophoresis (see Fig. 5–1). Antibodies directed against a specific antigen are prefixed by the term "anti," e.g. antibodies to the cytomegalovirus (CMV) are referred to as anti-CMV, while those directed against the syphilis-causing organism, *Treponema pallidum* are termed anti-*T. pallidum.* While each antibody has a unique specificity for antigen, antibodies possess structural and functional similarities which allow them to be grouped into classes called *immunoglobulins.* There are five major immunoglobulin classes, referred to as IgG, IgM, IgA, IgD, and IgE. The structure and function of each of these is discussed below.

IgG is the predominant immunoglobulin in the adult, constituting approximately 75% of the total immunoglobulins in the blood. In the clinical laboratory, IgG and other immunoglobulins are most commonly detected in the *serum,* or the liquid portion of the blood minus its coagulation factors. Serum concentrations of IgG, IgA, and IgM are listed in Figure 5–6. IgG molecules have a molecular weight of approximately 150,000 daltons and a sedimentation coefficient (i.e. sedimentation rate in an ultracentrifuge, expressed in Svedberg units of time, or 10^{-13} sec.) of 7S. The structure of IgG has been elucidated through biochemical treatments of the molecules and molecular analysis of homogeneous preparations of immunoglobulins derived from malignant plasma cell clones, and may serve as a prototype for the structure of immunoglobulins of the other classes.

Basically, antibodies of the IgG class may be depicted as symmetric "Y-shaped" molecules containing two identical polypeptide "heavy" chains, each with a molecular weight of about 50,000 daltons, and two identical polypeptide "light" chains, each with a molecular weight of about 25,000 daltons (Fig. 1–4). The heavy chains differ in each immunoglobulin class and are designated by Greek letters; those unique to IgG are called gamma (γ) chains. In contrast, the two light chain types, termed kappa (κ) and lambda (λ), are found in all immunoglobulin classes. A single antibody molecule contains either two kappa chains or two lambda chains, never a combination of one kappa and one lambda. The polypeptide chains of the immunoglobulin molecule are held together by a variety of molecular forces, including disulfide bonds, hydrogen bonds, hydrophobic forces, electrostatic forces, and van der Waals forces. Covalent bonds also link the amino acids to carbo-

hydrate moieties, which in the case of IgG, constitute approximately 4% of the molecule.

Laboratory treatment of the immunoglobulins with the enzymes papain or pepsin digests the molecule into discrete fragments commonly referred to by immunologists (Fig. 1–4). Papain cleaves the IgG molecule just above the set of disulfide bonds holding the two heavy chains together, creating at the amino terminal, two identical *Fab* fragments, which each contain an *a*ntigen *b*inding site, and at the carboxyl terminal, one *Fc* fragment, which *c*rystallizes spontaneously at 4° C in some species and is responsible for many of the biologic functions of the molecule (see below). Pepsin cleaves the molecule just below the disulfide bonds connecting the two heavy chains together, resulting in the production of one major fragment, $F(ab')_2$, which contains two antigen binding sites.

After comparing amino acid sequences of different antibody molecules, it was found that the first 110 amino acids at the amino terminal of the molecule showed much variability. This region is thus called the *variable* region, and contains the domains, V_H (on heavy chains) and V_L (on light chains) (Fig. 1–4). The unique amino acid sequence here and its resulting three-dimensional conformation are essential to the formation of the antigen binding site and give the molecule its specificity for antigen. Because of its symmetry, IgG contains two antigen binding sites, or a valency of 2. The remaining portion of the molecule contains a relatively constant amino acid sequence from one antibody to the next, and is referred to as the *constant* region. This region includes the C_L region (on light chains) and the C_H region (on heavy chains); the latter is further divided into the C_{H1} domain in the Fab region and the C_{H2} and C_{H3} domains, in the Fc region. Differences in the constant regions have been used to further divide IgG into four subclasses—IgG1, IgG2, IgG3, and IgG4. In addition, the amino acid sequences of the immunoglobulins are classified into

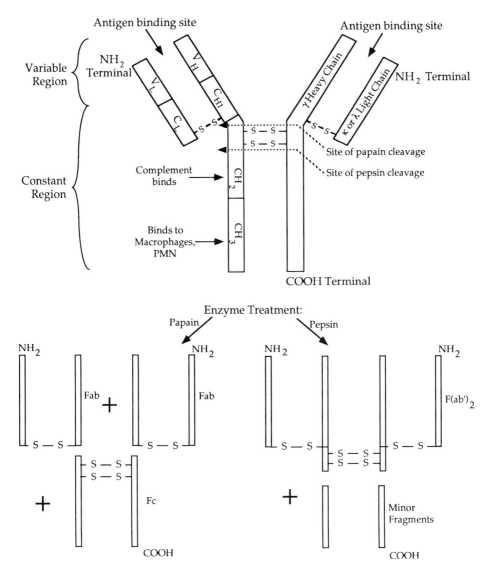

Fig. 1–4. Structure of IgG as related to function and fragments created by enzyme treatment.

three major groups as follows: (1) *isotypes* are defined as amino acid sequences, present in the constant regions of the heavy and light chains, which are identical in all members of a given species; (2) *allotypes* are genetically controlled sequences in the constant regions of the heavy and light chains, which are shared by some members of a species, but differ in other members (e.g. Gm allotypes on IgG heavy chains); and (3) *idiotypes* are unique amino acid sequences in the variable regions of the heavy and light chains, which contribute directly to the antigen binding specificity of the antibody molecule.

While the antigen specificity lies within the Fab portion of the antibody molecule, the Fc portion is responsible for many of the biologic functions of the antibody important to host defense against antigens. The major functions of IgG are:

1. *Binding of complement.* Complement is a group of proteins, found in the blood and

other body fluids, which can interact with antigen-antibody complexes in a series of steps called the Classical Pathway of Complement, to produce lysis of certain antigens (e.g. bacteria) and a number of other biologic effects (e.g. chemotaxis, enhanced phagocytosis, enhanced inflammation) (see Chap. 6 for details). The initial step of this process involves the binding of the C1q component of complement to the Fc portions of two adjacent IgG molecules which have already bound to antigen (Fig. 1–5a). Of the IgG subclasses, the IgG3 subclass is best able to bind complement, followed by IgG1 and IgG2; IgG4 is unable to bind complement.

2. *Opsonization.* Opsonization, or the enhancement of phagocytosis, can occur when IgG serves as a bridge between the antigen and the phagocytic cell (Fig. 1–5b). The Fab portion of the molecule binds to the antigen, while the Fc region binds to receptors on the surface of macrophages and PMN for the Fc portion of IgG. The resulting contact increases the efficiency of phagocytosis. The IgG1 and IgG3 subclasses are able to mediate this function. Opsonization may also occur as a result of complement activation by IgG-antigen complexes, with subsequent binding of the C3b component of complement to receptors on the surface of macrophages or PMN (Fig. 1–5b).

3. *Antibody dependent cellular cytotoxicity (ADCC).* In the process of ADCC, binding of antigen to the Fab portion of IgG is followed by binding of the Fc portion of the molecule to receptors on the surface of macrophages or natural killer cells (Fig. 1–5c). Enzymes are released from granules of the effector cells and destroy the antigen. In this situation, the natural killer cell is often referred to as a killer cell.

4. *Neutralization of toxins.* Binding of specific antibody (i.e. anti-toxin) to a bacterial toxin antigen can result in inactivation of that toxin, or inhibition of its pathologic effects (Fig. 1–5d).

5. *Crossing the placenta.* IgG is the only immunoglobulin that is capable of crossing the placenta. While all subclasses of IgG can mediate this function, IgG2 is least efficient. This function is important in the transferring of immunity from mother to infant and lasts for approximately the first 6 months after birth, as the level of maternal IgG decreases with the half-life of this molecule (about 23 days). In the meantime, the infant's own immune system has begun to produce IgG (Fig. 1–6).

6. *Agglutination and precipitation.* Functions observed in vitro, such as the agglutination of particulate antigens, or the precipitation of soluble antigens, occur when a large number of antibody molecules complex with their corresponding antigen to form a lattice-like structure (see Precipitation and Agglutination, Chap. 3). These processes may also have significance in vivo under certain physiologic conditions.

IgM is the largest of the immunoglobulins, with a molecular weight of about 900,000 daltons and a sedimentation coefficient of 19S. It is a pentamer, consisting of five basic subunits (i.e. two heavy chains bound to two light chains); the subunits are linked together by a protein called the J ("joining") chain (Fig. 1–7a). The heavy chains of IgM are called mu (μ) chains, and are longer than the γ heavy chains of IgG, because they contain an additional domain, C_{H4}, located at the carboxy terminal of the peptide chain. IgM has two subclasses, IgM1 and IgM2, and is highly susceptible to chemical reduction by 2-mercaptoethanol, which digests the numerous disulfide bonds found in the molecule. Functions of IgM include the following:

1. *Binding of complement.* Of all the immunoglobulin classes, IgM is the most efficient in performing this function, because of its numerous Fc portions. Only one IgM molecule is required for complement activation.

2. *Neutralization of toxins* (see above).

3. *Agglutination.* IgM is much more efficient than IgG in performing this function, since it has five functional antigen binding sites (theoretically there are ten but in real-

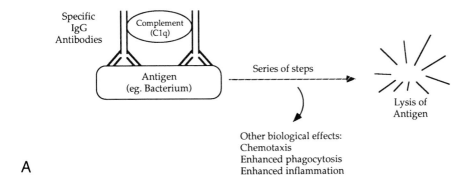

A

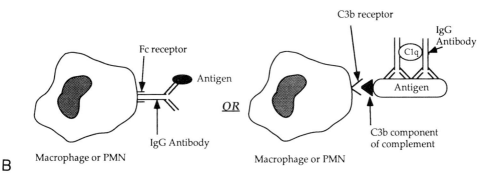

B

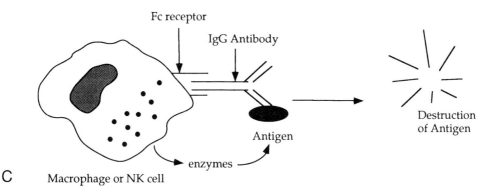

C

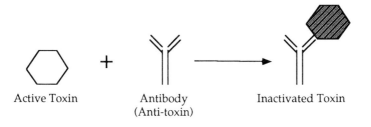

D

Fig. 1–5. Functions of IgG. (A) Binding of complement; (B) Opsonization; (C) Antibody-dependent cellular cytotoxicity (ADCC); (D) Neutralization of toxins.

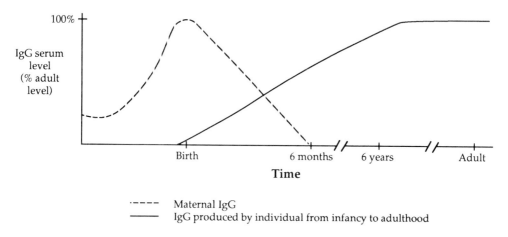

<!-- Legend -->
----- Maternal IgG
——— IgG produced by individual from infancy to adulthood

Fig. 1–6. Serum IgG levels during human development.

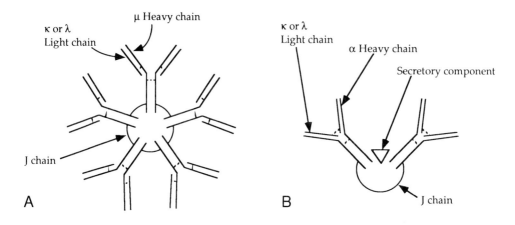

Fig. 1–7. Structures of IgM (A) and secretory IgA (B).

ity, only five of these sites are functional, probably because of the steric hindrance created when multiple antigens are bound).

4. *Early production.* IgM is the first immunoglobulin to be produced by an individual following exposure to an antigen (Fig. 1–11). IgM is also the first immunoglobulin to be produced by the infant during its development. Since maternal IgM cannot cross the placenta, IgM in the infant's serum is known to have originated solely from the infant (unlike IgG, which is primarily maternal in early infancy); detection of IgM antibodies in infant serum is therefore a valuable diagnostic aid in suspected cases of congenital infection, in which the infant will produce IgM antibodies in response to a pathogen.

IgA is present in the serum as a monomer, or one basic subunit of two heavy chains bound to two light chains. It has a molecular weight of about 170,000 daltons and a sedimentation coefficient of 7S. The heavy chains of IgA are called alpha (α) chains.

More importantly, IgA is the predominant immunoglobulin in the body's secretions, e.g. the saliva, tears, sweat, and breast milk, as well as the respiratory, intestinal, and genital secretions. Its main function, therefore, is thought to be binding of antigens at potential portals of entry into the body and preventing their adherence to mucous membranes and subsequent invasion into the body. In addition, ingestion of IgA in breast milk confers immunity from mother to infant.

In the body secretions, IgA occurs primarily as a dimer, or two basic subunits, held together by the J chain (Fig. 1–7b). This molecule has a molecular weight of about 390,000 daltons and a sedimentation coefficient of 9S. In addition, the dimer contains a protein known as the *secretory component* or *transport (T) piece,* synthesized by epithelial cells in the mucous membranes. The secretory component is thought to protect the IgA dimer from destruction by proteolytic enzymes and aid in its transport across mucous membranes and into the secretions. There are two subclasses of IgA, IgA1 and IgA2; IgA2 is the predominant immunoglobulin in the secretions, and unlike the other immunoglobulin classes, has disulfide bonds which link its light chains, rather than its heavy chains, together.

IgD exists as a monomer, with delta (δ) heavy chains, a molecular weight of about 150,000 daltons, and a sedimentation coefficient of 7S. It is found in low levels in the serum (approximately 3 to 5 mg/dL), and its function there is unknown. Like other immunoglobulin classes, IgD is also found on the surface membranes of B lymphocytes, where it serves as a receptor for antigen (see below).

IgE exists as a monomer with epsilon (ε) heavy chains, a molecular weight of about 200,000 daltons, and a sedimentation coefficient of 8S. It has the lowest serum concentration of any immunoglobulin class, comprising only about 0.004% of the total serum immunoglobulins (concentration, 17 to 450 ng/mL). Like the μ chain of IgM,

the ε chain of IgE contains an additional domain, C_{H4}. The ε C_{H4} region is capable of binding to Fc receptors on mast cells and basophils, an interaction that stimulates the development of Type I allergic reactions (see Chap. 10). IgE is also thought to play a role in defense against parasitic infections, and is elevated in the serum of individuals with parasitic infections or Type I allergic disorders.

The specificity of the antibody molecule for a particular antigen is determined at the level of the gene.[6,27,51] Within the undifferentiated stem cell exist a set of genes capable of coding for an estimated 10^6 to 10^8 antibody molecules. The genes coding for the immunoglobulin heavy chains are present on chromosome 14 and are organized into the three sets of genes coding for the variable portion of the immunoglobulin—approximately 500 to 1000 *Variable* (Vh) genes, approximately 5 *Diversity* (D) genes and approximately 5 *Joining* (J) genes—and a separate set of *Constant* (C) genes coding for the constant region of each type of heavy chain (Fig. 1–8). (The constant gene regions can be further divided into separate genes coding for each immunoglobulin subclass.) During the process of B cell maturation, most of these genes are deleted at the DNA and RNA levels through DNA recombinations and RNA splicing, so that in the mature B lymphocyte, a rearranged gene sequence exists such that one Vh gene is linked to one D gene, one J gene, and one C gene (Fig. 1–8). The order of recombinations is as follows: (a) D + J = DJ; (b) Vh + DJ = VhDJ; (c) VhDJ + C_μ = VhDJC$_\mu$. Through analysis of these rearrangements, one can determine the stage of B cell maturation, a laboratory observation which has been extremely useful in the typing of B cell malignancies. Each mature B cell then, is capable of producing one type of antibody molecule with a single specificity for antigen. Since the C_μ gene is located closest to the J region, VhDJ will first combine with C_μ to produce the μ heavy chain; thus, IgM is the first antibody to be

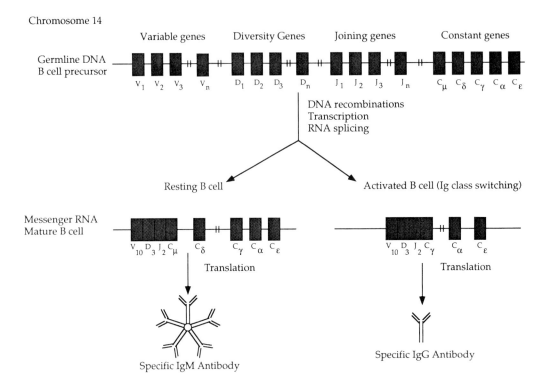

Fig. 1–8. Schematic diagram of genes coding for the immunoglobulin heavy chains.

produced. During B cell activation by antigen, differentiation continues, and the genes may undergo further rearrangement, resulting in the placement of the J gene next to a C gene coding for a different heavy chain; consequently, immunoglobulin production switches from IgM to another immunoglobulin class. Similar gene organizations and rearrangements occur for the immunoglobulin light chains, except that D genes are not present. Genes for the kappa chain are present on chromosome 2, and include Vκ genes, J genes, and one Cκ gene; genes for the lambda chain are on chromosome 22 and include Vλ genes, J genes, and one Cλ gene. Kappa gene rearrangements occur prior to lambda gene rearrangements.

The large variety of possible V,J, (D), and C gene combinations, coupled with somatic gene mutations, and various possible combinations of heavy and light chains at the protein level, create the diversity necessary for the body to respond to the estimated 10^8 antigens in our environment, without overwhelming the body's DNA load.

Each B lymphocyte will express immunoglobulin of the appropriately coded specificity on its surface membrane prior to its exposure to antigen. This surface immunoglobulin (sIg) serves as a receptor for its corresponding antigen. According to the clonal selection theory,[3] following exposure of the body to an antigen, the antigen will selectively bind to B cells possessing the appropriate sIg, stimulating those B cells to proliferate into a clone of identical cells and to differentiate into plasma cells that secrete the antibody specific for the inducing antigen into the body environment.

Activation of the B lymphocyte by antigen can occur by one of two different mechanisms:

1. *T cell independent antibody responses.* These are characterized by three major features: (a) no requirement for T cell "help," (b)

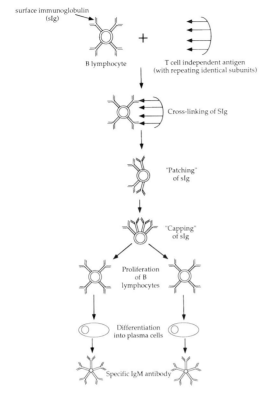

Fig. 1-9. Mechanism of T cell independent antibody response.

production of IgM antibody only, and (c) failure to develop a memory response. This T cell independent mechanism can be induced only by certain antigens, notably large polymers with repeating identical subunits. Many of these antigens function as polyclonal activators (mitogens) capable of stimulating many clones of B lymphocytes (e.g. lipopolysaccharide, *Staphylococcus aureus*—strain Cowan I). The mechanism of T cell independent antibody production is illustrated in Figure 1-9. Briefly, the subunits of the antigen bind to antigen binding sites on the sIg. Cross-linking of the sIg molecules stimulates the B cells to proliferate into a clone of identical cells and mature further into plasma cells. This process is thought to involve "patching" and "capping" of sIg receptors to one pole of the cell (Fig. 1-9), and subsequent ingestion or shedding of the sIg molecules by the cell.

Plasma cells thus lack sIg but contain cytoplasmic immunoglobulin, and secrete IgM antibody molecules into the body fluids.

2. *T cell dependent antibody responses.*[31,50] The vast majority of antigens stimulate antibody production by this mechanism, whose major features are (a) requirement of "help" from T helper lymphocytes, (b) production of antibody of any immunoglobulin class, and (c) induction of immunologic memory. The steps of this mechanism are illustrated in Figure 1-10 and outlined below.

a. *Processing of the antigen by the macrophage.*[4] Initial contact with the antigen is performed by macrophages, which process the antigen into a form which is more presentable to T lymphocytes. Antigen processing is thought to involve: (1) phagocytosis of the antigen by the macrophage, followed by (2) partial degradation of the antigen by macrophage enzymes, in order to expose parts of the antigen (*antigenic determinants* or *epitopes*) which can bind to lymphocyte receptors, and (3) placement of the partially degraded antigen on the macrophage cell surface adjacent to a genetically determined marker called HLA-D (or Ia) (see Chap. 13).

b. *Presentation of the processed antigen to a T helper lymphocyte.* Next, the macrophage presents the complex of processed antigen/Ia to a T helper lymphocyte. Specificity is achieved through binding of the complex to a specific T cell receptor (TcR) for antigen, found in association with the CD3 molecule (see Chap. 4) on the T cell surface membrane. The TcR is a glycoprotein dimer which contains structural similarities to the immunoglobulin molecule, with variable and constant domains.[2,30] The TcR dimer found on mature T cells consists of a 49 kilodalton alpha chain linked to a 43 kd beta chain through disulfide bonds. These chains are coded for by V, D, J, and C genes on chromosomes 7 and 14, and undergo rearrangements at the DNA and RNA levels similar to those of the immunoglobulin genes to

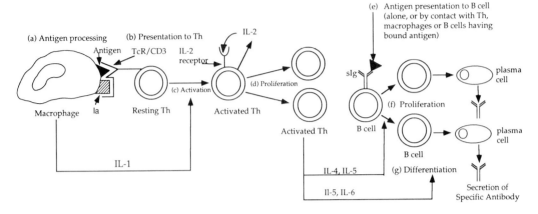

Fig. 1–10. Mechanism of T cell dependent antibody response.

create diversity among T cell clones, each clone bearing specificity for a single antigen.[14]

c. *Production of the monokine, Interleukin-1 (IL-1) by the macrophage* (see also Chap. 7—Cytokines). IL-1 induces T helper cells (Th) that have bound processed antigen to transform from a "resting" to an "activated" state. In the activated state, Th undergo a series of biochemical changes,[25] produce large quantities of lymphokines, including Interleukin-2 (IL-2), and acquire surface membrane receptors for IL-2, as well as surface Ia molecules. Activated Th also secrete other lymphokines that stimulate B cells (see below).

d. *Proliferation of the activated Th.* Binding of IL-2 to receptors for IL-2 on the membrane of the Th, causes the Th to proliferate in an autocrine stimulatory response. The result is the production of a clone of identical Th specific for the inducing antigen, and thus, amplification of the response.

e. *Contact of B cells with the antigen.* This contact may occur through direct binding of the antigen to sIg molecules on B cells with the appropriate antigen specificity, or by presentation of the antigen to the B cell sIg by contact with Th, macrophages, or other B cells which have bound the antigen on their surface.

f. *Proliferation of B lymphocytes.* The B cell that has contacted antigen is stimulated to proliferate into a clone of identical cells specific for the inducing antigen, under the influence of the Interleukin-4 (IL-4) and Interleukin-5 (IL-5) lymphokines, released from activated Th.

g. *Differentiation of B cells into plasma cells and secretion of immunoglobulin.* This occurs under the influence of the lymphokines, IL-5 and Interleukin-6 (IL-6), released from activated Th. Patching, capping, and internalization or shedding of sIg may be involved in triggering B cell proliferation and differentiation, as described above (see T cell independent antibody responses). The resulting plasma cells produce and secrete antibody molecules specific for the inducing antigen into the body environment, where they can participate in bringing about elimination of specific antigens via the mechanisms of humoral immunity discussed above.

Instead of differentiating into plasma cells, some of the stimulated B cells will develop into mature, long-lived "memory" cells, which can be activated rapidly upon a second or subsequent exposure to the same antigen. The effectiveness of this memory response, also referred to as the secondary or anamestic response, provides long-lived protection to the individual against disease caused by that antigen. The pattern of antibody development in a typical memory response is illustrated in Figure 1–11, and is compared to that seen in the primary response, which occurs after an individual's first exposure to the antigen. In the primary response, the time required for lymphocyte activation after initial exposure to the antigen results in a lag period before any antibody is produced. The length of the lag will vary with the type and dose of the antigen, as well as with host-related factors, but is usually about 3 to 4 days. The first immunoglobulin to be produced is IgM, which quickly peaks and plateaus, then decreases over the next few weeks. The production of IgG begins about 1 to 2 weeks after exposure, rises to higher levels, peaks within a few weeks, and decreases gradually over the next few months. In the secondary response, a shorter lag period is observed. The development and subsequent decline of IgM are about the same as in the primary response, but IgG reaches much higher levels, which decrease very gradually, often

over a period of several years. The antibodies in the secondary response also have a higher affinity (or binding ability) for antigen.

The typical responses described above are central to the detection of serum antibodies in the clinical laboratory. Because IgM is produced early and is of short duration, the presence of IgM antibody to a particular antigen (e.g. the hepatitis A virus), usually indicates a current exposure to the antigen (e.g. acute hepatitis A). IgG antibody, which decreases gradually over time, may signify either a current or a past exposure. Acute disease is strongly suspected, though, if there is a 4-fold increase in IgG antibody concentration in different serum samples collected over time, or if a high IgG antibody concentration is present in a single sample. If the serum sample is taken too early after antigen exposure, the specific antibody may be absent and yield false negative results, suggesting the absence of a particular disease when it is actually present.

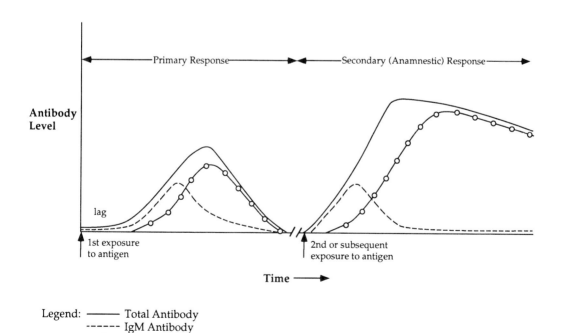

Fig. 1–11. Primary and secondary antibody responses.

CELL-MEDIATED IMMUNITY[16,29,44]

Cell-mediated immunity (CMI) involves effector mechanisms carried out by T lymphocytes and their products (lymphokines). CMI responses are critical to defense against infectious organisms, rejection of foreign grafts, tumor immunity, and delayed type hypersensitivity reactions.

Cytotoxic T cells (Tcx) are principal effectors of immunity against viruses, graft rejection, and tumor immunity. The mechanism of Tcx activation involves a series of steps which culminate in lysis of the appropriate target cells (e.g. virus-infected cells, graft tissue, tumor cells), as follows (Fig. 1–12):

1. Processing of the antigen and presentation to Th. This step is essentially the same as that discussed under *Humoral Immunity, T cell dependent antibody responses*, and may be stimulated by cell-bound antigens released from target cells into the body environment.

2. Release of IL-1 by the antigen-exposed macrophages.

3. Activation of Th and release of IL-2.

4. Binding of IL-2 to receptors on the surface of activated Th, resulting in proliferation of the activated Th and amplification of the response.

5. Generation of mature Tcx. The maturation of Tcx occurs under the influence of IL-2.

6. Direct cell-cell contact between the Tcx and the target cell. This contact is mediated through binding of an antigen specific TcR on the Tcx surface membrane to the appropriate antigen on the target cell. The binding is strengthened by simultaneous binding of the CD8 molecule on the Tcx surface membrane to a Class I HLA molecule on the surface of the target cell (see Chap. 13). Binding of the CD8 positive Tcx is restricted to target cells bearing the same type of Class I HLA molecule as that present in the host from which the Tcx were derived. Rarely, CD4(+) Tcx have been described which bind to self Class II HLA molecules on target cells.[7]

7. Release of cytolytic proteins from the Tcx. Binding of the Tcx to its target cell stimulates the release of cytolytic proteins (e.g. perforin, lymphotoxins, serine dependent proteases) from cytoplasmic granules within the Tcx, into the immediate environment of the target cell.[16] These proteins mediate destruction of the target cell by

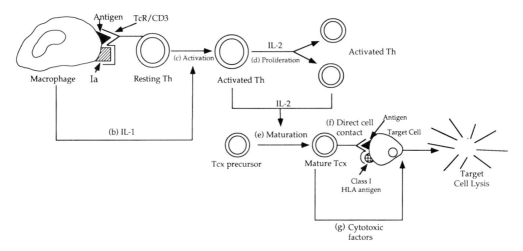

Fig. 1–12. Mechanism of cytotoxic T cell responses.

producing pores in the target cell membrane, causing alterations in cell permeability and osmotic swelling, and target cell lysis.

Cell-mediated immunity can also involve delayed type hypersensitivity T cells (Td), which release lymphokines that produce an inflammatory response important in defense against a variety of infectious organisms. This response can also cause pathologic consequences to the host under certain circumstances. The mechanism of this response is discussed below under *Hypersensitivity Reactions.*

NATURAL KILLER CELL ACTIVITY[10,16,29,36,49]

Like Tcx, NK cells are effector cells which mediate cytolysis of tumor cells, virus-infected cells, and foreign graft cells. Unlike Tcx, however, NK cells do not require previous sensitization to target cell antigens in order to perform this function. The cytolytic mechanism of NK cells is similar to the final steps of Tcx-mediated cytolysis and involves the following (Fig. 1–13):

1. Direct binding of the NK cell to the target by as yet unidentified recognition structures on the surface membranes of the NK cell and target cell;

2. Release of cytotoxic factors (e.g. natural killer cytotoxic factors (NKCF), serine dependent proteases, perforin) from NK cell granules into the target cell environment; and

3. The formation of pores within the target cell membrane, leading to a change in permeability, and ultimately, target cell lysis.

A more recently identified cell type, termed LAK (lymphokine activated killer cell) can be generated by pretreatment of peripheral blood lymphocytes with IL-2. LAK cells bear similarities to NK cells, but may be more clinically relevant because they display a higher cytotoxic capability and are able to lyse freshly derived tumor cells from patients, whereas NK cells can only lyse tumor cells that have been maintained in in vitro continuous cell lines.[21,42,43]

IMMUNOREGULATION[9,23,39,44]

Regulation of the immune system is thought to occur via a variety of mechanisms. A lengthy discussion of these mechanisms is beyond the scope of this discussion. Briefly, they are:

1. *Positive regulation by Th and negative regulation by Ts,* as mentioned above. These cells mediate their functions via networks of cellular interactions and soluble mediators,[18-20,50] and serve as a check and balance system for each other. Specific suppression of the immune system toward a particular antigen is called *immunologic tolerance.*[9,23,39,44]

2. *Regulation by cytokines.* These soluble factors are released by lymphocytes, monocytes, NK cells, and PMN.[15,50] Their effects

(a) Binding of NK cell to target cell

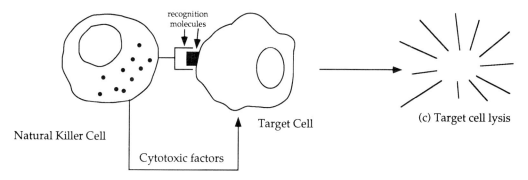

Fig. 1–13. Mechanism of natural killer cell mediated cytolysis.

are discussed in detail in *Cytokines*, Chapter 7.

3. *Anti-idiotypic antibodies.*[26] Activation of an immune response is thought to result in the production of antibodies to the idiotype portion of the newly produced antibody molecules. These anti-idiotype antibodies can bind to sIg on the appropriate B cells and to TcR on the appropriate T cells, and depending on their precise structure, may either (a) inhibit continuation of the immune response by blocking the attachment of antigen to these receptors; or (b) enhance the immune response by producing the same effects as bound antigen. This type of check and balance system is thought to involve a complex network of cellular interactions.

ACQUISITION OF IMMUNITY[9,46]

In general, humoral and cell-mediated immune responses can be acquired by one of three ways:

1. *Active Immunity.* This type of immunity is acquired by direct stimulation of an individual's own immune system, either by natural exposure to an antigen or by artificial exposure induced by vaccination. This type of immunity requires time to develop after exposure, but once produced, is long-lived, since memory cells are generated during the process.

2. *Passive Immunity.* This type of immunity is acquired through transfer of soluble mediators of immunity (i.e. antibodies, cytokines) from an immune individual to a nonimmune individual. It may occur naturally, from mother to infant (i.e. passive transfer of IgG antibodies through the placenta, or IgA antibodies through breast milk), or artificially (e.g. administration of gamma globulin containing Hepatitis A antibodies to an individual recently exposed to the Hepatitis A virus in order to prevent development of the disease). This type of immunity offers immediate protection to the nonimmune recipient, but is temporary, declining over time with the half-life of the soluble mediator.

3. *Adoptive Immunity.* This type of immunity is acquired through the passive transfer of lymphocytes from an immune individual, or lymphocytes immunized in vitro, to a nonimmune individual (e.g. thymic grafts to patients with T cell immune deficiencies, LAK cell administration to tumor patients[42,43]). It provides immediate, potentially long-lived immunity to the recipient.

DISEASES OF THE IMMUNE SYSTEM

Immunodeficiency Diseases[38,40,41,46,48]

Immunodeficiency diseases are diseases in which an individual is deficient in one or more of the following basic components of the immune system: (1) B lymphocytes, (2) T lymphocytes, (3) phagocytic cells, (4) the complement system. The diseases may be classified as (1) *primary*, i.e. congenitally derived, or (2) *secondary*, i.e. acquired as a result of other factors (e.g. infection, malignancy, autoimmune disease, protein losing states, malnutrition, burns, diabetes, immunosuppressive treatments). A partial list of immunodeficiency diseases is found in Table 1–2. Some of these diseases are discussed throughout this manual.

Immunoproliferative Diseases[13,22,28,46]

Immunoproliferative diseases are diseases in which there is a malignant proliferation of one of the key cells of the immune system. Immunoproliferative diseases include: (1) leukemias, or malignancies involving T or B lymphocytes, null cells, or monocytes in the blood, (2) lymphomas, or malignancies involving lymphoid cells within solid tissue, and (3) monoclonal gammopathies, which involve proliferation of malignant plasma cells and production of a large quantity of homogeneous immunoglobulin protein (i.e. monoclonal antibody; paraprotein) from the clone of malignant cells. The classification of leukemias and lymphomas[12,13,17,45] has been greatly aided by the identification of cell surface markers on the malignant cell type, as discussed in Chapter

Table 1–2. Examples of Immunodeficiency Diseases

Primary Component of Immune System Affected	Examples
B Cells	Bruton's congenital hypogammaglobulinemia Selective IgA deficiency Transient hypogammaglobulinemia of infancy Common variable immunodeficiency[a]
T Cells	DiGeorge syndrome Chronic mucocutaneous candidiasis
Complex (B and T cells)	Acquired immunodeficiency syndrome (AIDS) Severe combined immunodeficiency disease Ataxia telangiectasia Nezelof's syndrome Wiskott Aldrich syndrome
Phagocytic	Chronic granulomatous disease Chediak Higashi syndrome Job's syndrome Myeloperoxidase deficiency
Complement	Congenital deficiencies in individual complement components (e.g. C3 deficiency, C8 deficiency) Hereditary angioedema Acquired deficiencies in individual complement components

[a] May also involve T cell abnormalities.

Table 1–3. Monoclonal Gammopathies and Their Associated Paraproteins

Disease	Monoclonal Protein
Multiple myeloma	IgG or IgA; free κ or λ light chains; rarely, IgD or IgE
Waldenström's macroglobulinemia	IgM; some cases also have free κ or λ light chains
Heavy chain diseases	γ, α, or μ heavy chains

4. Essential to the clinical evaluation of monoclonal gammopathies is the identification of monoclonal proteins, as discussed in Chapter 5. A list of monoclonal gammopathies and their associated paraproteins can be found in Table 1–3.

Hypersensitivity Reactions[5,8,11,39,44,47]

In contrast to the immunodeficiency diseases in which immunologic function is subnormal, hypersensitivity reactions are characterized by a heightened state of immune responsiveness. While the basic mechanisms underlying hypersensitivity reactions are essential aspects of host defense, chronic activation of these mechanisms or direction of the mechanisms toward an in-appropriate antigen can result in hypersensitivity with pathologic consequences to the host.

Four basic mechanisms of hypersensitivity have been classified by Gell and Coombs[11] as follows:

Type I—Anaphylactic Hypersensitivity

Type II—Antibody Dependent Cytotoxic Hypersensitivity

Type III—Complex Mediated Hypersensitivity

Type IV—Cell Mediated Hypersensitivity

Types I, II, and III hypersensitivity involve antibodies, are manifested within a few minutes to a few hours after exposure to the inducing antigen, and are classified as *immediate hypersensitivity reactions.* Type IV hypersensitivity involves T cells, is observed 24 to 48 hours after antigen exposure, and is therefore classified as *delayed type hypersensitivity.*

Some examples of clinical conditions occurring as a result of the hypersensitivity mechanisms are listed in Table 1–4. Each of these mechanisms is outlined below.

TYPE I HYPERSENSITIVITY. The basic mechanism of type I hypersensitivity is il-

Table 1–4. Examples of Clinical Conditions Associated with Hypersensitivity Reactions

Hypersensitivity Type	Clinical Condition
Type I (Anaphylactic)	Allergic rhinitis Allergic (extrinsic) asthma Allergic urticaria Systemic anaphylaxis
Type II (Antibody dependent cytotoxic)	Erythroblastosis fetalis Autoimmune hemolytic anemia Autoimmune thrombocytopenic purpura Hashimoto's disease Graves' disease Goodpasture's syndrome
Type III (Complex mediated)	Arthus reaction Farmer's lung Pigeon fancier's disease Serum sickness Rheumatoid arthritis Systemic lupus erythematosus
Type IV (Cell mediated; delayed type)	Contact dermatitis Tuberculosis Delayed type skin testing responses

lustrated in Figure 1–14. The mechanism is outlined briefly below and discussed in more detail in Chapter 10. Basically, type I hypersensitivity involves:

1. Stimulation of specific IgE antibody production by the inducing antigen (allergen).

2. Binding of IgE to Fc receptors on mast cells and basophils.

3. A subsequent exposure to the allergen with binding of the allergen to the cell-bound IgE molecules, causing a cross-linking of these IgE receptors.

4. Release of chemical mediators (e.g. histamine, bradykinin, leukotrienes) from

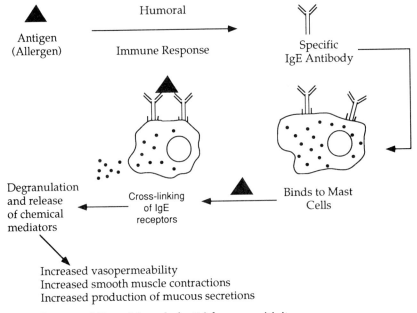

Fig. 1–14. Mechanism of Type I (anaphylactic) hypersensitivity.

granules within the mast cells and basophils.

5. Effects of the chemical mediators: increased vasopermeability, increased smooth muscle contractions, increased production of mucous secretions.

TYPE II HYPERSENSITIVITY. The basic mechanism of type II hypersensitivity is illustrated in Figure 1–15. Briefly, the steps of this mechanism involve:

1. Stimulation of specific IgG and IgM antibody production by the inducing antigen.

2. Possible effects:

a. Agglutination of antigen particles.

b. Opsonization and subsequent phagocytosis of the antigen.

c. Binding of complement and lysis of the antigen.

d. Antibody dependent cellular cytotoxicity (ADCC).

All four effects listed above inhibit the function of cells containing the target antigen. Conversely, if the antigen is a cell surface receptor, the antibody may bind to the receptor, imitating the natural ligand for that receptor, and stimulate the cell (Fig. 1–15). While frequently classified under type II hypersensitivity, the mechanism in this situation has sometimes been referred to as type V, or *stimulatory hypersensitivity.*

TYPE III HYPERSENSITIVITY. The basic mechanism of type III hypersensitivity is illustrated in Figure 1–16 and outlined briefly below:

1. Production of specific IgG or IgM antibodies and binding of the antibodies to their corresponding antigen (e.g. infectious organisms, self antigens) to form antigen-antibody complexes.

2. Binding of complement by the immune complexes.

3. Activation of the complement pathways with release of the following complement components and manifestation of their biologic activities:

C3a—increased vasodilation and vasopermeability.

C5a—increased vasodilation and vasopermeability, chemotaxis.

C3b—opsonization.

4. Binding of immune complexes to platelets, with consequent platelet aggregation, release of vasoactive amines and increase in vasopermeability.

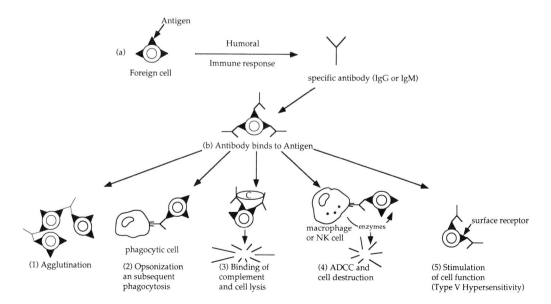

Fig. 1–15. Mechanism of Type II (antibody-dependent, cytotoxic) hypersensitivity.

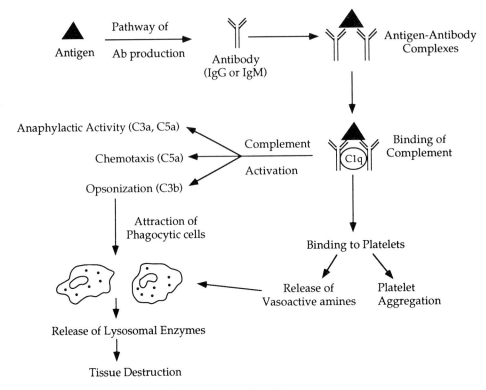

Fig. 1–16. Mechanism of Type III (complex-mediated) hypersensitivity.

5. Attraction of phagocytic cells (PMN and macrophages) to the site of immune complex deposition.

6. Release of lysosomal enzymes by the phagocytic cells into the surrounding environment. This can occur as a result of the process of phagocytosis or after death of the short-lived PMN. The released lysosomal enzymes mediate destruction of the surrounding tissues.

This mechanism is thought to be involved in the pathogenesis of rheumatoid arthritis and systemic lupus erythematosus and is also discussed in Chapter 11 under these disease headings.

TYPE IV HYPERSENSITIVITY. The basic mechanism of type IV hypersensitivity is illustrated in Figure 1–17, and outlined briefly below.

1. Processing of the antigen by macrophages and presentation of the antigen to Th.

2. Release of IL-1 by the macrophages, activation of the Th and subsequent release of IL-2 by the Th.

3. Effects of IL-2:

a. Activation of Td. Td effector cells release lymphokines which attract macrophages and PMN, thus promoting an inflammatory response. Macrophage chemotactic factor (MCF) attracts macrophages to the area, Macrophage Inhibition Factor (MIF) inhibits their migration from the area once they have arrived, and Macrophage Activation Factor (MAF, or gamma interferon) enhances the function of the macrophages. Chemotactic factors for PMN are also released. Chronic effects of inflammation, such as granuloma formation, may be seen.

b. Activation of Tcx. Activation of Tcx by IL-2 may also occur, with subsequent binding and lysis of appropriate target cells. This mechanism was described previously.

Antigen Processing and Presentation to Th

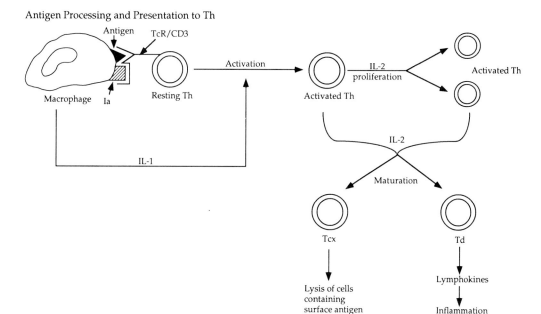

Fig. 1–17. Mechanism of Type IV (cell-mediated) hypersensitivity.

Type IV hypersensitivity is central to the procedure of delayed skin testing, as discussed under *Skin Testing: Assessment of Delayed Type Hypersensitivity*, Chapter 4.

Autoimmune Diseases[9,44,46,54]

In autoimmune diseases, changes in normal immunoregulatory mechanisms are thought to occur, resulting in inappropriate immune responses directed toward self antigens, with consequent harm to the host. These immune responses may involve both humoral immunity, with the production of autoantibodies, and cell-mediated immunity. While the precise causes of autoimmunity are unknown, several inducing fac-

Table 1–5. Examples of Autoimmune Diseases and Their Predominant Autoantibodies

Disease	Autoantibody Directed Against
Addison's disease	Adrenal cells
Autoimmune hemolytic anemia	Red blood cells
Autoimmune thrombocytopenic purpura	Platelets
Chronic active hepatitis	Smooth muscle
Goodpasture's syndrome	Renal basement membrane
Graves' disease	Thyroid stimulating hormone receptor, thyroglobulin, microsomal fraction
Hashimoto's thyroiditis	Thyroglobulin, microsomal fraction
Juvenile insulin-dependent diabetes	Islet cells
Mixed connective tissue disease	Nuclear antigens
Myasthenia gravis	Acetylcholine receptors
Pernicious anemia	Gastric parietal cells, intrinsic factor
Polymyositis dermatomyositis	Nuclear antigens; IgG
Primary biliary cirrhosis	Mitochondria
Progressive systemic sclerosis	Nuclear antigens
Rheumatoid arthritis	IgG, nuclear antigens
Sjögren's syndrome	IgG, nuclear antigens, salivary duct antigens
Systemic lupus erythematosus	Nuclear antigens, IgG, lymphocyte antigens

tors have been hypothesized.[9,44,46] Table 1–5 lists examples of autoimmune diseases and their predominant autoantibodies. Some of these diseases are discussed in Chapter 11.

REFERENCES

1. Abbas, A.K.: Immunol. Today, *9*:89, 1988.
2. Acuto, O., and Reinherz, E.L.: N. Engl. J. Med., *312*:1100, 1985.
3. Ada, G.L., and Nossal, G.: Sci. Am., *257*:62, 1987.
4. Allen, P.M.: Immunol. Today, *8*:270, 1987.
5. Aloisi, R.M.: *Principles of Immunology and Immunodiagnostics.* Philadelphia, Lea & Febiger, 1988.
6. Alt, F.W., et al.: Immunol. Rev., *89*:5, 1986.
7. Bach, F.H., and Sachs, D.H.: N. Engl. J. Med., *317*:489, 1987.
8. Barrett, J.T.: *Textbook of Immunology.* 5th ed. St. Louis, C.V. Mosby Co., 1988.
9. Bellanti, J.A.: *Immunology III.* Philadelphia, W.B. Saunders Co., 1985.
10. Bonavida, B., and Wright, S.C.: J. Clin. Immunol., *6*:1, 1986.
11. Coombs, R.R.A., and Gell, P.G.H.: In *Clinical Aspects of Immunology.* Edited by P.G.H. Gell, R.R.A. Coombs, and P.J. Lachmann. Oxford, Blackwell Scientific, 1975.
12. Cronenberger, J.H., and Jennette, J.C.: *Immunology: Basic Concepts, Diseases, and Laboratory Methods.* Norwalk, Conn., Appelton and Lange, 1988.
13. Davey, F.R., and Nelson, D.A.: In *Clinical Diagnosis and Management by Laboratory Methods,* 17th ed. Edited by J.B. Henry. Philadelphia, W.B. Saunders Co., 1984.
14. Davis, M.M.: Hosp. Pract., *23*:157, 1988.
15. Dinarello, C.A., and Mier, J.W.: N. Engl. J. Med., *317*:940, 1987.
16. DiNome, M.A., and Young, J.D.-E.: Hosp. Pract., *22*:59, 1987.
17. Foon, K.A., Gale, R.P., and Todd, R.F.: Semin. Hematol., *23*:257, 1986.
18. Gatenby, P.A., et al.: J. Exp. Med., *156*:55, 1982.
19. Germain, R.N., and Benacerraf, B.: Scand. J. Immunol., *13*:1, 1981.
20. Gershon, R.K.: Contemp. Top. Immunobiol., *3*:1, 1974.
21. Grimm, E.A., et al.: J. Exp. Med. *155*:1823, 1982.
22. Hong, R.: In *Manual of Clinical Laboratory Immunology.* 3rd ed. Edited by N.R. Rose, H. Friedman, and J.L. Fahey. Washington, D.C., American Society for Microbiology, 1986.
23. Hyde, R.M., and Pathode, R.A. (eds.): *The National Medical Series for Independent Study: Immunology.* New York, John Wiley and Sons, 1987.
24. In house reference values, Division of Clinical Pathology, SUNY Health Science Center at Syracuse, Syracuse, N.Y.
25. Isakov, N., Scholz, W., and Altman, A.: Immunol. Today, *7*:271, 1986.
26. Kennedy, R.C., Melnick, J.L., and Dreesman, G.R.: Sci. Am., *255*:48, 1986.
27. Korsmeyer, S.J., and Waldmann, T.A.: J. Clin. Immunol., *4*:1, 1984.
28. Kyle, R.A.: In *Manual of Clinical Laboratory Immunology.* 3rd ed. Edited by N.R. Rose, H. Friedman, and J.L. Fahey. Washington, D.C., American Society for Microbiology, 1986.
29. Lanier, L.L., and Phillips, J.H.: Immunol. Today, *7*:132, 1986.
30. Marrack, P., and Kappler, J.: Sci. Am., *254*:36, 1986.
31. Meuer, S.C.: Proc. Natl. Acad. Sci. U.S.A., *81*:1509, 1984.
32. Moller, G.: Scand. J. Immunol., *27*:247, 1988.
33. Nelson, D.A., and Davey, F.R.: In *Clinical Diagnosis and Management by Laboratory Methods,* 17th ed. Edited by J.B. Henry. Philadelphia, W.B. Saunders Co., 1984.
34. Porth, C.M.: *Pathophysiology: Concepts of Altered Health States,* 2nd ed. Philadelphia, J.B. Lippincott Co., 1986.
35. Price, S.A., and Wilson. L.M.: *Pathophysiology: Clinical Concepts of Disease Processes,* 3rd ed. New York, McGraw-Hill, Inc., 1986.
36. Reynolds, C.W., and Ortaldo, J.R.: Immunol. Today, *8*:172, 1987.
37. Ricardo, M.J., and Tomar, R.H.: In *Clinical Diagnosis and Management by Laboratory Methods,* 17th ed. Edited by J.B. Henry. Philadelphia, W.B. Saunders Co., 1984.
38. Roberts, R., and Gallin, J.I.: Ann. Allergy, *51*:330, 1983.
39. Roitt, I.: *Essential Immunology,* 5th ed. Oxford, Blackwell Scientific Publications, 1984.
40. Rosen, F.S., Cooper, M.D., and Wedgwood, R.J.P.: N. Engl. J. Med. *311*:235, 1984.
41. Rosen, F.S., Cooper, M.D., and Wedgwood, R.J.P.: N. Engl. J. Med. *311*:300, 1984.
42. Rosenberg, S.: J. Natl. Cancer Inst., *75*:595, 1985.
43. Rosenberg, S.A.: N. Engl. J. Med., *313*:1485, 1985.
44. Sell, S.: *Immunology Immunopathology and Immunity,* 4th ed. New York, Elsevier Science Publishing Co., Inc., 1987.
45. Simmons, A.: *Hematology: A Combined Theoretical and Technical Approach.* Philadelphia, W.B. Saunders Co., 1989.
46. Stites, D.P., Stobo, J.D., and Wells, J.V.: *Basic and Clinical Immunology,* 6th ed. Norwalk, Conn., Appelton and Lange, 1987.
47. Tomar, R.H.: In *Clinical Diagnosis and Management by Laboratory Methods,* 17 ed. Edited by J.B. Henry. Philadelphia, W.B. Saunders Co., 1984.
48. Tomar, R.H., Bellanti, J.A., and Kadlec, J.V.: In *Clinical Diagnosis and Management by Laboratory Methods,* 17th ed. Edited by J.B. Henry. Philadelphia, W.B. Saunders Co., 1984.
49. Trinchieri, G., and Perussia, B.: Lab. Invest., *50*:489, 1984.
50. Vitetta, E.S., et al.: Adv. Immunol., *45*:1, 1989.
51. Waldmann, T.A.: Hosp. Pract., *21*:69, 1986.
52. Ward, P.A.: In *Principles of Pathology,* 3rd ed. Ed-

ited by R.B. Hill and M.F. Lavia. New York, Oxford University Press, Inc., 1980.

53. Weiss, L.: *The Blood Cells and Hematopoietic Tissues,* 2nd ed. New York, Elsevier, 1984.

54. Zweiman, B., and Lisak, R.P.: In *Clinical Diagnosis and Management by Laboratory Methods,* 17th ed. Edited by J.B. Henry. Philadelphia, W.B. Saunders Co., 1984.

Chapter

2

SPECIMEN PREPARATION AND HANDLING

SERUM SEPARATION

PRINCIPLE. Whole blood, obtained by venipuncture, is allowed to clot, and the serum is removed for testing.

EQUIPMENT AND MATERIALS

1. Venipuncture Materials: Vacuum blood collection system, or syringe and needle, as desired; blood collection tubes
2. Clean, dry pour off tube, with label
3. Tube sealer (e.g., cork)
4. Centrifuge
5. Pasteur pipet

PROCEDURE

NOTE: See *Universal Precautions for Specimen Handling* below.

1. Obtain whole blood by standard venipuncture technique, allowing blood to flow directly into the tube (Vacutainer system) or transferring it aseptically into a tube after syringe collection.
2. Allow about 1 hour for the clot to retract. This may be done at either room or refrigerator temperature for all procedures except cold agglutinins and cryoglobulins. Increased yields of cryoglobulins are seen when allowed to clot at 37° C. Cold agglutinins must be at room temperature before centrifuging and separating sample.
3. Remove the tube top, loosening the clot if it adheres, and, using an applicator stick, rim the clot to prevent adhesion to the sides of the tube. Restopper tube.

4. Centrifuge for 10 minutes at approximately 9000 × g.
5. Label a test tube with accession number, tests requested, and the patient's name.
6. Using a pasteur pipet, transfer the serum to the labeled tube, and dispose of the clot by following correct specimen disposal protocol. Observe serum for cellular material. Repeat steps 4 to 6 if debris is noted.
7. Place a cork, or other appropriate seal, on the tube.
8. Test immediately, or place at −20° C for subsequent testing unless test procedure indicates otherwise.

QUICK-FREEZING

PRINCIPLE. Various proteins have poor stability at room temperature. They have increased stability when stored at −70° C or less. Protein yield is increased if specimen is brought to −70° C as quickly as possible.

EQUIPMENT AND MATERIALS

1. Dry ice
2. 95% ethanol
3. Plastic storage tubes with tight fitting seals (Vanguard International)
4. Small bowl
5. −70° C freezer
6. Thermal gloves
7. Freezer box filing system for subsequent identification of frozen samples

PROCEDURE

1. Following serum separation procedure, process specimen as soon as possible after venipuncture.

2. Log specimens in "freezer" log book, noting the number, row, and column of the freezer box to be used for the specimen. Label plastic storage tubes to correspond.

3. Transfer specimen to the tube.

4. Place a small block of dry ice in a bowl. Smash to smaller chunks.

5. Add 95% ethanol. NOTE: This mixture will "smoke" at first as CO_2 gas is released.

6. Gently swirl the specimen(s) to be frozen in the dry ice-ethanol mixture. The specimen will become opaque as it freezes.

7. Immediately place in the $-70°$ C freezer in the appropriate box, column and row.

NOTE: Because of the low temperature and freezer frost, it is important to clearly designate where frozen specimens are to be found and to maintain an accurate record.

INACTIVATION

PRINCIPLE. Inactivation is a process by which complement activity is removed from a patient or control specimen. Inactivation of body fluids is accomplished by heating to $56°$ C for 30 minutes.

Complement is known to interfere with the reactions of certain syphilis tests, although the mechanism is unknown. C_{1q} can cause agglutination in assays such as the Cryptococcal latex antigen test, and complement may cause lysis of the indicator cells in hemagglutination assays, e.g., heterophile tests. C_{1q} also interferes with the anti-DNA procedure. Removal of complement activity from the test specimen prior to assay prevents these interferences.

EQUIPMENT AND MATERIALS

1. Water bath, set at $56°$ C

2. Specimens

PROCEDURE. Place tubes containing specimens to be inactivated in a $56°$ C waterbath. Remove after 30 minutes. NOTE: When greater than 4 hours has elapsed since inactivation, a specimen can be reinactivated by heating to $56°$ C for 10 minutes.

UNIVERSAL PRECAUTIONS FOR SPECIMEN HANDLING

The following recommendations were developed by the Centers for Disease Control (CDC) for use in health care settings.[1,2] These guidelines assume that *all* specimens are potentially infectious.* The guidelines should be followed in all health care settings in which persons may be exposed to blood or other body fluids and should be in place for the protection of the health care worker.

1. Wear:

a. Gloves—to avoid skin contact with blood, blood-soiled items, body fluids, excretions, and secretions, as well as surfaces, materials, and objects exposed to them. Change gloves and wash hands after completion of specimen processing and after contact with each patient.

b. Gowns or lab coats—to avoid soiling with blood, body fluids, excretions, or secretions.

c. Masks and protective eyewear—if mucous-membrane contact with blood or body fluids is anticipated, i.e., splashing or aerosolation of specimen. NOTE: Alternatively, plastic workshields may be used to avoid contact with splashes.

2. Wash hands immediately if they become contaminated with blood, other body fluids, or tissue.

3. Take extraordinary care to avoid accidental wounds from sharp instruments contaminated with potentially infectious material and to avoid direct contact with blood, other body fluids, or tissue.

4. Promptly place needles and syringes in puncture-resistant containers for their disposal. Do *not* bend needles after use. Do

*NOTE: The Centers for Disease Control have revised their recommendations for universal precautions to apply to blood, other body fluids containing visible blood, semen, vaginal secretions, and certain body fluids for which the risk of transmission is unknown.[2] The precautions need not apply to feces, nasal secretions, sputum, sweat, tears, urine, or vomitus, unless they contain visible blood, since the risk of transmission with these fluids is thought to be negligible.

not re-insert needles into their original sheaths before being discarded into the container, since this is a common cause of needle injury.

5. Transport specimens in a well-constructed container with a secure lid or in a sealed plastic bag in order to prevent leaking. Take care when collecting each specimen to avoid contaminating the outside of the container and the lab form accompanying the specimen.

6. Clean blood spills promptly with a disinfectant solution, e.g. sodium hypochlorite (household bleach) diluted with water to concentration ranging from 1% (500 ppm) to 10% (5000 ppm).

7. Use mechanical pipetting devices for the manipulation of all liquids in the laboratory. Never mouth pipet.

8. Place specimens or articles soiled with blood in an impervious bag prominently labeled "Blood/Body Fluid Precautions" before being sent for reprocessing or disposal. Alternately, such contaminated items may be placed in plastic bags of a particular color designated solely for disposal of infectious wastes by the hospital. Disposable items should be incinerated or disposed of in accord with the hospital's policies for disposal of infectious wastes. All liquid waste containing body fluids should be mixed with a sodium hypochlorite solution giving a final concentration of 1% when the container is full.

9. Reprocess reusable items in accord with hospital policies for hepatitis B virus-contaminated items. Decontaminate all potentially contaminated materials used in laboratory tests, preferably by autoclaving, before disposal or reprocessing. Decontaminate and clean scientific equipment that has been contaminated with blood or body fluids prior to reuse.

10. Perform all procedures and manipulations of potentially infectious material carefully to minimize the creation of droplets and aerosols. Biological safety cabinets and other primary containment devices (e.g. centrifuge safety cups) are advised whenever procedures are conducted that have a high potential for creating aerosols or infectious droplets. These include centrifuging, blending, sonicating, vigorous mixing, and harvesting infected tissues from animals or embryonated eggs.

11. Decontaminate laboratory work surfaces with a disinfectant, such as sodium hypochlorite solution (see #6 above), following any spill of potentially infectious material and at the completion of work activities. Use absorbent disposable materials on work surfaces when applicable.

12. Wash hands following completion of laboratory activities and remove protective clothing before leaving the laboratory.

REFERENCES

1. Centers for Disease Control: MMWR, 36(suppl 2S):1s, 1987.
2. Centers for Disease Control: MMWR, 37:377, 1988.

Chapter | **3**

INTRODUCTION TO SEROLOGIC METHODS

TECHNICAL INSTRUCTION

Simple and Serial Dilutions; Titers

Many assays performed in the clinical immunology or serology laboratory involve the preparation of simple dilutions or serial dilutions. To prepare a simple dilution, a given volume of the substance to be diluted, or the *concentrate,* is added to a fixed volume of *diluent,* the medium in which the concentrate is diluted. Frequently, the concentrate consists of a serum specimen, while the diluent used is saline or a buffered solution. A given volume of a desired dilution of concentrate may be prepared using the following mathematical formula:

$$\text{Dilution} = \frac{\text{Volume of concentrate}}{\text{Total volume}}$$

where the dilution is expressed as a fraction (1/x) and the total volume is equal to the volume of concentrate plus the volume of diluent.

EXAMPLE 1

What volumes of patient serum and diluent are required in order to prepare 10 ml of a $\frac{1}{5}$ dilution of patient serum?

SOLUTION

Let x = volume of patient serum. Substituting the above values into the equation provides the solution:

$$\frac{1}{5} = \frac{x}{10}$$

$$5x = 10$$

$$x = 2 \text{ ml} = \text{volume of}$$

patient serum needed

Volume of diluent needed = Total volume

− volume of

patient serum

= 10 − 2 ml = 8 ml diluent

Therefore, in order to prepare 10 ml of a $\frac{1}{5}$ dilution of patient serum, one must add 2 ml of patient serum to 8 ml of diluent.

In serologic tests, estimates of the volume of antibody in a clinical specimen are often managed by a semiquantitation technique known as *titering*. This technique involves (1) preparing serial dilutions of the antibody solution (e.g. serum), and (2) adding a constant volume of antigen suspension to each dilution. Serial dilutions are prepared

31

by diluting the antibody sample in test tubes or microtiter plate wells by progressive, regular increments, resulting in a series of dilutions in which each dilution is less concentrated than the preceding dilution by a constant amount, "N." In an **N-fold** serial dilution system, the antibody concentration in each dilution is $\frac{1}{N}$ of the preceding dilution. Most commonly, serial dilutions are "two-fold"; that is, each dilution is $\frac{1}{2}$ as concentrated as the one immediately before it.

The dilution fold of a system can be determined by using the following formula:

$$\frac{1}{\text{Dilution Fold}} = \frac{\text{Volume transferred}}{\text{Total Volume}}$$

where volume transferred is equal to the constant volume transferred from one tube to the next in a serial dilution system, and the total volume is equal to the volume being transferred plus the volume of diluent already in the tube.

EXAMPLE 2

What is the dilution fold of the following serial dilution system, consisting of 10 test tubes? The following amounts of diluent have been added to the tubes: 1.0 ml to tube 1 and 1.5 ml to tubes 2 to 10. Next, 1.0 ml of patient serum is added to tube 1, and 0.5 ml is serially transferred through tube 10. Finally, 0.5 ml is discarded from tube 10.

SOLUTION

Let x = the dilution fold. Substituting the values given in the example into the above equation provides the solution:

$$\frac{1}{x} = \frac{0.5}{0.5 + 1.5}$$

$$\frac{1}{x} = \frac{0.5}{2.0} = \frac{1}{4}$$

$$x = 4$$

Thus, this is a fourfold serial dilution system.

After the dilution fold is known, the dilution in a given test tube or microtiter well

(n) in a serial dilution system may be calculated as follows:

Dilution of sample #n in a serial dilution system

$$= \frac{\text{Dilution of}}{\text{sample \#1}} \times \left[\frac{1}{\text{Dilution fold}}\right]^{(n-1)}$$

EXAMPLE 3

What is the dilution of patient serum in tube 3 in Example #2 above?

SOLUTION

Let x = dilution of tube 3. The solution is obtained by substituting the values given in the example into the above equation:

$$x = \frac{1.0}{1.0 + 1.0} \times \left[\frac{1}{4}\right]^{(3-1)}$$

$$x = \frac{1}{2} \times \left[\frac{1}{4}\right]^2 = \frac{1}{2} \times \frac{1}{16} = \frac{1}{32}$$

Thus, the dilution of patient serum in tube 3 is $\frac{1}{32}$.

When performing titers, the total volume in each test tube or microtiter well should be the same. The addition of antigen to a serial dilution increases the total volume in each sample, thus changing the dilution of the concentrate. Unfortunately, investigators disagree over whether the final dilution reported should be considered the dilution before or after the addition of antigen.

The dilution in a given sample in a serial dilution system after the addition of antigen may be calculated using the following mathematical formula:

$$\text{Dilution of sample \#n after addition of antigen} =$$

$$\frac{\text{Dilution of sample \#n before addition of antigen}} \times \frac{\text{Total volume in sample \#n before addition of antigen}}{\text{Total volume in sample \#n after addition of antigen}}$$

Note that in determining the total volumes, one must take into consideration the fact that a given volume has been transferred out of each sample and into the next sample of the series prior to the addition of antigen.

EXAMPLE 4

What would the new dilution of patient serum in tube 3 in Example 3 above be if 1.5 ml of antigen were subsequently added to the tube?

SOLUTION

Let x = dilution in tube 3 after the addition of antigen. The solution is obtained by substituting the values given in the example into the above equation:

$$x = \frac{1}{32} \times \frac{1.5 + 0.5 - 0.5}{(1.5 + 0.5 - 0.5) + 1.5}$$

(Note: The volumes subtracted above represent the 0.5 ml that was transferred out of tube 3 and into tube 4 prior to the addition of antigen).

$$x = \frac{1}{32} \times \frac{1}{2} = \frac{1}{64}$$

Thus, the dilution in tube 3 after the addition of 1.5 ml of antigen is $\frac{1}{64}$.

Finally, the concentration of antibody in the serially-diluted sample is expressed as the antibody *titer*, which is the reciprocal of the last dilution in the series to demonstrate the desired test result. For example, when performing an agglutination test, the antibody titer is commonly reported as the reciprocal of the dilution of the last sample in which agglutination is observed. The titer of tube 3 in Example 4 above would be the reciprocal of $\frac{1}{64}$, or simply, 64. A reference range of titers is established by the laboratory for each serologic assay, and is used to interpret patient results.

Preparation of Erythrocyte Cell Suspensions

PRINCIPLE

Erythrocytes are washed and standardized for use in various serologic procedures.

EQUIPMENT AND MATERIALS

1. Erythrocytes: Whole human blood may be obtained in an appropriate anticoagulant, e.g., Versene. Sheep erythrocytes are obtained commercially in Alsever's solution.

2. Test tubes or conical centrifuge tubes

3. Volumetric or Erlenmeyer flasks large enough to contain the final volume of cell suspension desired

4. Saline or diluent used for testing

PROCEDURE

1. Washing procedure:
    a. Place erythrocytes in a tube large enough to hold at least twice the volume of the erythrocytes.
    b. Add saline, or the appropriate diluent (see *Antistreptolysin O, CH₅₀*), to within $\frac{1}{2}$ inch of the tube surface. Parafilm and mix with an end-over-end motion.
    c. Serofuge for 3 minutes.
    d. Decant or evacuate the supernate using a Pasteur pipet attached to a vacuum source.
    e. Repeat steps a through d. (When using human erythrocytes, steps a through d are repeated twice).

2. Standardization of erythrocytes: Volumetric technique.
    a. Select a volumetric or Erlenmeyer flask large enough to contain or quantitate the total volume desired.
    b. For a volumetric flask, add a small amount of diluent to the flask. Add the volume of packed erythrocytes, calculated as follows:

% Suspension × Total Volume = Volume of packed cells

Qs to the total volume desired, using diluent.
    c. For an Erlenmeyer flask, calculate the volume of packed cells and the volume of diluent to be used as follows:

% Suspension × Total Volume = Volume of packed cells

The volume of diluent = the total volume minus the volume of packed cells. Pipet the diluent, then the packed cells, into the flask.

3. Standardization of erythrocytes: spectrophotometric technique. (See *CH₅₀ Procedure: standardization of erythrocytes.*)

4. Prepared suspensions of erythrocytes are labeled according to type of cell, % suspension, date, and technologist initials. Flasks should be tightly stoppered to prevent evaporation and/or contamination. Store at 2 to 8°C. (*NOTE:* For length of storage and special considerations, see individual procedures).

Use of Microtiter Equipment

PRINCIPLE

The process of titration is accomplished in wells of a polyethylene plate by the use of minute amounts of reagents and micropipets.

EQUIPMENT AND MATERIALS

1. Microtiter plates (Dynatech): U- or V-shaped wells, 6 mm wide; capacity volume: 0.125 ml.

2. Pipet droppers, 0.025 and 0.05 ml (Dynatech): Equipped with suction-filter adapter and disposable cellulose-acetate filter, to allow pipet to be filled by suction from automatic pipeter or syringe bulb. Droppers are calibrated to deliver ± 2% of the specified amount in each drop when using a 0.85% saline solution. Drop rate is controlled by finger pressure. May be autoclaved.

3. Microdiluters (Dynatech): Calibrated to pick up and deliver 0.025 or 0.05 ml (± 2%) of a 0.85% saline solution. Handles are specially tapered to give the same spacing as that found between the plate wells. May be autoclaved, but usually cleaned by flaming.

4. Go-no-go delivery tester (Dynatech): Made of special blotter material marked with circles. May be purchased for use with 0.025- and 0.05-ml amounts. Determines whether the microdiluters are delivering properly.

5. Plate-sealing tape (Dynatech): Transparent tape that seals microtiter plates and prevents evaporation.

6. Test-reading mirror (Dynatech): Provides magnification and high definition of test results.

PROCEDURE

1. Preparation of microdiluters: (NOTE: The following should be performed just prior to use to effect maximum use of surface tension.)
   a. Flame microdiluters with a Bunsen burner until the yellow sodium flame develops.
   b. Cool in distilled water.[1]
   c. Roll dry on the go-no-go delivery tester.

d. Place the appropriate go-no-go blotter on a smooth, nonabsorbent surface.
   e. Pre-wet a microdiluter by touching it to the surface of clean, distilled water.[1] Touch the microdiluter to the marked center of one of the circles on the blotter.
   f. Observe the dampened area within the circle. A properly prepared microdiluter will deliver all contained fluid, sufficient to immediately dampen the area within the circle. Do not use diluter if it does not function as indicated. (NOTE: The tester determines whether a diluter is delivering properly. It is not intended as a calibration check.)

2. Wipe the underside of the plates to be used, using a damp cloth or paper towel.[2]

3. Perform the test procedure (see MHA-TP; Thyroid Antibody Titers), using the following specifications:
   a. Fill pipet droppers with the desired solution, wipe with gauze, and hold vertically for delivery. Allow drops to fall onto gauze until rate is established.
   b. Fill the diluters with sample by lightly touching the surface. Transfer to the desired well. (NOTE: Do not touch the sides of the wells, as this may cause uneven dilution.)
   c. Mix without excessive downward pressure by rotating the tops of diluters between fingertips. A rate of 30 back-and-forth motions in 8 seconds is recommended.[1]
   d. Move all diluters to successive wells by stabilizing the bases between the first and second fingers of one hand, lift directly upward, and transfer by dropping straight down into the next row of wells. Avoid touching the sides of wells.
   e. Place microdiluters in distilled water.
   f. Seal plates if reactions are to be incubated in the plates.

4. Cleaning equipment:
   a. Microdiluters should be rinsed; flamed, as in step 1a; and cooled in clean, distilled water. Empty on a go-no-go blotter. Store with prongs upward.
   b. Place pipet droppers in a diluted 7X detergent solution, rinse thoroughly in tap water, then in distilled water, and air-dry.

DISCUSSION

Reproducibility of the microtiter system (± one two-fold dilution), was found to be 94.8% in one study,[2] as compared to 99.1% for macrodilutions.

Cooper et al. determined the percent error of Cooke Engineering (Dynatech) micropipeters at 9.9%.[1] Using the aforementioned specifications and properly calibrating their equipment, these authors project this microtiter system to be both reliable and reproducible.

REFERENCES

1. Cooper, H.A., Bowie, E.J.W., and Owen, C.A., Jr.: Am. J. Clin. Pathol., *57*:332, 1972.

2. Gavan, T.L., and Town, M.A.: Am. J. Clin. Pathol., *53*:880, 1970.

Quality Control Protocol

Patient sera and control sera are tested and interpreted according to the instructions for each individual procedure.

TUBE TITERS

Assayed values for most tube titer controls are supplied by the manufacturer with each lot produced. Each change in control lot number is recorded on the quality control sheet and the new expected control value is noted.

The control for each tube titer must titer to the same dilution as stated on the control records. The confidence range for tube titers is plus or minus one tube from the stated expected value. If the control fits within the confidence limits, the patient values can be reported. Control values are recorded for each set of tests completed.

R.I.D.

Commercial controls are available from manufacturer. The package insert provides confidence limits (± 2 SD) for all the R.I.D. procedures. Each control value must fall within these limits before the run can be accepted. Control values are recorded and plotted on Levy-Jennings graph.

COLD AGGLUTININS

Commercial control sera are not presently available for this procedure. Sera from an outdated unit of blood are harvested and then augmented if needed with appropriate positive sera. A control value giving a mid-range positive is desired. All control pools are tested for Hepatitis B surface antigen and antibody to HIV before proceeding further. Each pool of control is developed when 15 aliquots remain in the old pool. The new pool is tested simultaneously with the old

control for at least 10 runs. The mean and two standard deviations are calculated and the acceptable ranges are set. A control is run with each patient run. The reading from the control must fall within the confidence range set for the pool.

ELISA TECHNIQUES, FLUORESCENT ASSAY, AND POLARIZED IMMUNOFLUORESCENCE

Commercial controls are supplied by the manufacturer with each kit. If the controls are within the acceptable limits determined by the manufacturer, the run is accepted. Otherwise the run will be repeated. Control values are recorded appropriately.

OTHER TESTS (I.E. ANTI-DNA, NBT, AND LYMPHOCYTE SUBSETS)

Refer to individual test procedures for control preparation and treatment.

If the control run is not within the confidence limits set, a senior technologist is consulted and the patient run is rejected and discarded. Patients and controls are repeated with the next specimen run. If the run is again rejected, all test parameters involved must be investigated and corrected if needed. These include:

Incubation temperatures
Reagent outdate
Lot number changes
Pipette malfunction
Equipment malfunction
Following procedure incorrectly

All changes and corrective action must be documented on worksheet and/or equipment maintenance logs.

KIT COMPARISON BETWEEN LOT NUMBER CHANGES

To ensure that the same sensitivity is maintained between reagent lot number changes, a comparison should be run when a new reagent lot number is introduced.

A stock of weakly positive serum is stored at −20° C for this purpose. This stock includes sera for:

Anti-Streptolysin O Latex Screen
Rheumatoid Factor Latex Screen
Mononucleosis Screen

For all other procedures, control reagents, particularly the weakly positive control, from old and new lot numbers are used concurrently before using the last of the in use kit. For the new lot number to be acceptable, it must have the same sensitivity as the old in use lot number.

If kits do not agree, corrective replacement action should be taken. Comparison results and technician's initials should also be documented.

SEROLOGIC METHODS

Sensitivity, Specificity, and Predictive Value

A variety of serologic methods are currently available to the clinical laboratory. These methods possess inherent differences in *sensitivity, specificity*, and *predictive value.*

Sensitivity and specificity can be described in terms of both analytic performance, or the susceptibility of an assay to systematic error, and diagnostic performance, or the accuracy of a method in determining a correct diagnosis.[3]

The *analytic sensitivity* of a method is defined as its lower detection limit, or the lowest concentration of antibody or antigen capable of being detected by the method. Analytic sensitivity values for currently available methods range from 0.1 to 10 mg/dl for precipitation tests, to less than 1 pg/dl for radioimmunoassay.[3]

The *analytic specificity* of a serologic assay is defined as the ability of the method to detect only the antibody or antigen for which it is designed. Detection of cross-reacting substances will decrease the specificity of the test and create false-positive results.

The terms sensitivity and specificity can also be utilized to describe the ability of an assay to establish an accurate diagnosis. The *diagnostic sensitivity* of a method refers to the percentage of positive results produced by a laboratory test in individuals with a particular disease, and can be calculated by the following equation:[2]

$$\text{Diagnostic Sensitivity (\%)} = \frac{\text{\# true positive results}}{\text{\# true positive results} + \text{\# false negative results}} \times 100$$

Thus, a test which has a diagnostic sensitivity of 95%, for example, will produce positive results in 95 out of every 100 individuals tested who have the disease in question, but will yield false-negative results for every $^5\!/_{100}$ individuals who have the disease.

The *diagnostic specificity* of a method is the percentage of negative results produced by a laboratory test in individuals in which a particular disease is not present, and can be calculated as follows:[2]

$$\text{Diagnostic Specificity (\%)} = \frac{\text{\# true-negative results}}{\text{\# true-negative results} + \text{\# false-positive results}} \times 100$$

Thus, a test with a diagnostic specificity of 95%, for example, will produce a negative test result in 95 out of every 100 individuals tested who do not have the disease in question, but will yield false-positive results for every $^5\!/_{100}$ individuals tested who do not have the disease.

While the sensitivity and specificity are relatively fixed values for a given test, the *predictive value* of a test is influenced by the prevalence of a disease in the population tested, and describes the performance of the test in that population.

The *predictive value of a positive result* describes the likelihood that a positive test result represents a true positive, and is defined as follows:[2]

$$\text{Predictive value of a (+) result} = \frac{\#\ \text{true positives}}{\#\ \text{true positives} + \#\ \text{false positives}} \times 100$$

The predictive value of a positive result increases as the prevalence of a particular disease increases in the population being tested.

The *predictive value of a negative test result*, or the likelihood that a negative result is truly negative, may be calculated as follows:[2]

$$\text{Predictive value of a (−) result} = \frac{\#\ \text{true negatives}}{\#\ \text{true negatives} + \#\ \text{false negatives}} \times 100$$

The predictive value of a negative test result is higher in populations with a lower prevalence of a particular disease than in populations with a higher frequency of individuals with that disease.

The importance of predictive values to the diagnostic accuracy of a laboratory test is illustrated in a hypothetical situation described by the Centers for Disease Control[1] in which a screening test to detect HIV infection was employed: using an ELISA test for HIV antibody with a sensitivity of 99% and a specificity of 99.5%, the predictive value of a positive test was determined to be only about 28% in a population where the prevalence of infection was 0.2%, while the predictive value climbed to over 98% when the prevalence of infection was 20%. Depending on the population assayed, the accuracy of a laboratory test may thus be low even if sensitivity and specificity values are high. The diagnostic accuracy in the above example is greatly improved by the addition of a confirmatory test procedure.

In conclusion, the performance of a laboratory test is influenced by factors intrinsic to that test, such as methodology, reagents utilized, and lot number, as well as external variables, including technical expertise and population tested. The effects of these factors are reflected in the sensitivity, specificity, and predictive values of the laboratory test. Clinical laboratories will want to consider these values in choosing assays that will be best suited to meet their individual needs.

REFERENCES

1. Centers for Disease Control: MMWR *36* (suppl 2S):1s, 1987.
2. Galen, R.S.: In *Manual of Clinical Laboratory Immunology.* 3rd ed. Edited by N.R. Rose, H. Friedman, and J.L. Fahey. Washington, D.C., American Society for Microbiology, 1986.
3. Stites, D.P., and Channing Rodgers, R.P.: In *Basic and Clinical Immunology.* 6th ed. Edited by D.P. Stites, J.D. Stobo, and J.V. Wells. Norwalk, Appelton and Lange, 1987.

Monoclonal Antibodies

In the normal humoral immune response to an antigen, large numbers of heterogeneous B cell lines are produced, each in response to a single epitope, or antigenic determinant, on the inciting antigen. According to the clonal selection theory of Burnet,[2] each cell is capable of making only a single antibody, homogeneous in its chemistry, physical characteristics, and immune specificity. Multiple cells undoubtedly respond to a single epitope and most antigens are comprised of multiple epitopes. The sum of the antibody products of all the cells that respond is released into the serum to form the collective antibody pool.

In practice, serologists have depended on antibody pools, produced by axenic animals (i.e., animals raised in a germ-free environment) in response to an available source of injectable antigen for the antisera used in diagnostic testing. Antiserum preparations were unpredictable and relatively impure despite immunologists' best efforts to remove interfering antibodies. Cross-reactions were common features of the antisera available, and constant surveillance was required to ensure reasonable equality in the concentration strengths of antisera from different lot numbers, e.g., from different animal sources or the same animal but produced and collected at different times. Dissection of an antiserum into constituent groups, based on either the antibody class, its antigenic specificity, or both, was difficult and resulted in only small amounts of antibody, often with weak avidity.[18]

The work of Köhler and Milstein, published in 1975,[13] created a revolution in laboratory medicine. Recognizing that cells in tissue culture sometimes fuse spontaneously, they theorized that surfactants such as polyethylene glycol (PEG) might be used to fuse antibody-producing B cells with a more stable cultured cell line, resulting in the production of a *hybridoma,* or somatic cell hybrid: a homogeneous permanent cell line with potential for unlimited production of antibody. In effect, a clone of these hybrid cells would produce *monoclonal antibody,* homogeneous in nature and capable of reacting with only a single epitope.

In principle, production of hybridomas is relatively simple. In practice, the procedure is demanding, tedious, and labor-intensive. The steps to be followed are basically the same, regardless of the nature of the antigen used as a stimulus. (See discussion below and Fig. 3–1.) Most of the hybridomas in current use are the products of cell fusion between antibody-producing B cells (mouse) and a myeloma cell line (mouse).

Myelomas are naturally occurring malignancies that are characterized by continuous proliferation of a single clone of B cells. Usually, but not always, myeloma cell lines are prolific in their production of a monoclonal immunoglobulin, usually of unde-

termined specificity. Myeloma cell lines that are useful in hybridoma technology are those that do not inherently synthesize an immunoglobulin of their own.[5,10,16] The chosen myeloma must, in addition, be genetically deficient in the enzyme hypoxanthine guanine phosphoribosyl transferase (HGPRT), rendering it unable to grow in a medium containing hypoxanthine, aminopterin, and thymidine (HAT medium).[10,12,16] HAT medium can then be used in the separation phase of hybridoma production.

Antibody-producing B cells to be used in fusion are obtained by repeated injection of the chosen antigen into a mouse.[5] After several days, the spleen of the mouse is removed, minced, and prepared as a single cell suspension which should include B cell populations involved in producing antibody to many epitopes of the inducing antigen.

In the fusion phase of hybridoma production, the appropriate myeloma cells and spleen cells are mixed in culture medium to which PEG is added. Immediate fusion products, referred to as heterokaryons, are cells which contain more than two nonidentical nuclei. Often these nuclei subsequently fuse to form synkaryons containing a single nucleus with genomes from both parental cells. Some of these form stable hybrids that can multiply normally in culture.[5,10,16] In practice, 1 hybrid in 2×10^5 cells, or 300 to 500 hybrids per spleen, will be produced by a single producedure.[10] Only a few of these are likely to form antibody against the antigen of interest.

Cells that result from the fusion phase of hybridoma production are placed in culture, using HAT medium. Normal B cells, unable to grow well in culture, will be depleted, as will nonhybrid HGPRT-deficient myeloma cells. Hybrids that inherited HGPRT from the parental lymphocyte genome grow rapidly in the medium. Hybrid cells are diluted and plated into microtiter wells, further incubated, then screened to identify clones which are producing the desired antibody. Along with antigenic specificity, the class

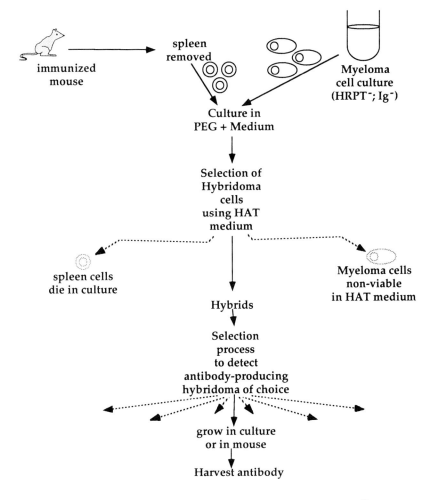

Fig. 3-1. Monoclonal antibody production: Mouse hybridoma technique.

of antibody and its avidity may be parameters for consideration.

The tedious process of separating viable cells and identifying cells producing antibody of a specific isotype has been facilitated by use of the fluorescence activated cell sorter (FACS).[12]

Methods used for purification and characterization of monoclonal antibodies include ion-exchange, gel filtration, immunoadsorbent chromatography, and delipidation techniques.[9,16] Multispecificity is not generally a property of monoclonal antibodies, although occasionally cross-reactions do occur.[16]

Hybridomas may be maintained in cell culture or may be injected into the peritoneal cavity of an appropriate mouse for growth and subsequent antibody harvest.[5,10]

The production of monoclonal antibodies has revolutionized diagnostic testing, not only in the clinical laboratory,[5,8,18] but also in histology and anatomic pathology,[8] and in radiologic diagnosis of cancer.[7,8,14] In vitro testing in immunology, immunohematology, clinical chemistry, hematology, and microbiology is rapidly undergoing replacement of reagents as monoclonal counterparts are developed. Certain assays whose usage was previously limited (e.g. immunoradiometric assays, or IRMA) are experiencing reemergence in their adaptations. Identification of HLA antigens[17,19] has been refined and simplified by development of monoclonal anti-HLA reagents, although the inherent specificity of monoclonal antibodies may be too restrictive for generalized use in this capacity. Monoclonal anti-lymphocyte reagents have been standardized[4] and are being used to phenotype leukemias and lymphomas, as well as to study changes in lymphocyte populations in different diseases.

Research into the mechanisms of immune responses has been facilitated by use of monoclonal antilymphocyte antibodies to selectively manipulate the immune system, both in vivo and in vitro.[20,23]

Use of monoclonal antibodies in therapeutic treatment of disease has been hampered somewhat by the slow development of human hybridoma technology. Human hybridomas have a special importance in treatment not only for their clinical relevance, but also for avoidance of adverse reactions that are often experienced when mouse antibodies are used.[11]

Human hybridoma production has been far less successful than that of mice in part because of problems with derivation of permanent human myeloma cell lines, and in part because the source of B cells (e.g. fresh spleens) is limited.[1,13,16] Studies continue, nonetheless. Alternatives such as immortalization of B cells by Epstein-Barr virus (EBV hybridomas)[11,22] have been developed; however, these too have experienced difficulties.

Many therapeutic monoclonal antibodies have been used in clinical trials. They have, for example, been used in treatment of transplant rejection,[15,24] where they may have the potential to facilitate induction of tolerance. Monoclonal antibodies against infectious agents or their products,[8,18] e.g. tetanus and diphtheria toxoids, as well as those which react with antigens involved in autoimmune diseases,[8,18] e.g. rheumatoid arthritis, systemic lupus erythematosus, have been tested.

The most widely used therapeutic applications of monoclonal antibodies have been in the treatment of cancer,[3,6,7,18,26] where they may be used alone, or as a means of targeting the actions of radionucleotides, toxins, chemotherapeutics, or other drugs.[25]

REFERENCES

1. Abrams, P.G. et al.: Methods Enzymol., 121:107, 1986.
2. Burnet, F.M.: *The Clonal Selection Theory of Acquired Immunity.* Vanderbilt and Cambridge University Press, 1959.
3. Campbell, A.M., Whitford, P., and Leake, R.E.: Br. J. Cancer, 56:709, 1987.
4. Chan, J.K.C., Ng, C.S., and Hui, P.K.: Histopathology, 12:461, 1988.
5. Diamond, B.A., Yelton, D.E., and Scharff, M.D.: N. Engl. J. Med., 304:1344, 1981.
6. Embleton, M.J.: Br. J. Cancer, 55:227, 1987.
7. Goldenberg, D.M.: Arch. Pathol. Lab. Med., 112:580, 1988.
8. Gordon, D.S. (Ed.), *Monoclonal Antibodies in Clinical Diagnostic Medicine,* New York, Igaku-Shoin, Pub., 1985.
9. Hardy, R.R.: In *Handbook of Experimental Immunology I,* Edited by D.M. Weir. Oxford, Blackwell Scientific Publications, 1986.
10. Hood, L.E., Weissman, I.L., Wood, W.B., and Wilson, J.H.: *Immunology.* 2nd ed., Menlo Park, The Benjamin/Cummings Publishing Co., 1984.
11. James, K., and Bell, G.T.: J. Immunol. Methods, 100:5, 1987.
12. Kipps, T.J., and Herzenberg, L.A.: In *Applications of Immunological Methods in Biomedical Sciences IV,* 4th ed. Edited by D.M. Weir. Oxford, Blackwell Scientific Publications, 1986.
13. Kohler, G., and Milstein, C.: Nature, 256:495, 1975.
14. Kupchik, H.Z. (Ed.): *Cancer Diagnosis in Vitro Using Monoclonal Antibodies,* New York, Marcel Dekker, Inc., 1988.
15. Luke, R.J.: National Kidney Foundation Conference: Am. J. Kidney Dis., 11:85, 1988.
16. Milstein, C., In *Handbook of Experimental Immunology IV.* Edited by D.M. Weir, Oxford, Blackwell Scientific Publications, 1986.
17. Pistillo, M.P.: Hum. Immunol., 21:265, 1988.
18. Price, B.J.: Ann. Otol. Rhinol. Laryngol., 96:497, 1987.
19. Radka, S.F.: CRC Crit. Rev. Immunol., 8:23, 1987.
20. Seaman, W.E., and Wofsy, D.: Annu. Rev. Med., 39:231, 1988.
21. Springer, T.A. (Ed.): *Hybridoma Technology in the Biosciences and Medicine,* New York, Plenum Press, 1985.
22. Strelkauskas, A.J. (Ed.): *Human Hybridomas: Diagnostic and Therapeutic Applications,* New York, Marcel Dekker, Inc., 1987.
23. Waldmann, H. et al.: Ciba Found. Symp., 129:194, 1987.

24. Waldmann, H.: Am. J. Kidney Dis., *11*:154, 1988.

25. Weinstein, J.N. et al.: Ann. N.Y. Acad. Sci., *507*:199, 1987.

26. Zalutsky, M.R. (Ed.): *Antibodies in Radiodiagnosis and Therapy,* Boca Raton, CRC Press, 1988.

Precipitation

When soluble antigen reacts with antibody, also in solution, a visible product may appear. This reaction product, or "precipitate," is formed by the process known as precipitation, and consists of insoluble antigen-antibody complexes.

On a molecular level, antigen-antibody reactions involve the combination of individual binding sites on antibody (the Fab portion) with single ligand sites, or epitopes, on an antigen. Such reactions are reversible and occur within milliseconds. For a given antigen-antibody reaction to progress to the formation of precipitate, several conditions must exist: First, both antigen molecules and antibody molecules must have multiple binding sites specific for one another. Secondly, the relative concentration of antigen and antibody in the mixture must be optimal for that system, usually corresponding to approximately equivalent amounts of antigen and antibody. Dean and Webb[3] approached the question of optimal reaction concentrations by mixing varying amounts of antigen in tubes containing antibody at constant (alpha method) levels. Ramon[17] added different antiserum concentrations to tubes containing fixed amounts of antigen (beta method). Heidelberger and Kendall[7,8] performed the classic quantitative precipitation reactions, establishing the lattice theory of precipitation; i.e., that precipitate is formed as a result of random, reversible reactions, where each antibody binds to more than one antigen and vice versa, eventually forming a "lattice" of antigen and antibody that exceeds the critical volume for solubility. Figure 3–2 illustrates basic tenets of the quantitative precipitation curve and the lattice theory. It should be noted that although this theory is easily understood and

generally accepted, it is likely an over-simplification of an extremely complex process.

Whether precipitation reactions are performed via alpha or beta methods, antibody excess (*"prozone"*) and antigen excess (*"prezone"* or *"postzone"*) usually result in suboptimal formation of precipitate, or in the partial or total dissolution of previously formed aggregates.

Other factors that affect the degree of precipitate formation include reaction time, temperature, mobility of the reactants in solution, electrolyte concentrations in the surrounding milieu, and pH.[15]

Precipitation is perhaps the simplest method of detecting antigen-antibody reactions. Most, but not all, antibodies are capable of precipitation, but not all antigens precipitate in the presence of the corresponding antibody. In solution, precipitation reactions get progressively turbid until, under optimal conditions, precipitate forms and drops out of solution. Capillary tubes have been used to mix antigen and antibody solutions and observe visible reactions. Examples include the Lancefield grouping method for streptococci[10] and the tube method for detection of C-reactive protein.

Gels have been widely used as the medium for performance of precipitation since the work of Oudin in 1946.[16] Gels, such as agar, agarose, and polyacrylamides, reduce the several anomalies observed with tube methods;[15] for example, they act to stabilize liquids and prevent the formation of convective currents. They provide a mesh-like structure where, if the pore size is greater than the particle size of the diffusing substance, and the substance does not react physically or chemically with the gel, free diffusion[15] will occur. Agar consists of a mixture of two polysaccharides, agarose and agaropectin, and is obtained by partial hydrolysis of seaweed. Preparation of agar at varying concentrations changes the pore size of the medium, e.g. a 0.3 to 1.5% agar gel concentration establishes a pore size large enough to allow diffusion of most reactants, but when precipitates form, molecular size

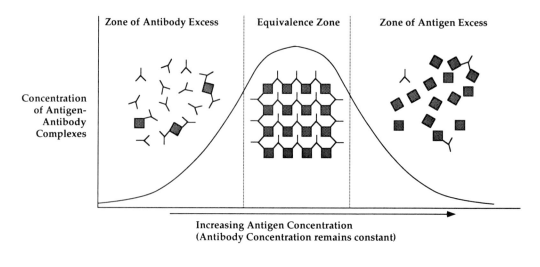

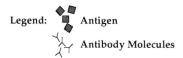

Fig. 3–2. Precipitation curve.

exceeds the dimensions of the agar pores, and diffusion stops. Agar has a strong negative charge, which is advantageous in electrophoresis (see below), but renders the use of basic dyes for staining difficult. In addition, positively charged substances may react with agar, inhibiting free diffusion in the medium and thereby obstructing precipitation reactions.

Agarose, the most widely used medium in gel diffusion tests, is prepared by removing agaropectin from agar. In contrast to agar, it has practically no charge, complexes with fewer antigens, is clearer, and permits the formation of sharper, better-defined, precipitation bands. Because it gels at a lower temperature than agar, it can be used at lower concentrations.

The rate of diffusion of a substance is dependent on molecular size (assuming it is sufficiently smaller than the pore size of a gel medium), temperature, gel viscosity, hydration, and any interaction between the substance and the gel matrix. The rate of diffusion, in turn, affects both the rate of reaction and the location of the precipitate in the gel.[9] In effect, concentration gradients are established by each reactant placed in a gel, such that highest concentrations may be found closest to the site of introduction of the reactant. As the distance from that site increases in any direction, the concentration of reactant decreases proportionately, following the equation for free diffusion.[15]

Under the principles of precipitation, visible precipitate will occur as a result of appropriate reactants being present in approximately equal concentrations under optimal conditions. When antigen and/or antibody are allowed to diffuse through a gel, the formation of precipitate at the point of equivalence indicates the presence and the relative concentration of both reactants. This technique is known as *immunodiffusion.* *Passive immunodiffusion* procedures are those where reactions are allowed to proceed without the addition of an electric field. They are slow, usually requiring days to perform, and are relatively insensitive. They are, however, simple and require no equipment or extensive training of personnel (see discussion of single and double immuno-diffusion, below). *Active immunodiffusion* combines immunodiffusion with electrophoresis, thereby shortening the time required for results and enhancing sensitivity, while increasing the need for equipment and technical expertise (see electroimmunodiffusion techniques described below).

Single diffusion techniques are those where only one reactant, usually antigen, is allowed to diffuse into a medium containing a lower concentration of corresponding antibody. One dimensional, single diffusion (*Oudin technique*) is performed in tubes (Fig. 3–3). In the original experiment,[16] antibody was mixed with agar at 60° C, then allowed to cool in a test tube. Antigen, the lone diffusing reactant, was overlaid on the cooled agar. In this system antigen can diffuse in only a single dimension (downward), and precipitate rings will form where equivalence between antigen and antibody occurs. Multiple antigen-antibody reactions, if present concurrently, will result in precipitin bands that form independently of one another.

Single immunodiffusion in two dimensions (*radial immunodiffusion*) involves incorporation of one reactant, again usually antibody, into gel that is subsequently poured into a flat plate (Fig. 3–4). Addition of the corresponding reactant, either by placing it in a circular well or on the gel surface, produces an advancing circular concentration gradient. As the molecules move outward from the point of application, precipitate stabilizes in the form of a precipitin ring, which forms at the site of approximate equivalence.

Two methods of radial immunodiffusion are commonly employed in clinical laboratories. The Fahey and McKelvey method[5] states that antigen concentration is approximately proportional to the rate of diffusion in a gel. In practice, the Fahey method is timed, and the diameter is plotted logarithmically against the concentration. The Mancini method[12] employs the principle that the area of a precipitin ring, hence, the diameter, is directly proportional to the concentration of antigen. In the Mancini technique, the reactant antigen is allowed to diffuse to completion, and antigen concentration is plotted on a linear graph against the square of the diameter.

Double immunodiffusion techniques (Fig. 3–5) are those where both antigen and antibody are allowed to diffuse through a neutral gel matrix. Each reactant diffuses independently at a rate dictated by its diffusion equation and by the parameters of the surrounding medium. Precipitates form at the equivalence points of the advancing fronts of the reactants. Unlike single diffusion, double diffusion precipitates tend to remain stationary after initial formation unless large disproportions exist, gaining only in intensity as more antigens and antibodies reach the site.

Two-dimensional double immunodiffusion, or the *Ouchterlony technique* (Fig. 3–5), was originally described by Ouchterlony,[13] and, simultaneously by Elek.[4] It is a highly versatile technique, useful for identifying and characterizing precipitating antigen-antibody systems. In practice, a neutral gel, allowed to solidify in a flat plate, is used as the diffusion matrix. Reactants may be

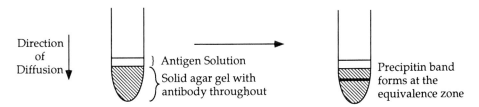

Fig. 3–3. Oudin technique. Single diffusion, one dimension.

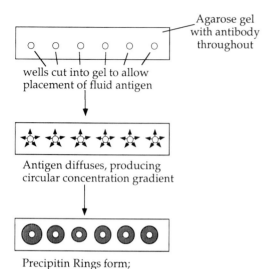

wells cut into gel to allow
placement of fluid antigen

Antigen diffuses, producing
circular concentration gradient

Precipitin Rings form;
Ring size is related to antigen concentration

Fig. 3–4. Radial immunodiffusion (RID).

placed in wells cut into the media or placed on its surface. Optimal well size and shape (if wells are used), and the distance and configuration of application points for antigen and antibody vary for each test system. Each reactant diffuses radially from the point of application and, as in one dimensional double diffusion, precipitin bands form at approximately the point of equivalence, between reacting antigen and antibody and perpendicular to the axis line between application points. The position of each precipitin band will then appear between the reactants in a position relative to each concentration, e.g. nearer the antigen well in conditions of antibody excess. When using circular wells, the precipitin bands are straight only when the molecular weights of the reactants are comparable. If antigen, for example, has a higher molecular weight than antibody, its rate of diffusion will be slower, and the precipitin band will be concave around the antigen well, but still in a position dictated by the relative concentration of the reactants.

Ouchterlony increased the versatility of double immunodiffusion by recognizing that reactants in the wells diffuse radially and hence are capable of reacting in any direction.[14] This introduces two common variations. Arranging wells equidistant around a center well allows the placement of decreasing concentrations of one component (e.g., antibody) around the radially diffusing center well, and makes titering, or determining a relative strength for the antibody solution, possible. Or, through the use of more than two wells, antigen or antibody solutions can be compared. Simply stated, if three wells are equidistant from one another, solutions with the same or different antigens can be placed in two wells, antibody in the third, and the nature of the antigens can then be observed. If the antigens are identical with respect to their reaction with antibody, their precipitin bands will fuse at their junction, as shown in Figure 3–6A. This is called a line of identity or, more correctly, a line of fusion. The high concentration of antigen in the area between the two wells prohibits the formation of precipitate beyond the point of fusion.

Lines of nonidentity, or lines of intersection, result within the same system when sample A and sample B do not contain identical antigens. Thus, they independently form their precipitates with anti-serum, as shown in Figure 3–6B.

A third possibility exists if sample A and sample B are somewhat alike, or if they share some of their molecular composition. This results in a pattern known as partial identity, or partial intersection, when one antigen and the antibody form a homologous pair, and the other antigen cross-reacts. Fusion of the two lines still occurs, but a spur forms, pointing toward the cross-reacting antigen, representing the reaction between homologous antigen and those antibodies that do not combine with the cross-reacting antigen. Hence, they diffuse past each other, as in Figure 3–6C where sample B contains a cross-reacting antigen. Partial intersection may also result when two identical solutions are used in highly disproportionate concentrations. For a more thorough discussion of the many applications of this technique, see Reference 15.

Top View

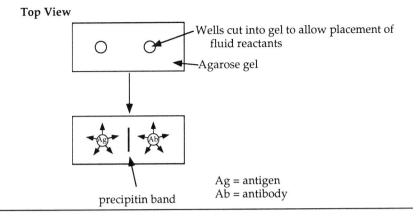

Wells cut into gel to allow placement of fluid reactants

Agarose gel

Ag = antigen
Ab = antibody

precipitin band

Side View

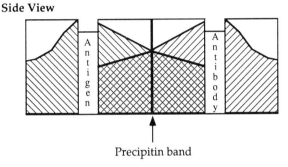

Precipitin band

Fig. 3–5. Ouchterlony technique.

Electrophoresis is the use of an electric current to induce the migration and separation of charged proteins in an electric field. In practice, electrophoretic procedures are usually stabilized by a porous material, e.g. agar, agarose, or cellulose acetate. Agarose and cellulose acetate are theoretically inert as supports for this technique, while agar possesses an electronegative charge in relation to buffer, a result of its agaropectin component. Although agarose and cellulose acetate are preferable for most electrophoresis procedures, agar is useful when endosmosis is desired (see below).

Many factors affect the migration of proteins in an electric field: the charge, size and shape of particles, the concentration, ionic strength and pH of the solvent, and the temperature and viscosity of the medium. The character and intensity of the electric field also play a role.

In the *zone electrophoresis* technique, fluid samples are placed on the medium and

placed in an electric field. Normal human serum, separated by this process, migrates into 5 distinct electrophoretic bands, i.e. albumin, $\alpha_1$globulin, $\alpha_2$globulin, β-globulin and γ-globulin. Zone electrophoresis is performed clinically as an aid in the diagnosis of human paraprotein disorders, such as multiple myeloma. (See *Characterization of Paraproteins*, Chap 5.)

Electroimmunodiffusion, or active immunodiffusion as defined above, combines electrophoresis with immunodiffusion techniques. Although many adaptations of these procedures exist,[2,9,15] we will describe only those most often employed in clinical settings. Electroimmunodiffusion, like immunodiffusion, may be classified as single or double diffusion in one- or two-dimensions. One-dimensional electrophoresis of a single component (the "rocket technique" developed by Laurell in 1966)[11] is an adaptation of radial immunodiffusion. Two-dimen-

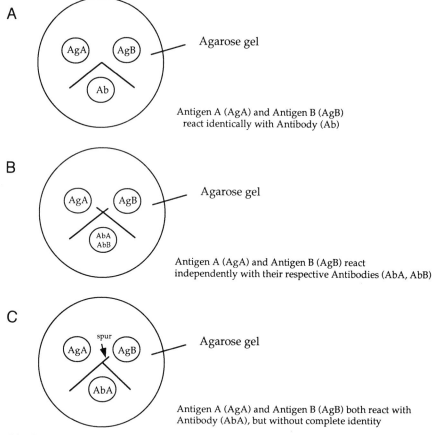

Fig. 3–6. (A) Reaction of identity; (B) Reaction of nonidentity; (C) Reaction of partial identity.

sional double diffusion ("crossed immu-noelectrophoresis")[15] is employed as a qual-itative and quantitative tool, primarily in research situations.

One-dimensional double diffusion, also known as *counter immunoelectrophoresis* (CIEP; Fig. 3–7) is based on the principle of end-osmosis. As described above, commercially available agar forms a gel with a negative electrical charge. When this type of gel is used for electrophoresis, a current of buffer is established in the direction opposite to the electrophoretic migration. This slows migration and, in the case of small or elec-trically neutral molecules, may actually cause cathodal migration. Counter immu-noelectrophoresis exploits this anomaly. In this technique, antigen and antibody are placed in appropriate, adjacent wells (an-tibody in anodal well; antigen in cathodal

well). If antigen has a relative negative charge, and antibody is neutral under test conditions, electric current will force the reactants to migrate toward one another, and precipitate forms as they meet. Endos-motic flow, in this example, is performed by the antibody.

Immunoelectrophoresis, developed by Grabar and Williams,[6] combines electrophoretic protein separation with immunodiffusion in an ingenious method of analyzing and iden-tifying serum proteins. Serum, placed in an appropriate medium (cellulose acetate, agar, agarose), is electrophoresed to separate its constituents according to their electropho-retic mobilities; albumin, the most nega-tively charged in basic buffers, moves the farthest distance toward the anode, fol-lowed by the alpha$_1$, alpha$_2$, beta, and gam-ma globulins. Following electrophoresis,

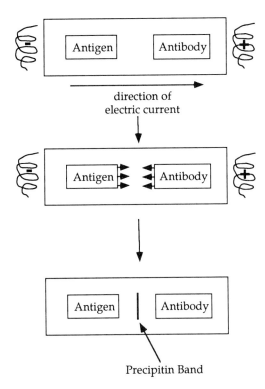

direction of
electric current

Precipitin Band

Fig. 3–7. Counter immunoelectrophoresis.

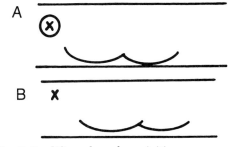

Fig. 3–9. Wing-shaped precipitin arcs.
a. Fusion of precipitin arcs.
b. Partial fusion of arcs.

trenches, or troughs, on each side of and parallel to the line of electrophoresis, are filled with antiserum, polyvalent, or mon-ovalent. Incubation allows double immu-nodiffusion to take place; each antiserum diffuses outward, perpendicular to its trough, and each serum protein diffuses outward from its point of electrophoresis (Fig. 3–8). Precipitin bands form approxi-mately at the equivalence point of antigen and antibody, as in conventional double im-munodiffusion. However, the shape and placement of the precipitate tell a great deal

about the proteins in question. In all, greater than 30 proteins can be differentiated in normal sera using this method.

The position and shape of precipitin bands after immunoelectrophoresis of hu-man serum are relatively stable and repro-ducible. Virtually any deviation is abnor-mal. A common technique is to compare arc shape, intensity, and location to normal ser-um treated the same way. It may be ob-served, for example, that excess serum pro-tein (antigen) forms precipitate nearer to the trough, and the arc is denser, with a sharp edge on the sample side, whereas the trough side is diffuse. With gross antigen excess, the precipitate may move into the trough, leaving visible only the tips of the band. Low levels of serum protein, con-versely, cause precipitate to form farther from the trough and to be more diffuse.

Heterogeneous serum proteins of a given type (e.g., normal IgG of smoothly gradated differences in electrophoretic mobilities) produce precipitin bands of moderate cur-vature. Homogeneous proteins (e.g. albu-min) form markedly curved bands, the re-sult of radial diffusion from a single point of electrophoresis.

An electrophoretically abnormal protein will be displaced from the position it would normally occupy. Occasionally, wing, or gull-wing, formation is noted, a result of fusion of precipitin bands (Fig. 3–9A) or of partial fusion (Fig. 3–9B), indicating the presence of proteins immunologically iden-

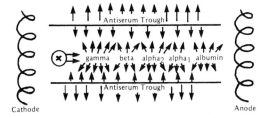

Cathode   Anode

Fig. 3–8. Principle of Immunoelectrophoresis.

tical, or similar but electrophoretically distinct.

The most useful clinical application of immunoelectrophoresis is in detection and identification of M-component paraproteins due to multiple myeloma, Waldenstrom's macroglobulinemia, benign monoclonal gammopathy, malignant lymphoma, Bence-Jones proteinemia or proteinuria, Franklin's disease, cold agglutinin disease, and other lympho-proliferative disorders. Immunoelectrophoresis can be used to identify proteins in most body fluids. (See also *Monoclonal Gammopathies; Characterization of Paraproteins.*)

Immunofixation electrophoresis, first described by Alper and Johnson,[1] is similar to immunoelectrophoresis, except that antiserum is applied to the surface of the gel, after electrophoresis. Strips of cellulose acetate or agarose, saturated with specific antisera, are often used.[18] Because immunodiffusion in this system will occur in both directions, either the gel or the cellulose acetate may be stained and observed for reactants. Major advantages of this adaptation include shortened immunodiffusion times and significantly higher resolution in many systems.[9] (See also *Characterization of Paraproteins.*)

REFERENCES

1. Alper, C.A., and Johnson, A.M.: Vox Sang., *17*:445, 1969.
2. Bier, O.G.: In *Fundamentals of Immunology,* 2nd ed. Edited by Bier, O.G., Dias da Silva, W., Gotze, D., and Mota, I., Berlin, Springer-Verlag, 1986.
3. Dean, H.R., and Webb, R.A.: J. Pathol. Bacteriol. *29*:473, 1926.
4. Elek, S.D.: Br. Med. J., *1*:493, 1948.
5. Fahey, J.L., and McKelvey, E.M.: J. Immunol. *94*:84, 1965.
6. Grabar, P., and Williams, C.A. Jr.: Biochim. Biophys. Acta, *10*:193, 1953.
7. Heidelberger, M., and Kendall, F.E.: J. Exp. Med., *61*:563, 1935.
8. Heidelberger, M., and Kendall, F.E.: J. Exp. Med., *62*:467, 1935.
9. Johnson, A.M.: In *Manual of Clinical Laboratory Immunology.* 3rd ed. Edited by N.R. Rose, H. Friedman, and J.L. Fahey. Washington, D.C., American Society for Microbiology, 1986.
10. Lancefield, R.C.: J. Exp. Med., *57*:571, 1933.
11. Laurell, C.B.: Anal. Biochem., *15*:45, 1966.
12. Mancini, G., Carbonara, A.O.: and Heremans, J.F.: Immunochemistry, *2*:235, 1965.
13. Ouchterlony, O.: Acta. Path. Microbiol. Scand., *25*:186, 1948.
14. Ouchterlony, O.: Acta. Path. Microbiol. Scand., *32*:231, 1953.
15. Ouchterlony, O.: and Nilsson, L.A. In *Handbook of Immunology I,* Edited by D.M. Weir. Oxford, Blackwell Scientific Publications, 1986.
16. Oudin, J.: C. R. Hebd. Séanc. Acad. Sci., *222*:115, 1946.
17. Ramon, G.: C. R. Séanc. Soc. Biol., *86*:661, 1922.
18. Ritchie, R.F., and Smith, R.: Clin. Chem., *22*:1735, 1976..

Agglutination

Agglutination is the observable clumping of particles which occurs as a result of specific interaction between an "agglutinin," usually antibody, and an "agglutinogen" or antigen. Agglutination is a two-phase reaction. The primary phase, where antibody reacts with single antigenic determinants on or close to the particle surface, is a rapid, reversible molecular reaction similar in nature to covalent chemical bonding (Fig. 3–10). The secondary phase is a result of the stabilization of antigen-antibody reactions in solution such that multivalent reactions occur, e.g., a single antibody molecule binds to antigenic determinants on adjacent particles. In equilibrated solutions, under appropriate conditions and over time, particles remain connected and interconnected by antibody bridges (Fig. 3–11) and visible aggregation occurs.

The secondary phase of an agglutination reaction depends on the physical state of the antigen, the relative concentrations of antigen and antibody, and environmental conditions. For a secondary, or agglutination reaction to occur, antibody must first be able to bridge the gap between particles so that at least one Fab portion is attached to an antigenic determinant on each of two adjacent particles. Because particulate antigens have net surface electrostatic charges resulting, at least in part, from surface chemical groupings that are completely or partially ionized, and because particles in a homologous reaction are virtually identical,

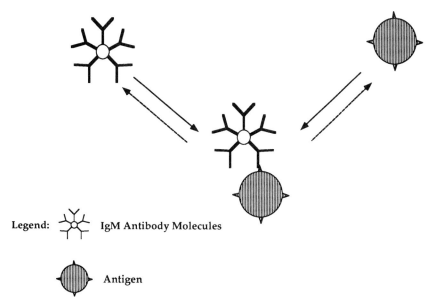

Fig. 3–10. Primary phase antigen-antibody reaction.

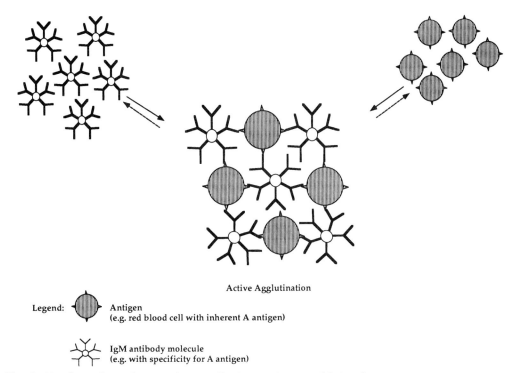

Fig. 3–11. Secondary phase antigen-antibody reaction, equilibriated.

these charges tend to repel one another, the net effect of which is to keep particles apart. In addition, ions in solution around a particle form an "ionic cloud" which increases the degree of repulsion. Electrolytes are crucial to agglutination reactions,[2] apparently because saline solution neutralizes net negative charges and tends to nullify these repulsive forces. Most agglutination reactions are optimal at near neutral pH and at physiologic salt concentrations (0.15 M NaCl).[1]

The viscosity of the fluid environment may also affect the degree of secondary reaction. Albumin or other agents (e.g. enzymes) act to enhance environmental pressure and may be needed to improve the likelihood of secondary reaction.

The optimal temperature required varies among agglutination reactions, and the reaction may be enhanced by changing the temperature during incubation. Agitation, centrifugation, or other physical manipulations may act to enhance agglutination in in vitro situations.

With the exception of those in vitro reactions where monoclonal antibody interacts with antigen, agglutination actually results from the sum of interactions among a mixture of heterogeneous antibodies and multiple antigenic determinants on a particle.

Antibodies involved in in vitro reactions are said to be *complete* if they are capable of both primary and secondary-stage interactions with antigen in normal saline solution. *Incomplete* antibodies effect primary but not secondary binding. Because IgM antibodies agglutinate far better than IgG, by 750-fold in one study,[7] most antibody-induced agglutination is probably due to IgM, as indicated in Figure 3–12. In practice, the presence of IgG in test samples may have the effect of *blocking* the agglutinating ability of IgM, by occupying needed binding sites on the antigen (Fig. 3–12).

Prozone, or absence of agglutination at higher antibody concentrations, may be due to a number of factors. The presence of blocking antibodies at low titers may be responsible. Inaccessible antigenic determinants (see below) or weak avidity (the sum of the association constants of antigens with antibody) may characterize the reaction. Or, as in precipitation, antibody excess may allow each antibody to occupy only a single site on the antigen surface such that cross-linkage, hence, secondary reaction, is improbable.[2]

Hemagglutination is the agglutination of red blood cells as a result of antibody or microbial (e.g. viral) interaction with antigenic determinants on the red cell surface. Hemagglutination reactions tend to be temperature-dependent, due, at least in part, to structural changes in the red cell membrane as temperature fluctuates, allowing antigens to "hide" or become exposed. (See discussion on cold agglutinins.) Incomplete hemagglutinating antibodies (IgG) commonly demonstrate warm antibody behavior.[8]

Agglutination reactions have the advantages of simplicity, a wide range of applicability, and relative sensitivity,[8] to the order of .003 μg/mL in some systems.[2] However, they are usually only semi-quantitative. Agglutination procedures are performed in test tubes or microtiter plates. Single tube (or well) reactions may be performed and the reaction *graded* (e.g. 4+, 3+, etc.), or one of the reactants (usually antibody) may be serially diluted with the subsequent addition of its counterpart (antigen) to all tubes, resulting in a *titer*. (See *Technical Instruction: Serial Dilutions and Titers.*) In titered assays, the reciprocal of the last dilution still exhibiting the predetermined reaction or reaction strength is considered the titer. Observation may be accomplished by eye, with the use of a magnifying lens, with a microscope, or, more recently, by turbidimetric or nephelometric instrumentation. In some systems, reactions result in three-dimensional agglutinates that may be graded, if desired, by size and the proportion of particles involved in the reaction, e.g. 4+ is one solid aggregate; 1+ is small aggregate with turbid background. In other assays, particles are allowed to settle and the sed-

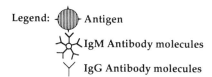

IgG and IgM
in serum

IgG binds to antigenic sites
and blocks the ability of IgM
molecules to cross-link antigens

Legend: ◉ Antigen

✹ IgM Antibody molecules

Y IgG Antibody molecules

Fig. 3–12. Effect of blocking antibodies.

iment pattern is subsequently observed. An even carpet of particles in this system indicates a 4+ reaction; a button results from no reaction at all. Intermediate reactions are graded 3+, 2+, etc. Instrumental analysis of agglutination reactions, referred to as Particle-Enhanced Immunoassay, is one of the newer technologies, serving to enhance the sensitivity of agglutination assays (see below). Use of smaller particles (e.g. latex) in some assays has enhanced sensitivity,[6,13] while employing monoclonal antibodies has improved both the sensitivity and the specificity of many systems.

One of the disadvantages inherent to agglutination procedures is their inability to quantitate antigen or antibody. Strict standardization is usually required and the relative sensitivity may depend on the reagents used and the technical performance of the test. In some assays, agglutination may result from cross-reactions caused by the presence of antibodies capable of binding to antigens similar in structure, e.g. Brucella and Francisella. The presence of heterophile antibodies in sera may cause false-positive reactions in those assays where red cells are obtained from a nonhuman source. Rheumatoid factors, if present in serum, may effect agglutination of particles in virtually any system, once antibody is attached to the particle. And, autoagglutination of particles may occur in some assays under certain conditions. Specific information regarding difficulties that may be encountered with individual assays are furnished in the text following the test description.

Agglutination reactions may be active (direct), passive (indirect), or reverse passive. Each of these classifications is described below. Discussions of agglutination inhibition, antiglobulin-mediated (Coomb's), and particle-enhanced immunoassays are also included.

ACTIVE AGGLUTINATION (FIG. 3–11)

Active, or direct, agglutination occurs when the antigenic determinant is inherent to the particle itself. Examples include use of anti-A or anti-B antisera to detect A and/ or B antigens on human red blood cells, or use of antigen from Brucella to detect Brucella antibody in sera from exposed individuals.

In many cases, as in the examples above, active agglutination occurs without augmentation. This implies the presence of "complete" antibodies (usually IgM) capable of cross-linking adjacent particles. However, if "incomplete" (usually IgG) antibodies are present or predominate, or where strongly repulsive antigen particles are used, enhancement of the reaction may be needed. Commonly used enhancers[9] include the addition of bovine albumin to test medium, which acts to increase environmental viscosity, and use of Low Ionic-Strength Salt Solutions (LISS), which provide hypotonic suspensions. Enzymes such as bromelin, papain, and ficin may act to enhance certain active agglutination reactions.

PASSIVE AGGLUTINATION (FIG. 3–13A)

Passive, or indirect, agglutination results when inert particles are coated with soluble antigen, creating antigens known as *passive agglutinogens,* which may then react with antibody. Polystyrene latex, red blood cells, bentonite, and charcoal are commonly employed as particles. Many substances, most notably polysaccharides and proteins, may spontaneously absorb to latex,[6,10] to erythrocytes[11] or to bentonite.[4] Many proteins, however, require some manipulation for optimal antigen-binding. Pretreatment of erythrocytes with tannic acid[3] enhances attachment of antigens, as do several covalent-bonding methods,[2,11] such as trypsin, bisdiazotized benzine (BDB), carbodiimide (CDI), or glutaraldehyde treatment.[13] Metallic bridges, using $Cr+$ ions or immunologic bridges, where antibody serves to adhere antigen, may also aid in antigen attachment to particles.[2] Latex particles used for passive agglutination are relatively large, 0.77 to 0.81 mm in diameter, and may require special techniques for covalent-bonding.[6] Smaller particles are used in the particle-enhanced immunoassays, described below. When erythrocytes are used for bonding, they are often stabilized in formaldehyde, glutaraldehyde, or an alternate fixative before storage.[13] Sera to be tested with erythrocyte-bound antigen may first require adsorption with antigen-free red cells to remove interfering substances (e.g. heterophile antibodies) that might cause false positive tests.

REVERSE PASSIVE AGGLUTINATION (FIG. 3–13B)

Reverse passive agglutination involves the adherence of antibody to inert particles, which can then be used to detect the presence of antigen. Because of the protein nature of antibody, adsorption may occur spontaneously, or may require manipulation as described above. *Reverse Passive Hemagglutination* (RPHA) assays are available for the detection of several antigens, including rubella, *Hemophilus influenzae, Neisseria meningitidis,* group B Streptococci, and several therapeutic drugs.

AGGLUTINATION INHIBITION / HEMAGGLUTINATION INHIBITION

In principle, agglutination inhibition involves interference, by antigen or antibody, with an antigen-antibody reaction which would have resulted in agglutination, if interference had not occurred. The technique is called hemagglutination inhibition if the particle employed in the reaction is an erythrocyte. Two agglutination inhibition techniques are currently applicable in clinical situations. The first (Fig. 3–14A) is used to detect soluble antigen (e.g. Hepatitis B surface antigen, human chorionic gonadotropin, Factor VII). In these procedures, patient sample, potentially a source of the antigen, is added to a limited amount of agglutinating antibody. In the absence of a particle, this reaction, if it occurs, will have no visible results. The addition of an antigen-coated particle (e.g. latex, red blood cells) will result in agglutination, if no antigen is present in patient sample. No agglutination would be seen if the patient sample contained antigen. Newer adaptations of agglutination inhibition technique involve the use of colloidal dye particles (Disperse Dye Immunoassay or DIA), or inorganic colloidal particles, known as "Sols" (Sol Particle Immunoassay or SPIA).[13]

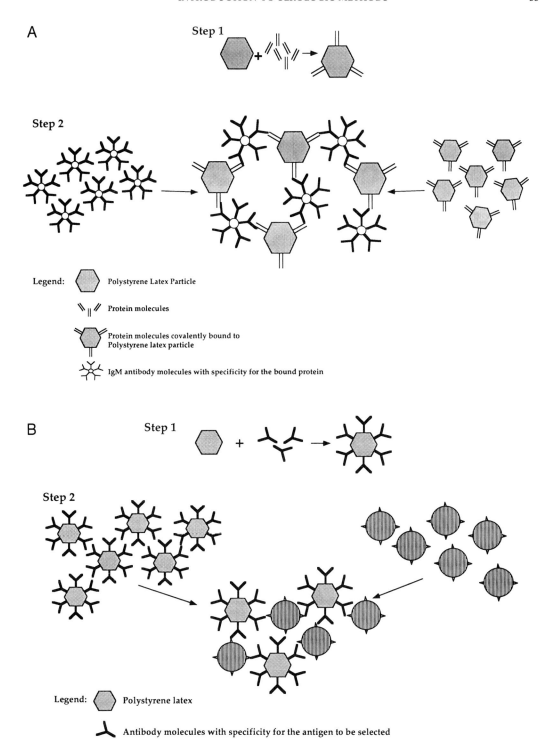

Fig. 3–13. (A) Passive agglutination. (B) Reverse passive agglutination.

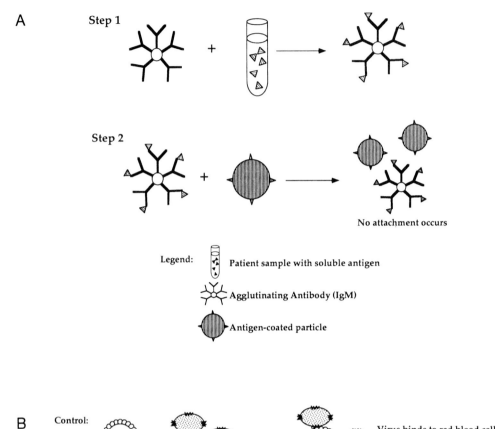

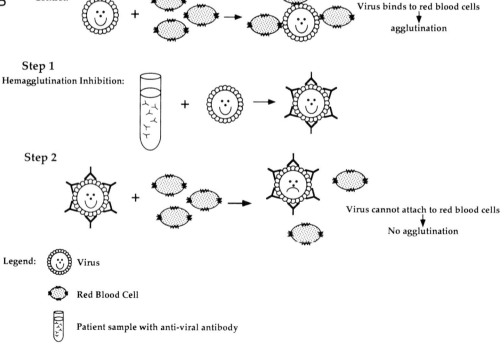

Fig. 3–14. (A) Agglutination inhibition. (B) Viral hemagglutination inhibition.

Several viruses have the ability to induce hemagglutination when combined in vitro with erythrocytes from specific animal sources,[12] for example, rubella virus can agglutinate red cells from newborn chickens. This phenomenon forms the basis for the second application of the agglutination inhibition technique (Fig. 3–14B). Antibody to a hemagglutinating virus can be detected by first reacting the patient sample (possibly containing antibody) with virus, then subsequently adding the appropriate erythrocytes in suspension. If inhibiting antibody is present in patient sample, agglutination will not occur. If antibody is absent, agglutination will be evident. A classic hemagglutination inhibition assay detects antibody to rubella, and requires several time-consuming pretreatment and standardization steps. Although the rubella HI remains as the comparison standard for rubella antibody, the technical difficulty of HI procedures has limited their application.

ANTIGLOBULIN (COOMB'S)–MEDIATED AGGLUTINATION

Antiglobulin-mediated agglutination, or Coomb's testing, involves the use of a second antibody, directed against immunoglobulin or complement, which acts as a bridge between molecules of antibody or complement on the cell surface. For *Direct Antiglobulin (Coomb's)* reactions (Fig. 3–15A), Coomb's antisera (usually anti-IgG, anti-C_{3d}, or both) is added to cells, in order to detect in vivo sensitization (attachment) of immunoglobulin or complement, as might occur in individuals with autoimmune hemolytic anemias, (e.g. anti-Rh antibodies) or hemolytic disease of the newborn (Rh disease). *Indirect Antiglobulin (Coomb's)* procedures (Fig. 3–15B) are usually performed to detect nonagglutinating ("incomplete") antibody in serum. Cells with known antigen(s) are reacted with patient serum, a source of nonagglutinating or "incomplete" antibody. Coomb's reagent (anti-IgG, anti-C_{3d}) is subsequently added to effect agglutination of the red cells, indicating the presence of antibody or complement activation.[9]

Indirect Coomb's tests are used to detect and identify potentially dangerous antibodies in candidates for transfusion (Antibody Screen and Identification), and currently to detect antibody to donor antigens in the antiglobulin phase of compatibility testing (the Cross-Match).[9]

PARTICLE-ENHANCED IMMUNOASSAY

The in vitro combination of a soluble antigen with antibody results in a secondary phase reaction (precipitation) only if optimal relative concentrations and sufficient quantities of each reactant are present to allow the reaction to be detected. The inherent insensitivity of soluble antigen reactions with antibody has been the basis of many adaptations, among them the particle-enhanced immunoassays.

Probably the simplest particle-enhanced assays are the passive and reverse passive agglutination reactions described above, where attachment of antigen (passive) or antibody (reverse passive) to a particle enhances sensitivity, and, in many cases, the ease of performance of an assay. Direct detection of antibody (e.g. rheumatoid factors, antibody to rubella) or of antigen (e.g., *Hemophilus influenzae, Neisseria meningitidis* in blood or spinal fluid) is easily accomplished by a manual kit method, often on a slide, and in a relatively short time period.

Further enhancement of sensitivity may be approached with the principle of agglutination inhibition, which essentially involves setting up a competition, either serially or spontaneously, between a known antigen or antibody with its identical counterpart in patient sample, as described above.

Over the past several years, the principles of light-scattering (nephelometry) and light-absorption (turbidimetry) have been applied to particle-enhanced reactions. Nephelometry has classically been used to enhance the detectability of soluble antigen-antibody reactions, achieving a sensitivity on the order of 1 to 10 $\mu g/ml$. The attachment of a small particle to either antigen or antibody enhances the sensitivity to ng/ml

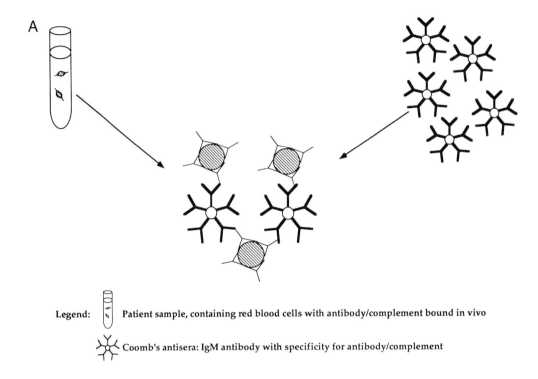

A

Legend: Patient sample, containing red blood cells with antibody/complement bound in vivo

Coomb's antisera: IgM antibody with specificity for antibody/complement

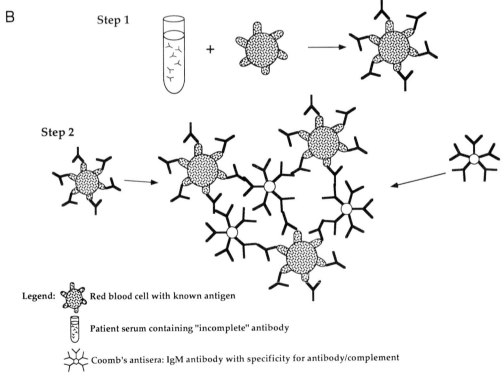

B

Step 1

Step 2

Legend: Red blood cell with known antigen

Patient serum containing "incomplete" antibody

Coomb's antisera: IgM antibody with specificity for antibody/complement

Fig. 3–15. (A) Direct antiglobulin (Coomb's) reactions. (B) Indirect antiglobulin (Coomb's) reactions.

in some systems. Latex particles[5] with diameters of 0.1 to 0.2 μm have been found to result in high sensitivity, and are commonly used,[6] often with monoclonal antibodies to improve specificity.[13]

PETINA, or particle-enhanced turbidimetric inhibition immunoassays, are being used to detect drugs (gentamicin, digoxin, and theophylline) and proteins in serum. In these assays, particles coated with the drug or protein are placed in competition with the unknown in patient serum for a limited amount of antibody reagent. Turbidimetric detection of particle aggregation is used to measure the degree of reaction. In this system, increases in turbidity are inversely proportional to the amount of the unknown in patient sample.

Particle-counting immunoassays (PACIA) and particle-enhanced quasi-elastic light-scattering spectroscopy (QUELS) are both adaptations based on the ability of nephelometry to recognize aggregated particles.[8] (See also *Nephelometry*.)

REFERENCES

1. Berzofsky, J.A., and Berkower, I.J.: In *Fundamental Immunology*. Edited by W.E. Paul. New York, Raven Press, 1984.

2. Bier, O.G.: In *Fundamentals of Immunology*. 2nd ed. Edited by O.G. Bier, W.D. deSilva, D. Götze, and I. Mota. New York, Springer-Verlag, 1986.

3. Boyden, S.V.: J. Exp. Med., *93*:107, 1951.

4. Bozeccvich, J. et al.: Proc. Soc. Exp. Biol. Med., *97*:180, 1958.

5. Craig, A.R. et al.: Clin. Chem. *30*:1489, 1984.

6. Galvin, J.P: In *Manual of Clinical Laboratory Immunology*. 3rd ed. Edited by N.R. Rose, H. Friedman, and J.L. Fahey. Washington, D.C., American Society for Microbiology, 1986.

7. Greenbury, C.L., Moore, D.H., and Nunn, L.A.C., Immunology 6:421, 1963.

8. Nichols, W.S., and Nakamura, R.M.: In *Manual of Clinical Laboratory Immunology*. 3rd ed. Edited by N.R. Rose, H. Friedman, and J.L. Fahey. Washington, D.C., American Society for Microbiology, 1986.

9. Pittiglio, D.H.: *Modern Blood Banking and Transfusion Practices*. Philadelphia, F.A. Davis, 1983.

10. Singer, J.M., and Plotz, C.M.: Am. J. Med., *21*:888, 1956.

11. Stites, D.P., and Channing Rogers, R.P.: In *Basic and Clinical Immunology*. 6th ed. Edited by D.P. Stites, J.D. Stobo, and J.V. Wells. Norwalk, Appleton and Lange, 1987.

12. Stott, E.J., and Tyrrell, D.A.J.: In *Handbook of*

Table 3–1. Agglutination Reactions

Active (Direct)
Passive (Indirect)
Reverse Passive
Agglutination—Inhibition
Antiglobulin-Mediated (Coomb's)
Particle-Enhanced Immunoassay

Experimental Immunology IV. Edited by D.M. Weir, Oxford, Blackwell Scientific Publications, 1986.

13. vanHell, H., Leuvering, J.H.W., and Gribnau, T.C.J.: In *Alternative Immunoassays*. Edited by W.P. Collins, London, John Wiley & Sons, 1985.

Complement Fixation

Antigen-antibody reactions that activate complement components may be detected by a serologic method known as complement fixation, or CF. In principle, complement fixation techniques may be used to detect either antigen or antibody; in clinical practice, however, they are most often used for establishing the presence of elevated antibody levels in patient samples. IgM and IgG, subclasses 1, 2, and 3, are capable of activating complement when they attach to antigen in most, but not all situations,[2] while the other classes of antibody apparently are not.

Because of the natural amplification that occurs during sequential complement component activation, complement fixation methods are among the more sensitive of serologic assays, tending to be more sensitive than standard agglutination and precipitation tests, but less sensitive than radioimmunoassay, immunofluorescence, or enzyme immunoassays. Although complement fixation assays are theoretically simple procedures, they are complicated in practice and are not routinely performed in most clinical immunology laboratories. Their usefulness in documentation of acute clinical infection with organisms such as viruses, rickettsia, and the dimorphic fungi, however, provides impetus for their continued performance in specialized laboratories.

In principle, complement fixation tests involve a competition between two antigen-antibody systems—a test system and an indicator system—which are each potentially capable of complement activation (Fig. 3–16). Initially, antigen and inactivated patient sample (the source of antibody) are reacted with a standardized, limited amount of reagent complement. If the specific, complement-activating antibody to the antigen is present in the serum, complement will be activated, or "fixed", and the components that are used will be depleted. Sheep red blood cells (SRBC), coated with anti-SRBC antibody (referred to as hemolysin, or amboceptor), are added as the indicator system. If complement components remain after the first reaction, they will be activated by the indicator (referred to as *Erythrocyte/Antibody*, or EA), resulting in hemolysis of the sheep red blood cells. The presence of antibody in the patient sample, then, is indicated by a decrease, or by the total absence, of hemolysis.

In practice, accurate results in complement fixation assays depend on appropriate use of each of the reagents involved, e.g.

the amount, purity and type of antigen, the concentration and reactivity of the complement used, the concentration of red blood cells, and the quantity and quality of hemolysin. Certain physical parameters of the reaction system, such as the ionic strength, pH, incubation times and temperatures, may affect the results as well. Careful preparation, standardization, and quality control of each reagent is imperative to ensure accuracy of results. In laboratories where complement fixation techniques are used with some regularity, the same basic procedure, and many of the same reagents and working dilutions, may be applied routinely to several antigen-antibody test situations.

It is necessary to run controls for each component of the test system during performance of complement fixation assays. Of particular theoretical interest is the control that is designed to detect anticomplementary factors in the patient sample which could interfere with the ability of the reagent complement to hemolyze. Addition of

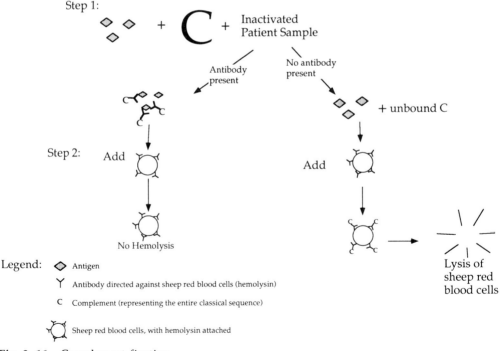

Fig. 3–16. Complement fixation.

inactivated patient sample to reagent complement, with the subsequent addition of the sheep erythrocyte-antibody suspension (EA) is used to detect any anticomplementary activity that may be caused by factors such as bacterial contamination or lipids.

Procedural guides for performance of both macro- and microtechniques for complement fixation are available.[2-4]

Detection of complement-binding antigen-antibody reactions may be accomplished by adaptation of Enzyme-Linked Immunosorbent Assay (ELISA). This combination technique, referred to as COMP-ELISA,[1] can be read photometrically, and requires fewer preliminary steps than do the more traditional complement fixation assays.

REFERENCES

1. Hincliffe, P.M., and Robertson, L.: J. Clin. Pathol., *36*:100, 1983.

2. Kabat, E.A., and Mayer, M.: *Experimental Immunochemistry*. 2nd ed. Springfield, Charles C Thomas, 1964.

3. Palmer, D.F.: *A Guide to the Performance of the Standardized Diagnostic Complement Fixation Method and Adaptation to Micro Test*. Atlanta, Centers for Disease Control, 1981.

4. Palmer, D.F., and Whaley, S.D.: In *Manual of Clinical Laboratory Immunology*, 3rd ed. Edited by N.R. Rose, H. Friedman, and J.L. Fahey. Washington, D.C., American Society for Microbiology, 1986.

Enzyme Inhibition

Enzymes are proteins produced by living cells that can cause detectable changes in substrates. As proteins, enzymes may also be antigenic, inducing the production of antibody in the heterologous, immunocompetent host. In many cases, the reaction of a specific antibody with an enzyme inhibits the enzyme's ability to react with its substrate molecule, a phenomenon known as enzyme inhibition.

In vitro assays have been developed that utilize the known inhibitory effects of antibody on the extracellular toxins produced by streptococci, e.g., streptolysin O, DNAse, and hyaluronidase. These are known as enzyme inhibition assays. In practical use, enzyme inhibition assays are performed by first reacting patient serum (the potential source of antibody) with reagent enzyme. After appropriate incubation, the substrate is added. In the presence of antibody to the enzyme, the enzyme-substrate reaction is inhibited and no changes will be observed in the substrate. In the absence of antibody, the substrate will be altered by free enzyme, and the alterations can be detected.

Nephelometry[1]

When a beam of light passes through a solution, alterations in the nature of the beam will occur as a result of its collision with suspended particles of varying sizes and shapes within the solution. Waves of light within the beam may be reflected, absorbed, or scattered by contact with these particles. In practice, much can be deduced about the nature of soluble particles by observing the degree of reflection, absorption, or scatter of incident light.

In the clinical laboratory, two practical applications of this principle are in common use: turbidimetry and nephelometry. *Turbidimetry*[2] measures the turbidity, or "cloudiness" of a solution. The detection device, referred to as a turbidimeter, is placed such that it is in direct line with the incident light and the solution, and collects the beam after passage through the solution (Fig. 3–17A). Turbidimetric readings, then, measure the reduction in light intensity that has occurred as a result of the combination of reflection, absorption, or scatter of the incident light. Turbidimetry is recorded in "absorbance units," which reflects the ratio of incident to transmitted light.

Nephelometry measures only the light that is scattered to a previously determined angle from the incident beam (Fig. 3–17B). Results of nephelometric assays are recorded in arbitrary units, e.g. "relative light scatter," or may be directly extrapolated by computer and recorded in mg/dl or IU/ml, based on the established values of the standards used. Controls are run concurrently with the test to establish the amount

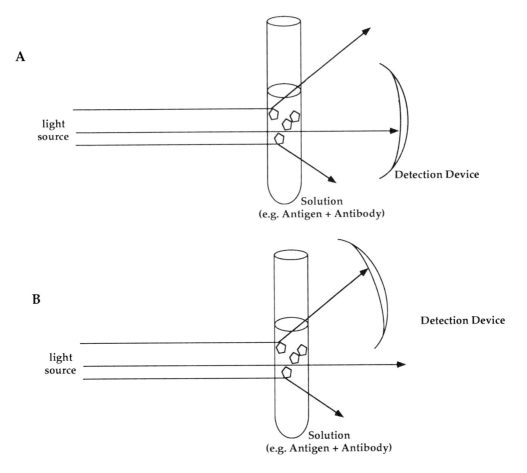

Fig. 3–17. (A) Turbidemetry; (B) Nephelometry.

of background scatter in reagents and test samples.

Both turbidimetry and nephelometry are viable principles in clinical immunology, owing at least in part to the relative success of each in different situations.[1,2]

In practical application, nephelometry may be used to measure either antigen or antibody in solution. Most commonly, an antibody reagent is used to detect antigen in patient sample, e.g.

reagent antibody +

    patient sample ⟶ measurement of
      (antigen)   light scatter

The amount of light scattered by antigen-antibody complexes in the solution will be affected by the complex shape and size, the refractive index of the media, the wavelength and intensity of incident light and the angle of detection.[3,4] In general, light scatter increases as the number and size of immune complexes increases. Once stabilization of the latter variables is assured within a nephelometric system, light scatter becomes an accurate reflection of the antigen-antibody complexes formed, and thus, of the unknown in patient sample, if the concentration of reagent antibody is controlled.

Use of nephelometry for detection of antigen-antibody complexes involves application of the principles of precipitation (see *Precipitation*), wherein approximate equivalence of antigen and antibody will result in optimal precipitation. From the curve derived by Heidelberger, it becomes evident that, if antigen is kept constant, the addition of increasing concentrations of antibody will induce gradual increases in the size of antigen-antibody complexes, until the equivalence zone is reached. The opposite also applies, i.e. when antibody is kept constant and antigen is added in increasing concentrations, similar results can be expected. In either case, if the antigen used is soluble, complexes increase in size only to the molecular weight applicable to Raleigh-Debye scatter (i.e. to approximately 3×10^6.[1,4] Use of a polymer such as polyethylene glycol (PEG) tends to enhance and stabilize the precipitates, thereby aiding in control of particle size for optimal light deflection. Significant excess of either antigen or antibody results in decreased immune complex formation, and therefore, decreased light scatter.

In its earlier stages, nephelometric instruments were designed to detect 90° light scatter, and they employed fluorimeters whose excitation and emission wavelength were the same, or nearly so. More recently developed nephelometers measure forward light scatter at angles ranging from 10 to 70° and use such sources as helium-neon lasers or quartz-iodide for incident light. Intensity of light is important in these assays and should be routinely monitored.[3]

In *end-point nephelometry*,[1] antigen and antibody concentrations are chosen to effect slight antigen or antibody excess, depending on which of the reactants is being detected. Reactions are allowed to proceed to completion, and results are determined. In the more widely used *kinetic nephelometric assays*, referred to as "rate nephelometry",[4] the reagents are incubated for a short period of time, and the rate of light scatter increase is measured. These assays are applicable for the detection and quantitation of a wide range of proteins (e.g. immunoglobulins, complement components, and acute phase reactants) and therapeutic drugs.

REFERENCES

1. Deaton, C.: Am. J. Med. Technol., *48*:657, 1982.
2. Foster, R.C., and Ledue, T.B.: In *Manual of Clinical Laboratory Immunology*. 3rd ed. Edited by N.R. Rose, H.H. Friedman, and J.L. Fahey. Washington, D.C., American Society for Microbiology, 1986.
3. Salkie, M.L.: Clin. Chim. Acta, *152*:363, 1985.
4. Sternberg, J.C.: In *Manual of Clinical Laboratory Immunology*, 3rd ed. Edited by N.R. Rose, H.H. Friedman, and J.L. Fahey. Washington D.C., American Society for Microbiology, 1986.

Labeling Techniques

Among the most useful techniques available to the clinical laboratory are three that involve labeling, or tagging antigen-antibody reactions in order to detect and/or quantitate the presence of one of the reactants: *Immunofluorescence* (IFA) uses a fluorescent label, *radioimmunoassay* (RIA) uses a radionucleotide label, and *enzyme immunoassay* (EIA) employs an enzyme as label.

Immunofluorescence, the first of these to be developed, had been somewhat restricted in applicability and sensitivity, until recent advances in theory and technology merged to foster its re-emergence with a wider range of applications.

Radioimmunoassay, developed in the early 1960s, moved quickly into a place of prominence in clinical and research aspects of medicine, a result of its extreme sensitivity to picogram (10^{-12}) range, and large number of applicable variations.

Because of its sensitivity, simplicity, wide applicability, and ease of operation, the newest of the labeling techniques, *enzyme immunoassay,* has rapidly emerged as an assay system of choice for many test systems.

Immunofluorescence Assays[8,11,15,21]

FLUORESCENCE IMMUNOASSAYS

Immunofluorescence assay (IFA) or fluorescence immunoassay (FIA) are generic terms used to include an increasingly large number of immunoassay techniques[2,8] that use fluorescent probes to label antigen-antibody reactions. The use of fluorescent compounds in this manner was initiated in

1941 by Coons et al.,[3] who labeled an antibody with a blue fluorescent compound, then used this as a reagent to detect the presence of the corresponding antigen in tissue.

The phenomenon known as fluorescence is the ability of certain molecules or compounds (fluorochromes or fluorophores) to absorb energy, usually from an incident light source, and convert that energy into photons of light of a different, characteristic wavelength within approximately 10^{-8} seconds. Most fluorescent compounds are organic molecules and each has a characteristic optimal absorption range and quantum efficiency yield. Fluorescein is the most frequently used probe in the clinical laboratory because of its inherent characteristics, which include a high fluorescence intensity, good photostability, high quantum efficiency yield, and an emission wavelength that is usually distinguishable from the background, under the conditions used.[8]

In practice, fluorescein is usually prepared as an isothiocyanate to facilitate its subsequent coupling with antigen or antibody. Fluorescein isothiocyanate (FITC), when combined with antigen or antibody, is referred to as a "conjugate."

Fluorescein + isothiocyanate $\longrightarrow$ FITC;

FITC + Antibody $\longrightarrow$ Conjugate

Other fluorescent probes, for example the rhodamine derivatives, porphyrins, phycoerythrin, and fluorescamine, may be more adaptable to certain assay systems than is fluorescein, depending on the parameters of the test being employed.[8]

As with radioimmunoassay and enzyme immunoassay, immunofluorescence assays may be categorized as homogeneous or heterogeneous. Heterogeneous assays are those that include a step for separation of labeled from unlabeled reactants. They may also be referred to as "solid-phase" reactions, as they are commonly performed, for example, on a bead, in plastic tubes or on a microscope slide. Homogeneous assays, by contrast, do not require a separation step and are carried out in solution. These are called "fluid-phase" reactions.

HETEROGENEOUS IFA

Solid-phase IFA may be performed using several techniques; the most common among them are the direct, indirect, competitive, and sandwich variations. Immunofluorometric assays (IFMA) and separation fluoroimmunoassays (Sep FIA) are a further modification of these techniques.[2,8,15]

Direct solid-phase IFA (Fig. 3–18A) may be used to identify an unknown antigen that can be attached to a solid phase. The antigen is reacted with a known, labeled antibody, the test is incubated, nonreacting molecules are washed away, and the solid phase is observed for attached fluorescence, which would indicate a reaction between the known antibody and the fixed antigen.

Direct solid phase IFA reactions include those reactions where labeled antibody is used to identify markers, e.g. CD antigens, on cell surfaces (see Chap. 4). In this case, the cell itself serves as the solid phase. The analysis of fluorescence on single cell suspensions has been greatly advanced by the use of flow cytometry (see *Methods of Lymphocyte Quantitation*, Chap. 4, for discussion).

Indirect solid-phase IFA (Fig. 3–18B) is used to search for the presence of antibody with a chosen specificity in a patient's serum. A known antigen is attached to the solid phase, then reacted with patient serum. An incubation period is allowed, then the reaction is washed. A fluorochrome-labeled antihuman immunoglobulin is subsequently incubated with the remaining reactants, followed again by washing. Observation of fluorescence indicates that antibody, specific for the antigen used, was present in the patient sample.

Indirect solid phase IFA may also be used to detect cellular antigens by incubation of test cells with an antibody specific for the marker to be identified, followed by addi-

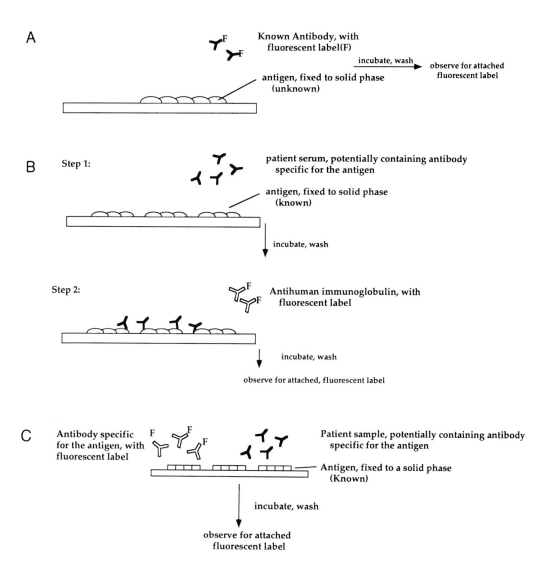

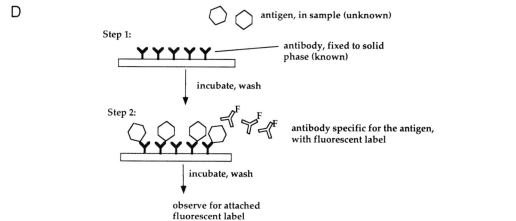

Fig. 3–18. Heterogeneous IFA. (A) Direct solid-phase IFA; (B) Indirect solid-phase IFA; (C) Competitive binding IFA; (D) Sandwich IFA.

tion of a fluorochrome-labeled antiimmunoglobulin (see Chap. 4).

In *competitive binding IFA,* labeled and unlabeled antibody are allowed to compete for a limited number of antigen sites fixed to a solid phase (Fig. 3–18C). After incubation and washing, the reaction is observed for fluorescence. With this technique, an inverse relationship occurs between the presence of patient antibody and the fluorescence observed, i.e. patient antibody, if present, interferes with the ability of the labeled reagent to bind to the antigen.

Separation fluoroimmunoassays (Sep FIA),[8] based on the principle of competitive binding, involve competition between labeled and unlabeled reagent, e.g. antigen, for limited amounts of their counterpart, e.g. antibody. Most often, one of the antigens is labeled with a fluorophore and the antibody is attached to the solid phase. In some assays, however, solid-phase antigen competes with fluid-phase antigen for limited sites on labeled antibody.

In *sandwich assays* (Fig. 3–18D), known antibody is usually attached to the solid phase. Subsequently, the sample is added, which is being tested for antigen. After incubation and washing, a fluorochrome-labeled antibody is added, followed by an additional incubation and wash. If fluorescence is detected in this method, it is indication of the presence of antigen in the sample.

Immunofluorometric assays (IFMA)[8] are solid-phase sandwich-type assays in which attached antibody is used to capture antigen from a solution. The immobilized antigens are then quantitated by the use of labeled antibodies.

Classic immunofluorescence assays, performed on a microscope slide, fall among the heterogeneous assays and are described below (Fluorescent Microscopy). Many of these are still in common use in clinical laboratories.

HOMOGENEOUS IFA

Homogeneous, or fluid-phase, immunofluorescence assays are those that do not

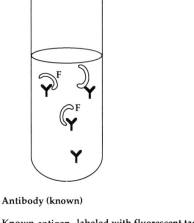

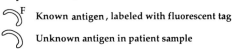

Y   Antibody (known)

Known antigen, labeled with fluorescent tag

Unknown antigen in patient sample

Fig. 3–19. Homogeneous IFA (prototype).

require a separation procedure before observing results. As such, they tend to be rapid, simple assays to perform, although they are historically somewhat limited in application. In most instances, homogeneous assays involve competitive binding of reactions, and can only be applied to reactions where binding of antibody to labeled antigen causes some change in the fluorescent label,[8] e.g. in its wavelength, rotational freedom, polarity, or dielectric strength. Figure 3–19 suggests a prototype of a homogeneous IFA reaction, wherein a direct relationship would exist between the amount of fluorescence observed (i.e. not altered by antibody) and the amount of antigen in the patient sample.

In practice, many adaptations of homogeneous assays have been developed[2,8,15] to address the limitations of these procedures, e.g. their relative insensitivity and the interference which can occur as a result of impurities in the sample. Among these adaptations are fluorescence enhancement immunoassays, fluorescence quenching immunoassays, indirect quenching immunoassays, fluorescence excitation transfer immunoassays (FETIA), release fluoroimmunoassays, and fluorescence polarization immunoassay, or FPIA (see below). Many of these have required the development of instrumentation which specifically detects the changes being created.

FLUORESCENT MICROSCOPY[20]

Many of the immunofluorescence assays currently in use in clinical laboratories employ microscope slides as the solid-phase. Results of such assays can then be observed under a specially adapted microscope referred to as a fluorescent microscope. Detection of treponemal antibodies, antibodies to *Toxoplasma gondii*, and antinuclear antibodies may be accomplished, for example, by fixing antigen to a slide, reacting with patient sample, then washing (heterogeneous assay). Subsequent addition of antihuman immunoglobulin with an attached fluorescent probe, followed by incubation and wash, will result in detectable fluorescence if the patient sample contains the appropriate antibody.

The schematics of a fluorescent microscope (Fig. 3–20) can be studied not only for an understanding of this aspect of IFA, but also as a window into the phenomenon of fluorescence. An incident light source is chosen that is capable of emitting appropriate wavelengths for evoking optimal fluorescence from the fluorochrome to be used. Filters are placed between the light source and the test slide, such that refinements can be made in the nature of the incident light. Heat filters may be used, for example, to diminish transmittance of longer wavelengths, and excitor or pass filters are chosen to eliminate extraneous wavelengths that could diminish efficiency of the fluorochrome. A condenser, dark or light field, is chosen for optimal concentration of light beams on the specimen.

As the incident light contacts the specimen, excitation of any fluorochrome present will occur. Incident light beams continue to pass through the specimen, while the new, longer wavelength beams are emitted. Both sets of beams would pass unhindered to the observer, if not for the use of a barrier, or secondary, filter, chosen to remove the incident light while allowing the light produced by the fluorochrome to pass through to the observer. In total, this prototype of a fluorescent microscope may serve as a model for initial understanding of other detection systems used in IFA.

Principal difficulties that arise in fluorescent microscopy are those inherent to IFA itself,[8] e.g., nonspecific or autofluorescence in reagents or background, imprecision in fluorochrome and fluorochrome labeled reagents,[19] quenching of fluorescence by environmental factors or by self quenching,[8,12] the relative insensitivity of the original IFA techniques as compared to radioimmunoassay and enzyme immunoassay, and the resistance of the technique to quantitation.

FLUORESCENCE POLARIZATION IMMUNOASSAY[21]

Only more recently have IFA techniques been developed that circumvent these in-

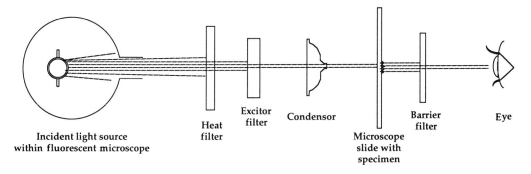

Incident light source within fluorescent microscope   Heat filter   Excitor filter   Condensor   Microscope slide with specimen   Barrier filter   Eye

Fig. 3–20. Schematic of a fluorescent microscope.

herent problems. One such assay system is fluorescence polarization immunoassay (FPIA). Through deployment of more complex physics and instrumentation, this system is among those that have revolutionized the use of immunofluorescent assays in recent years.

The principle of FPIA was pioneered by Perrin in 1926,[16] and applied to the physiochemical behavior of proteins by Weber.[22] Dandliker et al., developed the technique for use in the quantitation of proteins and haptens.[4-6] Maeda[14] is credited with the application of FPIA to proteolytic and enzymatic reactions.

In principle, FPIA makes use of competitive binding, and measures the binding of the tracer (fluorochrome) directly, without requiring a separation step (homogeneous assay). For fluorescence polarization to occur, incident light must be resolved (polarized) with a fixed, polarizing lens or prism, such that the electron vectors in the beam are aligned in a single plane. When fluorochromes in solution are excited by this polarized light, they emit partially polarized fluorescence, which is detected at right angles to the incident beam by a rotating polarizer.

Polarization of the fluorochrome emission depends on the relationship between its molecular orientation and its absorption and emission characteristics. Although the absorption and emission characteristics are inherent to the fluorochrome chosen for the assay, the molecular orientation of the fluorescent emission will depend on the size of the emitting particle; e.g. a small fluorescent hapten or antigen (m.w. 1,000 to 10,000) will have rapid movement, but binding of that molecule to antibody (m.w. 160,000) slows the rotational time. Addition of antibody to the fluorochrome, then, would increase polarization.

In fluorescence polarization immunoassay, a fluorochrome labeled antigen or hapten is chosen that is identical to the antigen to be tested. Labeled antigen is incubated with a known antibody and patient sample.

Any antigen present in this sample will compete with the fluorochrome-labeled antigen for antibody binding sites. The amount of unbound fluorochrome-labeled antigen, with rapid movement, increases proportionally to the amount of antigen in the sample, and is reflected by a decrease in polarization. In practice, then, the degree of polarization detected is inversely proportional to the amount of added, unlabeled antigen in patient sample.

Several mechanical innovations have resulted in the technology currently in use with FPIA. An automated flow cell polarization fluorometer was developed by Spencer et al.,[19] a photon counting polarization photometer was introduced by Jameson et al.,[10] and Smith et al.[18] devised a system for computing the degree of polarization on a time-shared basis. Finally, Popelka et al.[17] and Jolley et al.[13] were responsible for development of an instrument for quantitative FPIA (Prototype in Fig. 3–21) useful in clinical laboratories.

An inherent difficulty with FPIA has been its inability to detect reactions with larger molecules. Addition of a nephelometer (DeGrella et al.)[7] has expanded the capabilities of this technology.

REFERENCES

1. Chantler, S., and Batty, I.: Ann. N.Y. Acad. Sci., *420*:68, 1983.

2. Cobb, M., and Gotcher, S.: Am J. Med. Technol., *48*:671, 1982.

3. Coons, A.H., Creech, H.J., and Jones, R.N.: Proc. Soc. Exp. Biol. Med., *47*:200, 1941.

4. Dandliker, W.B., and Feigen, G.A.: Biochem. Biophys. Res. Commun., *5*:299, 1961.

5. Dandliker, W.B. et al.: Immunochemistry, *1*:165, 1964.

6. Dandliker, W.B. et al.: Immunochemistry, *10*:219, 1973.

7. DeGrella, R.F. et al.: Clin. Chem., *31*:1474, 1985.

8. Hemmilä I.: Clin. Chem., *31*:359, 1985.

9. Holborow, E.J., and Johnson, G.D.: Ann N.Y. Acad. Sci., *420*:62, 1983.

10. Jameson, D.M. et al.: Rev. Sci. Instrum. *49*:510, 1978.

11. Johnson, G.D., and Holborow, E.J.: In *Handbook of Experimental Immunology I.* Edited by D. M. Weir. Oxford, Blackwell Scientific Publications, 1986.

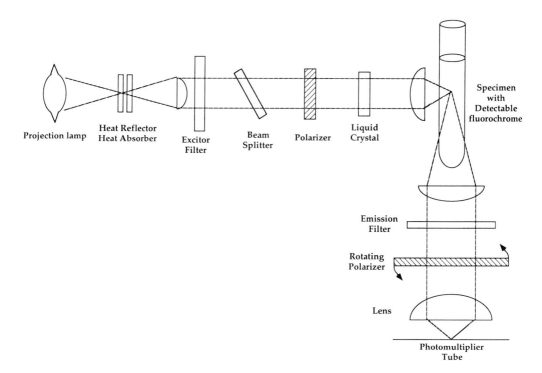

Fig. 3–21. Fluorescent polarization analyzer.

12. Johnson G.D. et al.: J. Immunol. Methods, 55:231, 1982.

13. Jolley, M.E. et al.: Clin. Chem., 27:1575, 1981.

14. Maeda, H.: Anal. Biochem., 92:222, 1979.

15. Nakamura, R.M., and Robbins, B.A.: In *Manual of Clinical Laboratory Immunology*. 3rd ed. Edited by N.R. Rose, H. Friedman, and J.L. Fahey. Washington, D.C., American Society for Microbiology, 1986.

16. Perrin, F.: J. Phys. Radium, 7:390, 1976.

17. Popelka, S.R. et al.: Clin. Chem., 27:1198, 1981.

18. Smith, J.C., Graham, N., and Chance, B.: Rev. Sci. Instrum., 49:1491, 1978.

19. Spencer, R. et al.: Clin. Chem., 19:838, 1973.

20. Stites, D.P., Stobo, J.D., and Wells, J.V. (eds.) *Basic and Clinical Immunology*. 6th ed., East Norwalk, Appleton and Lange, 1987.

21. Watanabe, F., and Miyai, K.: In *Nonisotypic Immunoassay*. Edited by T.T. Ngo. New York, Plenum Press, 1988.

22. Weber, G.: Adv. Protein Chem., 8:415, 1953.

Radioimmunoassay

Radioimmunoassay, or RIA, is a method by which a radionucleotide label, or *tracer,* is used to assess the concentration of biologic molecules. First developed in 1960,[11] RIA is one of the most widespread, useful, and precise techniques available. Its extreme sensitivity[9] is rivaled to date only by enzyme immunoassay (EIA) and some of the newer immunofluorescent assays (IFA).

In clinical laboratories, tritium (^{3}H), or ^{131}I, or ^{125}I may be chosen for detection of haptens or for proteins and polypeptides respectively; ^{125}I, however, has become the radionucleotide of choice.[3,7] Its half life of 60 days is shorter than that of ^{3}H, the counting rate is higher, and the total counting time required is less than with the other nucleotides. ^{125}I emits gamma radiation that may be counted with use of a solid crystal gamma counter or an alternate method.[9]

As it was originally proposed, radioimmunoassay involves use of a miniscule amount of radiolabeled antigen (Ag^*) in solution with a high affinity antibody (Ab) to that antigen. Patient sample, potentially containing unlabeled antigen (Ag), may be added to this system and will compete with labeled antigen for binding sites on the antibody. The concentration of unknown antigen will be reflected by a relative decrease in the amount of labeled antigen bound. Figure 3–22 illustrates the principle of this *competitive binding* assay.

A variation of the classic RIA procedure may be used where antibody is to be detected, i.e., radiolabeled antibody (Ab*) and its specific antigen (Ag) may be combined with patient sample. Again, the concentration of unknown antibody in the patient sample will correspond with a relative decline in the amount of labeled antibody bound to the antigen.

Among the most critical technical requirements[2,3,5] of RIA is development of an appropriate method to distinguish free from bound tracer. Enormous errors may accompany an ineffective technique. When antigen is sufficiently smaller than antibody, e.g. of molecular weight < 30,000, precipitation of antibody-bound antigen may be accomplished by use of concentrated solutions of either ammonium sulfate or polyethylene glycol (PEG).[2,4] In either case, essentially all bound reactants will be precipitated from the solution.

When antigen is larger, e.g. of molecular weight > 30,000 to 400,000, or when it is not globular in shape, alternative methods must be employed. For example, if the antibody used to detect large antigens is of a certain IgG subclass, Staphylococcus protein A may be used as a high affinity adsorbent, often bound to a sepharose bead to facilitate precipitation.[2] Alternately, a second antibody, an anti-immunoglobulin raised in another species may be used to precipitate antibody. In either case, both bound and free antibody will be removed from solution, along with any bound antigen.

With certain antigens, agents such as activated charcoal, or talc, may be used to adsorb free antigen, leaving bound antigen in solution. While these methods are inexpensive and rapid, they have specific physical requirements.[2]

Solid phase RIA, or *immunoradiometric* assay (IRMA), developed by Miles and Hales in 1968,[6] involves immobilization of one of the reactants of a competitive binding assay onto a solid surface, e.g. a sepharose bead, or the wall of a test tube or microtiter well. Attachment to the solid phase facilitates separation of bound from free reactants; simply washing removes free reactants. As originally developed, monospecific labeled antibody was used, rather than labeled antigen. Difficulty in preparation of monospecific antibody, however, hampered wide

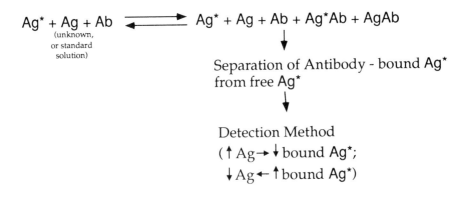

Legend: Ag* = radiolabelled antigen (RIA) or enzyme labelled antigen (EIA)

Ag = unknown antigen in patient sample (or in solution of standards)

Ab = high affinity antibody

Fig. 3–22. Classic competitive binding assay (RIA or EIA).

adaptation of IRMA until the development of monoclonal antibodies.[3]

A two-site, or *sandwich,* variation of IRMA assays was developed simultaneously by Wide[10] and by Addison and Hales.[1] In this procedure, illustrated in Figure 3–23, antibody is attached to the solid phase. Subsequent addition of the unknown sample, potentially containing antigen, allows for specific attachment. A washing step removes unbound antigen. Monospecific, radiolabeled antibody, specific for the antigen is then added and allowed to react. A final wash removes any unbound radiolabeled antibody, and the solid phase can be assayed for bound radiolabel.

Multiple variations of solid phase RIA have been developed,[7] including that of detection of unknown antibody by use of bound, then radiolabeled antigen.

IRMA assays have significantly wider applicability than fluid phase RIA, and use smaller amounts of reagent. Their use also allows a 10-fold increase in sensitivity over the traditional method.[3,7]

Data generated by RIA or IRMA techniques are usually expressed as counts per minute, usually of bound reactants. If standards with known concentration are included with each run, a linear curve may be plotted of cpm (bound) vs. concentration of the standard.[7] The concentration of the unknown may then be read from the curve. There are many equally valid alternative methods for data analysis.[2,3,5,9]

Beyond meticulous requirements for preparation of reagents to be used in RIA,[2,3,12] controls must be included to determine background binding of normal serum and to establish a baseline for immunologically inactive radiolabel.[2,8,9]

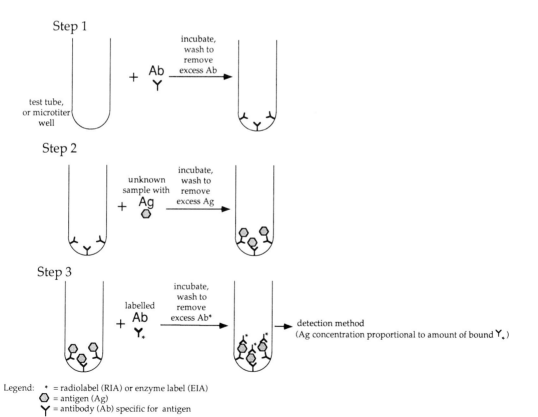

Legend: * = radiolabel (RIA) or enzyme label (EIA)
⬡ = antigen (Ag)
Y = antibody (Ab) specific for antigen

Fig. 3–23. Sandwich assay (RIA or EIA).

The major disadvantages of RIA and IRMA are inherent to the use of radioactive compounds which have limited shelf life and carry requirements for special handling and staff training. Waste disposal of radioactive compounds and its cost has become a major problem. Because of their potential as a health hazard, radiation monitoring of the laboratory site and employees is required. Counting radioactive emissions requires expensive equipment and is time-consuming. Nonetheless, with increasing use of monoclonal antibodies as reagents, both techniques are likely to retain their important role in clinical laboratories.

REFERENCES

1. Addison, G.M., and Hales, C.N.: Hormone Metab. Res. *3*:59, 1971.
2. Berzofsky, J.A., and Berkower, I.J.: In *Fundamental Immunology.* Edited by W.E. Paul. New York, Raven Press, 1984.
3. Bolton, A.E., and Hunter, W.M.; In *Handbook of Experimental Immunology I.* Edited by D.M. Weir. Oxford, Blackwell Scientific Publications, 1986.
4. Desbuquois, B., and Aurbach, G.D.: J. Clin. Endocrinol. Metab., *33*:732, 1971.
5. Larsen, J., and ODell, W.D.: In *Manual of Clinical Laboratory Immunology*, 3rd ed. Edited by N. R. Rose, H. Friedman, and J. L. Fahey. Washington, DC, American Society for Microbiology, 1986.
6. Miles, C.E.M., and Hales, C.N.: Nature, *219*:186, 1968.
7. Newby, C.J., Hayakawa, K., and Herzenberg, L.A.: In *Handbook of Experimental Immunology I.* Edited by D. M. Weir. Oxford, Blackwell Scientific, 1986.
8. Schioler, V.: Scand. J. Clin. Lab Invest., *172*:87, 1984.
9. Stites, D. P., and Channing Rodgers, R. P.: In *Basic and Clinical Immunology,* 6th ed. Edited by D. P. Stites, J. D. Stobo, and J. V. Wells. Norwalk, Appelton and Large, 1987.
10. Wide, L.: Acta Endocrinol. Suppl., *142*:207, 1969.
11. Yalow, R.S., and Berson, S.A., J. Clin. Invest., *39*:1157, 1960.
12. Zollinger, W.D., Dalrymple, J.M., and Artenstein, M.S.: J. Immunol., *117*:1788, 1976.

Enzyme Immunoassay

Enzymes are efficient, naturally occurring molecules that function as catalysts of certain biochemical reactions.[16] The inherent ability of enzymes to act on multiples of substrate molecules, without being themselves consumed in the reaction, results in amplification; i.e. the presence of a relatively small amount of enzyme can react with much larger amounts of substrate to produce detectable levels of substrate breakdown products. In laboratory practice, enzymes are usually chosen that induce chromogenic, fluorescent, or luminescent changes in their substrates; thus, enzyme "labels" such as those used in histology or, more recently, in enzyme immunoassay, react with their substrates to yield products which can be detected either visually or by instrumentation.

Enzyme immunoassay (EIA) was reported simultaneously by Engvall and Perlmann[6] and by von Weeman and Schuurs[31] in 1971. Both groups sought to employ an alternative label for antigen-antibody reactions; one that would circumvent many of the inherent difficulties of using radionucleotides as labels. Difficulties with such radioimmunoassay (RIA) techniques include[3,12,30] the short shelf life of radioactive reagents, their cost, the stringent regulatory environment which encompasses their use, the potential for hazard to health, the requirement for expensive equipment for detection of radioactive decay, and the requirement for staff training which accompanies safety procedures. By contrast, the use of enzyme labels[13,16,19,30] offers the potential for longer storage (the half life of peroxidase, for example, is 9 years at 4°C),[17] relative simplicity and ease of use, a wider range of apparatus for detection of end products (the human eye will do, in many cases), and greater flexibility. Since 1971, enzyme immunoassay has supplanted many of the traditional techniques in diagnostic medicine, including RIA, and surpassed others with its versatility and seemingly unlimited applications.

Nomenclature in current use in enzyme immunoassay is somewhat confusing and requires clarification. While some authors use the term enzyme-linked immunosorbent assay (ELISA) to refer to all EIA procedures, or to only those performed on a solid surface (solid phase), others confine that term to those solid-phase assays used to detect specific antibody.[6,20,28] The latter terminology will be used here, while the phrase "enzyme immunoassay," or EIA, will serve as the broader term to encompass all techniques where enzymes are used to label antigen-antibody reactions.

Enzyme immunoassays can be divided into two rather broad categories based on whether the reaction is carried out entirely in solution (*homogeneous assays*) or whether separation steps are required (*heterogeneous assays*).

In principle, homogeneous assays are based on the ability of antibody (Ab) to mediate a change in the activity of an enzyme (E) bound to its specific antigen (Ag), i.e.

$$Ag^E + Ab \longrightarrow \text{altered enzyme activity}$$

In the most common type of homogeneous EIA, marketed under the trademark EMIT (Enzyme-Multiplied Immunoassay; Syva Co., Palo Alto, California), antigen in patient sample is allowed to compete with enzyme-labeled antigen for a limited amount of antibody in a simple form of *competitive binding assay* (Fig. 3–24). Once enzyme labeled antigen is bound by antibody, enzyme activity decreases detectably. In practical use, EMIT-type assays are currently limited to detection of low molecular weight antigens such as therapeutic drugs, hormones, and a few antimicrobials.[16] With use of a standard curve, the rate of enzymatic activity may be detected,[15] which is directly proportional to the concentration of unknown antigen, over a limited range. These assays are simple to perform, but lose some of the inherent sensitivity of EIA to background "noise" which is retained in the solution;[16] at that, the sensitivity is in the range of $\mu g/ml$.[29,32]

Many modifications of the homogeneous assay have also been developed.[13,19,20,29]

Heterogeneous EIA is analogous to radioimmunoassay (RIA) in its requirement for separation of bound from free reactants. In EIA, this may be performed by use of a second, precipitating antibody,[3,19] followed by centrifugation and separation, or, far more commonly, by attachment of one of the reactants to a solid phase. Regardless of the procedure used, separation must be rapid, complete, and reproducible.[3]

Many types of materials have been used as the matrix for solid-phase, heterogeneous EIA procedures.[3,11,13,22] Plastics, e.g. polystyrene, are most often used, molded into beads, tubes, or especially, into 96-well microtiter plates. Glass rods, frosted glass beads, suspendable microbeads, and sepharose have been employed. More recently, strips of nitrocellulose, nylon,[2] or activated paper[3,4,33] have been adapted to the so-called DOT immunoassays (see below). The porous nature of the latter substances allows for an appreciable increase in the amount of antigen that can be bound per square millimeter.[2] Whatever the material chosen for use as the matrix, careful attention must be given to ensure optimal, reproducible adsorption of antigen (or antibody) to the matrix surface.[30]

Heterogeneous EIA techniques may be divided into three rather broad categories: competitive binding techniques, indirect techniques, and sandwich assays.

Competitive binding EIA is analogous to the classic RIA technique developed by Yalow and Berson (Fig. 3–22). In this procedure, patient sample (potentially containing antigen) is added to an antibody immobilized on a solid phase. Simultaneously or sequentially,[3] enzyme-labeled antigen is added. After incubation, the surface is washed (separation phase), and the enzyme activity remaining on the solid phase is analyzed by addition of the appropriate substrate. Activity of bound enzyme in this case is inversely proportional to the concentration of unlabeled antigen in the sample.

Indirect EIA procedures are patterned after the original work of Engvall and Perlmann.[6] Designated *enzyme-linked immunosorbent assays* (*ELISA*), these assays are used to detect specific antibodies in test samples (Fig. 3–25). Antigen, attached to the solid phase, is re-

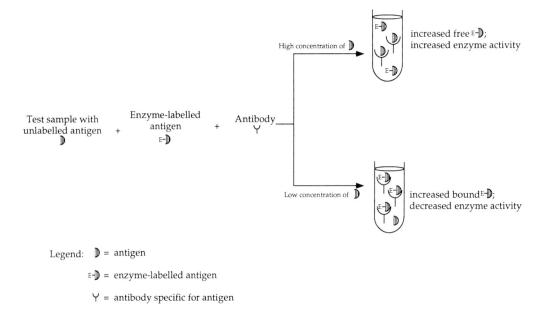

Legend: $\mathbb{D}$ = antigen

E-$\mathbb{D}$ = enzyme-labelled antigen

Y = antibody specific for antigen

Fig. 3–24. Homogeneous enzyme immunoassay (EMIT).

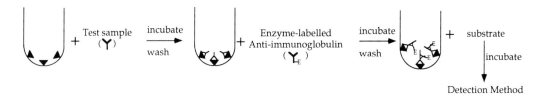

(Amount of bound E proportional to antibody concentration in test sample)

Legend: ▼ = Antigen bound to solid phase

Y = Antibody in test sample

Y_E = Enzyme-labelled anti-immunoglobulin

Fig. 3–25. Enzyme-linked immunosorbent assay (ELISA, Indirect EIA).

acted with the test sample, which potentially contains antibody. The reactants are incubated, and the surface washed. Subsequently, an enzyme-labeled anti-immunoglobulin is added, incubation is allowed, and the surface is again washed. Retention of enzyme on the surface is detected upon addition of the appropriate substrate and indicates the presence of the antibody being sought. The amount of enzyme detected is, in fact, directly proportional to the concentration of antibody in the sample.

It should be noted that use of an enzyme-labeled antibody directed toward a specific immunoglobulin class (e.g. anti-IgM) may be helpful in some instances. Alternately, *class capture assays*[12,14,30] may be used for the same effect. In class capture assays, the solid phase is coated with a specific anti-immunoglobulin (e.g. anti-IgM). The test sample is added, the reaction is incubated, and the surface washed; immunoglobulins of the desired class remain bound to the solid phase. Subsequently, enzyme-labeled antigen (e.g. rubella antigen) is added, and the incubation and wash are repeated. Enzyme which remains on the solid-phase in these assays is indicative of specific antibody in the test sample to that antigen (e.g. IgM anti-rubella antibodies).

Sandwich EIA[4] is alternately referred to as double antibody EIA, or immunoenzymetric assay (IEMA) in deference to its similarity to immunoradiometric assays (IRMA) (Fig. 3–23). In sandwich EIA procedures, antibody is immobilized on the solid phase. Subsequently, the test sample, potentially containing the bi- or polyvalent antigen, is added, and the reaction is incubated and washed to separate non-reactants. Enzyme-labeled antibody is than added to the surface, and the incubation and wash are repeated. Enzyme present on the surface after the final wash is directly proportional to the amount of antigen in the sample, and is detected by addition of the appropriate substrate.

In general, competitive binding heterogeneous assays are used to quantitate relatively high concentrations of drugs or hormones,[15] while sandwich assays are chosen to detect low concentrations of antigen.[3,15] If an antigen is difficult to purify, the sandwich technique would also be preferred. Indirect heterogeneous assays are applicable to a wide range of situations where detection of antibody or assessment of immunity is the goal.[3]

Innumerable variations of the above techniques exist, largely for research purposes.

The sensitivity and specificity that are achieved by use of heterogeneous EIA is approximately equivalent to that of RIA for the same assays.[1,6] In combination with IFA,[9] enzyme amplification methods,[10,24] or RIA,[26] the level of sensitivity may further increase.

In enzyme immunoassays, the results are visualized by use of the action of the enzyme label on a chosen substrate.[16] In the simplest form of EIA, chromogenic substrates can be chosen in which color is generated that is visible to the eye or to a spectrophotometer. Peroxidase enzymes[25] (e.g. horseradish peroxidase) are suitable for this purpose, with a long list of potential substrates.[13,29] The choice of enzyme/substrate for use in any particular EIA[20] may be made on the basis of stability, availability, absence from the biologic fluid being tested, and ease of preparation, as well as by the detection method to be used. Alkaline phosphatase is comparatively expensive and insensitive; however, it is useful in many situations.[13] β-galactosidase is a good enzyme choice if fluorimetric detection methods are used.[6,30] Alternative labeling methods that have been designed include the use of prosthetic groups[18] e.g. the apoenzyme reactivation immunoassays or ARIS,[18] the use of multiple selected enzymes that activate sequentially,[13] and use of redox reactions (e.g. NBT) to shorten reaction time.[7]

Inherent to enzyme/substrate interaction is continuation of the reaction for as long as substrate molecules remain available. In some enzyme immunoassays (e.g. homogeneous assays) the test is measured at timed intervals while enzyme/substrate interaction continues.[15] This is termed the kinetic, or rate method of measurement. Alternately, the enzyme/substrate interaction may be halted at an established time by use of a "stopping solution." In this case, end point measurements result.

An impressive array of instrumentation has been developed for commercial use in the performance, analysis, and evaluation of EIAs.[15,16] Both rate and end point spectrophotometry are used and are the most common means of analysis.

Enzyme immunoassays may be used to detect the presence or absence of antigen or antibody, they may be used to semiquantitate by titering the unknown, or they may be quantitative by use of standards and a standard dose-response curve,[8] where the standard concentrations, for example, are plotted vs. the enzymatic activity (e.g. absorbence). This adaptability allows the technique to be useful in a wide variety of divergent situations: in the field, for home monitoring, in developing countries, or in the most sophisticated laboratory where sensitivity and specificity are prerequisite requirements.

Among the difficulties[12,16,20] encountered using EIA techniques are the "background noise" (e.g. in homogeneous assays) from impure solutions, nonspecific protein binding, variability in reagent composition, and instrument variation. Inherent to EIA is the susceptibility of enzymes to environmental conditions, e.g. temperature. The techniques are not immune from technical problems.[12] Conscientious quality control[30] is a must with all immunoassays.

Notable innovative uses of enzyme-labeling techniques include DOT immunoassays (DOT ELISA; DOT Immunobinding) which are simple, solid-phase assays for detection of antibody, usually employing nitrocellulose strips,[1,2,21,33] and the use of enzymes to label DNA probes.[14] ELISA plaque assays (ELISA Spot) are used for detection of antibody-producing cells in vitro.[5,23]

REFERENCES

1. Boctor, F.N. et al.: J. Parasitol., 73:589, 1987.
2. Bordier, C., and Ryter, P.: Anal. Biochem., 152:113, 1986.
3. Bruni, J.F., and Maggio, E.T.: In Clinical Immunochemistry. Edited by R.C. Boguslaski, E.T. Maggio, and R.M. Nakamura. Boston, Little, Brown, & Co., 1984.
4. Butler, J.E. et al.: Mol. Immunol., 23:971, 1986.
5. Czerkinsky, C. et al.: In ELISA and Other Solid Phase Immunoassays. Edited by D.M. Kemeny, and S.J. Challacombe. London, John Wiley and Sons, 1988.
6. Engvall, E., and Perlmann, P.: Immunochemistry, 8:871, 1971.
7. Franci, C. et al.: J. Immunol. Methods, 88:225, 1986.
8. Hamilton, R.G., and Adkinson, N.F., Jr.: In ELISA and Other Solid Phase Immunoassays. Edited by D.M. Kemeny, and S.J. Challacombe. London, John Wiley & Sons, 1988.
9. Hemmilia, I.: Clin. Chem., 31:359, 1985.
10. Johannsson, A. et al.: J. Immunol. Methods, 87:7, 1986.
11. Kemeny, D.M., and Challacombe, S.J.: In ELISA and Other Solid Phase Immunoassays. Edited by D.M. Kemeny, and S.J. Challacombe. London, John Wiley & Sons, 1988.
12. Kemeny, D.M., and Chantler, S.: In ELISA and Other Solid Phase Immunoassays. Edited by D.M. Kemeny, and S.J. Challacombe. London, John Wiley & Sons, 1988.
13. Kurstak, E.: Bull. WHO, 63:793, 1985.
14. Kurstak, E. et al.: Bull. WHO, 64:465, 1986.
15. Lucas, D.H.: In Clinical Immunochemistry. Edited by R.C. Boguslaski, E.T. Maggio, and R.M. Nakamura. Boston, Little, Brown & Co., 1984.
16. Maggio, E.T.: In Clinical Immunochemistry. Edited by R.C. Boguslaski, E.T. Maggio, and R.M. Nakamura. Boston, Little, Brown & Co., 1984.
17. Montoya, A., and Castell, J.V.: J. Immunol. Methods, 99:13, 1987.
18. Morris, D.L.: In Clinical Immunochemistry. Edited by R.C. Boguslaski, E.T. Maggio, and R.M. Nakamura. Boston, Little, Brown & Co., 1984.
19. Nakamura, R.M., Voller, A., and Bidwell, D.E.: In Handbook of Experimental Immunology I. Edited by D.M. Weir. Oxford, Blackwell Scientific Publications, 1986.
20. O'Sullivan, M.J., In Practical Immunoassay. Edited by W. R. Butt, New York, Marcel Dekker, Inc., 1984.
21. Penner, E., Goldenberg, H., Meryn, S., and Gordon, J.: Hepatology, 6:381, 1986.
22. Polson, A., vanHeerdon, D., and vander-Merwe, K.J.: Immunol. Invest., 14:223, 1985.
23. Sedgwick, J.D., and Holt, P.G.: J. Immunol. Methods, 57:301, 1983.
24. Stanley, C.J., Johannsson, A., and Self, C.H.: J. Immunol. Methods, 83:89, 1985.
25. Sternberger, L.A.: Immunocytochemistry, 3rd ed. New York, John Wiley & Sons, 1986.
26. Stites, D.P., and Channing Rogers, R.P.: In Basic and Clinical Immunology. 6th ed. Norwalk, Appleton and Lange, 1987.
27. Towbin, H., Staehlin, T., and Gordon, J.: Proc. Natl. Acad. Sci. U.S.A., 76:4350, 1979.
28. Voller, A., Bidwell, D.E., and Bartlet, A.: The Enzyme Linked Immunosorbent Assay (ELISA), Micro Systems, Ltd., Vale, Guernsey, Summerfield House, 1979.
29. Voller, A., and Bidwell, D.E.: In Alternative Immunoassays. Edited by W.P. Collins. London, John Wiley & Sons, 1985.
30. Voller, A., and Bidwell, D.: In Manual of Clinical Laboratory Immunology. 3rd ed. Edited by N.R. Rose, H. Friedman, and J.L. Fahey. Washington, D.C., American Society for Microbiology, 1986.
31. vonWeeman, B.K., and Schuurs, A.: FEBS Lett., 15:232, 1971.
32. Warren, C., and Phillips, I.: J. Antimicrob. Chemother., 17:255, 1986.
33. Wiedbrauk, D.L. et al.: Am. Clin. Lab., 21:16, 1989.

LYMPHOCYTE QUANTITATION AND FUNCTION

Evaluation of lymphocytes in the clinical laboratory is performed by quantitation of the lymphocytes and their subpopulations, and by assessment of their functional activity. These laboratory analyses have become an essential component of the clinical assessment of a variety of disorders, and are particularly useful in the following areas:[11,61,64,71]

1. *Diagnosis of lymphoproliferative malignancies.* Characterization of the malignant cell in terms of lineage and stage of differentiation has provided valuable information with regard to prognosis and administration of the appropriate therapy;[21]

2. *Diagnosis of primary immunodeficiency diseases.* Diagnosis and indications for therapy have been aided by classification as B cell (e.g. Bruton's hypogammaglobulinemia), T cell (e.g. DiGeorge syndrome) or complex (e.g. Severe Combined Immunodeficiency Disease) disorders;[3,29]

3. *Diagnosis of acquired immunologic abnormalities.* Evaluation of alterations in the immune system secondary to infection (e.g. AIDS), autoimmunity (e.g. SLE), malignancy, other disorders, or treatment (e.g. organ transplantation) has been useful in the di-

agnosis and/or monitoring of patients with these conditions.[3]

METHODS OF LYMPHOCYTE QUANTITATION

Methods of lymphocyte quantitation and characterization are based on the detection of cell surface markers, cytoplasmic components, or nuclear material. Our discussion will focus primarily on the first of these, because surface markers are the most commonly detected in the routine clinical laboratory.

Lymphocyte quantitation is most frequently performed on cells of the peripheral blood, although other specimens (e.g. lymph nodes or bone marrow) may be used when indicated. Prior to analysis of peripheral blood, red blood cells are removed by lysis with a reagent such as ammonium chloride.[28,34,50] Alternatively, mononuclear cells may be isolated by Ficoll Hypaque density gradient centrifugation.[7,34,51] (See *Ficoll Hypaque Separation of Mononuclear Cells from Peripheral Blood*). The erythrocyte lysis procedure has the advantages of being far less time consuming, especially in the analysis of numerous samples, it minimizes biohazardous exposure because less manipulation of the samples is needed, and it requires a smaller volume of blood (particularly useful in patients with a low lymphocyte count).[34] The Ficoll Hypaque method removes granulocytes and any nucleated erythrocytes, and requires less sophisticated cellular analysis.[34] Comparable results are generally obtained with both methods,[23,44] although destruction of abnormal cells in the lysis procedure[71] and selective removal or enrichment of certain lymphocyte populations with Ficoll Hypaque[15,16,56] have been observed.

Following either method of cell preparation, individual surface membrane markers are analyzed. Some of the more commonly detected markers on T and B lymphocytes and natural killer (NK) cells are listed in Table 4–1, and will be discussed below.

Traditionally, B cells have been identified by the presence of surface immunoglobulin, which serves as their receptor for antigen (see Chap. 1). The synthesis of immunoglobulins (Ig) varies with the stage of B cell maturation:[72] pre-B cells contain cytoplasmic μ chains, immature resting B cells have surface membrane IgM, mature activated B cells contain surface Ig of any class, and plasma cells have lost surface Ig but contain cytoplasmic Ig. Surface Ig thus serves as a marker for identification of B cells in the peripheral blood, and can be detected by immunofluorescence[13,52] or immunoenzymatic methods.[45,59] In these methods, the possibility of certain technical problems must be noted, but can be averted by the following measures:[4] (1) the reaction must be carried out at 4° C in order to prevent rapid loss of surface Ig through capping, shedding, and internalization, (2) passive adsorption of serum antibody or anti-Ig conjugate to cells bearing Fc receptors may occur in some patients, but can be reduced by treatment of cells to remove extrinsic Ig,[31,36,63,71] use of goat or mouse antibody (vs rabbit) in the conjugate, or use of a F(ab')$_2$ conjugate reagent.[2,4]

Hybridization with molecular probes to detect Ig rearrangements has been useful in identifying the stage of differentiation of B cell malignancies.[40,69]

B cells also contain receptors for the Fc portion of IgG and for the C3 component of complement. The Fc receptor has been detected by several assays, most notably by the binding of tagged, aggregated gamma globulin,[18,26] or via an erythrocyte-antibody (EA) rosette assay[27,42,71] (Fig. 4–1B). The C3 receptor has classically been detected by the EAC (erythrocyte-antibody-complement) rosette method[1,67] (Fig. 4–1C). The specificity of the EA and EAC rosettes, however, is not limited to B cells, because Fc receptors are also present on monocytes, polymorphonuclear cells (PMN), some T cells, and NK cells,[17,32,42,47] and C3 receptors are found on monocytes and PMN as well.[60,71] Different classes of Fc and C3 receptors can now be identified with the use of monoclonal antibodies.[61,71] In addition to the above, immature B cells spontaneously form rosettes when incubated with mouse erythrocytes.[25,63]

In recent years, the detection of lymphocyte markers has been revolutionized by the development of monoclonal antibodies and flow cytometry (see below) and the high levels of sensitivity and specificity they provide. Immunofluorescence tests employing these technologies are now being used in conjunction with or in lieu of traditional detection methods in many routine clinical laboratories. The rapidly escalating production of monoclonal antibodies against lymphocyte surface markers led to a confusing situation with multiple nomenclatures in use for many surface antigens; subsequently, International Workshops on Leukocyte Differentiation Antigens were organized by the World Health Organization, together with the International Union of Immunological Societies (IUIS) and the Medical Research Council, in order to resolve this problem. These workshops led to the grouping of monoclonal antibodies directed against the same white blood cell antigen into

Table 4–1. Some Commonly Detected Lymphocyte Surface Markers

Marker[a]	Location[b]	Comments
Surface Ig	B cells	
Fc receptor for IgG	B cells, MO, PMN, some T cells	Can be detected by EA rosette
C3 receptors	B cells, MO, PMN, NK cells	Can be detected by EAC rosette or monoclonal antibodies to CD35 (the CR1 receptor), CD21 (the CR2 receptor), and CD11 (the CR3 receptor)
HLA-DR	B cells, MO, activated T cells	HLA Class II antigen, also known as Ia
CD2 (T11, OKT11, Leu5b)	T cells, NK cells	Can also be detected by E rosette; is the sheep red blood cell receptor
CD3 (T3, OKT3, Leu4)	T cells	
CD4 (T4, OKT4, Leu3)	Helper/inducer T cells, MO	
CD8 (T8, OKT8, Leu2)	Suppressor/cytotoxic T cells; NK subset	
CD16 (Leu11)	NK cells, PMN	An IgG Fc receptor
CD19 (Leu12, B4)	B cells, CLL and pre B-ALL cells	
CD20 (Leu16, B1)	B cells	

[a] Alternate nomenclatures defined by commercially available monoclonal antibodies are indicated in parentheses for the appropriate markers.
Prefix: **T** or **B**, originated from Coulter Electronics
OKT, from Ortho Diagnostics
Leu, from Becton Dickinson
[b] MO = monocytes
PMN = Polymorphonuclear cells
NK = natural killer cells
CLL = chronic lymphocytic leukemia cells
ALL = acute lymphocytic leukemia cells

"clusters of differentiation" (CD).[10,62] Over 45 CD antigens have been established,[62] and the number will undoubtedly continue to grow.

Three antigens designated by this system as CD19, CD20, and CD21, are restricted primarily to cells of the B cell lineage and are present on the vast majority of B cells in the peripheral blood.[72] The CD23 antigen is present on activated but not on resting B cells,[65] and functions as the Fc receptor for IgE.[39] Several other CD antigens, as well as antigens defined by unclustered antibodies, have been identified on various stages of the B cell lineage.[72]

Monoclonal antibodies have been particularly helpful in the identification of T lym-phocytes and their subpopulations. The CD3 marker (previously designated as T3 or Leu 4) is acquired at the stage of the medullary thymocyte and is expressed on the vast majority of human peripheral blood T cells.[58,61] The CD3 polypeptides are complexed with the T cell antigen receptor (TcR) on the cell surface membrane, and are thought to play a role in signal transduction during the activation of T cells in response to antigen.[6,14,33] The CD2 marker (previously designated T11 or Leu 5) is present on all thymocytes, peripheral T cells, and most NK cells, and is thought to play a role in T cell activation, independent of TcR antigen recognition.[6] CD2 has also been identified as the receptor for sheep red

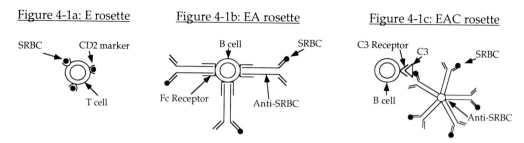

Figure 4-1a: E rosette   Figure 4-1b: EA rosette   Figure 4-1c: EAC rosette

Fig. 4–1. Lymphocyte Rosettes. These rosettes consist of a centralized cell (e.g. lymphocyte) surrounded by at least three peripheral red blood cells. They may be counted using phase-contrast or conventional light microscopy. The percentage of rosette forming cells (RFC) (i.e. the % of T or B lymphocytes) is calculated as % RFC = Number of RFC / Total number of lymphocytes counted, × 100. Three types of rosettes may be produced.
(A) E rosette. The E (erythrocyte) rosette is formed by incubating peripheral blood mononuclear cells with sheep red blood cells (SRBC). The SRBC bind to the CD2 marker on the surface of human T lymphocytes as shown;
(B) EA rosette. The EA (erythrocyte antibody) rosette is formed by incubating peripheral blood mononuclear cells with SRBC and an IgG anti-SRBC antibody. The complex binds to the Fc receptors on B lymphocytes as shown;
(C) EAC rosette. The EAC (erythrocyte antibody complement) rosette is formed by adding peripheral blood mononuclear cells to SRBC which have been preincubated with an IgM anti-SRBC antibody and complement deficient in the C5 component (in order to prevent lysis of the SRBC). The EAC complex binds to the C3 receptors on B lymphocytes as shown.

blood cells, a marker traditionally detected by the E rosette assay[5,35] (Fig. 4–1A).

T lymphocytes can be divided further into subpopulations on the basis of the CD4 and CD8 antigens. CD4 is expressed primarily by T helper/inducer cells and is thought to interact with Class II HLA molecules on the surface of antigen presenting cells.[6,55,58] The CD8 marker is found mainly on cytotoxic and suppressor T cells, and is thought to participate in intercellular adhesion through the recognition of Class I HLA molecules.[6,55,58] Approximately 55 to 70% of peripheral blood T cells are positive for the CD4 marker, while approximately 25 to 40% are positive for CD8;[58,68] cells coexpressing CD4 and CD8 are infrequent in peripheral blood.[61] Many laboratories report results in terms of the CD4/CD8 ratio, for which abnormalities have been described in a variety of disease states.[64] Using additional markers, the CD4(+) subset can be divided further into helper (Leu 8⁻, 4B4⁺) and suppressor inducer (Leu 8⁺, 2H4⁺) cells;[12,22,37,48,49] while the CD8(+) population can be sub-

divided into suppressor (Leu 15⁺) and cytotoxic (Leu 15⁻) T cells.[9,71]

Classification of T cell lymphoproliferative disorders and studies of T cell immunodeficiencies have also been aided by examination of TcR gene rearrangements via hybridization with DNA or RNA probes to define the stage of lymphocyte differentiation.[69]

The HLA-DR (Ia) marker is present on B cells, monocytes, and activated T cells[61] and is necessary for antigen presentation (see Chap. 1 and Chap. 13).

Natural killer cells have been defined as large granular lymphocytes with a CD3⁻, CD16⁺, Leu 19⁺ phenotype.[57] These cells also express the CD11 marker, and half are positive for the Leu 7 antigen.[11] Other effector cells exhibiting NK-like activity and different surface marker expressions have also been described.[57]

Monocytes possess Fc and C3 receptors, as well as a number of antigens defined by monoclonal antibodies, including CD11, CD13, and CD14.[61,62] Labeling with one of these antibodies or preincubation of cells with latex beads[71] may be helpful in excluding monocytes from lymphocyte analyses.

As mentioned above, lymphocyte markers are most commonly detected using immunofluorescence assays (IFA). These are available as either a direct staining method, where the fluorochrome is attached to the primary antibody (i.e. the antibody specific for the desired antigen), or the indirect method, in which the patient's white blood cells are incubated first with unlabeled primary antibody, followed by incubation with an antimouse immunoglobulin bound to the fluorochrome (because the primary antibodies are mouse monoclonal reagents (see also Chap. 3—*Immunofluorescence Assays*).

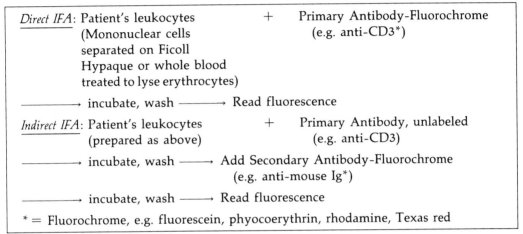

The direct method is subject to fewer interferences with nonspecific binding and saves time because it requires one less incubation step, while the indirect IFA provides the advantage of increased sensitivity because of larger conjugate formation.[34] The addition of biotin-avidin labeling allows for even greater sensitivity in the indirect system.[70]

The more recent introduction of dual immunofluorescence provides additional information by allowing for the simultaneous detection of two different surface markers on a single cell.[20,34,66] This is accomplished with a direct IFA employing two primary monoclonal antibodies, each labeled with a different fluorochrome. The differences in the emission spectra of fluorescein and phycoerythrin make these fluorochromes especially well suited for this method, and necessitate the use of only one laser in flow cytometry.[11,61] Modifications of this method have allowed for the simultaneous detection of as many as five cell subsets on a single aliquot of patients cells.[30] Systems using three-color immunofluorescence have also been described.[24,41] The use of multicolor analyses will likely be of great benefit in elucidating the relationships between lymphocyte subset values and various disease states.

IFA results may be read manually with a fluorescent microscope, or by automated analysis, using a flow cytometer (also known as the fluorescent activated cell sorter). Flow cytometry offers the advantages of increased sensitivity, accuracy of interpretation, and analytic speed, while manual reading allows for the preservation of cell architecture in tissue analysis, and is less expensive.[61] The principles of flow cytometry[43,52] are briefly described in Figures 4–2 and 4–3.

Benchtop, user-friendly instruments (e.g. the FACScan or Profile) are now commercially available and can be readily implemented into the routine clinical laboratory.[11] Some instruments also have the capability of cell sorting, or separating populations

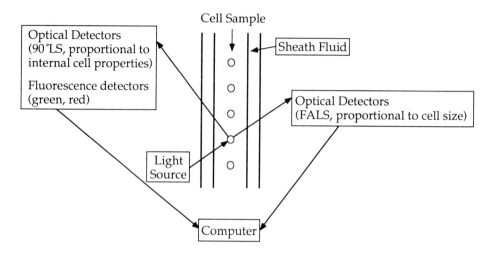

Fig. 4–2. Simplified principles of flow cytometry. Single cell suspensions of mononuclear cells or erythrocyte-lysed cells are prepared as described above in an isotonic medium or preserved in 1% paraformaldehyde prior to analysis. The sample is introduced into a flow cell surrounded by a pressurized isotonic sheath fluid. The differences between the pressures of the sheath fluid and the sample ~reates a laminar flow, or a stream of cells flowing in single file, allowing for analysis of individual particles. Each cell is met by a beam of light originating from a laser (argon, helium, neon, or krypton) or mercury arc lamp. The resulting light scatter (LS) is measured by optical detectors located at specific angles from the light source, and converted to electrical impulses by photomultiplier tubes. Forward angle LS (FALS), detected at 0° or 360° from the light source, is proportional to cell size, while 90° LS is proportional to certain properties of internal cell structure (e.g. granularity and membrane ruffling). Thus, FALS and 90° values can be used to characterize individual cell types and are related as follows: Erythrocytes and debris < lymphocytes < monocytes < polymorphonuclear granulocytes. On the basis of these LS parameters, electronic gates can be drawn around the cell population desired to be analyzed for fluorescence. The fluorescence of lymphocytes in the sample can then be selectively determined and plotted as a frequency distribution. All data are collected, calculated, and stored by a computer integrated with the system.

based on the presence or absence of a given surface marker.

Results of quantitation assays are reported both as a percentage of T or B lymphocytes and as the absolute number of T or B lymphocytes per defined volume (e.g. μl) of peripheral blood, where:

(1) % T or B lymphocytes $= \dfrac{\text{\# Fluorescent } (+) \text{ cells}}{\text{Total \# lymphocytes counted}} \times 100$

(2) Absolute # T or B lymphocytes =

(Absolute # white blood cells $\times$ % lymphocytes)[a] $\times$ % T or B lymphocytes (respectively)

[a]Obtained from cbc and differential

Reference ranges should be established by each individual laboratory keeping in mind that differences in lymphocyte subsets can occur in relation to age, race, sex, or environmental factors such as drugs, smoking, and season.[23] Diurnal variations, especially in CD4(+) cells, have also been reported.[46]

Immunoenzyme staining methods for detection of lymphocyte markers[19,38] are available as an alternative to immunofluorescence and are particularly useful in the analysis of tissue sections.[8]

REFERENCES

1. Aiuti, F., et al.: Scand. J. Immunol., *3*:521, 1974.
2. Alexander, E.L., and Sanders, S.K.: J. Immunol., *119*:1084, 1977.
3. Ammann, A.J.: In *Basic and Clinical Immunology.* 6th ed. Edited by D.P. Stites, J.D. Stobo, and J.V. Wells. Norwalk, Appleton and Lange, 1987.
4. Ault, K.A.: In *Manual of Clinical Laboratory Immunology.* 3rd ed. Edited by N.R. Rose, H. Friedman, and J.L. Fahey. Washington, D.C., American Society for Microbiology, 1986.
5. Bach, J.-F.: Transplant Rev., *16*:196, 1973.
*6. Bierer, B.E., et al.: Ann. Rev. Immunol., *7*:579, 1989.
7. Boyum, A.: Scand. J. Clin. Lab. Invest., *21* (suppl 97):77, 1968.
8. Chen, K., et al.: Lab. Invest., *56*:114, 1987.
9. Clement, L.T., Grossi, C.E., and Gartland, G.L.: J. Immunol., *133*:2461, 1984.
10. Committee on Human Leukocyte Differentiation Antigens, IUIS-WHO Nomenclature Subcommittee: Immunol. Today, *5*:158, 1984.
*11. Coon, J.S., Landay, A.L., and Weinstein, R.S.: Lab. Invest., *57*:453, 1987.
12. Damle, N.K., Mohagheghpour, N., and Engleman, E.G.: J. Immunol., *132*:644, 1984.
13. Davey, F.R., and Huntington, S.: Gerontology, *23*:381, 1977.
14. Davis, M.M.: Hosp. Pract., *23*:157, 1988.
15. DePaoli, P., et al.: J. Immunol. Methods, *61*:259, 1983 (letter).
16. DePaoli, P., et al.: J. Immunol. Methods, *72*:349, 1984.
17. Dickler, H.B.: Adv. Immunol., *24*:167, 1976.
18. Dickler, H.B., and Kunkel, H.G.: J. Exp. Med., *136*:191, 1972.
19. Endl, J., et al.: J. Immunol. Meth., *102*:77, 1987.
20. Fleisher, T.A., Marti, G.E., and Hagengruber, C.: Cytometry, *9*:309, 1988.
21. Foon, K.A., Gale, R.P., and Todd, R.F.: Semin. Hematol., *23*:257, 1986.
22. Gatenby, P.A., et al.: J. Immunol., *129*:1997, 1982.
23. Giorgi, J.V.: In *Manual of Clinical Laboratory Immunology.* 3rd ed. Edited by N.R. Rose, H. Friedman, and J.L. Fahey. Washington, D.C., American Society for Microbiology, 1986.
24. Glazer, A.N., and Stryer, L.: Biophys. J., *43*:383, 1983.
25. Gupta, S., Good, R.A., and Siegel, F.P.: Clin. Exp. Immunol., *25*:319, 1976.
26. Hallberg, T., et al.: J. Immunol. Methods, *4*:317, 1974.
27. Hallberg, T., Gurner, B.W., and Coombs, R.R.A.: Int. Arch. Allergy Appl. Immunol., *44*:500, 1973.
28. Hoffman, R.A., et al.: Proc. Natl. Acad. Sci. U.S.A., *77*:4914, 1980.
29. Hong, R.: In *Manual of Clinical Laboratory Immunology.* 3rd ed. Edited by N.R. Rose, H. Friedman, and J.L. Fahey. Washington, D.C., American Society for Microbiology, 1986.
30. Horan, P.K., Slezak, S.E., and Poste, G.: Proc. Natl. Acad. Sci. U.S.A., *83*:8361, 1986.
31. Horwitz, D.A., and Lobo, P.I.: J. Clin. Invest., *56*:1464, 1975.
32. Huber, H., and Fudenberg, H.H.: Int. Arch. Allergy Appl. Immunol., *34*:18, 1968.
33. Imboden, J.B., Weiss, A., and Stobo, J.D.: Immunol. Today, *6*:328, 1985.
*34. Jackson, A.L., and Warner, N.L.: In *Manual of Clinical Laboratory Immunology.* 3rd ed. Edited by N.R. Rose, H. Friedman, and J.L. Fahey. Washington, D.C., American Society for Microbiology, 1986.
35. Jondal, M., Holm, G., and Wigzell, H.: J. Exp. Med., *136*:207, 1972.
36. Jondal, M., Wigzell, H., and Aiuti, F.: Transplant Rev., *16*:163, 1973.
37. Kansas, G.S., et al.: J. Immunol., *134*:2995, 1985.
38. Karbowiak, I., and Appel, S.: J. Immunol. Methods, *112*:31, 1988.
39. Kikutani, H., et al.: Cell, *47*:657, 1986.
40. Korsmeyer, S.J., and Waldmann, T.A.: J. Clin. Immunol., *4*:1, 1984.
41. Lanier, L.L., and Loken, M.R.: J. Immunol., *132*:151, 1984.
42. LoBuglio, A.F., Cotran, R.S., and Jandl, J.H.: Science, *158*:1582, 1967.
*43. Lovett, E.J., et al.: Lab. Invest., *50*:115, 1984.
44. Macey, M.G., Hyam, C.J., and Newland, A.C.: Med. Lab. Sci., *45*:187, 1988.
45. Middleditch, P.R., et al.: J. Histochem. Cytochem., *27*:689, 1979.
46. Miyawaki, T., et al.: Clin. Exp. Immunol., *55*:618, 1984.
47. Moretta, L., et al.: J. Exp. Med., *146*:184, 1977.
48. Morimoto, C., et al.: J. Immunol., *134*:1508, 1985.
49. Morimoto, C., et al.: J. Immunol., *134*:3762, 1985.
50. Package Insert—FACS Brand Lysing Solution 10X Concentrate. Becton Dickinson Immunocytometry Systems, Mountain View, CA, 1988.
51. Package Insert—Ficoll-Paque, Pharmacia Fine Chemicals, Piscataway, NJ, 1979.
52. Patrick, C.W., et al.: Lab. Med., *15*:740, 1984.
53. Preud'homme, J.L., and Seligmann, M.: J. Clin. Invest., *51*:701, 1972.
54. Reinherz, E.L., et al.: Proc. Natl. Acad. Sci. U.S.A., *76*:4061, 1979.
55. Reinherz, E.L., et al.: J. Immunol., *124*:1301, 1980.
56. Renzi, P., and Ginns, L.C.: J. Immunol. Methods, *98*:53, 1987.
57. Reynolds, C.W., and Ortaldo, J.R.: Immunol. Today, *8*:172, 1987.
58. Romain, P.L., and Schlossman, S.F.: J. Clin. Invest., *74*:1559, 1984.
59. Rosenthal, S.H., Cassidy, J.T., and Soderstrom, S.: J. Lab. Clin. Med., *83*:584, 1974.
60. Ross, G.D.: Arch. Pathol. Lab. Med., *101*:337, 1977.

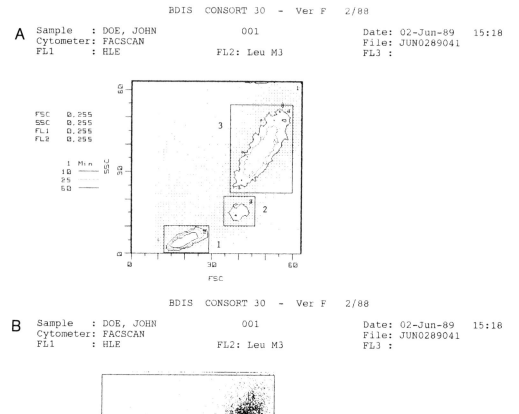

Fig. 4–3. Sample analyses from the FACScan Flow Cytometer (Becton Dickinson) (**A**) Contour plot of whole peripheral blood from a normal, healthy, control individual, pretreated to lyse erythrocytes. Drawn using BDIS Consort 30 Ver F software (Becton Dickinson). Contour levels show cell populations with varying degrees of fluorescence intensity. SSC = side scatter (i.e. 90° LS); FSC = forward scatter (0° LS). Box 1 contains lymphocytes, box 2 contains monocytes, and box 3 contains polymorphonuclear granulocytes; (**B**) Dot plot of same specimen analyzed in Figure 4–3A. Electronic gates have been drawn around the lymphocyte population in selection for subsequent fluorescence analysis; (**C**) (see next page) Fluorescence analysis of lymphocytes from a normal healthy control. Drawn using SimulSET Software, Version 2.1 (Becton Dickinson). Upper graph shows fluorescence using monoclonal Leu 12-phycoerythrin (PE) and Leu 4-fluorescein isothiocyante (FITC) antibodies. Quadrant #1 (upper left) contains Leu 4^-12^+ cells (i.e. B lymphocytes). Quadrant #4 (lower right) contains Leu 4^+12^- cells. (i.e. T lymphocytes). Quadrant #3 (lower left) contains cells negative for both markers. Lower graph shows fluorescence using monoclonal Leu 2-PE and Leu-3-FITC antibodies. Quadrant #1 (upper left) contains Leu 2^+3^- cells (i.e., cytotoxic/suppressor T cells). Quadrant #4 (lower right) contains Leu 2^-3^+ cells. (i.e. T helper cells). Quadrant #3 (lower left) contains cells negative for both markers.

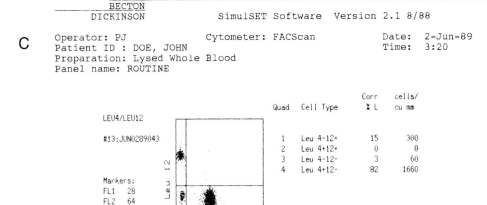

C

BECTON
DICKINSON   SimulSET Software   Version 2.1 8/88

Operator: PJ   Cytometer: FACScan   Date: 2-Jun-89
Patient ID : DOE, JOHN   Time: 3:20
Preparation: Lysed Whole Blood
Panel name: ROUTINE

| | | Corr | cells/ |
Quad	Cell Type	% L	cu mm
1	Leu 4-12+	15	300
2	Leu 4+12+	0	0
3	Leu 4-12-	3	60
4	Leu 4+12-	82	1660

LEU4/LEU12

#13:JUN0289043

Markers:
FL1 28
FL2 64

Leu 12 / Leu 4

FSC Mean 83   Events 2114
SSC Mean 21

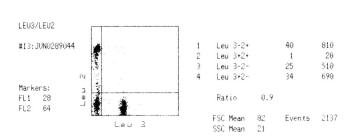

Quad	Cell Type	Corr % L	cells/ cu mm
1	Leu 3-2+	40	810
2	Leu 3+2+	1	20
3	Leu 3-2-	25	510
4	Leu 3+2-	34	690

LEU3/LEU2

#13:JUN0289044

Markers:
FL1 28
FL2 64

Leu 2 / Leu 3

Ratio   0.9

FSC Mean 82   Events 2137
SSC Mean 21

For research use only. Not for use in diagnostic or therapeutic procedures.

*61. Ryan, D.H., Fallon, M.A., and Horan, P.K.: Clin. Chim. Acta, *171*:125, 1988.

62. Shaw, S.: Immunol. Today, *8*:1, 1987.

63. Siegel, F.P., and Good, R.A.: Clin. Hematol., *6*:355, 1977.

64. Stites, D.P.: In *Basic and Clinical Immunology.* 6th ed. Edited by D.P. Stites, J.D. Stobo, and J.V. Wells. Norwalk, Appleton and Lange, 1987.

65. Thorley-Lawson, D.A., et al.: J. Immunol., *134*:3007, 1985.

66. Thornwaite, J.T., et al.: Am. J. Clin. Pathol., *82*:48, 1984.

67. Uhr, J.W., and Phillips, J.M.: Ann. N.Y. Acad. Sci., *129*:793, 1966.

68. vonBoehmer, H.: Ann. Rev. Immunol., *6*:309, 1988.

69. Waldmann, T.A.: Hosp. Pract., *21*:69, 1986.

70. Wilchek, M., and Bayer, E.A.: Immunol. Today, *5*:39, 1984.

*71. Winchester, R.J., and Ross, G.D.: In *Manual of Clinical Laboratory Immunology.* 3rd ed. Edited by N.R. Rose, H. Friedman, and J.L. Fahey. Washington, D.C., American Society for Microbiology, 1986.

*72. Zola, H.: Immunol. Today, *8*:308, 1987.

Lymphocyte Subset Analysis: Whole Blood Lysis Procedure[1]

PRINCIPLE

In this two-color, direct immunofluorescence method, lymphocytes in whole blood samples are incubated simultaneously with fluorescein (FITC) labeled and phycoerythrin (PE) labeled monoclonal antibodies. Following lysis of the red cells with FACS lysing solution, the samples are analyzed on the FACScan flow cytometer to determine the percentage of T cells, B cells, helper/inducer and suppressor/cytotoxic cells in the sample.

EQUIPMENT AND MATERIALS

1. Hanks Balanced Salt Solution without phenol red (1x: HBSS: Grand Island Biological). Store at room temperature. After opening, store at 2 to 8° C. May be used indefinitely unless contaminated

2. 10% sodium azide: Dissolve 10 g sodium azide (NaN_3) in 100 ml of distilled water. Store at 2 to 8° C. No expiration date

3. Washing Buffer: Add 5 ml of 10% sodium azide to 500 ml of HBSS. Store at 2 to 8° C. Discard if contaminated

4. Paraformaldehyde Solution:

a. Method 1—Place 100 ml of 0.9% saline solution in a sterile 100 ml glass bottle and place a stirring bar into it. Place bottle on heating block at medium temperature and medium speed. Add 1 g paraformaldehyde to saline solution. Stir and heat until dissolved. Do not let mixture boil. Cool. Store at 2 to 8° C. Stable for up to 1 week.

b. Method 2—Combine 1 g paraformaldehyde with 100 ml 0.9% saline solution in small bottle. Place in 56° C waterbath overnight. Cool and store at 2 to 8° C. Stable for 1 week.

5. 1% FACS Lysing Solution: (Becton Dickinson) Place 10 ml of 10x FACS lysing solution into 100 ml bottle. Add 90 ml distilled water. Invert to mix. Store at room temperature. Expiration: 1 month

6. Monoclonal Antibodies (Becton Dickinson)

a. Leukogate (CD45 FITC/CD14 PE); anti-Leucocytes/anti-Monocytes

b. Background (Mouse IgG1 FITC/Mouse IgG2 PE)

c. T & B cells (CD3 FITC/CD19 PE)—Leu-4/Leu-12

d. Helper/suppressor (CD4 FITC/CD8 PE)—Leu-3/Leu-2 Store at 2 to 8° C

7. Pipettor 20 μl and 100 μl with disposable tips

8. 12 × 75 plastic tubes (Falcon #2054 or #2052)

9. FACScan (Becton Dickinson) Flow Cytometer

10. Serofuge

11. Vortex

12. Biological safety cabinet

SPECIMEN COLLECTION AND PREPARATION

Blood must be collected in EDTA tubes. Volume requirements depend on the number of markers being tagged.

PROCEDURE

NOTE: All specimens must be processed in a biological safety cabinet.

1. Label 4 Falcon 2054 or 2052 tubes for each patient/control individual with patient name, and number 1 to 4. These tubes must be used to ensure a tight seal on the FACScan.

2. Place 20 μl of the following monoclonal antibodies into the corresponding tube:

Tube 1—Leukogate
Tube 2—Background
Tube 3—Leu-4/Leu-12
Tube 4—Leu-3/Leu-2

3. Add 100 μl of well-mixed EDTA blood.

4. Vortex.

5. Incubate at room temperature in the dark for 15 to 30 minutes.

6. Add 2 ml of 1% FACS lysing solution.

7. Vortex.

8. Let sit 5 minutes in the dark at room temperature. **Time is critical—do not lyse longer!**

9. Spin on high in serofuge for 3 minutes.

10. Pour off supernatant into waste bottle and gently blot tube on gauze. Approximately 50 μl of liquid will remain in tube.

11. Vortex tubes.

12. Add 2 ml of washing buffer.

13. Spin in serofuge on high for 3 minutes.

14. Decant and blot as in step 10.

15. Add 0.5 ml of 1% paraformaldehyde.

16. Store at 2 to 8° C until read on FACScan flow cytometer. Specimens can be stored for up to one week using fresh paraformaldehyde.

REPORTING

Reference ranges must be developed by each laboratory. The percentage of cells tagged and the absolute number of cells for each monoclonal marker are reported along with physician's interpretation of the data (see *Lymphocyte Reporting Sheet*).

REFERENCES

1. Package insert, FACS lysing solution, Becton-Dickinson Immunocytometry Systems, Mountain View, CA, 6/1988.

Ficoll Hypaque Separation of Mononuclear Cells from Whole Peripheral Blood[1]

PRINCIPLE

In a test tube, whole peripheral blood is gently overlaid onto a lymphocyte separation medium (LSM) having a specific gravity of 1.076 to 1.080 (e.g. Ficoll Hypaque).

LYMPHOCYTE REPORTING SHEET

Name:

Hospital Number:

Loc./DR.:

State University of New York
Health Science Center
Syracuse, New York 13210

Clinical Pathology
Immunology Report

Lymphocyte Subsets

Specimen Date: Acc. #

White blood cell count: _____ ×1,000/μL

Leukocyte:	relative # in %	absolute # in cells/μL	mean % (N = 20)	reference range in % (+/− 1 SD)
Total Lymphocytes				
Total B-lymphocytes (CD19)			13	8-18
Total T-lymphocytes (CD3)			73	66-80
Helper/Inducer T-lymphocytes (CD4)			46	38-54
Suppressor/Cytotoxic T-lymphocytes (CD8)			32	25-38
CD4/CD8 ratio (i.e. "Helper/Suppressor ratio")		> or = 1		

Comments:

_____

Immunology Director

Following centrifugation, five distinct layers are formed, from top to bottom: plasma, mononuclear cells and platelets, LSM, granulocytes, erythrocytes. Lymphocytes and monocytes may be recovered by harvesting and washing the mononuclear cell band.

EQUIPMENT AND MATERIALS

1. Lymphocyte separation medium (LSM; Ficoll-Hypaque from Bionetics Laboratory, or equivalent): Specific gravity 1.076 ± .001. Store at room temperature. May be used until the expiration date noted on the label

2. Pasteur pipets, 9 inch, disposable, sterile

3. Sterile plastic centrifuge tubes, 16 × 125 mm

4. 50-ml centrifuge tube (Falcon), sterile

5. Hanks' balanced salt solution (HBSS) 1 ×; (Grand Island Biological): Sterile. Store at room temperature. May be used indefinitely if no evidence of contamination occurs

6. White blood cell pipets and hemocytometer counting chambers or automated cell counter

7. Centrifuge

SPECIMEN COLLECTION AND PREPARATION

Specimen requirement is generally 5 to 10 ml of heparinized blood. Minimum volume depends on patient's lymphocyte count. Other types of anticoagulants may be used; however, Ca^{++} and Mg^{++} free Hanks' Balanced Salt Solution must be used in the procedure to prevent clotting. Blood must be kept at room temperature and used within 4 hours of collection.

PROCEDURE

NOTE: If cells are to be used in lymphocyte proliferation assays, the following should be performed using sterile technique.

1. Dilute whole blood approximately 1:2 with Hanks' Balanced Salt Solution (HBSS).

2. Pipet LSM into two 16 × 125 mm centrifuge tubes. The ratio of diluted blood to gradient should be approximately 2:1.

3. Carefully overlay the LSM in each tube with an equal volume of the blood sample by slowly adding blood down the side of the tube. The surface of the LSM must not be disturbed. If disturbance occurs, discard. The more care taken initially to layer the blood, the more distinct the lymphocyte band will be after centrifugation.

4. Place in centrifuge and turn up speed slowly to 400 × g. Centrifuge for 30 ± 5 minutes.

5. Immediately remove tubes from the centrifuge. Layers should appear as in Fig. 4-4.

6. Using a pasteur pipet, discard the plasma layer and harvest the mononuclear band from each tube at the interface between the plasma and LSM gradient. Transfer to a 50-ml tube.

7. Add HBSS to the 40-ml line to wash. Invert tube gently to mix and centrifuge at 100 × g for 15 minutes. Decant the supernate and repeat step #7.

8. Resuspend the cell button in 1 ml HBSS. (For lymphocyte transformation assays, resuspend in 1 ml RPMI with 5% fetal calf serum. If the cells are to be held overnight for testing the following day, add 2 ml RPMI with 5% fetal calf serum and store at room temperature).

9. Perform cell count and adjust lymphocyte suspension to desired cell concentration.

10. Modifications: Larger amounts of blood may be separated by the same method using larger tubes and larger amounts of gradient.

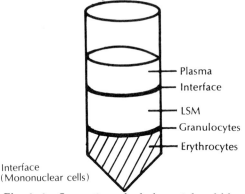

Interface
(Mononuclear cells)

Fig. 4–4. Separation of whole peripheral blood in Ficoll Hypaque.

LIMITATIONS OF THE PROCEDURE

Occasionally, a lymphocyte suspension will be contaminated with red blood cells that are not removed by centrifugation. These can be eliminated by diluting the cell suspension with HBSS, relayering it over new LSM, and repeating the centrifugation steps.

If contamination with platelets persists after the washing steps, the platelets can be removed by centrifugation in a 4 to 20% sucrose gradient layered over the LSM.[2]

REFERENCES

1. Boyum, A., Scan. J.: Clin. Lab. Invest., *21,* (suppl 97), 1968.
2. Peper, R.J., Tina, W.Z., and Mickelson, M.M.: J. Lab. Clin. Med., *72:*842, 1968.

TESTS OF LYMPHOCYTE FUNCTION

Functional assays of the immune system encompass evaluation of its major components: (1) T and B lymphocytes and natural killer cells, (2) phagocytic cells, and (3) complement. Tests of the last two components are discussed in Chapters 8 and 6, respectively. Common functional assays of T and B lymphocytes and NK cells are listed in Table 4–2. Some of these assays are discussed below.

Lymphocyte Proliferation Assays

Lymphocyte proliferation assays (also known as lymphocyte transformation assays) are in vitro tests used to assess the responsiveness of T or B lymphocytes to a given stimulus. These assays have a wide variety of clinical applications, including characterization and monitoring of congenital immunodeficiencies, detecting sensitization to infectious agents or other antigens, determination of histocompatibility in organ transplantation, and monitoring the effects of immunotherapy.[4,6,7]

The stimulants used in lymphocyte proliferation assays may be specific antigens, nonspecific polyclonal activators (i.e. mitogens), or allogeneic lymphocytes. The last of these is used in the mixed lymphocyte

Table 4–2. Commonly Employed Functional Assays of Lymphocytes

B lymphocytes	T lymphocytes	NK cells
Quantitation of immunoglobulim levels[a]	Skin tests (e.g. Anergy panel)	In vitro tests of NK cell cytotoxicity
Detection of specific antibodies[b]	Lymphocyte proliferation assays	
Detection of paraproteins[a]	Lymphokine assays	
Lymphocyte proliferation assays	In vitro tests of suppressor or cytotoxic cell function	

[a] See Chapter 5
[b] Usually involves detection of naturally occurring antibodies (e.g. isohemagglutinins) or antibodies to common environmental or vaccine antigens

culture test, which is discussed in detail in Chapter 13.

Specific antigens are used to detect previous sensitization of the immune system, e.g. to infectious agents, allergens, or autoantigens, or to determine the ability of an individual to respond to an antigenic challenge.[7] In the latter situation, the test commonly employs antigens ubiquitous to the environment, or antigens that have been routinely administered in vaccines.[7,11] In some diseases, a patient may be selectively unresponsive to a specific antigen while the rest of the immune system may be functional (e.g. Chronic Mucocutaneous Candidiasis is characterized by inability of T cells to respond to *Candida albicans,* and consequently, recurrent Candida infections).[1]

Antigen-induced proliferation, by nature, depends on an anamnestic response involving stimulation of a small number of previously sensitized cells and recruitment of some nonsensitized cells;[4] consequently, transformation is seen in 5 to 35% of the cell population tested.[9]

Conversely, mitogen-induced proliferation does not require previous exposure, and can be used to assess the responsiveness of T or B lymphocyte populations as a whole. Mitogens activate lymphocytes by binding to surface receptors that are distinct from antigen recognition receptors, and that are present on virtually all lymphocytes of a given type.[10] Consequently, mitogens induce transformation in a high percentage of lymphocytes (60 to 90%) tested in normal individuals.[9] Different mitogens may selec-

tively or preferentially activate T or B cell populations and may produce different responses in different species.[10] Some commonly used polyclonal activators of T and B cells are listed in Table 4–3.

Lymphocyte proliferation assays are performed by incubation of the patient's mononuclear cells (usually obtained by separation of whole peripheral blood on Ficoll Hypaque—see *Ficoll Hypaque Separation of Mononuclear Cells from Peripheral Blood*) with the appropriate mitogen or antigen under sterile conditions for a period of 3 to 6 days, depending on the stimulus. The procedure is routinely performed as a microtechnique using a 200 μl volume,[5,9] although microtechniques[3,7] or macrotechniques[8] using different volumes have also been described. During the incubation period, the stimulated lymphocytes are transformed into large blast-like cells that undergo DNA synthesis and mitosis.[2,7,8] Several methods have been employed to detect the degree or number of cells responding; among these are morphologic examination, incorporation of radiolabeled protein precursors (e.g. ^{3}H— leucine), and incorporation of a radiolabeled DNA precursor (e.g. ^{3}H— thymidine).[9] The last method is most often used because morphologic criteria depend on subjective interpretation, and leucine labeling, while more rapid and lacking a requirement for serum, is technically more difficult to standardize.

In routine procedure, ^{3}H— thymidine is added during the last 12 to 20 hours of incubation, and the cells are subsequently harvested onto glass fiber strips with a cell

Table 4–3. Commonly Employed Human B and T Cell Mitogens[a]

B Cell Mitogens Name	Abbreviation	Source
Pokeweed Mitogen[b]	PWM	Pokeweed plant
Epstein-Barr Virus	EBV	EBV-infected cell lines
Staphylococcus Protein A	SpA, SAC	Staphylococcus aureus, Cowan strain I

T Cell Mitogens[c] Name	Abbreviation	Source
Concanavalin A	Con A	Jack bean plant
Phytohemagglutinin	PHA	Kidney bean plant
Pokeweed Mitogen	PWM	Pokeweed plant
Leucoagglutinin	LA	Kidney bean plant
Soybean Agglutinin	SBA	Soybean plant

[a] Adapted from references 10 and 11
[b] Induces a T cell-dependent B cell response
[c] All T cell mitogens listed are lectins which bind to various sugar moieties on the T lymphocyte surface membrane[10]

harvester. The amount of $^3H-$ thymidine incorporation increases as the amount of DNA synthesis and cell proliferation increase in the population tested. The results are expressed as (1) net counts per minute (cpm) = cpm of stimulated cells minus cpm of unstimulated cells; (2) the stimulation index, SI = cpm of stimulated cells/cpm of unstimulated cells; or (3) the relative proliferation index RPI = net cpm of test individual/mean net cpm of at least three healthy, control individuals.[7] The third parameter is preferred because the RPI is less susceptible to changes in background cpm and variations among individual donors.[7]

Lymphocyte proliferation assays are highly susceptible to variations arising from a number of factors, including source of donor lymphocytes, type and concentration of stimulant, and slight changes in culture environment.[7] Attempts at standardization have been met with difficulty.[7] Each individual laboratory should therefore establish their own protocol and reference values, and follow rigorous quality assurance measures to minimize variability.[7]

REFERENCES

1. Ammann, A.J.: In *Basic and Clinical Immunology.* 6th ed. Edited by D.P. Stites, J.D. Stobo, and J.V. Wells. Norwalk, Appleton and Lange, 1987.

2. Douglas, S.D.: Int. Rev. Exp. Pathol., *10*:41, 1971.

3. Farrant, J., et al.: Immunol. Methods, *33*:301, 1980.

4. Fudenberg, H.H., et al.: Pediatrics, *47*:927, 1971.

5. Hartzman, R.J., et al.: Transplantation, *11*:268, 1971.

6. Hirschhorn, K.: Fed. Proc., *27*:31, 1968.

*7. Maluish, E., and Strong, D.M.: In *Manual of Clinical Laboratory Immunology.* 3rd ed. Edited by N.R. Rose, H. Friedman, and J.L. Fahey. Washington, D.C., American Society for Microbiology, 1986.

8. Nowell, P.C.: Cancer Res., *20*:462, 1960.

9. Oppenheim, J.J., and Schecter, B.: In *Manual of Clinical Laboratory Immunology.* 2nd ed. Edited by N.R. Rose and H. Friedman. Washington, D.C., American Society for Microbiology, 1980.

*10. Severinson, E., and Larsson, E.-L.: In *Handbook of Experimental Immunology.* Vol. 2. 4th ed. Edited by D.M. Weir. Oxford, Blackwell Scientific Publications, 1986.

11. Stites, D.P.: In *Basic and Clinical Immunology.* 6th ed. Edited by D.P. Stites, J.D. Stobo, and J.V. Wells. Norwalk, Appleton and Lange, 1987.

Lymphocyte Transformation:[1-7] PHA- or Candida-Induced Stimulation

PRINCIPLE

Antigens or mitogens are incubated with lymphocytes in a culture medium, allowing stimulation of lymphocyte activity to occur. Addition of a radioactive DNA precursor labels transforming cells for subsequent detection and indicates degree of cell proliferation.

EQUIPMENT AND MATERIALS

1. Stimulants:

a. Phytohemagglutinin P PHA; (Difco): A sterile, desiccated, purified protein

PHA. Store at 2 to 10° C without loss of potency. Rehydrate and dilute to 1:50; 1:100, and 1:500 with RPMI-HEPES before using.

b. *Candida albicans* (Hollister-Stier): Dermatophytin "0" antigen. Fungus extract prepared from Oidiomycin. Contains 0.45% phenol as a preservative. Store at 2 to 8° C. Do not freeze. May be used until expiration date noted on the label. Dilute 1:10, 1:30, and 1:100 in RPMI-HEPES before using.

NOTE: PHA and Candida are the only two stimulants in routine use in our clinical laboratory. Standardization of lymphocyte transformation with other stimulants can be developed.

2. HEPES (Gibco): N-2 hydroxyethyl-piperazine-N'-2-ethanesulfonic acid. Store at room temperature. No expiration date. To use, add 23.8 g HEPES to 70 ml of distilled water in a 100-ml volumetric flask. Adjust pH to 8.1 using approximately 13 ml NaOH. QS to 100 ml with distilled water. Pass through a millipore filter to sterilize. Store at 2 to 8° C. May be used indefinitely unless contamination becomes evident

3. RPMI-HEPES: Add 10 ml RPMI-1640 (Roswell Park Memorial Institute 1640; Grand Island Biological) to 0.3 ml HEPES. Store at 2 to 8° C. May be used up to 1 week

4. Millipore Filter (Sybron): Nalgene filter unit. Pore size 45 μm

5. Heparin (Fellows Testagar): 1000 U/ml. Contains no preservatives

6. Tritiated thymidine (^{3}H TdR; Amersham Corp.): 1 μCi/ml. Dilute 1:25 with RPMI-HEPES to 1 μCi/25 μl. Aliquot in approximately 3 ml amounts in plastic tubes. Store at $-20°$ C. May be used indefinitely. Thaw before use. Thawed aliquots may be stored at 2 to 8° C for subsequent use

7. Fetal bovine serum (Gibco): Heat inactivate prior to use

8. Scintillation fluid: Betafluor (National Diagnostics)

9. Cell harvester (Cambridge Technology)

10. Glass fiber strips (Cambridge Technology)

11. Beta scintillation counter

12. Pipets to deliver 25 μl, 12.5 μl, and 100 μl, with sterile, disposable tips

13. Laminar flow hood

14. Microtiter plates (Dynatech), flat bottom, with covers

15. 37° C incubator, with 5% CO_2

SPECIMEN COLLECTION AND PREPARATION

Aseptically collect 15 to 20 ml of blood from the patient and a normal, healthy control. Place into a sterile tube containing 0.1 ml preservative free heparin. Alternately, blood may be drawn into sterile heparin tubes.

PROCEDURE

NOTE: A normal control must be performed with each lymphocyte transformation assay.

1. Using sterile technique, separate mononuclear cells from patient and control following the *Ficoll Hypaque Separation of Mononuclear Cells from Whole Peripheral Blood* procedure.

2. Prepare RPMI-HEPES (see Equipment and Materials).

3. Resuspend each monolayer cell preparation in 1 ml RPMI-HEPES plus 5% fetal calf serum.

4. Adjust the mononuclear cell count to 4 × 10^6 cells/ml using the appropriate amount of RPMI-HEPES.

5. Reconstitute PHA to be used (see Equipment and Materials). Prepare the indicated dilutions in RPMI-HEPES for the stimulant to be used:

    PHA—1:50, 1:100, 1:500
    Candida—1:10, 1:30, 1:100

6. Label a flat-bottomed microtiter plate indicating one row for each antigen/mitogen for the patient and for the control. *NOTE:* PHA and Candida assays should be set up in separate microtiter plates if performed simultaneously.

7. Perform the following using sterile technique:

a. Place 100 μl of 4 × 10^6 cell/ml patient or control cell suspension into each well (1 to 12) of the appropriately labeled row.

b. Add 12.5 μl of fetal bovine serum to each well.

c. Add: 12.5 μl of RPMI-HEPES to wells 1 to 3.
    12.5 μl of PHA 1:500 (or Candida 1:100) to wells 4 to 6.
    12.5 μl of PHA 1:100 (or Candida 1:30) to wells 7 to 9.

12.5 μl of PHA 1:50 (or Candida 1:10) to wells 10 to 12.

8. Seal with microtiter cover.

9. Incubate at 37° C, 5% CO_2 for approximately 48 hours for PHA; 5 days for Candida.

10. After the appropriate incubation period, thaw an aliquot of ^3H TdR using gloves to prevent radiation contamination, and add 25 μl to each well.

11. Incubate at 37° C, 5% CO_2 for 12 to 20 hours (16 to 18 hours is optimal).

12. Aspirate cells onto glass fiber strips using a cell harvester.

13. Place glass fiber disk into scintillation vials.

14. Add 6 ml scintillation fluid to each disk in a scintillation vial.

15. Count on beta scintillation counter, using counts with 1% error or less.

CALCULATIONS

1. For each set of triplicates, calculate the following:

   a. The mean

   b. The standard deviation

   c. The standard error of the mean

   d. The stimulation index

$$\frac{\text{(mean of triplicate stimulated counts)}}{\text{(mean of control counts, i.e. wells 1 to 3)}}$$

   e. Net counts per minute (cpm) (mean of stimulated counts − mean of control counts)

2. In general, < 20% variation should occur among triplicate wells, and the normal control values should fall within the normal ranges for the assay.

REPORTING. For each mitogen or antigen dilution, report stimulation index and net counts per minute, along with the pathologist's interpretation.

INTERPRETATION OF RESULTS

Normal levels with age variation have been established for this laboratory by use of student's t test. Patient's lymphocyte transformation is compared to the normal levels for that age group. Extrapolation of normal values between laboratories must be avoided because of the degree of variation among techniques.

LIMITATIONS OF THE PROCEDURE

Total failure to incorporate radioisotope or inclusion of too much radioisotope may be the result of bacterial contamination or cell death caused by changes in the medium.

REFERENCES

1. Foad, B.S.I. et al.: Clin. Exp. Immunol., *17*:657, 1974.

2. Fudenberg, H.H. et al.: Pediatrics, *47*:927, 1971.

3. Kaplan, J.M., and Razzano, A.F.: Immunol. Commun., *2*:507, 1973.

4. Maluish, A.E. and Strong, A.M.: In *Manual of Clinical Immunology*. Edited by N.R. Rose, H. Friedman, and J.L. Fahey. Washington, D.C., American Society of Microbiology, 1986.

5. Nelson, D.S., and Penrose, J.M.: Clin. Immunol. Immunopathol., *4*:143, 1975.

6. Nowell, P.C.: Cancer Res., *20*:462, 1960.

7. Oppenheim, J.J. et al.: In *Laboratory Diagnosis of Immunological Disorders*. Edited by G.N. Vyas, and D.P. Stites. New York, Grune & Stratton, 1975.

SKIN TESTING: ASSESSMENT OF DELAYED TYPE HYPERSENSITIVITY

Delayed type hypersensitivity (DTH) is a cell-mediated immune response that develops after sensitization of a person to a specific antigen (see Chap. 1).[8] Formation of DTH necessitates not only a functioning anamnestic response by the afferent, central and efferent limbs of the cell-mediated immune system,[3] but an intact nonspecific inflammatory response as well.[5] On a cellular level, injection of an antigen causes an influx of mononuclear cells and polymorphonuclear granulocytes, resulting in detectable inflammation by 6 hours after exposure.[1,9,10] The reaction intensifies until a peak response is reached, usually at 24 to 48 hours.

Delayed hypersensitivity skin testing[1,12,13] is a well-recognized method for in vivo assessment of this cell-mediated immune response. In this procedure, a convenient site such as the volar surface of the forearm, is injected intradermally with antigens to which the individual has had a known or assumed previous exposure. Because some individuals may not have been exposed to a particular antigen, or may be unable to respond immunologically to a given antigen, the test generally employs a battery of common antigens known to elicit a response in most persons (e.g. tetanus toxoid, antigens from *Candida albicans,* products of Streptococcus bacteria).[1,6,13]

Evidence of an intact DTH response is indicated by the presence of a readily visible area of erythema and palpable induration located at at least one antigen site, 48 hours after exposure.

Skin testing is routinely used in conjunction with in vitro assays of immune function to evaluate immunologic status of the patient. *Anergy,* or failure of the immune system to respond to any of the common skin recall antigens used, may be seen in a variety of primary congenital cellular immunodeficiencies and in conditions in which the immune deficiency is acquired secondary to another disease state (e.g. infections, malignancies).[1,4,12]

Variations in skin reactions occur in association with geographic location and age of the patient, the strength and type of antigen used, and the criteria used to determine a positive reaction.[1,7,11-13] The test has limited value in children, who are more likely not to have had the appropriate antigen exposure,[2,9] and in the elderly (age >70 years), in whom decreased responsiveness has been observed.[14]

Proper technique is imperative in producing accurate results;[1,12,13] for example, administration of a subcutaneous injection results in rapid clearance of the antigen and false negative results.[12,13] Occasionally, interpretation of the reaction may be complicated by the occurrence of IgE-mediated hypersensitivity reactions (although these usually subside by 24 hours), or IgM and IgG-mediated Arthus reactions at 24 hours.[1]

If questionable results are obtained, other test strategies may be used, including sequential testing with a single antigen, sensitization and subsequent challenge with a contact allergen such as dinitrochlorobenzene, and application of an irritant such as croton oil to assess the nonspecific inflammatory response.[1,12,13] (see also *Anergy Panel for Cellular Hypersensitivity*).

REFERENCES

*1. Buckley, E.C.: In *Manual of Clinical Laboratory Immunology.* 3rd ed. Edited by N.R. Rose, H. Friedman, and J.L. Fahey. Washington, D.C., American Society for Microbiology, 1986.

2. Gaisford, W.: Br. Med. J., *2*:1164, 1955.

3. Golub, E.S.: *The Cellular Basis of the Immune Response.* Sunderland, Sinauer Associates, 1977.

4. Heiss, L.I., and Palmer, D.L.: Am. J. Med., *56*:323, 1974.

5. Johnson, M.W., Maibach, H.I., and Salmon, S.E.: J. Exp. Med., *284*:1255, 1971.

6. Package Insert, Multitest CMI, Merieux Institute, Inc., Miami, Florida, 1982.

7. Palmer, D.L., and Reed, W.P.: J. Infect. Dis., *130*:132, 1974.

8. Sell, S.: *Immunology Immunopathology and Immunity,* 4th ed. New York, Elsevier Science Publishing Co., Inc., 1987.

9. Smith, R.T.: Pediatr. Clin. North Am., *7*:269, 1960.

10. Sokal, J.E.: N. Engl. J. Med., *293*:501, 1975.

11. Stimpson, P.G., et al.: South. Med. J., *69*:424, 1976.

*12. Stites, D.P.: In *Basic and Clinical Immunology.* 6th ed. Edited by D.P. Stites, J.D. Stobo, and J.V. Wells. Norwalk, Appleton and Lange, 1987.

13. Urbaniak, S.J., et al.: In *Handbook of Experimental Immunology: Applications of Immunological Methods in Biomedical Sciences.* Vol. 4. 4th ed. Edited by D.M. Weir. Oxford, Blackwell Scientific Publications, 1986.

14. Waldorf, D.S., Willkens, R.F., and Decker, J.L.: JAMA, *203*:831, 1968.

Anergy Panel for Cellular Hypersensitivity[1]

PRINCIPLE

The delayed cutaneous responses associated with the antigens in the MULTITEST CMI battery appear to be typical cellular hypersensitivity reactions. A small amount of soluble antigen is introduced into the epidermis and superficial dermal tissue by puncture. Circulating T-cells (lymphocytes), sensitized to the antigen from prior contact, react with the antigens in the skin and induce a specific immune response that includes mitosis (blastogenesis) and the release of many soluble mediators (lymphokines). Some lymphokines initiate inflammation (vasculitis and edema) that is manifest after several hours. The intensity of the overall dermal inflammation reaches its peak 24 to 72 hours after antigen application, and is resolved within days or weeks.

EQUIPMENT AND MATERIALS

1. MULTITEST CMI (Merieux Institute, Inc.) disposable plastic applicator consisting of eight sterile test heads preloaded with the following antigens:

a. *Test Head No. 1—Tetanus Toxoid Antigen.* Tetanus Toxoid Antigen is a sterile, glycerinated solution containing Tetanus Toxoid prepared from the culture filtrate of *Clostridium tetani,* inactivated and detoxified with formaldehyde. Residual formaldehyde does not exceed 0.02%. Each ml of Tetanus Toxoid Antigen in 70% w/v glycerin is biologically equivalent to 550,000 Merieux Tetanus Units.

b. *Test Head No. 2—Diphtheria Toxoid Antigen.* Diphtheria Toxoid Antigen is a sterile glycerinated solution containing diphtheria toxoid prepared from the culture filtrate of *Corynebacterium diphtheriae,* inactivated and detoxified with formaldehyde. Residual formaldehyde does not exceed 0.02%. Each ml of Diphtheria Toxoid Antigen in 70% w/v glycerin is biologically equivalent to 1,100,000 Merieux Diphtheria Units.

c. *Test Head No. 3—Streptococcus Antigen.* Streptococcus Antigen is a sterile, glycerinated solution containing culture filtrate of Streptococcus (Group C) inactivated with phenol. Residual phenol does not exceed 0.5%. Each ml of Streptococcus Antigen in 70% w/v glycerin is biologically equivalent to 2,000 Merieux Streptococcus Units.

d. *Test Head No. 4—Tuberculin, old.* Tuberculin, old is a sterile glycerinated solution containing culture filtrates of *Mycobacterium tuberculosis* (C, D and PN) and *Mycobacterium bovis* (Vallee). Each ml of Tuberculin, Old in 70% w/v glycerin is biologically equivalent to 300,000 U.S. Tuberculin Units (TU).

e. *Test Head No. 5—Glycerin Negative Control.* Glycerin Negative Control is a 70% w/v sterile glycerin solution identical to the glycerin solution that serves as a vehicle for the skin test antigens.

f. *Test Head No. 6—Candida Antigen.* Candida Antigen is a sterile glycerinated solution containing culture filtrate of *Candida albicans* inactivated with phenol. Residual phenol does not exceed 0.5%. Each ml of Candida Antigen in 70% w/v glycerin is biologically equivalent to 2,000 Merieux Candida Units.

g. *Test Head No. 7—Trichophyton Antigen.* Trichophyton Antigen is a sterile glycerinated solution containing culture filtrate of *Trichophyton mentagrophytes* inactivated by the addition of phenol. Residual phenol does not exceed 0.5%. Each ml of Trichophyton Antigen in 70% w/v glycerin is biologically equivalent to 150 Merieux Trichophyton Units.

h. *Test Head No. 8—Proteus Antigen.* Proteus Antigen is a sterile glycerinated solution containing culture filtrate of *Proteus mirabilis* inactivated by the addition of phenol. Residual phenol does not exceed 0.5%. Each ml of Proteus Antigen in 70% w/v glycerin is biologically equivalent to 150 Merieux Proteus Units.

2. Marker

3. Millimeter Ruler

PRECAUTIONS

1. Do not apply at sites involving acneiform, infected, or inflamed skin. Although severe systemic reactions are rare to diphtheria and tetanus antigens, persons known to have a history of systemic reactions should be tested with MULTITEST CMI only after the test heads containing these antigens have been removed.

2. Epinephrine should be available in case of severe reactions.

3. Discard the MULTITEST CMI applicator after use. DO NOT REUSE.

4. The sterility of MULTITEST CMI is guaranteed only when the seals on the individual test heads are intact. Do not attempt to resterilize the applicator as this may result in transmission of hepatitis or other infections.

5. If periodic testing is done more frequently than every 2 months, then the test sites should be rotated so that retesting is

not conducted at the same site sooner than 2 months.

6. Reactivity to delayed hypersensitivity skin test antigens may decrease or disappear temporarily as a result of febrile illness, measles and other viral infections, or live virus vaccination including measles, mumps, rubella, and poliomyelitis vaccines.

7. Individuals may acquire skin testing sensitivity resulting from either immunization or infection.

8. Patients should be informed of the types of test site reactions that may be expected.

9. It is possible to observe loss of reactivity in patients undergoing treatment with drugs or procedures that suppress immunity such as: cortiocosteroids, chemotherapeutic agents, antilymphocyte globulin, and irradiation.

10. The effect of repeated skin testing on specific antibody levels is not yet known; consequently those doing in vitro testing must be cognizant of the fact that repeated skin testing may alter antibody levels.

11. Animal reproduction studies have not been conducted with MULTITEST CMI. It is also not known whether MULTITEST CMI can cause fetal harm when administered to a pregnant woman, or whether it affects reproduction capacity. MULTITEST CMI should be given to pregnant woman only if clearly needed. Pregnancy may result in a decreased level of sensitivity to the test antigens.

12. The safety and effectiveness of MULTITEST CMI in children below the age of 17 have not been established.

13. Vesiculation, ulceration, or necrosis may occur in highly sensitive subjects at the test site. Pain or pruritus at the test site may be relieved by topical glucocorticoids or ice pack.

14. Systemic reactions may occur in those persons sensitive to allergenic media components.

PROCEDURE

1. Remove MULTITEST CMI from refrigeration approximately 1 hour before use.

2. Select only test sites that permit sufficient surface area and subcutaneous tissue to allow adequate penetration of all points on all eight test heads. Preferred sites are the volar surfaces of the arms and the back. Skin of the posterior thighs may be used if necessary. If several tests are planned, alternating forearms is desirable. Avoid hairy areas when possible because interpretation of reactions will be more difficult.

3. Cleanse test site with alcohol and allow to dry completely before testing. Ether or acetone may also be used.

4. Tear off the foil strip covering the test heads.

5. Tap the device on a hard surface, foil side up, to release antigen from top of cap.

6. Remove the protective plastic cap on each preloaded test head by twisting cap clockwise and counterclockwise. Carefully lift cap away from points.

7. Point "T-bar" end of MULTITEST CMI toward a constant reference point such as the elbow or head of the subject being tested to eliminate later identification problems with antigens or the control. The antigens and control are numbered clockwise, 1 through 8, beginning top right on the round plastic platform supporting each test head.

8. Keep the skin at test site taut.

9. Press loaded unit into the skin with sufficient pressure to puncture the skin and allow adequate penetration of all points. Maintain firm contact for at least 5 seconds. During application the device should be "rocked" back and forth and side to side **without removing any of the test heads from the skin sites.** Bleeding rarely occurs with proper pressure.

10. If adequate pressure is applied, it will be possible to observe:

a. The puncture marks of the nine tines on each of the eight test heads.

b. An imprint of the circular platform surrounding each test head.

c. Residual antigen and glycerin at each of the eight sites.

If any of the above 3 criteria are not fully followed, the test results may not be reliable.

11. Identify the area of test sites by drawing one line above test sites No. 8 and No. 1, and another below test sites No. 5 and No. 4. The lines should be drawn about one-quarter inch from the puncture patterns and made with an indelible marker so that they will remain clearly visible on the skin for at least 48 hours.

12. Allow residual antigens and glycerin to remain on the skin surface for at least three minutes, then gently dab with a gauze pad so as not to cross-contaminate test sites with antigen.

13. Discard MULTITEST CMI applicator after use.

14. Reading should be done in good light. Read the test sites at both 24 and 48 hours, if possible. The largest reaction recorded from the two readings at each site should be used. If two readings are not possible, a single 48-hour reading is recommended. The time for maximal reactivity to the various antigens may vary in different people. This may depend on the presence of antibodies.

REPORTING

If the patient is anergic, report: Subject failed to develop a delayed skin test. If the patient responded to antigen, report: Subject responded to at least one of the antigens tested and therefore is *NOT* anergic.

INTERPRETATION OF RESULTS

Induration of 2 mm or greater from any of the seven delayed hypersensitivity skin test antigens is considered a positive reaction providing there is no induration at the negative control site. Fewer than 2% of healthy volunteers tested during clinical studies exhibited detectable induration from the glycerin negative control solution. Should induration occur at the negative control site, then indurated reactions from individual antigens must exceed the size of induration from the negative control solution by 2 mm or greater to be considered positive. Erythema without induration is of no significance. The size of the induration reactions with MULTITEST CMI may be smaller than those obtained with other intradermal procedures. Occasionally, a small and diffused reaction (2 to 3 mm) may be present at one time of testing and not at another. The disappearance or recurrence of such a reaction is probably not significant, providing positive reaction sizes to other antigens remaining relatively constant. However, the disappearance or substantial reduction in size of a larger, well-defined reaction may be significant, even though the total score is not appreciably affected.

REFERENCE

1. Package insert, MULTITEST CMI, Merieux Institute, Inc., Miami, FL, October, 1982.

IN VITRO CYTOLYTIC ASSAYS

In vitro cytolytic assays are performed to evaluate the functional activity of cytotoxic T lymphocytes (Tcx) or natural killer (NK) cells, and are based on the ability of the lymphocytes to lyse appropriate target cells (e.g. tumor cells and virus-infected cells).

Tcx are generated after sensitization of the immune system to a specific cell bound antigen[16] and bind directly to target cells containing that antigen (see Chap. 1). The bound Tcx are stimulated to release cytolytic lymphokines, which produce pores in the membranes of the target cells, causing changes in permeability and ultimately, cell lysis.[4,8] Cytolysis is conducted in an HLA-restricted fashion: CD8(+) Tcx may only bind to target cells containing self Class I antigens, while the less common CD4(+) Tcx bind only to target cells with self Class II antigens.[1,12]

The cytolytic function described is measured in vitro by the cell-mediated lympholysis (CML) assay,[6,9,10,14,17,18] and is most frequently performed in microtiter plates. This assay is a two-step procedure, as follows: in the first step, lymphocytes are usually sensitized in vitro to a particular antigen by incubation of peripheral blood mononuclear cells with virus-infected syngeneic cells, or with allogeneic cells in a mixed lymphocyte culture for 4 to 5 days (see Chap. 13); alternately, fresh lymphocytes from a patient may be used if determination of prior in vivo sensitization is desired. Sensitization of the cells is followed by incubation for 4 hours with target cells containing HLA antigens (usually Class I) identical to the original stimulating cells. PHA-stimulated blasts, virus-infected cell lines, or tumor cell lines are usually used as targets, because they possess the greatest sensitivity to cytolysis.[6,17] Assays are routinely performed by setting up triplicate cultures of various effector (Tcx): target cell ratios. Cytolytic activity of the Tcx is most commonly determined by labeling the target cells with radiolabeled sodium chromate (^{51}Cr) prior to use in the assay, and measuring the amount of ^{51}Cr released by killed target cells into the culture supernatant. The results are expressed as % cytotoxicity, calculated as follows:[6,9]

$$\% \text{ cytotoxicity} = \frac{\text{experimental cpm } - \text{ spontaneous cpm}}{\text{maximum cpm } - \text{ spontaneous cpm}} \times 100, \text{ where}$$

cpm = mean counts per minute of triplicate cultures, determined by a gamma counter;

experimental cpm = cpm from cultures of test cells plus target cells;

spontaneous cpm = cpm from cultures of target cells alone;

maximum cpm = cpm from cultures of target cells lysed with Triton detergent.

The results can also be expressed in terms of the lytic unit, equal to the number of effector cells required to lyse a defined % of target cells and determined graphically from the lytic responses at various effector:target ratios.[6,9]

Cytolysis mediated by NK cells is similar to that effected by Tcx;[5] however, previous antigen sensitization is not required, and killing is not HLA-restricted (see also Chap. 1). Cytotoxicity may, therefore, be determined by incubation of fresh peripheral blood mononuclear cells with target cells susceptible to NK lysis (e.g. the erythroleukemia line, K562, and the acute T cell leukemia line, MOLT-4).[11,20]

In the most commonly performed in vitro assay of NK cell activity, mononuclear cells are incubated with ^{51}Cr-labeled target cells in microtiter plates for 4 hours, and ^{51}Cr release is measured as described above for the CML.[11,13] Prior to assay, cell populations may be enriched for NK cells by using discontinuous Percoll density gradient centrifugation;[11,20] collection of plastic or nylon wool nonadherent cells, or E rosette positive cells may also be performed as part of a purification protocol for NK cells,[19,20] or selection may be accomplished on the basis of NK surface markers.[15,19,20] NK activity is enhanced by prior incubation with interleukin-2 or α, β, or γ interferon.[7,11,19] Another manifestation of NK cytotoxicity, known as killer cell activity, or ADCC (antibody-dependent cellular cytotoxicity),

can be assayed in vitro by incubation of NK cells with target cells coated with specific antibody.[11]

NK cytotoxicity may also be examined by the single cell cytotoxic assay, in which the frequency of lytic conjugates is determined microscopically after incubation of NK cells and target cells in agarose.[2,3]

REFERENCES

1. Bach, F.H., and Sachs, D.H.: N. Engl. J. Med., *317*:489, 1987.
2. Bonavida, B., Bradley, T.P., and Grimm, E.A.: Immunol. Today, *4*:196, 1983.
*3. Bonavida, B., Bradley, T.P., and Grimm, E.A.: Methods Enzymol., *93*:270, 1983.
4. Bonavida, B., Fan, J., and Hiserodt, J.C.: Immunol. Today, *5*:138, 1982.
*5. Bonavida, B., and Wright, S.C.: J. Clin. Immunol., *6*:1, 1986.
6. Carpenter, C.B.: In *Manual of Clinical Laboratory Immunology*. 3rd ed. Edited by N.R. Rose, H. Friedman, and J.L. Fahey. Washington, D.C., American Society for Microbiology, 1986.
7. Coon, J.S., Landay, A.L., and Weinstein, R.S.: Lab. Invest., *57*:453, 1987.
8. DiNome, M.A., and Ding-E. Young, J.: Hosp. Pract., May 30, 1987, p. 59.
9. Dubey, D.P., Yunis, I., and Yunis, E.J.: In *Manual of Clinical Laboratory Immunology*. 3rd ed. Edited by N.R. Rose, H. Friedman, and J.L. Fahey. Washington, D.C., American Society for Microbiology, 1986.
10. Hayry, P., and Defendi, V.: Science, *168*:133, 1970.
11. Herberman, R.B.: In *Manual of Clinical Laboratory Immunology*. 3rd ed. Edited by N.R. Rose, H. Friedman, and J.L. Fahey. Washington, D.C., American Society for Microbiology, 1986.
12. Lanier, L.L., and Phillips, J.H.: Immunol. Today, *5*:132, 1986.
13. Pross, H.F., Callewaert, D., and Rubin, P.: In *Immunobiology of Natural Killer Cells*, Vol. 1. Edited by E.

Lotzova and R.B. Herberman. Boca Raton, CRC Press, Inc., 1986.

14. Romano, P.J.: In *Manual of Clinical Laboratory Immunology*. 3rd ed. Edited by N.R. Rose, H. Friedman, and J.L. Fahey. Washington, D.C., American Society for Microbiology, 1986.

15. Ryan, D.H., Fallon, M.A., and Horan, P.K.: Clin. Chim. Acta., *171*:125, 1988.

16. Sell, S.: *Immunology Immunopathology and Immunity*. 4th ed. New York, Elsevier Science Publishing Co., Inc., 1987.

17. Simpson, E., and Chandler, P.: In *Handbook of Experimental Immunology*. Vol. 2, 4th ed. Edited by D.M. Weir. Oxford, Blackwell Scientific Publications, 1986.

18. Solliday, S., and Bach, F.H.: Science, *170*:1406, 1970.

19. Trinchieri, G., and Perussia, B.: Lab. Invest., *50*:489, 1984.

20. Wigzell, H., and Ramstedt, U.: In *Handbook of Experimental Immunology*. Vol. 2, 4th ed. Edited by D.M. Weir. Oxford, Blackwell Scientific Publications, 1986.

Natural Killer Cell Assay[1,2]

PRINCIPLE

Natural killer cell cytotoxic activity in peripheral blood is assessed by its action upon K562 target cells. The target cells are tagged with sodium chromate (Cr^{51}). As the natural killer cells destroy target cells, Cr^{51} is released into the supernatant. The amount of Cr^{51} released is quantified and reflects natural killer cell activity.

EQUIPMENT AND MATERIALS

1. RPMI 1640 with L-Glutamine (Flow Laboratories)

2. K-562 cell line grown in vitro, tumor cell line derived from patient with chronic myelogenous leukemia in blast crisis

3. Phosphate buffered ringer's solution (PBR)

4. Fetal calf serum (Gibco Laboratories)

5. Sodium Chromate (Cr^{51}) (Amersham Corp.), 50 to 400 mCi/mg

6. Microtiter plates, U bottom, Linbro, (Flow Laboratories)

7. Scintillation fluid: BetaFluor (National Diagnostics)

8. Test tubes, 13 × 100 mm

9. Pipettes

10. Pipettors and tips

11. 37° C shaking waterbath

12. Centrifuge

13. Laminar flow hood

14. CO_2 incubator with 5% CO_2

15. Titertek supernatant harvester (Flow Laboratories)

16. Glass fiber strips (Cambridge Technology)

17. Gamma counter

18. 10% Triton X-100 (Packard)

SPECIMEN COLLECTION

Specimen requirement is generally 5 to 10 ml of heparinized blood. Minimum volume depends on patient's lymphocyte count. Blood must be kept at room temperature and used within 4 hours of collection.

PROCEDURE

NOTE: Preparation and plating of effector and target cells should be performed under a sterile biohazard hood.

1. Prepare mononuclear cell suspension as described under *Ficoll Hypaque Separation of Mononuclear Cells from Peripheral Blood.* This is the effector cell population.

2. Resuspend cells from step 1 in RPMI to a concentration of 8 × 10⁶ cells/ml.

3. Labeling target cells

a. Place K562 cells in test tube and spin at 250 × g for 5 minutes.

b. Resuspend cells in 0.4 ml phosphate buffered ringer's solution (PBR) with 10% FCS and count cells. Adjust cells to a concentration of 20 × 10⁶ cells/ml in a final volume of 0.4 PBR with FCS.

c. Add 200 μl of CR^{51} if 20 × 10⁶ cells are used; adjust appropriately if not enough cells are available.

d. Incubate for 40 minutes in a 37° C shaking waterbath (100/200 oscillations/min.)

e. Centrifuge at 250 × g and wash three times in PBR with 10% FCS at 4° C.

f. Resuspend cells in RPMI with 40% FCS to a concentration of 2 × 10⁵ cells/ml.

4. Target cells are mixed with effector cells with resultant ratios of 80:1, 40:1, and 20:1. Plate labeled target cells and effector cells in triplicate using linbro U bottom microtiter plates as follows:

	80:1	40:1	20:1
RPMI	0.5 ml	.10 ml	.125 ml
Effector cells	.10 ml	.05 ml	.025 ml
Target cells	.05 ml	.05 ml	.050 ml

Autologous control—unlabeled target cells added in place of effector cells giving baseline release.

100% release Cr^{51} control—0.5 ml RPMI + 0.1 ml RPMI with 10% Triton X-100 + 0.05 ml target cells

5. Centrifuge microtiter plates for 5 minutes at 500 rpm.
6. Place in CO_2 incubator at 37° C for 4 hours.
7. Centrifuge microtiter plates for 5 minutes at 1500 rpm.

8. Harvest supernatant with titertek supernatant harvester.
9. Place in scintillation vial with scintillation fluid.
10. Count on gamma counter for 10 minutes per vial.

REPORTING

Calculate and report standard deviation, standard error from the mean, and the cytotoxic index (C.I.)

$$\text{C.I.} = \frac{(\text{mean CPM of test}) - (\text{mean CPM autologous control})}{(\text{mean CPM 100\% release}) - (\text{mean CPM autologous control})} \times 100$$

REFERENCES

1. Herberman, R.B.: In *Manual of Clinical Laboratory Immunology*. 3rd ed. Edited by N.R. Rose, H. Friedman, and J.L. Fahey. Washington, D.C., American Society of Microbiology, 1986.

2. In house procedure, Division of Clinical Pathology, SUNY Health Science Center at Syracuse, Syracuse, NY.

Chapter 5

IMMUNOGLOBULINS

QUANTITATION OF IMMUNOGLOBULINS

The basic biologic and chemical properties of the five immunoglobulin classes arediscussed in Chapter 1. Normative values of the serum immunoglobulins have been reported by numerous investigators,[1,3,5,20,23,34,42] and have been shown to vary with age,[5,7,45] as illustrated in the table of normal immunoglobulins used in our laboratory (Fig. 5–6). These values are also affected by the sex and race of the individuals tested, and by a variety of environmental factors, as reviewed by Maddison.[34] Serum levels of IgM, for example, appear to be particularly influenced by sex, being higher in females than in males.[6,40] In addition, IgG, IgA, and IgM levels are reportedly higher in individuals with pigmented skins than in Caucasians.[6,24,31]

Quantitation of serum immunoglobulins is indicated in a variety of disease states in which alterations in immunoglobulin levels are evident. Immunoglobulin concentrations significantly lower than normal are found in a number of congenital or acquired humoral immunodeficiency syndromes[4] or may occur secondary to other disease processes.[9] All immunoglobulin classes may be affected. The frequency of *agammaglobuline-*

mia is low, estimated at 1:50,000.[4] Alternatively, individuals may be selectively deficient in one immunoglobulin class; of these disorders, selective IgA deficiency is the most common, with incidence in healthy blood donors reportedly ranging from 1 in 3000 to 1 in 328.[4]

Hypergammaglobulinemia, or an increase in serum immunoglobulin levels, is associated with a variety of disease states, may involve one or more of the immunoglobulin classes, and may be either polyclonal or monoclonal in nature. A polyclonal increase in immunoglobulins results from the stimulation of several different immunoglobulin-producing cells, and is associated with certain immunodeficiency diseases, infections, liver diseases, pulmonary disorders, autoimmune disorders, and a number of miscellaneous conditions.[29,41] Hypergammaglobulinemia due to the production of a monoclonal immunoglobulin is believed to result from the expansion of a single immunoglobulin-producing lymphoid cell into a clone of cells producing identical immunoglobulin molecules. Disease states associated with monoclonal immunoglobulins are discussed under *Monoclonal Gammopathies,* and include multiple myeloma, Waldenströms's macroglobulinemia, chronic lymphocytic leukemia and other leukemias, lymphomas, "benign" monoclonal gammopathy, chronic liver diseases, and autoimmune disorders.[41] Frequently, patients with high concentrations of monoclonal immunoglobulins resulting from a lymphoid malignancy have decreased levels of normal immunoglobulins, and may thus actually be immunodeficient.[41] Quantitation of immunoglobulins is helpful in monitoring the concentration of the monoclonal immunoglobulin and the extent to which normal immunoglobulin production is suppressed during the course of disease. The detection of monoclonal immunoglobulins in the laboratory is discussed under *Characterization of Paraproteins.*

Most commonly, levels of IgG, IgA, and IgM are quantitated. Quantitation of IgD or IgE may be indicated in extremely rare cases in which IgD or IgE myelomas are suspected. The quantitation of IgE may also be used in the evaluation of allergic conditions, and is discussed in Chapter 10.

In addition to quantitating immunoglobulin classes, concentrations of immunoglobulin subclasses may also be determined. Proportions of the IgG subclasses relative to total IgG are: IgG1 (60 to 70%), IgG2 (14 to 20%), IgG3 (4 to 8%), and IgG4 (2 to 6%).[44] Values of the IgG subclass concentrations in normal populations of various age groups have been reported, but results of different clinical studies are difficult to compare because of differences in the methods used for quantitation and the genetic backgrounds of the populations studied.[38]

Studies on the distribution of the IgA subclasses indicate that IgA1 constitutes 65 to 95% of the total serum IgA, while IgA2 comprises 16 to 20%, depending on the methodology used.[36] In the external secretions, IgA1 is also the dominant subclass, but the percentage of IgA2 appears to be higher than that in serum.[36]

The role of the immunoglobulin subclasses in disease has been the focus of several recent studies and has been more extensively investigated for the IgG subclasses. Selective IgG subclass deficiencies are un-

common. Deficiencies involving more than one subclass are more frequent, and have been associated with a number of disorders, particularly with the presence of recurrent acute or chronic respiratory tract infections.[19,38] Numerous studies[43] have shown that different IgG subclasses may be preferentially produced in specific antibody responses, depending on the inducing antigen. Because of the differences in molecular structure and biologic function of the various subclasses, the distribution pattern of IgG subclasses in the antibody produced may play a profound role in host defense as well as in the pathogenesis of certain conditions, such as autoimmune phenomena.[43]

Quantitation of immunoglobulins in body fluids other than serum may also be indicated. Measurement of IgG in the cerebral spinal fluid (CSF) may be used to evaluate the permeability of the blood-CSF barrier or to detect increased immunoglobulin synthesis within the central nervous system (CNS). In normal individuals, the majority of CSF IgG is derived from diffusion of plasma across the blood-CSF barrier, with a smaller proportion synthesized by plasma cells of the CNS.[27] CSF concentrations, however, are much lower than those found in serum and are related to the diffusion coefficient of the individual immunoglobulin.[17,18] Various neurologic conditions,[13,14,21,22,28,30,32,33,48] most notably multiple sclerosis, neurosyphilis, subacute sclerosing panencephalitis (SSPE), and meningoencephalitis, may cause increased CSF immunoglobulin levels as a result of local synthesis[15] or increased diffusion from plasma. The latter may occur with increased serum levels, as in multiple myeloma[47] or with a breakdown in the blood-brain barrier.[18] To distinguish increased synthesis within the CNS from increases due to leakage of plasma proteins across the blood-CSF barrier, the CSF IgG may be expressed as a percentage of the CSF total protein, or as a ratio of CSF IgG:CSF albumin.[26,27] These ratios are thought to reflect the integrity of the blood-brain barrier because albumin is not produced within the CNS.[26,27] This information is commonly used in conjunction with detection of oligoclonal bands by high-resolution agarose gel electrophoresis to evaluate patients with multiple sclerosis and other neurologic disorders.[8]

Quantitation of immunoglobulins in other body fluids is less commonly performed but includes quantitation of salivary IgA in the evaluation of IgA deficiency, quantitation of urinary IgG in patients with nephrotic syndrome to distinguish between selective and nonselective proteinuria, determination of immunoglobulin concentrations in the synovial fluid of patients with collagen vascular diseases, and quantitation of immunoglobulins in tissue culture supernatants of pokeweed mitogen-stimulated lymphocytes in the evaluation of hypogammaglobulinemia.[8]

The most frequently used methods of quantitating immunoglobulins are rate nephelometry and radial immunodiffusion (RID); other techniques, such as solid-phase ELISA, solid-phase fluorescence immunoassays, and turbidimetric methods using fast analyzers are also available.[8] In nephelometry, patient specimens containing immunoglobulin are added to a constant amount of antibody directed against a specific immunoglobulin class; the extent of immune complex formation will increase as the concentration of immunoglobulin in the patient specimen increases, provided that the antibody in solution is present in excess. The light scattered by the particles in solution is measured at a specific angle to the incident light beam within the nephelometer, and will increase as the number of immune complexes increases. In endpoint nephelometry, the antigen-antibody reaction is allowed to reach completion. In rate nephelometry, the rate of light scatter increase is measured seconds after the reagents are mixed; the peak rate of scatter increases with increasing antigen concentration, as long as the antibody is present in excess. The principal advantage of rate

nephelometry is that interference by background scatter (caused by lipids, for example), which can greatly affect the endpoint method, is minimized.[37]

For RID, two techniques have been devised. In the method developed by Mancini et al.,[35] antibody in the agarose is present in excess, allowing the antigen-antibody reaction to reach equivalence. At the reaction endpoint, the area of the precipitin ring, hence the ring diameter squared, is directly proportional to the antigen concentration. In the Fahey-McKelvey, or timed diffusion method,[12] antibody in the gel matrix is not present in excess. Ring diameters are measured before equivalence, and the antigen concentration is approximately proportional to the rate of diffusion in the gel. Several authors have compared the two techniques and have found that although the Fahey-McKelvey technique is more rapid, the Mancini method is preferable for linearity of standards, reproducibility, accuracy, and lack of dependence on certain variables, e.g. temperature.[2,16,25]

Studies in our laboratory and reports in the literature comparing laser nephelometry and RID generally show good correlation between the techniques.[10,11,37,46] The major advantages of the RID method are its relative ease of performance and low cost of capital equipment.[8,37] Situations of marked antigen excess are easily recognized and may be dealt with by diluting the sample serum, while extremely low concentrations of antigen can be detected using low level RID plates. Disadvantages of the method include the time required to obtain results, strong dependence on antigen size, and possible production of double or triple rings due to paraproteins in excessively high concentrations, rheumatoid factor activity, or circulating immune complexes.[8,37,39]

With rate nephelometry, automation controls the operator functions, reducing the chances of operator error and making fast procurement of results possible.[37] Disadvantages of rate nephelometry include the initial and maintenance costs of the instrumentation, and high susceptibility to fluctuations in conditions such as temperature, buffer ionic strength, and mixing of reagents.[37] Consideration of these features is essential in determining which technique is most suitable for each individual laboratory.

REFERENCES

1. Becker, V.W. et al.: Z. Klin. Chem. Klin. Biochem., 6:113, 1968.

2. Berne, B.H.: Clin. Chem., 20:61, 1974.

3. Bradley, J.: J. Med. Genet., 11:80, 1974.

4. Buckley, R.H.: Clin. Immunol. Immunopathol., 40:13, 1986.

5. Buckley, R.H.: In Human Health and Disease. Edited by P.L. Altman and D.D. Katz. Federation of American Societies for Experimental Biology, Bethesda, 1977.

6. Cassidy, J.T., Nordby, G.L., and Dodge, H.J.: J. Chron. Dis., 27:507, 1974.

7. Cejka, J., Mood, D.W., and Kim, C.S.: Clin. Chem., 20:656, 1974.

8. Check, I.J., and Piper, M.: In Manual of Clinical Laboratory Immunology. 3rd ed. Edited by N.R. Rose, H. Friedman, and J.L. Fahey. Washington, D.C., American Society for Microbiology, 1986.

9. Church, J.A., and Schlegel, R.J.: In Immunology III. Edited by J.A. Bellanti. Philadelphia, W.B. Saunders Co., 1985.

10. Cloppet, H. et al.: Clin. Chem., 28:180, 1982.

11. Deaton, C.D. et al.: Clin. Chem., 22:1465, 1976.

12. Fahey, J.L., and McKelvey, E.M.: J. Immunol., 94:84, 1965.

13. Fischer-Williams, M.: Practitioner, 217:108, 1976.

14. Fischer-Williams, M. and Roberts, R.: Arch. Neurol., 25:526, 1971.

15. Glasser, L., Payne, C., and Corrigan, J.J.: Neurology, 27:448, 1977.

16. Grant, G.H.: J. Clin. Pathol., 24:89, 1971.

17. Grant, G.H., and Butt, W.R.: Adv. Clin. Chem., 13:383, 1970.

18. Green, N.M.: Adv. Immunol., 11:1, 1969.

19. Hanson, L.A., Soderstrom, T., and Oxelius, V.A. (eds): Monogr. Allergy, volume 20, 1986.

20. Hobbs, J.R.: Adv. Clin. Chem., 14:219, 1971.

21. Kabat, E.A. et al.: Am. J. Med. Sci., 219:55, 1950.

22. Kabat, E.A., Moore, D.H., and Landu, H.: J. Clin. Invest., 21:571, 1942.

23. Kalff, M.W.: Clin. Chim. Acta, 28:277, 1970.

24. Karayalchin, G., Rosher, F., and Sawitsky, A.: N.Y. State J. Med., 73:751, 1973.

25. Keil, L.B., DeBari, V.A., and Needle, M.A.: Clin. Biochem., 9:222, 1976.

26. Killingsworth, L.M.: Clin. Chem., 28:1093, 1982.

27. Kjeldsberg, C.R., and Krieg, A.F.: In Clinical Diagnosis and Management by Laboratory Methods. 17th ed. Edited by J.B. Henry. Philadelphia, W.B. Saunders Co., 1984.

28. Kolar, O.J.: Lancet, 1:864, 1977.

29. Lane, H.C., and Fauci, A.S.: Ann. Rev. Immunol., 3:477, 1985.

30. Laterre, E.C. et al.: Neurology, 20:982, 1970.

31. Lichtman, M.A., Vaughan, J.H., and Hames, C.G.: Arthritis Rheum., 10:204, 1967.

32. Link, H., and Moller, R.: Arch. Neurol., 25:326, 1971.

33. Link, H. et al.: Acta Neurol. Scand. (Suppl), 63:173, 1977.

34. Maddison, S.E., and Reimer, C.B.: Clin. Chem., 22:594, 1976.

35. Mancini, G., Carbonara, A.O., and Hereman, J.F.: Immunochemistry, 2:235, 1965.

36. Mestecky, J., and Russell, M.W.: Monogr. Allergy, 19:277, 1986.

*37. Normansell, D.E.: CRC Crit. Rev. Clin. Lab. Sci., 17:103, 1982.

38. Ochs, H.D., and Wedgwood, R.J.: Ann. Rev. Med., 38:325, 1987.

39. Product Insert—Behring Diagnostics, NOR-Partigen IgG, IgA, IgM (HC) Kits, 1984.

40. Rhodes, K. et al.: Br. Med. J., 3:439, 1969.

*41. Ricardo, M.J., and Tomar, R.H.: In Clinical Diagnosis by Laboratory Methods. 17th ed. Edited by J.B. Henry. Philadelphia, W.B. Saunders Co., 1984.

42. Ritzmann, S.E., and Daniels, J.C. (Eds): Serum Protein Abnormalities—Diagnostic and Clinical Aspects. Boston, Little, Brown & Co., 1975.

43. Shakib, F. (ed): Monogr. Allergy, volume 19, 1986.

44. Steinberg, A.G. et al.: J. Immunol., 110:1642, 1973.

45. Stoop, J.W. et al.: Clin. Exp. Immunol., 4:101, 1969.

46. Virella, G., and Fudenberg, H.H.: Clin. Chem., 23:1925, 1977.

47. Weiss, A.H. et al.: J. Lab. Clin. Med., 66:280, 1965.

48. Yahr, M.D., Goldensohn, S.S., and Kabat, E.A.: Ann. N.Y. Acad. Sci., 58:613, 1954.

Radial Immunodiffusion: Mancini Technique

PRINCIPLE. Serum is applied to a circular well cut in a gel containing antibody to a serum protein. After appropriate incubation, the square of the diameter of the precipitin ring formed can be plotted against the known protein concentration of a series of standards.

EQUIPMENT AND MATERIALS

1. RID plates (Mancini technique; Behring Diagnostics): Contain a thin layer of 2% agarose containing a monospecific antibody. Store at 2 to 8° C. Do not freeze. May be used until expiration date noted on each plate.

2. Micropipettes (Oxford) for delivering 5 μl and 20 μl.

3. Standard Sets I, II, and IV (Behring): Each set contains five vials, each containing 0.5 ml of a stabilized solution of human proteins. Refer to Table 5–1 to find standard set to be used for each determination. The standards contain 0.1% sodium azide as a preservative. Store at 2 to 8° C.

4. Protein Standard Plasma (PSP; Behring): A lyophilized human plasma. Store at 4 to 6° C. Reconstitute with 0.5 ml distilled water. Stable for 7 days at 4 to 6° C after reconstitution. Contains 1 mg/ml sodium azide. Expiration date is noted on the label.

5. Standard Human Serum (SSS; Behring): A stabilized, pooled normal human serum assayed for various proteins. Contains 1 mg/ml sodium azide. Store at 4 to 6° C. Expiration date is noted on the label.

6. C-reactive Protein Standard Serum (Behring): A stabilized preparation of human serum containing C-reactive protein. Store at 4 to 6° C. Do not freeze. Expiration date is noted on the label. Contains 1 mg/ml of sodium azide.

7. Control plasma (human; Behring): A lyophilized control plasma used to quality control quantitation of C_3 Activator. Store at 2 to 8° C. Expiration date is noted on the label. Reconstitute with the amount of distilled water noted on the label. After reconstitution, plasma is stable for 7 days at 2 to 8° C. Avoid extreme temperature changes.

8. Control Set I (Behring): Two vials each containing 0.5 ml of a stabilized solution of human proteins. Vial N is used for most tests and vial H is diluted and used for LC-IgG tests. Either control is suitable. Store at 2 to 8° C.

9. Viewer (Kallestad): With eyepiece calibrated to 0.1 mm.

10. Patient sample: Serum samples are required for all peripheral blood testing, as all normal values were obtained with the use of serum. Plasma, synovial fluid, pleural fluid, cerebral spinal fluid, etc., may be used

for testing; however, no normal values have been established.

11. Radial immunodiffusion worksheets (Behring).

PROCEDURE

The following general procedure may be used in conjunction with the accompanying table for all radial immunodiffusion assays performed in this laboratory:

1. Obtain an RID plate appropriate for the protein to be tested. Warm to room temperature.

2. If no standard curve has been established within the past month, the appropriate standards should be reconstituted with the amount of distilled water noted on the label, and diluted if required (Table 5–1). Standard curves are established with each new lot number of plates; subsequently, standard curves are run every 4 weeks and compared with the existing curve to ensure the quality of the curve. Aberrancies necessitate the use of the newer curve.

3. Control serum and patient serum samples should be diluted with saline solution if required (Table 5–1).

4. Fill out an RID worksheet for the assay, including the type of assay, the lot numbers of all standards, controls and plates used, and the names and accession numbers of patients.

5. An appropriate amount of each standard (or standard dilution), control (or dilution of control), and patient serum (or dilution thereof) (Table 5–1) is placed in designated wells.

6. Place on a flat surface at room temperature and allow to incubate for the amount of time designated in Table 5–1.

7. After incubation, ring diameters are read using the Kallestad viewer and the readings are squared and then recorded on the worksheet.

8. If standards have been prepared, they are plotted, diameter squared vs. concentration, on graph paper. For all assays using 5 μl of sample, the best straight lines on the graph must cross the y axis at 11 $\pm$ 2.5; for those using 20 μl, at 20 $\pm$ 3.5. Any standard curve not crossing within these ranges must be repeated.

9. Control readings are plotted on the graph, adjusted for dilution factor if any, and the results compared with the expected value established for that control with that assay (see Equipment and Materials #7 and #8). The control result must be $\pm$ 2 S.D. from the mean obtained upon repeated testing. Controls must be within range before the patient results can be reported. Record control and patient results.

10. Plot the results obtained from each patient sample on the graph to obtain the serum concentration.

Table 5-1. RID Protocol Sheet Clinical Immunology—Health Science Center

Protein	Serum Dilution	Volume Applied (μl)	Standards	Control	Incubation
Alpha$_1$ Antitrypsin	undil	5	Std. Set II	Control Set II	48 hours
Antithrombin III	undil	5	Std. Set IV	Control Set IV	48 hours
Ceruloplasmin	undil	5	Std. Set IV	Control Set IV	48 hours
C$_3$(β1A)	undil	5	Std. Set I	Control Set I	48 hours
C$_4$	undil	5	Std. Set I	Control Set I	48 hours
Factor B (C$_3$A)	1:3	20	PSP 1:1, 2, 4	Control Plasma 1:3	72 hours
C-reactive protein	undil	20	CRP 1:1, 2, 4	Pooled Positive Serum	48 hours
IgG	undil	5	Std. Set I	Control Set I	48 hours
IgA	undil	5	Std. Set I	Control Set I	48 hours
IgM	undil	5	Std. Set I	Control Set I	48 hours
LC-IgG, A, or M	undil	20	Std. Human Serum 1:1, 2, 4	Control Set I diluted appropriately	48 hours

NOTE: Values determined from diluted samples must be multiplied by the dilution factor to obtain the correct concentration.

REPORTING. Results are reported with appropriate units of measurement and normal values, as follows:

Protein	Normal Range
alpha$_1$ antitrypsin	116-384 mg/100 ml
antithrombin III	16-34 mg/100 ml
ceruloplasmin	18-51 mg/100 ml
C$_3$ (β1A)	54-112 mg/100 ml
C$_4$	15-49 mg/100 ml
Factor B (C$_3$A)	9-29 mg/100 ml
C-reactive protein	< 1.2 mg/100 ml
IgG (Adult)*	591-1965 mg/100 ml
IgA (Adult)*	77-400 mg/100 ml
IgM (Adult)*	50-311 mg/100 ml

*Pediatric normal ranges are on the IEP report sheet.

LIMITATIONS OF PROCEDURE. Normal ranges for all adult serum proteins were established in this laboratory or at the company providing the reagents.

Radial immunodiffusion measures the concentration of serum proteins without regard to their activity potential. Normally, the filtering mechanism of the kidneys depletes the serum of used components. However, in areas of the body where no efficient filtering mechanism exists, e.g. synovial fluids, cerebral spinal fluid, used as well as active components may be detected by RID.

C$_3$ and C$_4$ because of their relative instability and variations in the antigenicity of their breakdown products pose a problem when detected by radial immunodiffusion.[3,9,11,12] The C$_3$ (β1A) plates produced by Behring detect C$_{3c}$, an intermediate product produced by activation or deterioration of C$_3$.

Two methods have been devised for using the radial immunodiffusion technique: Fahey and McKelvey[4] devised the Fahey technique; Mancini, Carbonara, and Heremans,[10] the Mancini technique. Fahey employed the idea that the amount of antigen is approximately proportional to the rate of diffusion in a gel. The Mancini method allows the antigen-antibody reaction to reach equivalence, contending that the area of the precipitin ring, hence, the diameter squared, is directly proportional to the amount of antigen and inversely proportional to the antibody concentration. Several authors[2,5,8] have compared the two techniques and found that although the Fahey technique is more rapid, the Mancini technique is preferable for linearity of standards, reproducibility, accuracy and lack of dependence on certain variables, e.g. temperature.

Kalff[7] studied the reproducibility of Mancini radial immunodiffusion and found the coefficient of variation to be $\leq 8.5\%$. Hosty, et al.[6] compared commercially available kits from five companies and concluded Behring was the preferred vendor.

REFERENCES

1. Attwood, E.C.: Clin. Biochem., 8:279, 1975.
2. Berne, B.H.: Clin. Chem., 20:61, 1974.
3. Davis, N.C., West, C.D., and Ho, M.: Clin. Chem., 18:1485, 1972.
4. Fahey, J.L., McKelvey, E.M.: J. Immunol., 94:84, 1965.
5. Grant, G.H.: J. Clin. Pathol., 24:89, 1971.
6. Hosty, T., Hollenbeck, N., and Shane, S., Clin. Chem., 19:524, 1973.
7. Kalff, M.W.: Clin. Biochem., 3:91, 1970.
8. Keil, L.B., DeBari, V.A., and Needle, M.A.: Clin. Biochem., 9:22, 1976.
9. Kohler, P.F., and Muller-Eberhard, H.J.: J. Immunol., 99:1211, 1967.
10. Mancini, G., Carbonara, A.O., and Heremans, J.F.: Immunochem., 2:235, 1965.
11. Vladutiu, A.O., and Winiarski, B.M.: Clin. Chem., 22:267, 1976.
12. West, C.D. et al.: J. Immunol., 96:650, 1965.

MONOCLONAL GAMMOPATHIES

The monoclonal gammopathies, or para-proteinemias, are a group of disorders characterized by the presence of a monoclonal immunoglobulin protein in the serum or urine. This monoclonal protein, also referred to as a *paraprotein* or *M component,* is produced by a single homogeneous clone of immunoglobulin-producing cells undergoing excessive proliferation, and is often associated with a neoplastic process.

Normal B cells and plasma cells produce heavy and light chains in approximately equal numbers, assembling and secreting whole immunoglobulin molecules with only a small number of excess light chains, or incomplete subunits, elaborated, which are rapidly excreted in the urine (rate: 20 to 40 mg/24 hours). In most cases, cells hyper-proliferating in a monoclonal pattern continue to produce polypeptide chains virtually identical in composition and function,[17,25] to the normal immunoglobulin molecule; certain diseases, however, are characterized by increased production of variant proteins, e.g. heavy chains and light chains produced but not assembled, heavy chains or light chains produced exclusively, or only fragments of polypeptide chains elaborated.

Paraproteins are found in the serum and/or urine of patients with certain leukemias, notably chronic lymphocytic, hairy cell, and plasma cell leukemias, some lymphomas, including heavy chain diseases, amyloidosis, Waldenström's macroglobulinemia, a few assorted carcinomas, and with plasma cell dyscrasias such as multiple myeloma and light chain diseases. They are also observed in idiopathic cold agglutinin disease. (For discussion of paraproteins characteristic of idiopathic cold agglutinin disease, see *Cold Agglutinins.*) Additionally, over one-fourth of the M components identified occur in persons with various nonmalignant conditions,[2,25] including benign monoclonal gammopathy, also known as monoclonal gammopathy of undetermined significance (MGUS).[18]

Chronic lymphocytic leukemia (CLL)[4,5,10,24] is a lymphoproliferative disease characterized by accumulation in the lymphoid organs, bone marrow, and blood, of long-lived cells morphologically similar to small lymphocytes. CLL is the most commonly diagnosed leukemia in the Western countries, accounting for approximately 25% of all cases, with an overall incidence of 3 in 100,000. More males than females are affected (3:2), and the disease occurs predominantly in people over 60 years of age. Unlike acute leukemias, the rate of cell production is little, if at all, above normal in CLL, and increased cell concentrations probably reflect an elongated cellular life span. A significant number of cases are asymptomatic when diagnosed. Onset of symptoms is usually insidious with lymphadenopathy, weakness, fatigue, anorexia, low-grade fever, and weight loss. Frequently, hepatosplenomegaly, skin lesions, gastrointestinal infiltrate, and bone pain evolve. An absolute lymphocytosis with 80 to 90% small, normal-appearing lymphocytes is observed in blood smears. Ninety-five percent of CLL cases are of B cell lineage, and display surface immunoglobulin, usually IgM with or without IgG, receptors for mouse erythrocytes, the Fc receptor for IgG, complement receptors, Ia, and other B cell antigens, such as BA1, B1, B2, and B4.[7,22] Over 5% of CLL sera have a monoclonal protein, usually IgM, with or without associated hyperviscosity syndrome.[21]

Progressive infiltration of the bone marrow with CLL cells may result in neutropenia, thrombocytopenia, anemia, and hypogammaglobulinemia, with associated clinical manifestations, as the disease progresses. Death usually ensues as a result of bleeding or infection. The average life span for symptomatic CLL patients ranges from less than 2 years to over 7 years, and correlates with the stage of disease at diagnosis.[21]

Hairy cell leukemia is a rare disease characterized by the proliferation of morphologically distinct mononuclear cells with hairy-like cytoplasmic projections in the bone marrow, spleen, and blood.[5,12] Although the origin of hairy cell leukemia has been controversial, present evidence suggests that the neoplastic cells are typically mature B cells, displaying surface immunoglobulin, usually IgG, other B cell markers detected by monoclonal antibodies, and immunoglobulin gene rearrangements.[1,7,12] Rare cases of T cell variants of the disease have been associated with the retrovirus, HTLV-II.[16,27] Complications of hairy cell leukemia include anemia, granulocytopenia, monocytopenia, platelet dysfunction, immune defects, and susceptibility to infections. Paraproteins of the IgG or IgM class may be produced.[3,13] In a retrospective study, the median survival of patients with hairy cell leukemia was found to be 70 months;[14] as advances in diagnosis and therapy continue, the prognosis for these patients is expected to improve.[12]

Waldenström's macroglobulinemia[5,19,20,28] may be classified as either a malignant lymphoma or a plasma cell dyscrasia, and involves a generalized hyperproduction of cells of lymphoid or plasmacytoid morphology which are involved in IgM production. Macroglobulinemia occurs more commonly in persons over age 40, with the peak age between 60 and 70. Presymptomatic IgM paraproteins are sometimes noted ≤ 20 years prior to onset of clinical symptoms. Lymphadenopathy, splenomegaly, hepatomegaly, anemia, and an increased tendency for infection and/or bleeding are among symptoms shared with other immunoproliferative diseases. Macroglobulinemia, however, also produces clinical patterns associated with hyperviscosity syndrome:[21] visual disturbances, neurologic symptoms, impaired kidney function, congestive heart failure, and hemorrhage, a result of adherence of immunoglobulin molecules to platelets and/or complexing with clotting factors. Cryoglobulins are frequently present with associated symptoms. Bone pain and osteolytic lesions, hallmarks of other plasma cell dyscrasias, are rare. In the blood, only relative or slight lymphocytosis (plasmacytosis) usually accompanies marked rouleaux formation. Bone marrow is infiltrated with cells of morphology ranging from that of small lymphocytes to mature plasma cells. *Bence-Jones protein*, or free monoclonal light chains,[6] are detectable in urine from about 10% of patients. Waldenström's macroglobulinemia appears to be a variant of CLL, the differences arising from the greater degree of plasmacytoid maturation of the cell line.

Multiple myeloma[5,15,19,23] (plasma cell myeloma, myelomatosis) is a disease state resulting from a neoplastic proliferation in the bone marrow of plasma cells, manifesting in focal or widespread skeletal destruction. In most cases, a presymptomatic period, ranging ≤ 20 years and evidenced only by the presence of a persistent paraproteinemia, is followed, usually after age 40, by abrupt onset of clinical symptoms: skeletal pain, possibly associated with pathologic fracture, neurologic symptoms, and increased susceptibility to infections. Lymph nodes and spleen are only rarely enlarged. Roentgenograms often reveal "punched out" osteoporotic lesions, thought to develop as a result of myeloma cell proliferation and activation of osteoclasts, which destroy the bone.[19] Diffuse osteoporosis may be observed, causing generalized thinning of trabeculae, or only a single bone lesion, a solitary plasmacytoma, may be present. Skeletal destruction results in the release of bone salts into the vascular system, causing hypercalcemia with associated dehydration. In many patients, a few plasma cells are observed in the blood, and rouleaux formation is often seen, probably contributing to decreased life span of erythrocytes with associated clinical anemia. Bone marrow aspirates may range from less than 1% to over 90% plasmacytosis, depending on the site of aspiration.

An M component is observed in over 99% of patients with multiple myeloma.[19] In over half of the cases, the protein is IgG, about one-fifth are IgA, approximately 1% are IgD, and rarely, a patient with IgE myeloma is documented. About half of these M components are accompanied by the production of free light chains (*Bence Jones protein*),[6] which are apparently identical to the light chains of the immunoglobulin molecule. This free light chain is usually not seen in serum, as it is rapidly excreted in the urine. Bence Jones proteinuria is associated with the clinical development of decreased renal function. Commonly, coincident with increase in M component concentrations are corresponding decreases in normal immunoglobulin levels, probably a result of decreased synthesis because of macrophage suppression of polyclonal immunoglobulin production.[29]

Approximately one-fourth of patients with multiple myeloma have "light chain disease,"[5] with only free light chains produced by the proliferating plasma cell line. Immunoelectrophoresis of serum from these patients may reveal only hypogammaglobulinemia; urine samples demonstrate the paraprotein, which again is reflected in renal destruction.

Up to 15% of multiple myeloma patients develop amyloidosis,[11] which has been linked to deposition of light chains, or aminoterminal fragments of immunoglobulin, in various tissues of the body.

Each M protein possesses its own solubility, viscosity, thermostability, and reactivity with other proteins (e.g. cryoglobulins, clotting factors). Symptomatology varies accordingly.

The prognosis of multiple myeloma varies considerably with presenting symptoms.

Heavy chain diseases[5,8,19] have been described in which the M component is gamma, alpha, or mu polypeptide chains. The heavy chains secreted usually show structural abnormalities, with a deletion in the hinge or Fd regions.[5,19] Clinically, these diseases resemble lymphomas. *Franklin's disease*[5,9,19] is a relatively rare disorder resulting from the proliferation of plasmacytic or atypical lymphocytic cells producing only gamma chains. The paraproteins produced in the disease are primarily of the IgG1 subclass, and react with antibody to IgG, but not with anti-light chain reagents. Lymphadenopathy, splenomegaly, and hepatomegaly occur, with weakness, fever, weight loss, anemia, and increased susceptibility to infection. No skeletal destruction is evident. Proteinuria is usually present in variable amounts. Diagnosed patients survive 4 months to 5 years, usually succumbing to bacterial infection.

Seligmann's disease[5,19,26] is the most common of the heavy chain diseases. It is characterized by a hyperproduction of alpha chains, occurs somewhat more often than Franklin's disease, and usually involves a younger age group. In the vast majority of patients, the small bowel is affected. Malabsorption, diarrhea, and weight loss occur as a result of infiltration of the small intestines with lymphocytes and plasma cells; infiltration is progressive, usually leading to development of abdominal lymphoma. In a few cases, the respiratory tract rather than the gastrointestinal tract is affected. The bone marrow and other lymphatic organs are not involved. Alpha heavy chains are demonstrable in serum, urine, and saliva by immunoelectrophoresis, but usually not by protein electrophoresis, since the alpha chains tend to polymerize and appear as a smear, rather than a sharp peak.

Mu chain paraproteinemia[5,19] has been described in a few patients in association with clinical chronic lymphocytic leukemia. In most cases, kappa light chains have been demonstrated in the patient's urine; hence, a lack of assembly of the immunoglobulin molecule is implied.

REFERENCES

1. Al-Katib, A. et al.: Semin. Oncol., *13* (Suppl. 5):48, 1986.
2. Ameis, A., Ko, H.S., and Pruzanski, W.: Can. Med. Assoc. J., *114*:889, 1976.
3. Cawley, J.C. et al.: Br. J. Haematol., *43*:215, 1979.
4. Champlin, R., and Golde, D.W.: In *Harrison's Principles of Internal Medicine.* 11th ed. Edited by E. Braunwald et al. New York, McGraw-Hill Book Co., 1987.
*5. Davey, F.R., and Nelson, D.A.: In *Clinical Diagnosis by Laboratory Methods.* 17th ed. Edited by J.B. Henry. Philadelphia, W.B. Saunders Co., 1984.
6. Edelman, G.M., and Gally, J.A.: J. Exp. Med., *116*:207, 1962.
*7. Foon, K.A., Gale, R.P., and Todd, R.F.: Semin. Hematol., *23*:257, 1986.
8. Frangione, B., and Franklin, E.C.: Semin. Hematol., *10*:53, 1973.
9. Franklin, E.C. et al.: Am. J. Med., *37*:332, 1964.
10. Gale, R.P., and Foon, K.A.: Ann. Intern. Med., *103*:101, 1985.
11. Glenner, G.G., Terry, W.D., and Isersky, C.: Semin. Hematol., *10*:65, 1973.
12. Golde, D.W. et al.: Semin. Hematol., *23* (Suppl.1):3, 1986.
13. Golde, D.W., Saxon, A., and Stevens, R.H.: N. Engl. J. Med., *296*:92, 1977.
14. Golomb, H.M., Catovsky, D., and Golde, D.W.: Ann. Intern. Med., *99*:485, 1983.
15. Graziani, M.S., and Lippi, U.: Clin. Chem., *32*:2220, 1986.
16. Kalayanaraman, V.S. et al.: Science, *218*:571, 1982.
17. Kyle, R.A.: In *Manual of Clinical Laboratory Immunology.* 3rd ed. Edited by N.R. Rose, H. Friedman, and J.L. Fahey. Washington, D.C., American Society for Microbiology, 1986.
18. Kyle, R.A.: Am. J. Med., *64*:814, 1978.
*19. Longo, D.L., and Broder, S.: In *Harrison's Principles of Internal Medicine.* 11th ed. Edited by E. Braunwald, et al. New York, McGraw-Hill Book Co., 1987.
20. MacKenzie, M.R., and Fudenberg, H.H.: Blood, *39*:874, 1972.
21. McGrath, M.A., and Penny, R.: J. Clin. Invest., *58*:1155, 1976.
22. Minowada, J.: Lab. Med., *16*:305, 1985.
23. Pruzanski, W.: Can. Med. Assoc. J., *114*:896, 1976.
24. Rai, K.R., and Sawitsky, A.: In *Neoplastic Diseases of the Blood.* Edited by P.H. Wiernik, G.P. Canellos, R.A. Kyle, and C.A. Schiffer. New York, Churchill Livingstone, 1985.
*25. Ricardo, M.J., and Tomar, R.H.: In *Clinical Diagnosis by Laboratory Methods.* 17th ed. Edited by J.B. Henry, Philadelphia, W.B. Saunders Co., 1984.
26. Seligmann, M. et al.: Science, *162*:1396, 1968.
27. Wachsman, W., Golde, D.W., and Chen, I.S.Y.: Semin. Oncol., *11*:446, 1984.
28. Waldenström, J.: Acta Med. Scand., *117*:216, 1944.
29. Waldmann, T.A., and Broder, S.: Prog. Clin. Immunol., *3*:155, 1977.

CHARACTERIZATION OF PARAPROTEINS

Serum or urine specimens are commonly screened for the presence of an M-component by protein electrophoresis on a cellulose acetate membrane. The major fractions separated by serum protein electrophoresis (SPEP) are shown in Figure 5–1. Immunoglobulins are the major component of the gammaglobulin fraction, but also extend into the beta-gamma junction, and the beta and alpha regions.

In the normal individual, immunoglobulins are polyclonal, and therefore, heterogeneous in their antigen specificity, molecular structure, and electrophoretic mobility, appearing as a broad, diffuse band on SPEP. Monoclonal immunoglobulins comprise a homogeneous group of molecules derived from one clone of cells, and are therefore identical in molecular structure and antigen specificity. The monoclonal immunoglobulin has limited electrophoretic mobility, appearing as a narrow, discrete band or "spike," on SPEP. When such a band is observed, it is frequently indicative of a neoplastic process, such as multiple myeloma or Waldenström's macroglobulinemia, but may be present in a variety of non-malignant disorders (see *Monoclonal Gammopathies*). In some situations, including the presence of a small quantity of monoclonal immunoglobulin or Bence Jones proteinemia, SPEP on cellulose acetate may not be sensitive enough to detect a monoclonal band.[10] Electrophoresis on agarose appears

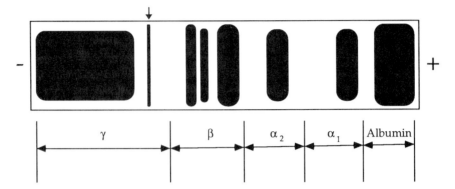

Fig. 5–1. Serum protein electrophoresis (SPEP) results in the formation of 5 major fractions:
1. Albumin
2. Alpha-1 globulins (alpha-1 antitrypsin, alpha-1 lipoprotein, and alpha-1 acid glycoprotein)
3. Alpha-2 globulins (alpha-2 macroglobulin, alpha-2 lipoprotein, haptoglobin, ceruloplasmin, and erythropoietin)
4. Beta globulins (beta lipoprotein, transferrin, C3, and hemopexin)
5. Gamma globulins (immunoglobulins and CRP)
Major proteins in each fraction are in parentheses. An arrow indicates the location of the specimen application slit.

to be a more sensitive procedure in detecting small monoclonal bands.[10]

If a monoclonal spike is observed on SPEP, or if a monoclonal gammopathy is suspected on the basis of the patient's immunoglobulin concentrations or clinical presentation, immunoelectrophoresis, or immunofixation electrophoresis should be performed in order to characterize the M-component in terms of immunoglobulin class and light chain type. Both procedures involve two major steps, whereby: (1) proteins within a clinical specimen (usually serum or urine) are first separated by electrophoresis in molten agar or agarose on a plastic or glass support, and (2) the separated proteins are analyzed by their reactivity with specific antisera to form a precipitate where the antigen and antibody meet in equivalent proportions. The procedures are routinely performed using the following antisera: anti-IgG (gamma), anti-IgA (alpha), anti-IgM (mu), antikappa, and antilambda. Uncomplexed proteins are removed by submersion of the agarose plate in saline. The plate is then stained and destained in order to facilitate visualization of the precipitin patterns.

In immunoelectrophoresis (IEP), the patient serum and a normal control human serum are applied in alternate wells lined up vertically on the agarose plate. Electrophoresis is performed, and specific antisera are placed in horizontal troughs cut into the agarose and located parallel to the line of electrophoretic migration. The separated protein components will react with the antisera in the troughs above and below, to produce arcs of precipitation. The precipitin arcs are analyzed in order to distinguish between monoclonal and polyclonal immunoglobulins.

Interpretation of the precipitin patterns requires experience and is sometimes difficult. Observation of the following characteristics are essential to accurate analysis of IEP results:[15]

1. *Shape* of the precipitin arc—The normal, polyclonal immunoglobulin produces a broad, elliptical shaped arc, whereas the monoclonal immunoglobulin, being homogeneous and of limited electrophoretic mobility, produces a more narrow, bowed or sharply peaked arc, shaped more like an arc of a circle.

2. *Thickness and intensity* of the precipitin arc and *distance from the antiserum trough*— These characteristics reflect the concentration of the immunoglobulin protein. A monoclonal immunoglobulin is often synthesized in high concentrations and will produce an arc that is thicker and more intensely stained than the corresponding arc produced by the normal control specimen. An increase in polyclonal immunoglobulins produces an arc that is thicker and more intense, but still retains its broad, elliptical shape. The increased thickness and peakedness of the arc produced by the monoclonal protein may result in the arc being positioned closer to the antiserum trough than an arc produced by normal serum and, in some cases, even diffusing into the trough.

3. *Electrophoretic position* of the precipitin arc—Paraproteins may have an altered electrophoretic mobility as compared to the corresponding normal immunoglobulin protein, and be positioned differently relative to the anode. A change in electrophoretic position may be a result of amino acid deletions in the M-component, a monoclonal band being comprised of a minor immunoglobulin subclass, the presence of monoclonal light chains unattached to heavy chains, or the formation of non-covalently linked light chain dimers.

4. *Light chain patterns*

a. *Kappa:lambda ratio*—High concentrations of a paraprotein will result in an excess of the light chain type incorporated in the M-component, and therefore, in a significant alteration in the normal kappa:lambda ratio of approximately 2:1.[9,11] The precipitin arc produced by the monoclonal light chain in these cases will thus be much darker and thicker than the arc produced by the other light chain type.

b. *Symmetry*—Polyclonal immunoglobulins produce light chain precipitin arcs which are symmetrical in shape. In contrast, symmetry is often lacking in the precipitates produced by monoclonal light chains. This dissymmetry can be the result of production of the monoclonal

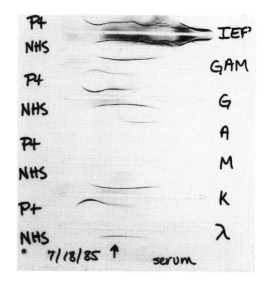

Fig. 5–2. Immunoelectrophoresis (IEP) on a clinical serum specimen reveals the presence of a monoclonal IgG-kappa protein. IgM and IgA are decreased in the patient. The patient specimen (Pt) and a normal human serum (NHS) control are placed in alternate vertical rows at the point of application indicated by the arrow. Antisera to whole human serum (IEP), gamma chains (G), alpha chains (A), mu chains (M), all three heavy chains (GAM), kappa chains (κ), and lambda chains (λ), were placed in individual troughs, as illustrated.

protein in addition to polyclonal light chains which occur as part of normal immunoglobulin molecules, or to the production of free monoclonal light chains, in addition to the monoclonal light chains occurring as part of the intact monoclonal immunoglobulin molecule. These situations can be distinguished by examination of the electrophoretic mobility of the light chain arcs with respect to that of the arcs produced in response to anti-IgG, anti-IgA, or anti-IgM.

An example of an IEP pattern from a clinical serum specimen tested in our laboratory is illustrated in Figure 5–2.

Although IEP has been the traditional method used by many laboratories in identifying and typing monoclonal proteins for many years,[4,5] the procedure has several limitations. Result turnaround time is slow (1 to 2 days), and in some cases, ambiguous results are produced, making it difficult to interpret the normality of the precipitin arcs.[7,12,13,17] In cases in which there are low concentrations of an IgM or IgA paraprotein, identification of the light chains contained in these proteins may be difficult. This phenomenon, referred to as the "umbrella effect," is caused by the masking of these monoclonal light chains by the reactivity of antikappa and antilambda sera with IgG,[16] which predominates in the serum and diffuses into the agarose more rapidly than the immunoglobulin classes of larger molecular weight. The light chains within a monoclonal IgM molecule may be revealed by pretreatment of the serum with reducing agents such as 2-mercaptoethanol or dithiothreitol prior to IEP, in order to break down the pentamer molecule into smaller, more rapidly diffusing subunits.[10,15]

Another method that can be used in the characterization of paraproteins is immunofixation electrophoresis (IFE). The application of IFE to the study of monoclonal immunoglobulins was first introduced in 1976.[1,17] Since then, a number of technical improvements have allowed this method to become commercially available, offering laboratories an additional procedure which can be used as an alternative to, or in conjunction with, IEP. In IFE, high resolution electrophoresis of the serum sample is followed by application of monospecific antisera directly over the separated proteins. This brings the antigen and antibody in direct contact, resulting in the formation of precipitin bands. Polyclonal bands are indicated by areas of diffuse staining, while monoclonal immunoglobulins produce sharp, discrete, and intensely stained bands.[20] A sample IFE performed on a clinical specimen in our laboratory is illustrated in Figure 5–3.

IFE has several advantages over IEP, including faster turnaround time for results (approximately 2 hours), and greater sensitivity, allowing the method to be used in the determination of oligoclonal bands in the CSF, as seen in multiple sclerosis,[1,6,8,20]

and facilitating detection of monoclonal immunoglobulin proteins present in low concentrations.[1,8,20] Several investigators have reportedly found IFE to yield results that are generally agreeable with IEP in routine clinical testing, and easier to interpret in special situations, such as the characterization of biclonal gammopathies and the identification of light chains in IgM and IgA paraproteinemias,[2,7,12,17-19] because the restricted area of diffusion in IFE eliminates the umbrella effect.[10,19,20]

Disadvantages of IFE include the need for a larger amount of concentrated technologist time than required for IEP, and dependence on critical immunoglobulin concentrations for optimal performance.[10,13,14,19] Failure to prepare the appropriate specimen dilutions in IFE may result in prozoning, whereby the bands produced contain a faded central area surrounded by stained margins.[8,17,20] In addition, when normal immunoglobulins in a sample are present in much higher concentrations than the monoclonal immunoglobulin of the same class, presence of the paraprotein may be obscured by the appearance of a diffuse band characteristic of polyclonal immunoglobulins.[19]

Another limitation associated with both IFE and IEP involves the antisera used in the procedures. Occasionally, these antisera may fail to react with the antigenic determinants present in an M-component. In cases where a suspected paraprotein is not revealed, and dilution of the specimen fails to resolve the problem, antisera directed against different epitopes may be used.[10,16]

In approximately 25% of multiple myeloma cases, only free monoclonal light chains are detected in the serum.[3] If these are revealed by IEP or IFE, antisera specific for delta or epsilon may be used to rule out the small possibility of an IgD or IgE myeloma.

As M-components are often excreted in the urine, analysis of urine from patients with monoclonal gammopathies by IEP or IFE should also be performed. Over 50% of myeloma patients excrete free monoclonal

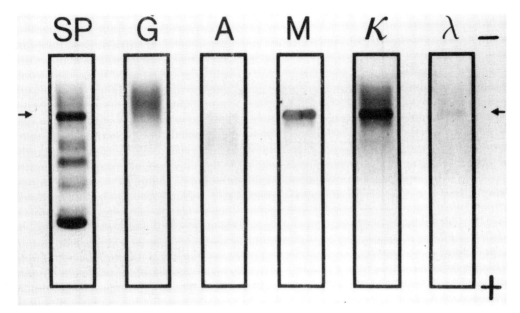

Fig. 5–3. Immunofixation electrophoresis (IFE) reveals the presence of a monoclonal IgM-kappa protein in a clinical serum specimen. Arrow indicates point of application of specimen. SP = Serum protein electrophoresis. IFE was performed on the remaining strips using antisera to gamma chains (G), alpha chains (A), mu chains (M), kappa chains (κ), and lambda chains (λ).

light chains in their urine,[15,16] often resulting in the obstruction of the nephrons. In patients with renal damage, whole immunoglobulin molecules and albumin are also found in the urine.[3] Testing should be performed on a urine sample collected for 24 hours in order to determine the amount of protein excreted per day.[10,11] The sample should be concentrated to a total protein content of approximately 25 mg/ml through selective membranes or by lyophilization for optimal detection of M-components.

IEP and IFE may be used by the laboratory as either alternative or complementary methods for the analysis of M-components in serum or urine samples. These procedures are helpful in making the initial diagnosis of a monoclonal gammopathy and in monitoring the course of disease. Disappearance of a monoclonal protein suggests therapeutic success in reducing the size of the tumor, while persistence of the M-component may indicate disseminated myeloma.[10] A complete laboratory investigation of the paraproteinemias should involve IEP and/or IFE

in conjunction with other laboratory tests, including bone marrow analysis, quantitation of immunoglobulins, serum viscosity, and routine hematology and chemistry tests.

REFERENCES

1. Cawley, L.P. et al.: Clin. Chem., *22*:1262, 1976.
2. Chu, S.Y. et al.: Clin. Chem., *33*:617, 1987.
3. Davey, F.R., and Nelson, D.A.: In *Clinical Diagnosis and Management by Laboratory Methods.* 17th ed. Edited by J.B. Henry. Philadelphia, W.B. Saunders Co., 1984.
4. Grabar, P., and Williams, C.A.: Biochim. Biophys. Acta, *17*:67, 1955.
5. Grabar, P., and Williams, C.A.: Biochim. Biophys. Acta, *10*:193, 1953.
6. Keshgegian, A.A.: Clin. Chem., *26*:1340, 1980.
7. Keshgegian, A.A., and Peiffer, P.: Clin. Chim. Acta, *110*:337, 1981.
8. Killingsworth, L.M., and Warren, B.M.: *Immunofixation for the Identification of Monoclonal Gammopathies.* Booklet from Helena Laboratories, 1986.
9. Kunkel, H.G.: Cancer Res., *28*:1351, 1968.
10. Kyle, R.A.: In *Manual of Clinical Laboratory Immunology.* 3rd ed. Edited by N.R. Rose, H. Friedman, and J.L. Fahey. Washington, D.C., American Society for Microbiology, 1986.
11. Kyle, R.A., and Greipp, P.R.: Mayo Clin. Proc., *53*:719, 1978.
12. Marshall, M.O.: Clin. Chim. Acta, *104*:1, 1980.
13. Miller, L.E., and Sgroi, J.M.: *Clinical Immunology*

Tech Sample No. CI-6. Chicago, American Society of Clinical Pathologists, 1985.

14. Normansell, D.E.: Am. J. Clin. Pathol., *84*:469, 1985.

*15. Penn, G.M., and Batya, J.: *ASCP Manual—Interpretation of Immunoelectrophoretic Patterns.* Chicago, American Society of Clinical Pathologists, 1978.

16. Ricardo, M.J., and Tomar, R.H.: In *Clinical Diagnosis and Management by Laboratory Methods.* 17th ed. Edited by J.B. Henry. Philadelphia, W.B. Saunders Co., 1984.

17. Ritchie, R.F., and Smith, R.: Clin. Chem., *22*:1982, 1976.

18. Schreiber, W.E., and Pudek, M.R.: Am. J. Clin. Pathol., *85*:532-11A (letter), 1986.

19. Sun, T., Lien, Y.Y., and Degnan, T.: Am. J. Clin. Pathol., *22*:5, 1979.

20. Warren, B.M.: *Immunofixation Electrophoresis: Methodology and Application.* Booklet from Helena Laboratories, Beaumont, Texas, 1983.

Immunoelectrophoresis Assay (IEP) (Serum or Urine)

PRINCIPLE. A technique combining immunodiffusion and electrophoresis is used to precipitate serum components for characterization and identification of certain immunodeficiency or immunoproliferative disorders.

EQUIPMENT AND MATERIALS

1. Corning Electrophoresis System (or equivalent) with the following components:

   a. Cell base with cover.

   b. Power supply: Operates on 110V AC, maintaining a constant output of 90 volts to the electrophoresis film. A red pilot light indicates the correct placement of the cell cover on the cell base.

   c. Corning Universal Electrophoresis Film[R] (or equivalent): Pre-packaged, ready to use agarose film fixed to a clear, plastic base, with protective cover. Contains a uniform layer, 0.015 inches thick, composed of 1% agarose, 5% sucrose and 0.035% disodium ethylenediamine tetraacetate (EDTA) in barbital buffer, pH 8.6. Sample wells and antiserum troughs are molded and are uniform in depth, width and length. Polarity is indicated on each film. The protective cover is removed just before use by gently peeling off the agarose-plastic film.

   d. Electrophoresis buffer kit containing: 0.05M barbital buffer, pH 8.6, consisting of approximately 17.7 g sodium barbital, 2.6 g barbital, 1.0 g sodium chloride and 0.70 g EDTA as a preservative. Stable at least 2 years if stored in a dry place at room temperature. Do not use if solidly caked. To use: Empty contents of one vial of sodium barbital into a 2000 ml volumetric flask which is about one-half filled with distilled water. Rinse the vial with distilled water and add rinse to flask. Dilute to volume. After reconstitution, buffer is stable for up to 4 months if stored at 2 to 8° C. Barbital buffer changes in pH on use, and should not be reused.

   e. Amido Black 10B Stain Set (Corning) or equivalent: A calorimetric stain. Store at 15 to 30° C. Stable for 2 years. Reconstitute by emptying vial (2.0 g) into a 1000 ml volumetric flask. QS to 1000 ml with 5% acetic acid, rinsing out vial well. Cover and mix by inversion. Store at 15 to 30° C in a closed container. Stable for 3 months.[3]

2. Acetic Acid: Prepare by adding 50 ml of glacial acetic acid to 950 ml distilled water in a 1000 ml cylinder. Stable indefinitely at room temperature

3. Microliter pipet, capable of delivering 0.8 μl

4. 20 μl disposable pipets, with bulbs

5. Staining dishes

6. Moist chambers

7. Incubator set at 37 to 60° C

8. 0.9% saline solution

9. Patient Sample:

   a. *Serum:* Serum for immunoelectrophoresis should be fresh, or frozen no more than once, before testing. Inactivated samples are not acceptable.

   b. *Urine Samples:* Urine samples are tested for total protein in the Microscopy laboratory before immunoelectrophoresis is done. Urines with >15 mg of protein per 100 ml are tested immediately. Those with <15 mg/100 ml, from patients who are known to have a monoclonal immunoproliferative disorder, are also tested immediately. Samples of <15 mg/100 ml with no immunoglobulin file are referred to a pathologist for evaluation before the film is run. Urines may be concentrated to a total protein content of approximately 25 mg/ml using a Minicon[R] concentrator according to the chart that follows (Fig. 5–4):[1]

10. Minicon-B Clinical Sample Concentrator (Amicon): Utilizes a membrane rated at 15,000 MW retention.[1] Store at room temperature. Fill using a 9-inch Pasteur pipet or syringe, taking care to avoid scratching the membrane. Extract concentrate using a 9-inch Pasteur pipet. Store used concentrator in a refrigerator for subsequent uses

11. Normal Human Serum (NHS): Serum from a person known to be free of immunopathologic abnormality (usually a technician) is aliquoted in 0.5 ml amounts. Store at −20° C. May be used indefinitely. A drop of bromophenol blue dye is added before using. Once thawed, an aliquot may be used up to 1 week, if kept refrigerated or frozen

12. Bromophenol Blue Dye 0.04% (Fischer Scientific): Store at room temperature. Expiration date is noted on the label

13. IEP Antiserum:

a. IEP antiserum (Meloy): Goat anti-whole human serum for immunoelectrophoresis. Store at 2 to 8° C. Expiration date is noted on the label.

b. Anti-IgG, -IgA, -IgM (Meloy): Goat antiserum to human immunoglobulin (IgG, IgA, IgM). Precipitin titer and expiration date are noted on the label. Store at 2 to 8° C.

c. Anti-IgG (Meloy): Goat anti-human IgG, absorbed to render monospecificity for gamma (γ) chains. May be stored at 2 to 5° C until the expiration date noted on the label.

d. Anti-IgA (Meloy): Goat anti-human IgA, absorbed to render monospecificity for alpha (α) chains. Store at 2 to

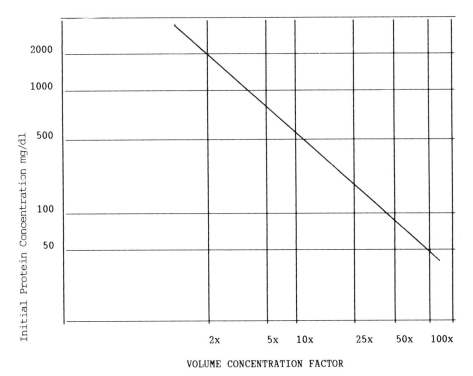

Fig. 5–4. Concentration chart to achieve 25 mg/ml.

5° C. May be used until the expiration date noted on the label.

e. Anti-IgM (Meloy): goat anti-human IgM, absorbed to render it monospecific for mu (μ) heavy chains. Store at 2 to 5° C. Expiration date is noted on the label.

f. Anti-IgD (Meloy): goat antiserum to human IgD, delta (δ) chain specific. Precipitin titer and expiration date are noted on the label. Store at 2 to 8° C.

g. Anti-IgE (Meloy): Goat antiserum to human IgE, epsilon (ϵ) chain specific. Precipitin titer and expiration date are noted on the label.

h. Anti-Kappa (Meloy): Burro antiserum to human kappa (κ) chain, specific for immunoglobulin-bound and free kappa chains. Prepared against urinary monoclonal kappa chains. Precipitin titer and expiration date are noted on the label. Store at 2 to 8° C.

i. Anti-Lambda (Meloy): Burro antiserum to human lambda (λ) chains, specific for immunoglobulin-bound and free lambda chains. Prepared against urinary monoclonal lambda chains. Precipitin titer and expiration date are noted on the label. Store at 2 to 8° C. *NOTE:* This laboratory keeps IEP antisera from at least two companies for an alternative in difficult testing situations.

PROCEDURE

1. Fill each chamber of the cell base with approximately 100 ml of barbital buffer. Equalize by tilting the cell base upward on one end until buffer flows freely from one chamber to the other. Blot cell base divider dry.

2. Plug cell base banana plugs into power supply unit. Press the two units firmly together until the washers behind the banana plugs are snugly pressed against the power supply. Leave cell base cover off. Plug power cord into 110V wall outlet.

3. Remove the plastic cover from the electrophoresis film and place the gel on a sheet of lined note-book paper, putting the vertical sample wells along one line of the sheet.

4. Using a microliter syringe, place 0.8 μl of the appropriate samples (Fig. 5–5) over the line of the notebook paper immediately to the right of the one bisecting the sample wells.

5. Allow the samples to soak into the media.

6. Slip the film, gel side up, into the overturned cell base cover, with the top of the film toward the everted end of the cover. Pull the side edges of the film up flush with the boundaries of the holder.

7. Gently place the cover on the cell base, everted end toward the power supply. The red pilot light will go on if the unit has been properly engaged.

8. Electrophorese for 35 minutes for Corning Power Source. After electrophoresis, observe for the bromophenol blue dye in the NHS, which should have migrated across the membrane. If the dye has not migrated, electrophoresis was not completed.

9. Remove the film carefully and blot excess moisture from the edges and back. Lay flat and allow to sit until all excess moisture has been evaporated or absorbed by the gel.

10. With a 20-μl capillary pipet and bulb, spread approximately 20 μl of the appropriate antisera (see template) evenly across the horizontal troughs. *Take care not to gouge gel, overfill, splash, or expel a bubble from the pipet tip.* Allow to absorb until no excess moisture is evident.

11. Place film in a humidity chamber (a container, closed tightly with a moistened gauze inside), lying flat. Cover and allow immunodiffusion to occur for 24 to 48 hours at room temperature.

12. Submerge film in 0.9% saline solution and allow elution of uncomplexed protein for 4 hours (with regular agitation) or overnight.

13. Remove film. Place in Amido black 10B stain (see *Equipment and Materials, # 1e,* for preparation) for 7 minutes. Remove. Rinse for 30 to 60 seconds in 5% acetic acid.

14. Remove and drain, blotting excess moisture from the edges and the back. Place on a gauze and dry in an incubator or drying unit until *completely* dry.

15. Rinse in two changes of acetic acid until all excess stain is removed. Blot excess moisture from edges and back of the film with gauze. Lay flat to dry or dry in an incubator or drying unit.

16. Label with magic marker. Include all components indicated on the template.

17. Observe for abnormalities in the precipitin bands.

REPORTING. In this laboratory, all immunoelectrophoresis films are evaluated and reported by a pathologist.

IEP results are compiled with immunoglobulin levels on a special report sheet (a copy is included for reference; Fig. 5–6). A photocopy is sent to the requesting physi-

SERUM* OR URINE*

```
                                                      ANTISERUM TO:

NHS        1 |_____        IEP

Patient    2 |_____        IgG, IgA, IgM

NHS        3 |_____        IgG

Patient    4 |_____        IgA

NHS        5 |_____        IgM

Patient    6 |_____        Kappa

NHS        7 |_____        Lambda

Patient    8 |


           Patient Name - Date - Source of Specimen
```

*Templates given for immunoelectrophoresis are those used for routine

diagnosis, and may be altered to include antiserum to IgD, IgE, Kappa,

Lambda, etc., when desired.

Fig. 5–5. Template—Immunoelectrophoresis, Clinical Immunology—SUNY Health Science Center at Syracuse.

cian. The original sheet and the IEP film are kept on permanent file in the laboratory.

LIMITATIONS OF THE PROCEDURE. Immunoelectrophoresis is a semiquantitative technique, and should be used in conjunction with immunoglobulin levels, as obtained by a quantitative method. Serum protein electrophoresis may also be desirable as an aid to diagnosis.

Occasionally, it is desirable to observe the effects of 2-mercaptoethanol treatment on immunoelectrophoresed protein. For that procedure, see 2-*Mercaptoethanol Treatment.*

The lower limits of sensitivity using this technique have been assessed in this laboratory at approximately 10 mg/100 ml for a given monoclonal protein.[2]

REFERENCES

1. Insert, Amicon Corporation. Minicon Macrosolute Concentrators, Amicon Corp. Davers, MA, 01923.

2. Insert, Antisera, Meloy Laboratories, Inc. Tarrytown, N.Y.

3. Inserts, Corning Electrophoresis Buffer and Stain sets, Corning Medical and Scientific., Palo Alto, Ca.

2-Mercaptoethanol Treatment

PRINCIPLE. Dissolution of IgM molecules is effected by treatment with 2-mercaptoethanol.[1]

EQUIPMENT AND MATERIALS

1. 2-mercaptoethanol (2-ME; Calbiochem): MW 78.1. Store at room temperature in a hood. Prepare 0.1M 2-mercaptoethanol in a fume hood by adding 0.1 ml 2-mercaptoethanol to 14.2 ml saline solution. *NOTE: 2-ME IS TOXIC.* Do not pipet by mouth. Store at room temperature

2. 0.9% saline solution

3. Serologic pipets, with bulbs

4. Fume hood

5. Glass test tubes

STATE UNIVERSITY HOSPITAL
Health Science Center at Syracuse

Clinical Pathology
Immunology Report

DIAGNOSIS:

All figures are in mg/dl.

	Date	Date	Date	Date	Date	Date
IgG						
IgA						
IgM						

NORMALS: mg/dl

Age:	(number)	IgG mean	IgG range	IgA mean	IgA range	IgM mean	IgM range
Newborns*		1000	600-1670	0	–	10	7-17
10-14 days	(4)	791	530-1035	2.5	0-10	19	6-35
1-6 mos.	(8)	452	104-696	40	12-61	60	18-119
9-18 mos.	(19)	591	243-1130	34	5-98	72	24-188
2-5 yrs.	(28)	652	130-2243	66	7-173	79	24-203
6-9 yrs.	(27)	930	226-1870	87	3-155	88	12-219
10-15 yrs.	(45)	965	609-2626	118	35-420	112	35-262
Adults		1278	591-1965	239	77-400	140	50-311

*Data from R. Buckley in Human Health and Disease

SERUM IMMUNOELECTROPHORESIS (Date):

URINE IMMUNOELECTROPHORESIS (Date):
                        (Original urine protein concentration):
                        (Concentrated X   ):

COMMENTS:

_____, M.D.
               Clinical Pathologist

Fig. 5-6. Immunoelectrophoresis report sheet.

PROCEDURE

NOTE: 2-mercaptoethanol is toxic. Do not pipet by mouth. Perform procedures in a fume hood.

1. Place 0.3 ml serum in a test tube.
2. Add 0.05 ml of 0.1M 2-ME.
3. Parafilm, shake to mix, and allow to stand until ready for use.

REFERENCE

1. Penn, Gerald, Personal Communication.

Immunofixation Electrophoresis[5](IFE)

PRINCIPLE. Immunofixation electrophoresis (IFE) is used for the diagnostic identification of immunoglobulins and abnormal proteins using high resolution protein electrophoresis and immunofixation in human serum, cerebrospinal fluid, and urine.

Proteins are first separated by electrophoresis. The separation depends on charge and size of the proteins, buffer, current applied, and gels used. Antisera is applied directly onto electrophoresed protein, allowing antigen-antibody precipitation. Free protein and antisera are removed by washing, and the fixed immunoprecipitin complexes are stained, allowing for pattern examination.[1,7]

EQUIPMENT AND MATERIALS

1. Titan Gel ImmunoFix Kit (Helena Laboratories):

a. Titan Gel IFE Plate

Each plate contains agarose in barbital solution with 0.1% sodium azide and 0.02% thimerosal added as preservatives. The plates are ready for use as packaged. The plates should be stored at room temperature (15 to 30° C) and are stable until the expiration date indicated on the package. The plates must be stored in the protective packaging in which they are shipped. DO NOT REFRIGERATE OR FREEZE.

b. Titan Gel IFE Buffer

The buffer contains barbital, calcium lactate, and 0.1% sodium azide as a preservative; pH 8.4 to 8.8. Dissolve one package of buffer in 1500 mL purified water. The buffer is ready for use when all material is completely dissolved. The packaged buffer should be stored at 15 to 30° C and is stable until the expiration date indicated on the package. Diluted buffer is stable 6 months stored at 15 to 30° C or 2 to 6° C. Discard packaged buffer if the material shows signs of dampness or discoloration. Discard diluted buffer if it becomes turbid.

c. Titan Gel IFE Stain

The stain contains amino black. Dissolve the dry stain in 250 mL methanol. Add 250 mL purified water and acidify with 50 mL glacial acetic acid. Filter before use if necessary. Total volume: 550 mL. The dry stain should be stored at 15 to 30° C and is stable until the expiration date indicated on the package. The diluted stain is stable for 6 months when stored at 15 to 30° C in a closed container. Used stain may be returned to the bottle and reused.

The diluted stain should be a homogeneous mixture free of precipitate.

d. Titan Gel IFE Protein Fixative

The fixative contains 10% sulfosalicylic acid and 10% acetic acid. The fixative should be stored at 2 to 6° C and is stable until the expiration date indicated on the vial. The fixative should be a clear yellow solution.

e. Antisera to Human IgG, IgA, IgM, Kappa Light Chain, and Lambda Light Chain

Antisera vials in the kit contain monospecific antisera to human immunoglobulin heavy chains, IgG, IgM, IgA and to human light chains, Kappa and Lambda. The antisera have been prepared in horse, sheep, or goat. Each vial or antisera contains sodium azide as a preservative.

The antisera are ready for use as packaged. The antisera should be stored at 2 to 6° C and are stable until the expiration date indicated on the vial. Extremely cloudy antisera may be indicative of product deterioration.

f. Sample templates

g. Antisera templates

h. Titan Gel Blotter A

i. Titan Gel Blotter C

j. Titan Gel wicks

2. Dialamatic microdispenser and tubes (1 to 10 μL) or equivalent

3. Dialamatic microdispenser and tubes (1 to 50 μL) or equivalent

4. Titan Gel chamber

5. EWS Dryer/Incubator or equivalent

6. Power supply

7. Titan blotter pads (100/box) or equivalent

8. Incubation chamber

9. Staining chamber

10. Development weights

11. Glacial acetic acid

12. Destaining solution: 5% acetic acid. Store at 15 to 30° C

13. 10% sodium chloride: dissolve 100 g in 1 L purified water.

14. Saline solution (0.85%)

15. Laboratory rotator

16. Cooling device

17. Methanol

SPECIMEN COLLECTION. The specimen may be serum, cerebrospinal fluid, or urine.

1. Serum Specimens

Specimen should be collected in a normal manner. Samples stored at 2 to 8° C for up to 72 hours can be used. If stored longer, keep at −20° C.

2. Urine Specimens

a. If necessary, concentrate urine sample to 100 mg/dL of total protein for detection of Bence Jones proteins (free kappa and lambda light chains).

b. Immunoglobulins: concentrate the urine specimen to 800 to 1000 mg/dL total protein for the detection of immunoglobulins. Use concentrated sample for all patterns.

3. Interfering factors

a. Evaporation of uncovered specimens may cause inaccurate results.

b. Plasma should not be used because the fibrinogen may adhere to the gel matrix, resulting in a band near the application point in all patterns across the plate.

4. Storage and Stability

a. Fresh serum, CSF, or urine are the specimens of choice.

PROCEDURE

1. Dilute the patient serum samples with 0.85% saline solution as follows:

1:2 for the serum protein pattern (SP)

1:10 for identification of all immunoglobulins

a. When typing minimonoclonal specimens, if the sample IgG level exceeds 1500 mg/dL, the sample should be diluted 1:20 for the IgG slot only.

b. When typing IgM or Lambda proteins in specimens containing minimonoclonal bands, a sample dilution of 1:5 is recommended for the IgM and Lambda patterns.

2. If necessary concentrate urine and cerebrospinal fluids.

3. Pour approximately 125 mL IFE buffer into each outer section of the Titan Gel chamber. Cover the chamber until ready to use to prevent evaporation. Store the cooling device in the refrigerator for at least 1 hour prior to use. Place it in the Titan Gel chamber immediately before placing the agarose plate in the chamber.

4. Remove the IFE plate from the protective packaging and remove the paper overlay.

5. Gently blot the plate at the area of application with Blotter A. The arrows on the plate edges indicate the sample application alignment.

6. Place the IFE sample template on the plate, aligning the application slits with the arrows on the plate edges. Apply slight fingertip pressure to the template, making sure there are no air bubbles between it and the plate.

7. Apply 3.0 µL of the appropriate serum sample dilution or concentrated urine or cerebral spinal fluid onto the template slots. Urine and CSF are used concentrated on all patterns.

8. Wait 5 minutes after the last sample has been applied to allow the samples to diffuse into the agarose. While the sample is absorbing into the plate, remove the cooling device from the refrigerator and place it in the center of the chamber. Wet the entire surface of the cooling device with a few drops of buffer.

9. After allowing the samples to absorb into the agarose, gently blot the template with a new Blotter A and carefully remove the template.

10. Quickly place the IFE plate in the electrophoresis chamber *agarose side up*, on top of the cooling device. The application point should be on the cathodic (−) side. Avoid trapping air bubbles between the agarose plate and glass of the cooling device. Run one plate per chamber. Prepare a wick for each side of the plate by placing three wicks together in two sets making two thick wicks. Evenly align the edge of each set of wicks and dip into the chamber buffer and then attach the wicks to each side of the plate parallel to the edge of the cooling device. Gently rub one finger across the plate at the wick contact area to ensure good contact and to displace trapped bubbles.

11. Place the cover on the chamber.

12. Electrophorese the plate at 250 volts for 15 to 18 minutes.

13. Remove the electrophoresed plate from the chamber.

14. Place the plate in the incubation chamber that has been lined with damp blotter paper or filter paper.

15. Align the antisera template on the plate so that the slits in the template are aligned over the antisera application areas on the plate. The holes on the bottom edge of the template match the black dots on the plate. Make sure the template makes good contact with the agarose on the sample plate.

16. Apply 70 µL of the IFE protein fixative to the "SP" position on the plate. This pattern will provide the complete electrophoresis pattern upon completion of staining.

17. Apply 70 μL of the appropriate antiserum to the template slots.

18. Close the incubation chamber and incubate the plate for 10 minutes at room temperature (15 to 30° C).

19. At the end of the incubation period, remove the antisera template and place the plate in a shallow dish containing sufficient 0.85% NaCl to achieve a level of approximately ½ inch. Place the dish on a laboratory rotator at slow speed.

20. Wash the plate in 0.85% NaCl for 10 minutes.

21. Remove the plate from the NaCl wash and press-dry for 10 minutes. The press-dry step is performed as follows: Place the plate on a blotter pad agarose up. Layer three blotter Cs and then three blotter pads on the plate. Place a development weight on top of the blotters and plate and allow to stand 10 minutes.

22. Repeat steps 20 and 21 once more for a total of two wash steps and two press steps.

23. Dry the plate at 56° C in a laboratory drying oven with forced air for 1 to 2 minutes or until completely dry.

24. Stain the plate for 4 minutes.

25. Destain the plate in two washes of 5% acetic acid, 1 minute each or until the background is clear.

26. Dry the plate for 5 minutes (or until dry) at 56° C. The completed, stained, and dried immunofixation plate is stable for an indefinite period of time.

INTERPRETATION OF RESULTS. A stained band represents a reaction between antisera and protein in the specimen. Most monoclonal proteins migrate in the cathodal (gamma) region of the protein pattern, but they may migrate anywhere within the globulin region on protein electrophoresis.

The monoclonal protein band on the immunofixation pattern will occupy the same migration position and shape as the monoclonal band on the reference protein electrophoresis pattern. The abnormal protein is identified by the corresponding antiserum used. When low concentrations of M-protein are present, the immunofixation band may appear on the stained background of the polyclonal immunoglobulin. A polyclonal increase produces a diffuse staining pattern with no sharp band delineations.

LIMITATIONS OF THE PROCEDURE

1. Prozoning in IFE is usually the result of an antigen excess (the patient sample needs to be further diluted). This will manifest itself as a clearing in the center of the band.

2. Monoclonal proteins, especially IgM, may occasionally adhere to the gel matrix. These bands will appear in all five antisera reaction areas of the gel. However, where the band reacts with the specific antisera for its heavy chain and light chain, there will be a significant increase in size and staining activity, allowing the band to be identified.

3. Serum samples which have a precipitin band with Kappa or Lambda light chain antisera but no corresponding band with IgG, IgA or IgM antisera may have a free light chain. Such sera should be tested with IgD and IgE antisera on an immunoelectrophoresis plate to rule out the presence of a monoclonal IgD or IgE immunoglobulin.

4. Cerebrospinal fluid may contain a nonimmunoglobulin band, referred to as gamma-trace, which migrates in the gamma region. Because gamma-trace is nonimmunoglobulin in nature, it will not react with antisera against human immunoglobulins. Gamma trace is often detected in normal cerebrospinal fluid.[3,6]

5. A CRP band may be detected in patients with an acute inflammatory response.[2,4] These specimens can be checked by performing a quantitative CRP.

REFERENCES

1. Cawley, L.P. et al.: Clin. Chem., 22:1262, 1976.
2. Jeppsson, J.E. et al.: Clin. Chem., 25:629, 1979.
3. Keshgegian, A.A.: Clin. Chem., 26:1340, 1980.
4. Killingsworth, L.M. et al.: Diag. Med. 3-15, Jan/Feb 1980.
5. Package Insert, Titan Gel Immunofix Kit, Helena Laboratories, Beaumont, TX, 1987.
6. Papadopoulos, N.M. et al.: Clin. Chem., 29:1842, 1983.
7. Ritchie, R.F., and Smith, R.: Clin. Chem., 22:1982, 1976.

COMPLEMENT

The complement system is a group of proteins, found in body fluids or on cell membranes, which are capable of specific, sequential interactions leading to a myriad of physiologic effects. Although disruption of microbial cell walls appears to be an evolutionary mainstay of this system, complement also plays a major role in the mediation of inflammation, in regulation of phagocytic activity, and in metabolism of immune complexes. When directed against inappropriate targets, e.g. apparently normal body cells or cellular elements, it may function as an integral component of the pathophysiology of disease.

Complement may be initiated by the presence of certain chemical activators (e.g. zymosan or lipopolysaccharide), by interaction of C-reactive protein with its substrate molecule, or by the complexing of some classes or subclasses of antibody (i.e. IgM, IgG1, IgG2, and IgG3) with specific antigen. In the latter case, complement constitutes a principal effector system for antibody, in that the antibody serves primarily to specifically target sites on the membranes of foreign cells, thus labeling them for lytic or phagocytic destruction. At different stages in the activation sequence, cleavage products (e.g. C3a and C5a) are formed that have profound effects on inflammation and phagocytosis.

Soluble components of the complement system circulate as inactive precursor proteins of molecular weights between 60,000D and 400,000D, electrophoretic mobilities from alpha-2 to gamma, and serum concentrations ranging from a high of 120 mg/dl (C3) to virtually undetectable levels (C2, C9, factor D). As a whole, they comprise 10 to 15% of the weight of all plasma proteins. Synthesis of soluble complement components occurs in mononuclear phagocytes,[31,33,34,35,69] hepatocytes,[1,28] fibroblasts,[28,32,46] and in endothelial cells of the umbilical vein.[91] Regulation of synthesis is a function of interleukin 1 (IL-1)[9] and of gamma,[31,52] alpha, or beta[31] interferons. The presence of endotoxins[29] or lipopolysaccharides[46] can also modulate production.

Many cell surface proteins have been identified that react with soluble complement components or their degradation products.[87] These proteins appear to control turnover of complement and/or regulate the behavior and growth of leukocytes. Some are designated "receptors" (Table 6–3) while others act as surface bound regulators of the system (Table 6–2).

Three of the complement components (C4,[6] C2, and factor B[5]) have been shown to be coded by genes in the Class III region of the human major histocompatibility complex (MHC) on chromosome #6.[7] MHC-linked complement genes occur in populations and segregate in families as single genetic complotypes. Molecular probes for at least 10 of the 20 known complement genes have been developed[9] and are being used to study complement synthesis and regulation in the body.

The terminal complement complex (TCC), known as the membrane attack complex (MAC) when it occurs on a cell surface, may be activated by either of two prior complement sequences, designated "classical" and "alternative" pathways (Fig. 6–1 and discussion below). The biologic consequences of both pathways such as anaphylaxis, opsonic adherence, and activation of the TCC, are virtually identical. It may be helpful to the reader to note that components included in the classical pathway and the TCC are usually designated by numbers (e.g. C3, C9), while components exclusive to the alternative system are indicated by letters (e.g. factor B) (Table 6–1).

THE CLASSICAL PATHWAY[28,80]

The steps of the classical pathway are summarized in Figure 6–1.

C1, the first component to be activated in the classical pathway, exists in serum as a Ca^{++} dependent complex of three different subunits, C1q, C1r, and C1s, having a $C1q,C1r_2,C1s_2$ composition.[49]

IgM and IgG, subsets 1,2,3, have receptors of C1q on the constant region of their heavy chains[85] which are exposed once the immunoglobulin has attached to its specific antigen. Activation of C1q is dependent upon cross-linkage of at least two of the molecule's six binding sites with these receptors. It is important to note that one molecule of IgM, by virtue of its pentameric structure, can cross-link and activate a molecule of C1q. However, side-by-side molecules of monomeric IgG must be available, necessitating close proximity between antigenic determinants and a sufficient quantity of IgG, before cross-linkage and activation of C1q can occur.

Ag-Ig (1 IgM or $\geq$ 2 IgG) + C1q → activated C1q

In addition, pentameric C-reactive protein, upon binding with its substrate molecule, can cause C1q activation.

By interaction with immunoglobulin or with C-reactive protein, C1q is sufficiently changed to induce the activation of $C1r_2$, which in turn splits $C1s_2$ by an intramolecular, autocatalytic mechanism.[10,97] The resulting molecule, designated C1 esterase (C1s), may continue the pathway by catalyzing the assembly of C3 convertase (see below), or it may be inactivated by the binding of C1 esterase inhibitor (C1s INH)[74] to C1r and C1s light chains, causing them to lose their attachment to C1q and thereby stopping the pathway.[50]

$$\text{Ag-Ig} + \text{C1 (C1q, C1r}_2\text{, C1s}_2\text{)} \longrightarrow \text{C1s} \xrightarrow{\text{C1s INH}}$$

C4 and C2, the next two components to become involved, tend to interact freely in solution to form an inactive, reversible complex. C1 esterase cleaves C4 into 2 fragments, designated C4a and C4b, and cleaves C2 into the fragments C2a and C2b. Fragments C4a and C2b are released into the surrounding environment. The remaining split product of C4 (C4b) acquires a short-lived ability to bind to immune complexes or to cells in its vicinity. Subsequent binding of C2a to C4b results in the formation of a reversible complex, C4b,2a, which functions as the C3 convertase of the classical pathway via its reaction with C3 (see below).

$$C1s + C4 \xrightarrow{\hspace{1.2cm}} \begin{array}{c} \longrightarrow C4a \\ C4b \end{array} \longrightarrow C4b, 2a(C3\ Convertase)$$

$$C1s + C2 \xrightarrow{\hspace{1.2cm}} \begin{array}{c} \longrightarrow C2b \\ C2a \end{array} \quad\nearrow\quad \begin{array}{c} \downarrow\uparrow \\ C4b + C2a \end{array}$$

The assembly and activity of C4b,2a may be regulated by the presence in plasma of C4 binding protein (C4bp)[29] or by membrane-bound proteins known as membrane cofactor protein (MCP)[87] and decay-accelerating factor (DAF).[61] In each case, interference of C4b-to-C2a binding is accomplished by direct binding of the regulatory protein with the C4 entity.[16,41] Both MCP and DAF are thought to play an important role in the protection of autologous cells from harmful complement activity via this mechanism.[87]

$$C4b + C2a \begin{array}{c} \nearrow\ C4bp,\ MCP,\ or\ DAF \\ \searrow\ C4b,\ 2a \end{array}$$

Inactivation of C4b may also be accomplished by factor I which cleaves the mol-

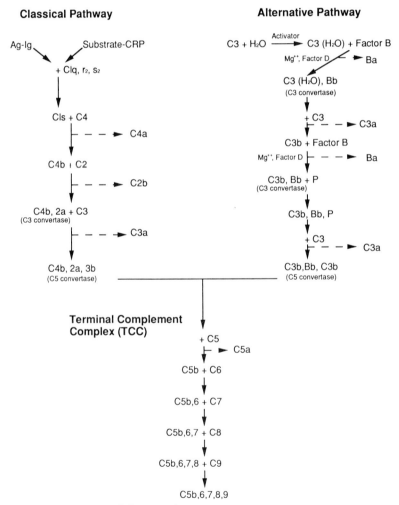

Classical Pathway

Ag-Ig ⟍   ⟋ Substrate-CRP

+ C1q, r₂, s₂

C1s + C4

⊢ – – ▶ C4a

C4b ι C2

⊢ – – ▶ C2b

C4b, 2a + C3
(C3 convertase)

⊢ – – ▶ C3a

C4b, 2a, 3b
(C5 convertase)

Alternative Pathway

$C3 + H_2O \xrightarrow{\text{Activator}} C3\ (H_2O) + Factor\ B$

Mg⁺⁺, Factor D ⟋   ▶ Ba

C3 (H₂O), Bb
(C3 convertase)

+ C3
⊢ – – ▶ C3a

C3b + Factor B

Mg⁺⁺, Factor D ⊢ – – ▶ Ba

C3b, Bb + P
(C3 convertase)

C3b, Bb, P

+ C3
⊢ – – ▶ C3a

C3b,Bb, C3b
(C5 convertase)

Terminal Complement Complex (TCC)

+ C5
⊢ ▶ C5a

C5b + C6

C5b,6 + C7

C5b,6,7 + C8

C5b,6,7,8 + C9

C5b,6,7,8,9

Fig. 6–1. Activation sequence of the complement system.

Table 6–1. Human Complement Components I

Effector Pathways	Component Name
Classical Pathway	C1 (C1q, C1r, C1s)
	C4
	C2
	C3
Alternative Pathway	C3
	Factor B
	Factor D
Terminal Complement Cascade	C5
	C6
	C7
	C8
	C9

ecule, yielding an inactive protein known as iC4b. In the presence of C4bp or the CR1 receptor (see *Complement Receptors*) as cofactors to this reaction, iC4b is further degraded into C4c and C4d fragments.[41]

$$\text{factor I} + \text{C4b} \longrightarrow \text{iC4b}$$

or

$$\text{factor I} + \text{C4b} \xrightarrow[\text{(CR1)}]{\text{(C4bp)}} \begin{array}{c} \nearrow \text{C4c} \\ \text{C4d} \end{array}$$

C4b, 2a, the C3 convertase, can rapidly activate and cleave many molecules of C3 into its split products, C3a and C3b.

$$\text{C4b, 2a} + \text{C3} \xrightarrow{} \begin{array}{c} \nearrow \text{C3a} \\ \text{C3b} \end{array}$$

C3a is released into the surrounding medium. The larger fragment, C3b, can bind via its metastable binding site either directly to the C4b,2a complex or to sites on adjacent cell membranes. When combined with the C4b,2a complex, the resulting molecule, C4b,2a,3b, functions as a C5 convertase and initiates formation of the terminal complement complex (TCC) (see below).

$$\text{C4b,2a} + \text{C3b} \rightarrow \text{C4b,2a,3b}$$
$$\text{(C5 convertase)}$$

When attached to a site on a cell membrane, C3b is also capable of alternative pathway activation.

Modulation of C3b is primarily achieved by factor I[21] which, in combination with the cofactor activity of factor H in plasma[66,75,80] or the CR1 receptor or MCP on cells, induces dissociation of C3b to iC3b.

$$\text{C3b} + \text{factor I} \xrightarrow[\substack{\text{(CR1)} \\ \text{(MCP)}}]{\text{(factor H)}} \text{iC3b}$$

The iC3b fragment, although capable of enhanced binding to complement receptors,[68] is hemolytically inactive, i.e. is incapable of activation of the terminal complement complex.

Cell-bound iC3b is slowly degraded by factor I and its cofactors into C3dg, which remains attached, and C3c, which is released and further degraded to C3e. Hydrolysis of C3dg eventually splits the molecule into C3d and C3g.

$$\text{factor I} + \text{iC3b} \xrightarrow[\text{(Cofactors)}]{} \begin{array}{c} \nearrow \text{C3c} \xrightarrow{} \text{C3e} \\ \text{C3dg} \longrightarrow \text{C3d} + \text{C3g} \end{array}$$

THE ALTERNATIVE PATHWAY[23,28,80]

The alternative pathway of complement activation suggests a natural mechanism for defense against microbial invasion, which can be activated by exposure, before antibody becomes available. Activators of this pathway include lipopolysaccharides from gram-negative bacteria, teichoic acid from the cell walls of gram-positive organisms, zymosan from the cell walls of fungi and yeasts, some viruses and virally-infected cells, certain parasites (e.g. trypanosomes), and some tumor cells. Therapeutic sulfhydryl compounds, e.g. those containing thiol compounds, can initiate this sequence,[100] as can several molecules and complexes[43,64] used in experimental situations. Controversy over whether IgA can initiate alternative pathway activation is unresolved, at present.[30,36,37]

Six plasma proteins comprise the activation sequence known as the alternative pathway; four of these, C3, factor B, factor D, and properdin (P), are involved in assembly of the alternative pathway C3 convertase while two, factor I and factor H, act as regulator proteins.

The steps of the alternative pathway are summarized in Figure 6–1: The pathway is initiated spontaneously by hydrolysis of the internal thioester of native C3 in a reaction with a molecule of water in the presence of one of the activators mentioned above.[28,65]

$$C3 + H_2O \xrightarrow[\text{(Activator)}]{} C3(H_2O)$$

Factor D, a serine esterase that circulates in plasma in active form, is capable of acting on its substrate, factor B, when the latter is modulated by C3 (H_2O) in a Mg^{++} dependent reaction.[73] Following factor D action, factor B is cleaved into two fragments designated Ba and Bb. Bb remains attached to the modulating molecule, C3(H_2O), forming C3(H_2O),Bb, which is capable of cleaving further molecules of C3, and hence is known as a C3 convertase.

$$C3(H_2O) + \text{factor B} \xrightarrow[\text{(Factor D)}]{(Mg^{++})} \overset{\text{Ba}}{\nearrow} C3(H_2O), \text{Bb (C3 Convertase)}$$

The action of C3 (H_2O),Bb on native C3 produces metastable C3b, which can covalently attach to the surface of cells and bind in a Mg^{++} dependent reaction with factor B, which again renders that molecule susceptible to cleavage by factor D. This phenomenon is called the amplification loop of the alternative pathway, and, in the absence of inhibitors, can result in continuous, spontaneous generation of C3b and C3b,Bb until either cell surfaces are saturated or the supply of complement components is depleted. Properdin (P) binds to C3b, Bb and acts to stabilize its action as a C3 convertase.[20]

$$C3(H_2O), \text{Bb} + C3 \xrightarrow{\overset{\text{C3a}}{\nearrow}} C3b + \text{factor B} \longrightarrow C3b, \text{Bb} + P \longrightarrow C3b, \text{Bb}, P$$

With the addition of only a single molecule of C3b to the existing C3 convertase, the enzyme becomes capable of C5 activation, in addition to its ability to continue to cleave available C3. Cleavage of C5 initiates the terminal complement cascade (see below).

$$C3b, \text{Bb} + C3b \longrightarrow C3b, \text{Bb}, C3b \text{ (C5 convertase)}$$

The activities of alternative pathway C3/C5 convertases are primarily restricted by factor I and factor H. Factor H complexes with C3b, whether in fluid or on a particle, and competes with factor B for appropriate binding sites.[86] In addition, C3b, when in combination with factor H, is accessible to factor I, which can cleave the alpha chain from C3b converting it to iC3b, a molecule which is inactive as a convertase, but maintains its ability to bind to receptors.

$$C3b + \text{factor H} \xrightarrow{\text{(factor I)}} iC3b$$

The CR1 receptor, as a cell bound molecule, can also act as a cofactor in the degradation of C3b.

$$C3b + \text{CR1 receptor} \xrightarrow{\text{(factor I)}} iC3b$$

Further degradation of the C3b molecule proceeds as described in the latter paragraphs of the discussion of the classical pathway.[21]

THE TERMINAL COMPLEMENT CASCADE[44,57,70]

(Membrane Attack Complex)

As described above, the terminal complement cascade (TCC) may be initiated by C5 convertases from the classical or the alternative pathways. In either case, cleavage of molecular C5 occurs as the last of the enzymatic steps in the complement sequences, resulting in the production of fragments designated C5a, which are released from the reaction, and C5b, which remain bound to the $-$C3b unit of convertase molecules.[70]

$$\text{C5 convertase} + \text{C5} \xrightarrow{\qquad} \begin{array}{l} \text{C5a} \\ \text{C5b} \end{array}$$

C5b is transiently capable of absorptive binding to C6, which subsequently serves as an acceptor for C7. With the binding of C7, the complex becomes increasingly hydrophobic, tending to insert itself into nearby membrane lipids.

$$\text{C5b} + \text{C6} \xrightarrow{\qquad} \text{C5b, 6} + \text{C7} \xrightarrow{\qquad} \text{C5b, 6, 7}$$

When C5b,6 is formed on a surface that is not part of an appropriate lipid membrane, or if there are no readily available C7 molecules in the environment, C5b,6 tends to dissociate from the surface and float free,[54] circulating as an active, stable complex. Subsequent attachment of C7 may induce attachment of the trimolecular complex (C5b,6,7) to an available bystander cell, or it may facilitate incorporation of S protein into the complex.[72] In the former case, membrane bound C5b,6,7 is responsible for subsequent C8 and C9 deposition. C5b,6,7,8,9 is known as the membrane attack complex or MAC (see below). In the latter case, addition of the regulatory S protein renders the complex hydrophilic, preventing further membrane attachment. The addition of S protein to C5b,6,7 also prevents polymerization of C9 by the complex, thus minimizing futile depletion of that important protein.[14,70,72]

Membrane-bound C5b,6,7 constitutes the receptor for C8, allowing for its insertion into the hydrocarbon core of the target membrane.[18]

$$\text{C5b,6,7} + \text{C8} \xrightarrow{\qquad} \text{C5b,6,7,8}$$

The C5b,6,7,8 complex forms small transmembrane channels in the target cell that can slowly lyse heterologous erythrocyte targets[44] and, at high multiplicity, may kill nucleated cells.[57] Its greatest effect, however, lies in its ability to facilitate polymerization of C9,[71] inducing the formation of an unfolding tubular structure[57] known as poly C9,[71] and its propensity to allow the polymerizing molecule to insert into the cell membrane. Transmembrane channels formed by C8/C9 interaction vary in size depending on the number of C9 subunits to a maximum of $\sim$100Å in diameter.[57]

Several mechanisms apparently contribute to the MAC-mediated destruction of cellular targets. Displacement of membrane constituents may contribute simply by effecting physical derangement of vital components of the cell.[70] Lysozyme destruction of the peptidoglycan layer may be facilitated by transmembrane pores.[70] Within minutes of complement activation, target cell membranes become permeable to small molecules,[67] resulting in an increased intracellular Ca^{++} concentration which may be harmful or may actually trigger the cell's defenses[57] (see below), while allowing the escape of vital ions such as Na^+ and K^+. Rapid depletion of cellular energy becomes evident,[15] and accompanies rapid dissipation of membrane potential. If the cell cannot maintain its osmotic pressure, it swells and may burst. Evidence suggests that the contribution of these and other factors may differ with each instance, depending in part on the nature of the target cell itself.

Recently, the mechanisms by which cells and organisms escape destruction by the

Table 6–2. Human Complement Components II: Regulators

	Component Name
of Classical Pathway:	C1 Esterase Inhibitor (C1INH)*
	C4 Binding Protein (C4bp)*
	Factor H*
	Factor I*
	Decay-Accelerating Factor (DAF)+
	Complement Receptor 1 (CR1)+
	Membrane Cofactor Protein (MCP)+
of Alternative Pathway:	Factor P (Properdin)*
	Factor I*
	Factor H*
	Nephritic Factor (C3Nef)*
	Decay-Accelerating Factor (DAF)+
	Complement Receptor 1 (CR1)+
	Membrane Cofactor Protein (MCP)+
of Terminal Complement Cascade:	S Protein*
	C8 Binding Protein (C8bp)*
	Homologous Restriction Factor (HRF)*
	Glycophorin+
of Anaphylatoxins/ Chemotaxins:	Anaphylatoxin Inactivator (ANA* INA; Carboxypeptidase N)
	Chemotaxic Factor Inactivator (CFI)*

* Components are proteins, present in human plasma
+ Components are cell bound molecules

MAC have been under scrutiny. Cells autologous to the activated complement appear to be protected from lysis[38] by proteins such as C8 binding protein (C8bp),[83] C9 binding protein (C9bp)[101] and/or homologous restriction factor (HRF).[57,101] Allogeneic cells such as yeast may be the target of early complement activation, yet they lack the lipid bilayers required for effective C5b,6,7 binding.[70] Other organisms have shielded lipid bilayers, such that they are protected from C5b,6,7 attachment. Glycophorins in cell membranes have been shown to inhibit attachment of C5b,6,7 to the membrane.[80] The lytic effect of complement may, in fact, depend on the ability of antibody to target vulnerable membrane

areas.[24] Some organisms[51] have the ability to shed,[24,70] or endocytose[55] the MAC, effectively removing it from the cell membrane. In some cases, thresholds of permeability to the MAC appear to occur,[67] wherein mild attacks may trigger repair and result in cell recovery while more intense attacks lead to destruction.[56]

COMPLEMENT RECEPTORS[76]

Many cells of the body carry surface proteins that act as receptor sites for cleavage products of complement activation (Table 6–3). Although several of these function as important components of host defense mechanisms,[84] these and some others may also function as regulators of immune responsiveness.[93]

The C1q receptor is found on mononuclear phagocytes, neutrophils, many subsets of lymphocytes, lymphoblastoid cell lines, platelets, endothelial cells, fibroblasts, and epithelial cells.[4,27] When the receptor recognizes the collagenous tail portion of free C1q, binding results in enhancement of IgG/Fc$_r$ receptor-induced phagocytosis,[4,53] i.e. when both receptors (C1qR and Fc$_\gamma$R) and both molecules (free C1q and IgG) are present, cooperative boosting of phagocytosis and triggering of a respiratory burst are evident.[76]

CR1 receptors, first definitively described by Nelson in 1953,[59] can be found on erythrocytes, B lymphocytes, some T lymphocytes, platelets, eosinophils, mast cells, null cells, follicular dendritic cells, and glomerular podocytes (epithelial cells).[19,21,99] The receptor binds reversibly to the C3c portion of C3b and iC3b and to C4b and iC4b fragments, whether they appear on foreign or altered cells, on immune complexes, or on microorganisms.

Although the physiologic importance of this receptor is still under investigation, some aspects of its function are apparent. For example, CR1 receptor binding is a poor inducer of ingestion by receptor-bearing phagocytes.[81] In conjunction with the Fc$_\gamma$ receptor and IgG, or in the presence of fi-

Table 6–3. Cell Receptors for Human Complement Components

Name of Receptor	Synonym(s)	Complement Component Bound	Cell Type
C1q Receptor[27]	------	C1q	mononuclear phagocytes, neutrophils, some lymphocytes, platelets, endothelial cells, fibroblasts, epithelial cells
CR1[21,81,99]	immune adherence receptor, C3b receptor	C3c portion of C3b, iC3b; C4b, iC4b	erythrocytes, B cells, some T cells, null cells, platelets, eosinophils, mast cells, follicular dendritic cells, glomerular podocytes
CR2[96]	C3d receptor	C3d portion of C3b, iC3b, C3dg and C3d	B cells, (others)
CR3[3,88]	iC3b receptor	iC3b, (C3dg, C3d)	mononuclear phagocytes, granulocytes, large granular lymphocytes
"CR4"[76,77]	P150,95	iC3b, C3dg, C3d	mononuclear phagocytes, neutrophils, NK and ADCC-effector lymphocytes
DAF[16]	------	C3b, C4b	erythrocytes, mononuclear phagocytes, T cells, B cells, neutrophils, platelets, endothelial cells
Factor H Receptor[58]	------	Factor H	B cells, neutrophils, mononuclear phagocytes
C3e Receptor	------	C3e	(implied on neutrophils, mononuclear phagocytes)
C3a Receptor[39,42]	------	C3a, C3e, C4a	mast cells, vascular endothelium, eosinophils, basophils
C5a Receptor[39,40,42]	------	C5a, C5a des Arg	neutrophils, mast cells, eosinophils, basophils, implied on mononuclear phagocytes, some T cells

bronectin, however, it becomes an effective stimulator of phagocytosis,[23,76] particularly of encapsulated organisms.[44] Coincident exposure of neutrophils to C5a greatly enhances the concentration of CR1 and CR3 receptors on the cells.[81] Stimulation of CR1 receptors on B cells may play a role in regulation of immunoglobulin synthesis.[13,87] On dendritic cells, antigen sequestering is probably enhanced by the presence of the receptor.[87]

On erythrocytes, the CR1 receptor functions as an important mediator of immune complex size and deposition[11,12] (see *Biologic Activity of Complement Components*). CR1 receptors on erythrocytes are reduced in numbers in patients with certain immune complex diseases,[28] in patients with AIDS related complex (ARC),[28] and in some types of infections.[28,89]

CR1 receptors apparently play an important role in protecting host cells from autologous lysis by complement, e.g. by enhancing factor I degradation of C3b[89] and C4b.[48,89]

CR2 receptors, previously referred to as C3d receptors, bind C3d at a site which is only poorly exposed prior to factor I cleavage of C3b to iC3b. Thus, the receptor binds poorly to C3b, but effectively to iC3b, C3dg, and C3d. The receptors are present on 80 to 90% of B cells,[76,96] particularly on mature cells, but are lost when differentiation to plasma cells occurs. There is also some evidence of the presence of CR2 on follicular dendritic cells and on a small set of the cells active in antibody-dependent cellular cytotoxicity (ADCC).[76]

CR2 is coincident with the membrane attachment point for Epstein-Barr virus,[22,60] although the virus apparently binds at a different site on the receptor.

The function of CR2 has not, as yet, been defined, although a modulatory effect on lymphocyte proliferation has been suggested.[58,68]

CR3 refers to a family of proteins,[3] found on monocytes, macrophages, granulocytes, and large granular lymphocytes (LGLS),[88] which play a role in surface adhesion, spreading and aggregation of phagocytic cells. As such, they are functionally and structurally similar to the Mac-1 and LFA-1 molecules described on phagocytes.[87,88] These molecules function as receptors for complement degradation products, particularly fixed iC3b. A lower affinity for C3dg and C3d is also apparent,[26] and the receptors can bind with certain polysaccharides capable of alternative pathway activation, e.g. zymosan. Unlike CR1 and CR2 ligand binding, CR3 binding requires both Mg^{++} and Ca^{++}.

Observations of patients who apparently lack CR3[2] define an impressive role for these molecules in phagocytic function.[88] Leukocytes of these patients are lacking a variety of adhesion-dependent functions, such as chemotaxis, surface adherence, and aggregation as well as demonstrating deficiencies in C3R-mediated phagocytosis and degradation of iC3b-opsonized particles.

Although not as well characterized, CR4 receptors, found on monocytes, neutrophils, and NK and ADCC effector lymphocytes, have also been shown to bind to and mediate clearance of iC3b-, C3dg-, and C3d-opsonized particles.[76,77]

Decay-accelerating factor (DAF) is a membrane protein which, with the CR1 receptor, acts to protect autologous bystander cells from complement activation.[16] DAF is present on erythrocytes,[64] monocytes, peripheral blood and tonsillar T and B lymphocytes, neutrophils, platelets, and endothelial cells,[16] where it binds reversibly to C3b or C4b fragments on cell membranes, and competitively inhibits C2 or factor B uptake. This action effectively blocks both

C3 convertases and subsequent pathway activation.

Receptors for factor H may be found on B lymphocytes, neutrophils, and monocytes.[58] Attachment of complex-associated or fluid phase factor H to these receptors on B cells triggers release of intrinsic factor I, as well as inducing blastogenesis of the cells with subsequent immunoglobulin synthesis.[76] Functional significance of factor H receptors on phagocytes has yet to be well defined.[76,87]

Receptors for C3e on neutrophils and monocytes are implied by the ability of C3e to induce leukocytosis and enzyme release from isolated neutrophils.[76]

For a discussion of C3a and C5a receptors, see *Biologic Activity of Complement Components*.

BIOLOGIC ACTIVITY OF COMPLEMENT COMPONENTS[28,81]

The lytic action of complement on target cells, while important in the defense against microbial invasion and in certain autoimmune disorders, represents only a portion of the physiologic effects mediated by the complement system. Sequential activation of the classical and/or alternative pathways, with subsequent involvement of the terminal cascade, results in several cleavage products which have biologic significance.

C4, C3, and C5 are homologous molecules, sharing not only physical, but also biologic properties. During sequential activation, or as a result of the action of noncomplement proteases such as trypsin,[8] these molecules are split, with the smaller fragments, C4a, C3a, and C5a, being released into the environment while the larger portions, C4b, C3b, and C5b, tend to bind and continue in the activation sequences. Collectively, these fragments have significant effects on phagocytes, on anaphylaxis, and in inflammation. They play a role in immunoregulation and are of major importance in the metabolism of immune complexes. C4a, C3a, and C5a are known as the *anaphylatoxins*,[8] in reference to their ability to cause smooth muscle contraction, enhance secretion of mucus by airway goblet cells, increase vascular permeability, and induce the release of histamine from basophils and mast cells.[39] C5a is the most potent anaphylatoxin; C4a the least effective.[8] The anaphylatoxin designation, although accurate, is not encompassing, given the other activities, described in the following paragraphs, which are attributed to these molecules.

Regulation of C4a, C3a, and C5a is the responsibility of an inactivator, found in serum, known as carboxypeptidase N or the anaphylatoxin inactivator. In the presence of this enzyme, C4a and C3a fragments rapidly lose the COOH-terminal arginine, converting them to inactive derivatives designated C4 des Arg and C3 des Arg, respectively.[42] In effect, the physiologic significance of C4a and C3a is probably limited in scope to only localized areas as a result of this regulatory mechanism. Although C5a is also targeted by carboxypeptidase N, a small proportion of the molecules may escape its action.[8] Additionally, the C5a des Arg formed by the enzyme's action on C5a retains the anaphylatoxin properties of the C5a molecule, albeit at a reduced level of activity.[8]

C4a, C3a, and C5a apparently function via high affinity attachment to specific receptors on cell surfaces. C3a and C4a bind to the C3a receptor (C3aR);[21,42] C5a and C5a des Arg, to the C5a receptor (C5aR).[39,40,42] These receptors have been described on neutrophils, eosinophils, basophils, monocytes to some extent, smooth muscle cells and vascular endothelium, platelets, and presumably certain T cell subsets.[28,42,81] The anaphylatoxin activity of these molecules apparently results in part from direct stimulation of receptors on mast cells, basophils, and/or vascular endothelium.[39,42] The anaphylatoxin activity of C5a des Arg, and to some degree C5a, is a function of its ability to stimulate neutrophils to release leukotrienes,[45,98] e.g. slow-reacting substance of anaphylaxis (SRS-A).[45,79,98]

The effects of complement split products[42,45] on phagocytosis are numerous and varied. Phagocytes, particularly neutrophils, are stimulated by attachment of C5a or C5a des Arg to the C5a receptor,[40] which is then internalized and degraded.[23] Similar activity may result transiently by the interaction of C3a, C4a, or C3e with the C3a receptor.[42] The cell responds with enhanced aggregation and adherence to surfaces such as endothelium, which, in turn, increases the ability of the cell to glide over such surfaces.[42]

Neutrophils, basophils, eosinophils and mononuclear phagocytes respond to C5a and C5a des Arg by directed locomotion (*chemotaxis*) toward the source of the activation. Lymphocyte derived chemotactic factors, e.g. eosinophil chemotactic factor of anaphylaxis, may act in synergism with C5a and C5a des Arg to enhance this activity. Simultaneously, phagocytes undergo an oxidative burst, resulting in increased production of factors such as IL-1 (monocytes),[63] hydrolytic enzymes, neutrophil chemotactic factor (monocytes), and platelet activating factors.[28] Degranulation occurs in granulocytes, e.g. neutrophils and basophils.[79] C3e may stimulate the release of neutrophils from bone marrow, and may itself induce leukocytosis.[79]

The fragments designated C4b, C3b, and iC3b may further stimulate phagocytic activity via a phenomenon known as *opsonization* or *immune adherence*. Complement activation, whether on immune complexes, particles, or target cells, generates and deposits these fragments which are subsequently capable of attachment to the CR1 receptor (see *Complement Receptors*) on phagocytes, erythrocytes, and platelets. Antigens which become attached to red blood cells or platelets are easier prey for mononuclear phagocytes in the liver or spleen,[23] while adherence of complement-coated antigen directly to phagocytes presumably enhances the probability of ingestion.

Complement-derived fragments also exert dynamic effects on T lymphocytes, simultaneously affecting both humoral and cell mediated immune responses.[42,95] The presence of C3a suppresses both specific (T-dependent) and polyclonal antibody formation, probably as a result of its effect on helper T lymphocytes. C5a and C5a des Arg, when present, counteract and override the effect of C3a working via helper cells to enhance these same activities.[42,94] Additionally, complement fragments may enhance proliferative responses of lymphocytes.[17,42]

Antibody-mediated cellular cytotoxicity (ADCC) by K cells may be enhanced by complement fragment binding of the target cell to the CR1 receptor on the K cell;[68] iC3b appears especially capable of this activity.

Immune complexes are formed in the body whenever such substances as soluble drugs, food, microbial, or host cell antigens react with appropriate antibody.[62] Activation of complement by such complexes serves to prevent formation of insoluble complexes by facilitating early disposal.[25,82] Current belief is that this is accomplished by the CR1 receptor on red blood cells. RBC-CR1 attachment to C3 fragments sequesters circulating immune complexes and transports them to the liver or spleen.[11,12,23,92] Complexes and the CR1 receptor are stripped, without damage to the red cell,[78] by macrophages in those organs. If complement is absent in situations where immune complexes form, deposition of those complexes in organs vulnerable to injury results.[92] The importance of complement as a mediator of tissue damage in immune complex diseases, e.g. systemic lupus erythrematosus (SLE), or in infections like leprosy or AIDS where cell-mediated immunity is impaired,[89] has been implied by significant decreases in CR1 receptors on the erythrocytes of patients with these disorders.[23,78,87]

REFERENCES

1. Alper, C.A., Johnson, A.M., Birtch, A.G., and Moore, F.D.: Science, 163:286, 1969.

2. Anderson, D.C. et al.: J. Infect. Dis., 152:668, 1985.

3. Arnaout, M.A., Pierce, M.W., Dana, N., and Clayton, L.K.: Methods Enzymol., 150:602, 1987.

4. Bobak, D.A., Gaither, T., Frank, M.M., and Tenner, A.J.: J. Immunol., 138:1150, 1987.

5. Campbell, R.D.: Br. Med. Bull., 43:37, 1987.

6. Carroll, M.C., and Alper, C.A.: Br. Med. Bull., 43:50, 1987.

7. Carroll, M.C. et al.: Proc. Natl. Acad. Sci. U.S.A., 84:8535, 1987.

*8. Chenoweth, D.E., In Immunobiology of the Complement System. Edited by G.D. Ross. London, Academic Press, 1986.

9. Colten, H.R., and Dowton, S.B.: Biochem. Soc. Symp., 51:37, 1986.

10. Colomb, M., and Arlaud, G.: J. Mol. Biol., 195:435, 1987.

11. Cornacoff, J.B., Hebert, L.A., Birmingham, D.J., and Waxman, F.J.: Clin. Immunol. Immunopathol., 30:255, 1984.

12. Cornacoff, J.F. et al.: J. Clin. Invest., 71:236, 1983.

13. Daha, M.R., Bloem, A.C., and Ballieux, R.E.: J. Immunol., 132:1197, 1984.

14. Dahlbach, B., and Podack, E.R.: Biochemistry, 24:2368, 1985.

15. Dankert, J.R., and Esser, A.F.: Biochem. J., 244:393, 1987.

16. Davitz, M.A.: Acta. Med. Scand. Suppl., 715:111, 1987.

17. Dierich, M.P. et al.: Immunol. Lett., 14:235, 1987.

18. DiScipio, R.G., Chakravarti, D.N., Muller-Eberhard, H.J., and Fey, G.H.: J. Biol. Chem., 263:549, 1988.

19. Fearon, D.T.: J. Exp. Med., 152:20, 1980.

20. Fearon, D.T., and Austen, K.F.: J. Exp. Med., 142:856, 1975.

21. Fearon, D.T.: Immunol. Today, 5:105, 1984.

22. Fingeroth, J.D., et al.: Proc. Natl. Acad. Sci. U.S.A., 81:4510, 1984.

*23. Frank, M.M.: N. Engl. J. Med., 316:1525, 1987.

24. Frank, M.M., Joiner, K., and Hammer, C.: Rev. Infect. Dis., 9 Suppl., 5:S537, 1987.

25. Fries, L.F., Siwik, S.A., Malbran, A., and Frank, M.M.: Immunology, 62:45, 1987.

26. Gaither, T.A., Vargas, I., Inada, S., and Frank, M.M.: Immunology, 62:405, 1987.

27. Ghebrehiwet, B.: Methods Enzymol., 150:558, 1987.

*28. Gigli, I.: Biochem. Soc. Symp., 51:1, 1986.

29. Gigli, I., Fujita, T., and Nussenzweig, V.: Proc. Natl. Acad. Sci. U.S.A., 76:6596, 1979.

30. Griffiss, J.M., and Jarvis, G.A.: Adv. Exp. Med. Biol., 216B:1303, 1987.

31. Hamilton, A.O., Jones, L., Morrison, L., and Whaley, K.: Biochem. J., 242:809, 1987.

32. Hartung, H.P., and Hadding, U.: Springer Semin. Immunopathol., 6:283, 1983.

33. Hetland, G., Johnson, E., and Aasebo, U.: Scand. J. Immunol., 24:603, 1986.

34. Hetland, G., Johnson, E., Royset, P., and Eskeland, T.: Acta Pathol. Microbiol. Immunol. Scand., 95C:117, 1987.

35. Hetland, G., Johnson, E., Falk, R.J., and Eskeland, T.: Scand. J. Immunol., 24:421, 1986.

36. Hiemstra, P.S. et al.: Adv. Exp. Med. Biol., 216B:1297, 1987.

37. Hiemstra, P.S. et al.: Eur. J. Immunol., *17*:321, 1987.

38. Houle, J.J., Hoffman, E.M., and Esser, A.F.: Blood, *71*:280, 1988.

39. Huey, R., Fukuoka, Y., Hoeprich, P.D., Jr., and Hugli, T.E.: Biochem. Soc. Symp., *51*:69, 1986.

40. Huey, R., and Hugle, T.E.: Methods Enzymol., *150*:615, 1987.

*41. Hughes-Jones, N.C.: In *Immunobiology of the Complement System*. Edited by G.D. Ross. London, Academic Press, 1986.

42. Hugli, T.E., and Morgan, E.L.: Contemp. Top. Immunobiol., *14*:109, 1984.

43. Ikeda, K. et al.: J. Biol. Chem., *262*:7451, 1987.

44. Joiner, K.A., Fries, L.F., and Frank, M.M.: Immunol. Lett., *14*:197, 1987.

45. Jose, P.J.: Br. Med. Bull., *43*:336, 1987.

46. Katz, Y., Cole, F.S., and Strunk, R.C.: J. Exp. Med., *167*:1, 1988.

47. Kim, S.H., Carney, D.F., Hammer, C.H.,and Shin, M.L.: J. Immunol., *138*:1530, 1987.

48. Kinoshita, T., Medof, M.E., Hong, K., and Nussenzweig, V.: J. Exp. Med., *164*:1377, 1986.

49. Lakatos, S.: Biochem. Biophys. Res. Commun., *149*:378, 1987.

50. Laurell, A.B., Martensson, U., and Sjoholm, A.G.: J. Immunol., *139*:4145, 1987.

51. Loos, M., (ed.): Bacteria and Complement, Curr. Top. Microbiol. Immunol., *121*:1985.

52. Lotz, M., and Zuraw, B.L.: J. Immunol., *139*:3382, 1987.

53. Mocharla, R., Mocharla, H., and Leu, R.W.: Cell. Immunol., *105*:127, 1987.

54. Mollnes, T.E., and Harboe, M.: Scand. J. Immunol., *26*:381, 1987.

55. Morgan, B.P., Dankert, J.R., and Esser, A.F.: J. Immunol., *138*:246, 1987.

56. Morgan, B.P., Luzio, J.P., and Campbell, A.K.: Cell Calcium, *7*:399, 1986.

57. Müller-Eberhard, H.J. et al.: J. Rheumatol. (14 Suppl.), *13*:28, 1987.

58. Myanes, B.L., and Ross, G.D.: Methods Enzymol., *150*:586, 1987.

59. Nelson, R.A., Jr.: Science, *118*:733, 1953.

60. Nemerow, G.R., and Cooper, N.R.: Proc. Natl. Acad. Sci. U.S.A., *81*:4955, 1984.

61. Nicholson-Weller, A., Burge, J., and Austen, K.F.: J. Immunol., *127*:2035, 1981.

62. Nydegger, U.E., and Kazatchkine, M.D.: Prog. Allergy, *39*:361, 1986.

63. Okusawa, S. et al.: J. Immunol., *139*:2635, 1987.

*64. Pangburn, M.K.: In *Immunobiology of the Complement System*, Edited by G.D. Ross. London, Academic Press, 1986.

65. Pangburn, M.K., and Müller-Eberhard, H.J.: Springer Semin. Immunopathol., *7*:163, 1984.

66. Pangburn, M.K., Schreiber, R.D., and Müller-Eberhard, H.J.: J. Exp. Med., *146*:257, 1977.

67. Patel, A.K., and Campbell, A.K.: Immunology,*60*:135, 1987.

68. Perlmann, H., Perlmann, P., Schreiber, R.D., and Müller-Eberhard, H.J.: J. Exp. Med., *153*:1592, 1981.

69. Petterson, H.B., Johnson, E., and Hetland, G.: Scand. J. Immunol., *25*:567, 1987.

*70. Podack, E.R.: In *Immunobiology of the Complement System*. Edited by G.D. Ross. London, Academic Press, 1986.

71. Podak, E.R., Tschopp, J., and Müller-Eberhard, H.J.: J. Exp. Med., *156*:268, 1982.

72. Preissner, K.T., Wassmuth, R., and Muller-Bershaus, G.: Biochem. J., *231*:349, 1985.

73. Pryzdial, E.L., and Isenman, D.E.: J. Biol. Chem., *263*:1733, 1988.

74. Ratnoff, O.D., Pensky, J., Ogston, D., and Naff, G.B.: J. Exp. Med., *129*:315, 1969.

75. Ripoche, J., Day, A.J., Harris, T.J.R., and Sims, R.B.: Biochem. J., *249*:593, 1988.

*76. Ross, G.D.: In *Immunobiology of the Complement System*. Edited by G.D. Ross. London, Academic Press, 1986.

77. Ross, G.D., and Medof, M.E.: Adv. Immunol., *37*:217, 1985.

78. Ross, G.D. et al.: Arthritis Rheum., *27*:S28, 1984.

79. Ross, S.C., and Densen, P.: Medicine, *63*:243, 1984.

*80. Rother, K., and Rother, U.: Prog. Allergy, *39*:8, 1986.

81. Rother, K., and Rother, U.: Prog. Allergy, *39*:24, 1986.

82. Schifferli, J.A.: Immunol. Lett., *14*:225, 1987.

83. Schönermark, G. et al.: J. Immunol., *136*:1772, 1986.

84. Schreiber, R.D.: Springer Semin. Immunopathol., *7*:221, 1984.

85. Shulman, M.J., Collins, C., Pennell, N., and Hozumi, N.: Eur. J. Immunol., *17*:549, 1987.

86. Schultz, T.F. et al.: Eur. J. Immunol., *16*:1351, 1986.

87. Sim, R.B., Malhotra, V., Day, A.J., and Erdei, A.: Immunol. Lett., *14*:183, 1987.

88. Springer, T.A., and Anderson, D.C.: Biochem. Soc. Symp., *51*:47, 1986.

89. Tausk, F.A., Schreiber, R.D., and Gigli, I.: Trans. Assoc. Am. Physicians, *97*:346, 1984.

90. Vukajlovich, S.W., Hoffman, J., and Morrison, D.C.: Mol. Immunol., *24*:319, 1987.

91. Warren, H.B., Pantazis, P., and Davies, P.F.: Am. J. Pathol., *129*:9, 1987.

92. Waxman, L.A. et al.: J. Clin. Invest. *74*:1329, 1984.

93. Weigle, W.O. et al.: Springer Semin. Immunopathol. *6*:173, 1983.

94. Weigle, W.O. et al.: Fed. Proc. *41*:3099, 1982.

95. Weiler, J.M.: In *Complement in Health and Disease*. Edited by K. Whaley. Lancaster, MTP Press Ltd., 1987.

96. Weis, J.J., Tedder, T.F., and Fearon, D.T.: Proc. Natl. Acad. Sci. U.S.A., *81*:881, 1984.

97. Weiss, V., Fauser, C., and Engel, J.: J. Mol. Biol., *189*:573, 1986.

98. Williamson, L.M., Sheppard, K., Davies, J.M., and Fletcher, J.: Br. J. Haematol., *64*:375, 1986.

99. Wong, W.W., and Fearon, D.T.: Methods Enzymol., *150*:579, 1987.

100. Zabern, I., and Nolte, R.: Int. Arch. Allergy Appl. Immunol., *84*:178, 1987.

101. Zalman, L.S., Wood, L.M., and Müller-Eberhard, H.J.: Proc. Natl. Acad. Sci. U.S.A., *83*:6975, 1986.

COMPLEMENT ABNORMALITIES

The genetic sites for the coding of complement components have been under investigation in recent years. Research in this area has resulted in the mapping of several of the genes responsible for component production; coding for C3, for example, is linked to that of the Lewis blood group system and the secretor ABH site on chromosome #19, while genetic sites for the determination of C2, factor B (Bf), and the two genes comprising the structure of C4 may be found in the major histocompatibility complex on chromosome #6, between the class I (HLA-A,B,C) and class II (HLA-D) loci.[1,8] (See also Chap 13.) In parallel with these observations, an understanding of structural polymorphism in the majority of complement components[1] is leading to intense study of genetic patterns of inheritance, genetic linkages, and their association with susceptibility to disease. Several aspects of this work appear to be especially promising: the location, nature, and inheritance patterns of deficiencies of individual complement components, the relationship of individual component deficiency states with observable disease associations, the effects of genetic alleles, or their expression, on complement activity and immune function, and the relationship between complement and autoimmune diseases.

Inheritance of allelic variants of all components appears to be autosomal codominant, with the exception of properdin,[41,53] which appears to be X-linked recessive.[1,2,43] For some components, particularly those comprising the C3 convertases (C4, C2, and Bf) and those affecting regulation, the degree of polymorphism is similar to that seen with the HLA A, B, and C loci. Linkages among these more highly polymorphic alleles[8,16] appear to be remarkably stable and may be associated with increased susceptibility to certain diseases.[3,28]

Congenital Abnormalities[1,2,45]

Deficiency states have been described for every human complement component[33,43,44,50] and cellular receptor.[5,29] In most instances, deficiency occurs as a result of a silent or "null" allele at the structural locus which encodes that component.[1] In other cases, abnormal alleles may appear as dysfunctional molecules.[33] Incomplete deficiencies, or reduced amounts of a component, may result from inheritance of a single null allele[30] or from some other as yet undescribed abnormality.[51] With components which are composed of multiple chains, e.g. C4, which has both an alpha and a beta chain in the normal individual, deficiency can result from the lack of coding for either unit.[1,30] It should be noted that in most cases of component deficiency states, only the concentration of the affected component is low or absent; in exceptional situations, however, defects may also be observed in other components.[2]

The frequency of component deficiencies in the general population is low.[30,43] Demonstrably higher frequencies can be seen among persons with collagen vascular disease or those with recurrent infections. Worldwide, disparities among ethnic groups have also been observed.[33,43] Among Americans of African descent for example, only C5–C8 deficiencies have been described to date. C2 deficiencies are relatively common among caucasoids, but are not seen in Japanese populations. By contrast, C9 deficiency is relatively common in Japan.[33]

Several good reviews of known complement deficiencies are available in the literature.[33,37,43,50]

Although some individuals with genetic dysfunctions or deletions of complement components enjoy good health over their lifetime, defects are often associated with an increase in the frequency of pyogenic infections.[33,43] In addition, strong associations may be made between deficiencies within functional groups of complement and certain disease states. Deficiency among components of the classical pathway, for example, are associated with autoimmune disorders, particularly systemic lupus erythematosus (SLE),[1,14,43,46] subacute cutaneous lupus erythematosus (SCLE),[7] discoid lupus, and glomerulonephritis,[43,50] suggesting a failure to effectively metabolize immune complexes in these patients.[6,32,33,46] C2 deficiencies appear twice as often as other defects; 1/10,000 are affected.[7,33,43,46] Even among heterozygous C2-deficient individuals, SLE or other autoimmune disorders occur with increased frequency.[33] Patients lacking appropriate coding for either of the structural chains which comprise C4 (C4A or C4B) have increased risk of developing SLE-like syndromes.[24] It may be significant that a high frequency of anti-Ro (SS-A) antibodies are associated with C4-deficient SLE syndromes.[24,46] Most individuals with homozygous C3 deficiency suffer the increased risk of bacterial infections and immune complex disease.[1,2,14]

Among the components of the alternative pathway, X-linked properdin (P) deficiencies are associated with recurrent meningococcal meningitis, which follow a fulminant course and have high fatality rates.[17,34] Deficiencies of Factor D are extremely rare but do appear to predispose patients to repeated infections.[33,50]

Deficiencies of Factor I or Factor H result in functional depletion of C3 and Factor B, due to excessive activation of the alternative pathway feedback, or amplification, loop.[50] Recurrent infections and immune complex diseases are common disease manifestations.[1,2,14,50]

Defects in the terminal complement components (C5–C9) induce an increased propensity for systemic Neisseria infections,[23,38,54] e.g. meningococcal meningitis or disseminated gonococcal disease.[1,2,23] Among this group, C9 deficiency carries the lowest risk for these infections.[36] Autoimmune disorders occur in these patients, albeit less frequently than in individuals with defects in early-acting components.[23,38,43,54]

Deficient phagocytosis by neutrophils often results from a genetic deficiency in that cell's CR3 receptor. Recurrent bacterial infections are associated with this defect.[42]

Hereditary Angioedema[31]

Hereditary angioedema (HAE), previously designated hereditary angioneurotic edema, is an inherited disorder induced by an inborn defect in the plasma protein known as C1 inhibitor (C1-INH). Clinically, HAE is characterized by recurrent attacks of acute, noninflammatory edema, which can occur in any tissue, but appears most often in subcutaneous and mucosal areas. Subcutaneous edema appears to spread outward from a single site, and may evolve to a few centimeters in diameter, or may progress to include an entire limb. Mucosal surfaces of the gastrointestinal tract are often affected (> 90% of cases),[1,31] manifesting as abdominal pain, usually with vomiting and diarrhea. Patients may appear to be suffering from food allergies, appendicitis, or acute gastrointestinal obstruction, and unnecessary surgery may result. The only known fatal complication of HAE is death by asphyxiation, a result of the respiratory obstruction that can occur when laryngeal or pharyngeal tissue is involved. Abdominal attacks may last 1 to 3 days to a week, while subcutaneous edema progresses for up to 48 hours, then subsides over a 48 to 72-hour period. Although many attacks are without apparent cause, local tissue trauma, especially of the head and neck region (tooth extraction, surgery), prolonged pressure or vibrations, emotional stress, and overexposure to sunlight have been noted as exacerbating attacks. Symptoms usually do not appear until late childhood, and may disappear with age.[2]

Normally, C1-INH is a glycoprotein molecule that migrates as an alpha-2 globulin and is maintained at plasma concentrations of 15 to 35 mg/100 ml. It is the only known inhibitor of C1r and C1s, two of the three initiating molecules of the classical pathway of complement. In addition, C1-INH inhibits enzymes involved in coagulation, fibrinolysis, and in kinin generation (e.g. activated Hageman factor, plasmin, kallikrein).[2,22,31] Although the precise role(s) of C1-INH in the latter metabolic systems are yet to be clarified, there is some evidence that a plasmin-modified fragment of C2 (C2-Kinin), or perhaps prekallikrein activation, is responsible for HAE symptoms.[2,18,25,31] In addition, local depletion of the C1-INH molecules at sites of complement activation favors continual cleavage of C4 and C2 molecules, with resultant activation, cleavage, and depletion of those components.[2,33] Association of HAE with systemic lupus erythematosus (SLE) or SLE-like syndromes in these patients may occur as a result of the consumptive depletion of the C4 and C2 components.[31] C3 levels in individuals with HAE are normal, perhaps because fluid phase activation of the complement system does not encourage formation of the C3 convertase.[3]

Two forms of hereditary angioedema have been described. Both appear to be due to point mutations inducing DNA rearrangement on one of the two structural genes for C1-INH.[9,21,49] Approximately 85% of the families reported have the "protein deficient" form of the disease which manifests as low concentrations (5 to 31%) of functionally normal C1-INH.[1,31] Decreased synthesis, rather than increased catabolism, induces the deficiency. The remaining 15% of kindreds have what is referred to as the "dysfunctional form," with normal to increased concentrations of antigenically normal C1-INH, most of which is, however, functionally abnormal.[21,31] Both are inherited in an autosomal dominant fashion; therefore, affected individuals are heterozygous for the defect they carry.

Clinical manifestations similar to those seen with congenital C1-INH deficiency have also been described in patients with an acquired, non-familial deficiency of the protein.[4,12,22,31,48] Associated with B cell abnormalities such as lymphosarcoma, Waldenström's macroglobulinemia, multiple myeloma, chronic lymphocytic leukemia and B cell lymphomas, acquired deficiencies appear to be the result of increased catabolism rather than of decreased synthesis, as is seen in congenital HAE. Patients with acquired C1-INH deficiency are usually elderly and may be asymptomatic, or symptoms of angioedema may precede evidence of the corresponding tumor by up to three years.[31]

Diagnosis of hereditary angioedema or of the acquired form of C1-INH deficiency must involve differentiation of these from the many other causes of angioedema. The absence of urticaria is a useful clinical indication, while a history of familial inheritance or coexistence with a B cell tumor may be helpful in the diagnosis of hereditary and acquired angioedema, respectively.[31] Altogether, C1-INH deficiency probably accounts for less than 1% of the cases of angioedema observed.[31] Most are idiopathic.

Differentiation among hereditary and acquired defects in C1-INH may be made with the use of immunochemical assays for complement components (e.g. radial immunodiffusion, nephelometry). In the protein deficient form of HAE, C1 and C3 levels are normal while C4 and C2 levels are decreased. C1-INH is found in low concentrations. The dysfunctional form differs from the protein deficient form in that C1-INH antigen levels remain normal. In cases of acquired C1-INH deficiency, C1 levels decrease in conjunction with C4, C2, C1-INH. Only C3 levels remain normal. Functional assays for C1-INH activity may also be helpful in the diagnosis.[31]

Prior to the advent of effective treatment for HAE, 25 to 54% of patients died, most commonly as a result of laryngeal edema.[31] More recently, administration of lyophilized C1-INH, or prophylactic treatment with androgenic steroids, for example, have made normal life expectancy possible.[10,31,33]

Acquired Abnormalities

Elevations in the serum concentration of certain complement components, e.g. C3, may occur in acute phase reactions, such as those that accompany inflammation, tissue damage, or infection. These acquired elevations are usually transient and concentrations return to normal when the inciting situation is resolved. An inherent difficulty in the interpretation of quantitative complement levels occurs when acute phase production of components, and catabolism due to pathway activation, happen simultaneously. In such situations, quantitative test results will reflect the influence of both processes.

Decreases in complement components are seen in many diverse situations. Components may, for example, be catabolized as a result of a genetic deficiency of a related inhibitory component, e.g. as C4 and C2 are often catabolized in the absence of C1-INH. Individuals who develop the disease known as paroxysmal nocturnal hemoglobinuria (PNH),[15,35] produce erythrocytes lacking decay-accelerating factor (DAF) and homologous restriction factor (HRF),[26] rendering the cells exquisitely sensitive to complement activation via the alternative pathway. Chronic activation in such diseases results in depressed levels of the components involved.

Immunoconglutinins (IK) are autoantibodies directed against components of the complement system which are "fixed," or bound to a surface.[13] While most of the immunoconglutinins described lack any association with disease,[13] autoantibodies directed against C3 convertases from both the classical and alternative pathways are related to pathologic conditions. C3 nephritic factor (C3NeF), for example, is an unusual IgG autoantibody directed against the amplification C3/C5 convertase.[13,40] The effect of IK is stabilization of the convertase, enhancing its resistance to inactivation by inhibitors.[39] Depletion of subsequent sequential components usually occurs as a result of IK activity. Diseases associated with C3NeF are membranoproliferative glomerulonephritis (MPGN) and partial lipodystrophy (PLD).[13] Immunoconglutinins which

react with classical pathway C3 convertase have been described in patients with several diagnoses, including systemic lupus erythematosus (SLE), where its concentration can be shown to increase during clinically active disease.[13,20]

There are many clinical situations where complement, recruited by atypical or inappropriate antigen-antibody reaction, plays an integral role in disease pathogenesis. In autoimmune hemolytic anemia (AIHA), for example, complement is activated by autoantibody reacting with antigen on the patient's own erythrocytes, resulting in intra- or extravascular lysis by complement or complement-mediated phagocytosis.[35] Similar reactions accompany introduction of alloantigen on red blood cells into a sensitized individual (transfusion reactions), transplacental passage of maternal antibody into a fetus whose erythrocytes carry the corresponding antigen (hemolytic disease of the newborn, Rh disease), and drug-sensitization of red blood cells in individuals who have drug-induced antibody (drug-induced hemolytic anemia).[35] Platelets may be the target of complement activation (autoimmune thrombocytopenic purpura or ATP) as may leukocytes (agranulocytosis). In all of these instances, pathogenesis is primarily mediated by type II immunopathologic processes, as described by Coombs and Gell,[11] and reduced levels of complement components may accompany active disease.

Type III immunopathologic reactions, according to the prototype developed by Coombs and Gell, involve reaction of soluble antigen with antibody and complement in the formation of immune complexes.[52] It appears that complement plays an integral role in maintaining the solubility of immune complexes in normal situations via its ability to bind them to receptors on cells such as erythrocytes and macrophages,[6,52] triggering their removal from the system. Individuals with atypical production of autoantibodies such as those with rheumatic diseases, or those with dysfunctional complement (as described above) or cellular complement receptors, overwhelm the ability of this mechanism to remove the complexes. Inappropriate vascular deposition of complexes results, promoting the influx of inflammatory cells and subsequent inflammation and tissue damage.[6,47] Although rheumatic diseases such as systemic lupus erythematosus (SLE) and rheumatoid arthritis (RA) are prototypic examples of this type of immunopathology, patients with RA typically demonstrate elevated rather than depressed systemic complement levels as a result of the inflammatory nature of the disease (see also Chap. 11).

Transient depressions in complement components may also accompany agent-induced diseases such as hepatitis or post streptococcal glomerulonephritis.

REFERENCES

1. Alper, C.A.: Ann. N.Y. Acad. Sci., 475:32, 1986.
2. Alper, C.A.: Immunol. Lett., 14:175, 1987.
3. Alper, C.A., Awdeh, Z., Raum, D., and Yunis, E.J.: Biochem. Soc. Symp., 51:19, 1986.
4. Alsenz, J., Bork, K., and Loos, M.: N. Engl. J. Med., 316:1360, 1987.
5. Anderson, D.C. et al.: J. Infect. Dis., 152:668, 1985.
6. Atkinson, J.P. et al.: In Immunobiology of the Complement System. Edited by G.D. Ross. London, Academic Press, 1986.
7. Callen, J.P. et al.: Arch. Dermatol., 123:66, 1987.
8. Carroll, M.C. et al.: Nature, 307:237, 1984.
9. Cicardi, M. et al.: J. Clin. Invest., 80:1640, 1987.
10. Colten, H.R.: N. Engl. J. Med., 317:43, 1987.
11. Coombs, R.R.A., and Gell, P.G.H.: In Clinical Aspects of Immunology. 2nd ed. Edited by P.G.H. Gell and R.R.A. Coombs. Oxford, Blackwell Scientific Publications, 1968.
12. Cullmann, W., and Opferkuch, W.: Prog. Allergy, 39:311, 1986.
13. Daha, M.R.: In Complement in Health and Disease. Edited by K. Whaley. Lancaster, MTP Press, Ltd., 1987.
14. Day, N.K.: Prog. Allergy, 39:267, 1986.
15. Davitz, M.A.: Acta. Med. Scand. Suppl., 715:111, 1987.
16. deCordoba, S.R. et al.: J. Exp. Med., 161:1189, 1985.
17. Densen, P., Weiler, J.M., Griffis, J.McL., and Hoffman, L.G.: N. Engl. J. Med., 316:922, 1987.
18. Donaldson, V.H., Rosen, F.S., and Bing, D.H.: Trans. Assoc. Am. Physicians, 90:174, 1977.
19. Downey, E.C. et al.: J. Trauma, 27:661, 1987.

20. Durand, C.G., and Burge, J.J.: J. Immunol. Methods, 73:57, 1984.
21. Frank, M.M.: J. Allergy Clin. Immunol., 78:848, 1986.
22. Frank, M.M.: N. Engl. J. Med., 316:1525, 1987.
23. Gianella-Borradori, A., Borradori, L., and Spath, P.: Arch. Intern. Med., 148:754, 1988.
24. Hauptmann, G., Goetz, J., Uring-Lambert, B., and Grosshans, E.: Prog. Allergy, 39:232, 1986.
25. Hentges, F. et al.: J. Allergy Clin. Immunol., 78:860, 1986.
26. Houle, J.J., Hoffman, E.M., and Esser, H.F.: Blood, 71:280, 1988.
27. Hunt, L.T., Elzanowski, A., and Barker, W.C.: Biochem. Biophys. Res. Commun., 149:282, 1987.
28. Kay, P.H., and Dawkins, R.L.: In Complement in Health and Disease. Edited by K. Whaley. Lancaster, MTP Press, Ltd., 1987.
29. Kazatchkine, M.D. et al.: Immunol. Lett., 14:191, 1987.
30. Kemp, M.E. et al.: Arthritis Rheum., 30:1015, 1987.
31. Kerr, M.A., and Yeung-Laiwah, A.A.C.: In Complement in Health and Disease. Edited by K. Whaley. Lancaster, MTP Press, Ltd., 1987.
32. Lachmann, P.J.: Br. J. Rheumatol., 26:409, 1987.
33. Lachmann, P.J., and Walport, M.J.: In Immunobiology of the Complement System. Edited by G.D. Ross. Orlando, Academic Press, 1986.
34. Lancet, 1:95, 1988.
35. Leddy, J.P., and Rosenfeld, S.I.: In Immunobiology of the Complement System. Edited by G. D. Ross. Orlando, Academic Press, 1986.
36. Lint, T.F., and Gewurz, H.: Prog. Allergy, 39:307, 1986.
37. Loos, M., and Heinz, H-P.: Prog. Allergy, 39:212, 1986.
38. McCarty, G.A., and Snyderman, R.: Prog. Allergy, 39:271, 1986.
39. Mollnes, T.E. et al.: Clin. Exp. Immunol., 65:73, 1986.
40. Ng, Y.C., and Peters, D.K.: Clin. Exp. Immunol., 65:450, 1986.
41. Nielson, H.E., and Koch, C.: Clin. Immunol. Immunopathol., 44:134, 1987.
42. Ross, G.D.: Prog. Allergy, 39:352, 1986.
43. Ross, S.C., and Densen, P.: Medicine, 63:243, 1984.
44. Rother, K.: Prog. Allergy, 39:202, 1986.
45. Rother, K., and Rother, U.: Prog. Allergy, 39:1, 1986.
46. Ruddy, S.: Prog. Allergy, 39:250, 1986.
47. Sanders, M.E., et al.: J. Immunol., 138:2095, 1987.
48. Sheffer, A.L., Melamed, J., Fearon, D.T., and Austen, K.F.: J. Allergy Clin. Immunol., 71:107, 1983.
49. Stoppa-Lyonnet, D. et al.: N. Engl. J. Med., 317:1, 1987.
50. Thompson, R.A.: In Complement in Health and Disease. Edited by K. Whaley. Lancaster, MTP Press, Ltd., 1987.
51. Wesnieski, J.J. et al.: Arthritis Rheum., 30:919, 1987.

52. Whaley, K.: In *Complement in Health and Disease.* Edited by K. Whaley. Lancaster, MTP Press, Ltd., 1987.

53. Wyatt, R.J.: Prog. Allergy, *39*:339, 1986.

54. Zeitz, H.J., Lint, T.F., Gewurz, A., and Gewurz, H.: Prog. Allergy, *39*:289, 1986.

CH$_{50}$ Test[1]

PRINCIPLE. The hemolytic ability of the patient's classical pathway of complement is determined by comparison with the activity of normal sera.[2] To determine the hemolytic ability of both patient and normal sera, dilutions of serum are incubated with sensitized sheep red blood cells. The dilution that lyses 50% of the red cells under the defined conditions of the test is known as the CH$_{50}$ value.

EQUIPMENT AND MATERIALS

1. Veronal Buffered Saline—Stock Solution (VBS;$5\times$)

   a. Add and dissolve:

   41.9 g NaCl

   5.1 g Na-5,5' diethyl barbiturate

   in approximately 800 ml of distilled water

   in a 1000 ml volumetric flask

   b. Mix well and pH to 7.35 $\pm$ .05 with 1N HCl.

   c. QS to 1 L with distilled water.

2. EDTA (0.1 M disodium ethylenediaminetetraacetate)—Stock solution

   a. Add and dissolve 3.72 g disodium ethylenediaminetetraacetate in approximately 80 ml of distilled water in a 100-ml volumetric flask.

   b. Mix well and pH to 7.65 $\pm$ .05 with 2N NaOH.

   c. QS to 100 ml with distilled water.

3. Metal ions—Stock solution

   a. Prepare a 1.0M MgCl$_2$, 0.15M CaCl$_2$ solution

4. Veronal buffered saline—Working solution (VBS^{++}, $1\times$)

   a. To a 1000-ml volumetric flask,

   Add: 200 ml stock VBS

   1.0 ml stock metal ion solution

   QS to 1 L with distilled water

   b. To approximately 200 ml of this solution, add 1 g gelatin. Heat to dissolve and recombine with the remainder of solution.

5. EDTA Buffer (.01 M EDTA VBS Buffer)

   To a 50-ml volumetric flask, add

   9 ml stock VBS

   5 ml stock EDTA

   QS with distilled water

   NOTE: All stock solutions and buffers should be stored at 2 to 8° C. May be used indefinitely. Discard if contamination becomes evident.

6. Hemolysin (Becton Dickinson): Store at 2 to 8 ° C. Reconstitute lyophilized hemolysin with 2-ml accompanying diluent. Hemolysin is difficult to dissolve; it is advisable to reconstitute it some time prior to use and refrigerate. Once dissolved, aliquot 0.5 ml to plastic screw top vials, quick freeze and store at −70° C for future use. Aliquots at −70° C will last indefinitely.

7. Guinea Pig Complement (Cordis): Store at 2 to 8° C. Reconstitute lyophilized complement with 5 ml *cold* distilled water. Reconstituted complement can be aliquoted in 0.5 ml amounts in plastic screw top vials, quick frozen, labeled, and stored at −70° C for future use. May be used indefinitely.

8. Sheep Red Blood Cells in Alsever's Solution: Store at 2 to 8° C. Cells 1 to 6 weeks old are acceptable for use, if they are not hemolyzed.

9. Serum Control: Normal control sera are assayed, aliquoted, quick frozen, and stored at −70° C for use in the CH$_{50}$ procedure.

10. Ice bath.

11. 37° C water bath.

12. Refrigerated centrifuge.

13. 12 $\times$ 75 mm and 13 $\times$ 100 mm test tubes.

14. Pipets.

15. Spectrophotometer, set at 541 nm.

16. Log-log graph paper (2 cycle by 3 cycle).

SPECIMEN COLLECTION AND PREPARATION. Allow blood to clot at room temperature. Separate serum from clot. Specimen must be aliquoted in 0.5 ml aliquots in plastic screw top vials, quick frozen, labeled and stored at $-70°$ C if it is not to be used within a few hours.

PROCEDURE FOR REAGENT PREPARATION

1. Preparation of standardized sheep red blood cell (SRBC) suspension:

a. Turn on spectrophotometer if warm-up time is necessary.

b. Serofuge about 10 ml of SRBC-Alsevers solution and discard the supernate and buffy coat.

c. Suspend packed cells in EDTA buffer. Incubate at $37°$ C for 10 minutes.

d. Wash cells once with EDTA, then $\times$ 3 with VBS^{++} (1$\times$).

e. Dilute packed cells approximately 1:18 in VBS^{++}.

f. Lyse 0.1 ml of this cell suspension in 2.4 ml distilled water. Check OD of the lysate at 541 nm. An OD of .420 corresponds to the ideal cell concentration of 1×10^9 cells/ml. If necessary, adjust the cell suspension to achieve this OD by adding more VBS^{++} to original suspension if OD $>$ .440, or more red blood cells if OD $<$ .400.

2. Hemolysin (anti-SRBC) Preparation: (perform in an ice bath).

NOTE: Titration of hemolysin need only be done once for each lot number reconstituted. For storage, see Equipment and Materials, #6.

a. Dilute reconstituted guinea pig complement 1:30 in VBS^{++}.

b. Dilute an aliquot of reconstituted hemolysin (see *Equipment and Materials* #6) 1:500 in VBS^{++}.

c. Prepare twofold dilutions of the 1:500 dilution by adding 1 ml of VBS^{++} to each of 5 tubes, placing 1 ml of the 1:500 dilution in the first tube, mixing, and serially diluting 1 ml through tube 5.

d. Set up a row of seven 13 $\times$ 100 mm tubes and label 6 for the twofold dilutions ranging 1:500 to 1:16000. The seventh tube will serve as the 100% hemolysin tube.

e. Add 0.5 ml SRBC suspension to each tube.

f. Transfer 0.5 ml of the appropriate hemolysin dilution to each of tubes 1 though 6, taking care to mix during addition.

g. Incubate for 10 minutes at $37°$ C.

h. Add 5.5 ml VBS^{++} to tubes 1 through 6 and 6.0 ml distilled water to tube 7.

i. Add 1 ml diluted guinea pig complement to each tube except tube 7. Incubate at $37°$ C for 1 hour. Turn on refrigerated centrifuge, set at $4°$ C.

j. Centrifuge for 5 minutes at 3000 rpm and read absorbance of supernate of each tube at 541 nm.

k. Calculate % lysis of each tube(y) by:

$$\frac{OD}{OD \text{ of } 100\% \text{ Tube}} \times 100 = \% \text{ Lysis}$$

1. Plot % lysis against the reciprocal of the dilution on 2 $\times$ 3 cycle log paper.

m. The highest dilution of hemolysin which in the presence of complement, can effect complete hemolysis is called one hemolytic unit. One to four hemolytic units may be used to prepare EA. We usually use two units, or one doubling dilution below the last tube showing 100% hemolysis.

3. Preparation of EA (Erythrocyte-antibody)

a. Make up the appropriate dilution of hemolysin in VBS^{++} to a volume greater than or equal to the volume of standardized sheep cell suspension prepared in Step 1.

b. In a large Erlenmeyer flask, add an equal volume of hemolysin dilution to the standardized SRBC suspension. Add antibody dropwise while swirling SRBCs.

c. Incubate at $37°$ C for 15 minutes. Store EA at 2 to $8°$ C. Discard if hemolysis or contamination become evident.

CH$_{50}$ TEST PROCEDURE

Set up in an ice bath

1. Dilute an aliquot of each serum and control 1:60 in VBS^{++} (add 0.2 ml of serum to 11.8 ml of VBS^{++}).

2. Set up and label a row of six 13 $\times$ 100 mm tubes for each serum/control to be tested. Place two additional tubes in the rack, one to be used as a cell/buffer (CB) control, the other as a 100% hemolysis tube.

3. Pipet VBS^{++}, EA and serum/control dilutions (in that order) into the appropriate tubes, according to:

Tube #	1	2	3	4	5	6(SB)	CB	100%
VBS^{++}	5.5	5.3	5.0	4.5	4.0	5.5	6.5	---
EA	1.0	1.0	1.0	1.0	1.0	---	1.0	1.0
Serum (1:60)	1.0	1.2	1.5	2.0	2.5	2.0	---	---
Distilled H$_2$O	---	---	---	---	---	---	---	6.5

4. Mix well and incubate for 1 hour at 37° C. Turn on refrigerated centrifuge, set at 4° C, and set the spectrophotometer at 541 nm.

5. Centrifuge for 5 minutes at 3000 rpm.

6. Read absorbance (OD) of the supernate of each tube at 541 nm and record on worksheet.

7. Correct absorbance of tubes 1 to 5 by subtracting the CB value and the serum/buffer (SB) tube (tube #6 of each row).

8. Correct absorbance of the 100% tube by subtracting the OD of the cell/buffer (CB) tube. Record corrected 100% on worksheet.

9. Calculate % hemolysis (y) of each tube:

$$y = \frac{\text{corrected OD}}{\text{corrected OD of 100\% hemolysis tube}} \times 100$$

10. Using the conversion table (Table 6–4), convert % hemolysis (y) to y/1−y. It is recommended that you convert only y values between 20% and 80%.

11. For each serum/control, plot the volume of serum dilution ("y" axis) against the y/1−y value ("x" axis) on 2 × 3 cycle log paper. Draw the best straight line between the points for each sample.

12. The CH_{50} value is determined by dividing the value of y when x = 1.0 into the dilution factor (60), as when y = 1.480 at 1:60 dilution: 60/1.480 = 40.5 CH_{50} units.

RESULTS. Report as CH_{50} units.

INTERPRETATION OF RESULTS. It is recommended that a baseline level be established for patients who are to be followed using this procedure. Normal range for this assay should be established within each laboratory.

REFERENCES

1. Gaither, T.A., Frank, M.M.: *Clinical Diagnosis and Management by Laboratory Methods.* 16th ed. Edited by J.B. Henry. Philadelphia, W. B. Saunders, Co., 1979.

2. Kabat, E.A. and Mayer, M.M.: *Experimental Immunochemistry*, 2nd ed. Springfield, Charles C Thomas, 1964.

C_1 Esterase Inhibitor Assay[1,2]

PRINCIPLE. Utilizing an Ouchterlony plate, dilutions of patient and normal control sera are reacted against Anti-C_1 esterase inhibitor. The resulting precipitin patterns are compared to determine if the patient's C_1 esterase inhibitor is immunochemically and quantitatively similar to that of the normal control.

EQUIPMENT AND MATERIALS

1. Ouchterlony plate with three sets of five concentric wells around a center well (Technicon). Store at 2 to 8° C.

2. Capillary pipets, or a 20-μl micropipet.

3. Anti-C_{1s} Inhibitor (Rabbit; Behring): Store at 4 to 6° C. May be used until expiration date noted on the label, unless contamination becomes evident.

4. Control Serum: A fresh serum known to be normal for C_1 esterase inhibitor is used.

5. Moist chamber for incubation.

6. 12 × 75 mm test tubes and pipets for preparing dilutions of patient and control sera.

7. 0.9% (w/v) saline solution.

SPECIMEN COLLECTION AND PREPARATION. Serum should be fresh, or quick frozen and stored at −20° C or −70° C before use.

PROCEDURE

1. Make 1:2, 1:4, 1:8, and 1:16 dilutions of patient serum and control serum in saline.

2. Fill wells of an Ouchterlony plate as diagrammed below. Use one set of wells for patient serum and one set for normal control.

1:2
○

Patient or Control Serum
Undiluted ○   ○1:4

○
Anti-C_{1s}
Inhibitor

1:16   ○   ○1:8

Prepare an Ouchterlony worksheet noting the patient data, the placement of the patient and control sera, and the date set up.

3. Incubate for 3 days, observing daily for precipitin lines and recording your observations.

4. After the 3-day observation, stain as follows: flood plate with 7.5% acetic acid, let stand for a few minutes, and rinse in tap water. Observe again for precipitin lines. Precipitin lines formed between dilutions of patient serum and anti-C_1 esterase inhibitor are compared with those formed by the control, observing both presence of precipitation at each dilution and distance of each from the well. Resulting dilutions are recorded on the worksheet.

Table 6–4. y/1-y Values

	0	.1	.2	.3	.4	.5	.6	.7	.8	.9
10	0.111	0.112	0.114	0.115	0.116	0.117	0.119	0.120	0.121	0.122
11	0.124	0.125	0.126	0.127	0.129	0.130	0.131	0.133	0.134	0.135
12	0.136	0.138	0.139	0.140	0.142	0.143	0.144	0.145	0.147	0.148
13	0.149	0.151	0.152	0.153	0.155	0.156	0.157	0.159	0.160	0.161
14	0.163	0.164	0.166	0.167	0.168	0.170	0.171	0.172	0.174	0.175
15	0.176	0.178	0.179	0.181	0.182	0.183	0.185	0.186	0.188	0.189
16	0.190	0.192	0.193	0.195	0.196	0.198	0.199	0.200	0.202	0.203
17	0.205	0.206	0.208	0.209	0.211	0.212	0.214	0.215	0.217	0.218
18	0.220	0.221	0.222	0.224	0.225	0.227	0.229	0.230	0.232	0.233
19	0.235	0.236	0.238	0.239	0.241	0.242	0.244	0.245	0.247	0.248
20	0.250	0.252	0.253	0.255	0.256	0.258	0.259	0.261	0.263	0.264
21	0.266	0.267	0.269	0.271	0.272	0.274	0.276	0.277	0.279	0.280
22	0.282	0.284	0.285	0.287	0.289	0.290	0.292	0.294	0.295	0.297
23	0.299	0.300	0.302	0.304	0.305	0.307	0.309	0.311	0.312	0.314
24	0.316	0.318	0.319	0.321	0.323	0.325	0.326	0.328	0.330	0.332
25	0.333	0.335	0.337	0.339	0.340	0.342	0.344	0.346	0.348	0.350
26	0.351	0.353	0.355	0.357	0.359	0.361	0.362	0.364	0.366	0.368
27	0.370	0.372	0.374	0.376	0.377	0.379	0.381	0.383	0.385	0.387
28	0.389	0.391	0.393	0.395	0.397	0.399	0.401	0.403	0.404	0.406
29	0.408	0.410	0.412	0.414	0.416	0.418	0.420	0.422	0.425	0.427
30	0.429	0.431	0.433	0.435	0.437	0.439	0.441	0.443	0.445	0.447
31	0.449	0.451	0.453	0.456	0.458	0.460	0.462	0.464	0.466	0.468
32	0.471	0.473	0.175	0.477	0.479	0.481	0.484	0.486	0.488	0.490
33	0.493	0.495	0.497	0.499	0.502	0.504	0.506	0.508	0.511	0.513
34	0.515	0.517	0.520	0.522	0.524	0.527	0.529	0.531	0.534	0.536
35	0.538	0.541	0.543	0.546	0.548	0.550	0.553	0.555	0.558	0.560
36	0.563	0.565	0.567	0.570	0.572	0.575	0.577	0.580	0.582	0.585
37	0.587	0.590	0.592	0.595	0.597	0.600	0.603	0.605	0.608	0.610
38	0.613	0.616	0.618	0.621	0.623	0.626	0.629	0.631	0.634	0.637
39	0.639	0.642	0.645	0.647	0.650	0.653	0.656	0.658	0.661	0.664
40	0.667	0.669	0.672	0.675	0.678	0.681	0.684	0.686	0.689	0.692
41	0.695	0.698	0.701	0.704	0.706	0.709	0.712	0.715	0.718	0.721
42	0.724	0.727	0.730	0.733	0.736	0.739	0.742	0.745	0.748	0.751
43	0.754	0.757	0.761	0.766	0.767	0.770	0.773	0.776	0.779	0.783
44	0.786	0.789	0.792	0.795	0.799	0.802	0.805	0.808	0.812	0.815
45	0.818	0.822	0.825	0.828	0.832	0.835	0.838	0.842	0.845	0.848
46	0.852	0.855	0.859	0.862	0.866	0.869	0.873	0.876	0.880	0.883
47	0.887	0.890	0.894	0.898	0.901	0.905	0.908	0.912	0.916	0.919
48	0.923	0.927	0.931	0.934	0.938	0.942	0.946	0.949	0.953	0.957
49	0.961	0.965	0.969	0.972	0.976	0.980	0.984	0.988	0.992	0.996
50	1.000	1.004	1.008	1.012	1.016	1.020	1.024	1.028	1.033	1.037
51	1.041	1.045	1.049	1.053	1.058	1.062	1.066	1.070	1.075	1.079
52	1.083	1.088	1.092	1.096	1.101	1.105	1.110	1.114	1.119	1.123
53	1.128	1.132	1.137	1.141	1.146	1.151	1.155	1.160	1.165	1.169
54	1.174	1.179	1.183	1.188	1.193	1.198	1.203	1.208	1.212	1.217
55	1.222	1.227	1.232	1.237	1.242	1.247	1.252	1.257	1.262	1.268
56	1.273	1.278	1.283	1.288	1.294	1.299	1.304	1.309	1.315	1.320
57	1.326	1.331	1.336	1.342	1.348	1.353	1.358	1.364	1.370	1.375
58	1.381	1.387	1.392	1.398	1.404	1.410	1.415	1.421	1.427	1.433
59	1.439	1.445	1.451	1.457	1.463	1.469	1.475	1.481	1.488	1.494

Table 6–4. y/1-y Values (Cont'd)

	0	.1	.2	.3	.4	.5	.6	.7	.8	.9
60	1.500	1.506	1.513	1.519	1.525	1.532	1.538	1.545	1.551	1.558
61	1.564	1.571	1.577	1.584	1.591	1.597	1.604	1.611	1.618	1.625
62	1.632	1.639	1.646	1.653	1.660	1.667	1.674	1.681	1.688	1.695
63	1.703	1.710	1.717	1.725	1.732	1.740	1.747	1.755	1.762	1.770
64	1.778	1.786	1.793	1.801	1.809	1.817	1.825	1.833	1.841	1.849
65	1.857	1.865	1.874	1.882	1.890	1.899	1.907	1.915	1.924	1.933
66	1.941	1.950	1.959	1.967	1.976	1.985	1.994	2.003	2.012	2.021
67	2.030	2.040	2.049	2.058	2.067	2.077	2.086	2.096	2.106	2.115
68	2.125	2.135	2.145	2.155	2.165	2.175	2.185	2.195	2.205	2.215
69	2.226	2.240	2.247	2.257	2.268	2.279	2.289	2.300	2.311	2.322
70	2.333	2.344	2.356	2.367	2.378	2.390	2.401	2.413	2.425	2.436
71	2.448	2.460	2.472	2.484	2.497	2.509	2.521	2.534	2.546	2.559
72	2.571	2.584	2.597	2.610	2.623	2.636	2.650	2.663	2.676	2.690
73	2.704	2.717	2.731	2.745	2.759	2.774	2.788	2.802	2.817	2.831
74	2.846	2.861	2.876	2.891	2.906	2.922	2.937	2.953	2.968	2.984
75	3.000	3.016	3.032	3.049	3.065	3.082	3.098	3.115	3.132	3.149
76	3.167	3.184	3.202	3.219	3.237	3.255	3.274	3.292	3.310	3.329
77	3.348	3.367	3.386	3.405	3.425	3.444	3.464	3.484	3.505	3.525
78	3.545	3.566	3.587	3.608	3.630	3.651	3.673	3.695	3.717	3.739
79	3.762	3.785	3.808	3.831	3.854	3.878	3.902	3.926	3.950	3.975
80	4.000	4.025	4.050	4.076	4.102	4.128	4.155	4.181	4.208	4.236
81	4.263	4.291	4.319	4.348	4.376	4.405	4.435	4.464	4.495	4.525
82	4.556	4.587	4.618	4.650	4.682	4.714	4.747	4.780	4.814	4.848
83	4.882	4.917	4.952	4.988	5.024	5.061	5.098	5.135	5.173	5.211
84	5.250	5.289	5.329	5.369	5.410	5.452	5.494	5.536	5.579	5.623
85	5.667	5.711	5.757	5.803	5.849	5.897	5.944	5.993	6.042	6.092
86	6.143	6.194	6.246	6.299	6.353	6.407	6.463	6.519	6.576	6.634
87	6.692	6.752	6.813	6.874	6.937	7.000	7.065	7.130	7.197	7.264
88	7.333	7.403	7.475	7.547	7.621	7.696	7.772	7.850	7.929	8.009
89	8.091	8.174	8.259	8.346	8.434	8.524	8.615	8.709	8.804	8.901
90	9.000	9.101	9.204	9.310	9.417	9.526	9.638	9.753	9.870	9.989

REPORTING. Patient's results are reported as less than, equal to, or greater than normal control.

INTERPRETATION OF RESULTS. Precipitin lines of a normal patient will resemble the control. Deficiencies of C_1 esterase inhibitor will be demonstrated by absence of precipitate, precipitation at low dilutions only, or by proximity of the precipitate to the antigen well.

LIMITATIONS OF THE PROCEDURE. This technique will not detect functional abnormalities of C_1 esterase inhibitor (see *Complement Abnormalities*).

REFERENCES

1. Fong, J.S., Good, R.A., and Gewurz, H.: J. Lab. Clin. Med., *76*:836, 1970.
2. In lab modification of procedure of Fong, Good, and Gewurz.

Chapter 7

OTHER SERUM PROTEINS

ACUTE PHASE PROTEINS

Acute phase proteins[1,9] are plasma proteins, produced primarily by hepatocytes (liver parenchymal cells),[2,4,6] whose concentrations significantly and independently increase during the acute phase of an inflammatory process, whether induced by injury, infection, neoplastic or other inflammatory stimuli. Among the proteins known to be altered in concentration,[4,8] several have been designated "acute phase proteins" as a result of their appreciable increase during acute-phase reactions (Table 7–1). Among these, the fibrinogen concentration is primarily responsible for the increased erythrocyte sedimentation rate (ESR),[5,7] which is also associated with acute phase responses, and C-RP and SAA are known to increase proportionally with the amount of injury or inflammation.[12]

Several proteins have been shown to decrease in concentration during acute phase reactions,[3,4,12] e.g. albumin and transferrin, and have been designated "negative acute phase proteins," or "concentration depressed acute phase proteins."

Although the mechanisms have not been entirely determined,[4] increased production of acute phase proteins may be initiated, and are normally mediated by[4,12] mononu-

Table 7–1. Acute Phase Proteins

Plasma Protein	Extent of Increase[4,7]
C-Reactive Protein (C-RP)	20-1000 fold
Serum amyloid A protein (SAA)	20-1000 fold
Alpha₁ proteinase inhibitor (alpha₁ antitrypsin)	2-5 fold
Alpha₁ acid glycoprotein	2-5 fold
Alpha₁ antichymotrypsin	2-5 fold
Haptoglobin	2-5 fold
Fibrinogen	2-5 fold
Alpha₂ antiplasmin 1	30-60%
C₁ inactivator	30-60%
Ceruloplasmin	30-60%
C₃	30-60%

clear (or alternate)[4] cell production of interleukin 1, which is released within 3 hours[4,12] in response to an inflammatory stimulus.[3,10,12] Unless irritation persists or acute phase reactions occur repeatedly, as in chronic inflammation, an acute phase reaction usually resolves in 2 to 3 days.[12]

Although increases or decreases in the acute phase proteins are nonspecific in nature, correlations have been made among patterns of these proteins and many human disease states.[4] The importance of their detection in monitoring disease activity during therapy of rheumatic diseases is widely accepted. Erythrocyte sedimentation rates (ESR) and C-reactive protein (C-RP) levels are most often tested. A rapid, reliable method for serum amyloid A protein (SAA) detection is not yet available.

REFERENCES

1. Abernethy, T.J., and Avery, O.T.: J. Exp. Med. 73:173, 1941.

2. Benson, M.D., and Kleiner, E.: J. Immunol., 124:495, 1980.

3. Bornstein, D.L.: Ann. N.Y. Acad. Sci., 389:323, 1982.

*4. Gordon, A.H., and Koj, A. (Eds.): The Acute-Phase Response to Injury and Infection. Amsterdam, Elsevier, 1985.

5. Kushner, I.: In Textbook of Rheumatology. 2nd ed. Edited by W.N. Kelly et al. Philadelphia, W. B. Saunders, 1985.

6. Kushner, I., and Feldmann, G.: J. Exp. Med., 148:466, 1978.

7. Kushner, I., Gewurz, H., and Benson, M.D.: J. Lab. Clin. Med., 97:739, 1981.

8. Kushner, I., Volankis, J.E., and Gewurz, H. (Eds.): Ann. N.Y. Acad. Sci., 389: 1982. Publisher-New York Academy of Sciences, New York, N.Y.

9. MacLeod, C.M., and Avery, O.T.: J. Exp. Med., 73:183, 1941.

10. Pepys, M.B., and Baltz, M.L.: Adv. Immunol., 34:141, 1983.

11. Selinger, M.J. et al.: Nature, 285:498, 1980.

12. Sipe, J.D.: In Rheumatology and Immunology. 2nd ed. Edited by A.S. Cohen and J.C. Bennett. Orlando, Grune & Stratton, 1986.

C-Reactive Protein (CRP)

C-reactive protein (CRP) is a protein[1] constituent of normal serum and serous fluids, first described by Tillet and Francis in 1930.[19,32] It is a cyclic, homogeneous molecule, comprised of 5 identical subunits[22,23] and having a molecular weight of 118,000 D.[33] Evidence suggests that synthesis occurs only in hepatocytes.[12,16] In man, CRP is the classical and most dramatic acute phase reactant, with levels rising as much as 1000-fold from the reference range[3,24] within 1 to 2 days as a result of active tissue-damaging processes, then falling rapidly with cessation of the stimulus. CRP has extensive homology with serum amyloid P component (SAA; SAP).[22]

Substrates for the CRP molecule include phosphocholine (PC),[10] galactose,[34] and galactosamine[11] in Ca^{++} dependent reactions, and various polycations[4,10] in reactions that are inhibited by Ca^{++}.

Reaction of C-reactive protein with its substrate molecules results in activation of the classical system of complement,[5,14] generating all known complement-dependent reactivities, including classical component consumption, immune adherence, enhanced phagocytosis and cytolysis.[10] Two molecules of CRP are required to initiate C1q activation.[5]

In recent years, there has been renewed interest in C-reactive protein and its role in disease. There is evidence of a strong association between increases in CRP and microbial infections;[20] for example, in neonates,[7,29] and in patients with acute leukemias.[31] C-reactive protein may help with differentiation of viral from bacterial meningitis[25,28,29] and with monitoring of antibiotic therapy in meningitis or septicemia.[28,29] Increased levels have been reported useful in differentiation of upper from lower urinary tract infections,[9,20] and of bacterial pneumonia and bronchitis from COPD.[20] Fisher et al.[8] describes increased CRP as an indicator of postoperative infection; Angerman, et al.[2] found it useful in evaluation of antibiotic therapy in pelvic infections.

C-reactive protein levels correspond with CK MB values,[6] rising rapidly after myocardial infarction.[15] Levels of CRP are high in certain rheumatic diseases, most notably rheumatoid arthritis, but are normal to slightly elevated in others, such as SLE, progressive systemic sclerosis, and generalized osteoarthritis.[13]

C-reactive protein has been used to predict onset and termination of renal allograft rejection up to 4 days before other signs occur,[36] and to indicate the existence of metastases in a broad spectrum of neoplastic diseases.[35]

Laboratory tests for detection of CRP include precipitation by the C-polysaccharide of pneumococcus,[32] crystallization,[18] tube precipitation using anti-CRP,[17] complement fixation,[27] Ouchterlony,[21] latex agglutination,[30] radioimmunoassay,[3] radial immunodiffusion,[21] and fluorescence polarization.

(See also *Acute Phase Reactants, Complement, Fluorescence Polarization*)

REFERENCES

1. Abernethy, T.J., and Avery, O.T.: J. Exp. Med., *73*:173, 1941.
2. Angerman, N.S. et al.: J. Reprod. Med., *25*:63, 1980.
3. Claus, D.R., Osmand, A.P., and Gewurz, H.: J. Lab. Clin. Med., *87*:120, 1976.
4. Claus, D.R. et al.: J. Immunol., *118*:83, 1977.
5. Claus, D.R. et al.: J. Immunol., *119*:187, 1977.
6. DeBeer, F.C. et al.: Br. Heart J., *47*:239, 1982.
7. Felix, N.S., Nakajima, H., and Kagan, B.M.: Pediatrics, *37*:270, 1966.
8. Fisher, C.L. et al.: Am. J. Clin. Pathol., *66*:840, 1976.
9. Jodal, U., and Hansen, L.A.: Acta Pediatr. Scand., *65*:319, 1976.
*10. Gewurz, H. et al.: Adv. Internal Med., *27*:345, 1982.
11. Higgenbotham, J.D., Heidelberger, M., and Gotschlich, E.C.: Proc. Natl. Acad. Sci., *67*:138, 1970.
12. Hurlimann, J., Thorbecke, G., and Hochwald, G.: J. Exp. Med., *123*:365, 1966.
13. Hutton, C.W. et al.: Br. J. Rheumatol., *24*:86, 1985.
14. Kaplan, M.H., Volanakis, J.E.: J. Immunol., *112*:2135, 1974.
15. Kushner, I., Broder, M.L., and Karp, D.: J. Clin. Invest., *61*:235, 1978.
16. Macintyre, S.S., Schultz, D., and Kushner, I.: Ann. N.Y. Acad. Sci., *389*:76, 1982.
17. MacLeod, C.M., and Avery, O.T.: J. Exp. Med., *73*:183, 1941.
18. McCarty, M.: J. Exp. Med., *85*:491, 1947.
19. McCarty, M.: Ann. N.Y. Acad. Sci., *389*:1, 1982.
20. Morley, J.J., and Kushner, I.: Ann. N.Y. Acad. Sci., *389*:406, 1982.
21. Nilsson, L.A.: Int. Arch. Allergy, *33*:16, 1968.
22. Oliveira, E.B., Gotschlich, E.C., and Liu, T.-Y.: J. Biol. Chem., *254*:489, 1979.
23. Osmand, A.P. et al.: Proc. Natl. Acad. Sci., *74*:739, 1977.
24. Palosus, T. et al.: Acta Med. Scand., *220*:175, 1986.
25. Peltola, H.O.: Lancet, *1*:980, 1982.
26. Pepys, M.B., and Baltz, M.L.: Adv. Immunol., *34*:141, 1983.
27. Rapport, M.M., and Graf, L.: Proc. Soc. Exp. Biol. Med., *93*:69, 1956.
28. Sabel,K.G., and Hansen, L.A.: Acta Pediatr. Scand., *63*:381, 1974.
29. Sabel, K.G., and Wadsworth, C.: Acta Pediatr. Scand., *68*:825, 1979.
30. Singer, J.M. et al.: Am. J. Clin. Pathol., *28*:611, 1957.
31. Starke, I.D. et al.: Eur. J. Cancer Clin. Oncol., *20*:319, 1984.
32. Tillet, W.S., and Francis, T.: J. Exp. Med., *52*:561, 1930.
33. Volanakis, J.E., Clements, W.L., and Schrohenloher, R.E.: J. Immunol. Methods, *23*:285, 1978.
34. Volanakis, J.E., and Narkates, A.J.: Fed. Proc., *39*:702, 1980.
35. Weinstein, P.S. et al.: Scand. J. Immunol., *19*:193, 1984.
36. White, J., Meyer, E., and Hardy, M.A.: Transplant Proc., *13*:682, 1981.

C-Reactive Protein Quantitation by Fluorescence Polarization Immunoassay

PRINCIPLE. The TDX C-Reactive Protein system utilizes fluorescent polarization for the quantitative measurement of C-reactive protein (CRP). CRP in patient serum competes with CRP bound to a fluorescein tracer for anti-CRP. The fluorescence polarization of the tracer, as measured by an optical detection system, increases as the amount of tracer bound to antibody increases, and is inversely related to the concentration of CRP in the patient serum. CRP is elevated in the serum of many patients with acute phase reactions.

EQUIPMENT AND MATERIALS

1. No. 9550-20, C-Reactive Protein Reagent Pack (Abbott Diagnostics, Inc.):

P Pretreatment Solution
Surfactant in buffer (3 mL).
Preservative: 0.1% sodium azide

S C-reactive protein antiserum (sheep) in buffer with protein stabilizer (3 mL)
Preservative: 0.1% sodium azide

T C-reactive protein—Fluorescein tracer in buffer with stabilizer (3 mL)
Preservative: 0.1% sodium azide

2. No. 9550-01, C-reactive protein calibrators (Abbott Diagnostics, Inc): Six vials with accurately measured amounts of human C-reactive protein in protein stabilizers to give the following concentrations on the TDX Analyzer:

Vial	CRP Concentration on TDX* (mg/dL)	Actual CRP Concentration (mg/dL)
A	0	0
B	4.0	1.0
C	8.0	2.0
D	12.0	3.0
E	18.0	4.5
F	26.0	6.5

Preservative: 0.1% sodium azide

*NOTE: TDX C-reactive protein calibrators are supplied at $\frac{1}{4}$ the concentrations specified in the assay parameters (53.7–53.12). Four times the sample volume, or 32 μL of the calibrators are dispensed during a calibration run.

3. No. 9500-10, C-reactive protein controls (Abbott Diagnostics, Inc.): Two vials of human C-reactive protein in protein stabilizers should read within the following ranges:

Vial	CRP Concentration on TDX* (mg/dL)	Actual CRP Concentration (mg/dL)
L	2.5– 3.5	3.0
H	13.5–16.5	15.0

Preservative: 0.1% sodium azide

4. TDX Analyzer System, (Abbott Diagnostics, Inc.) including the following:

Cuvettes No. 9518-06

Dilution buffer No. 9519-02

Sample carousel

Calibration carousel

TDX sample cartridges

5. Precision pipettes to deliver 75 μL and 50 μL

STORAGE. TDX C-reactive protein reagent pack, calibrators and controls are stored at 2 to 8° C and must be brought to room temperature before use.

SPECIMEN COLLECTION AND PREPARATION. Serum specimen is required for assay. Re-move serum from red cells to avoid hemolysis. Levels of protein up to 9.5 g/dL, lipid hemoglobin and bilirubin result in less than 10% error in quantitating a sample with the TDX C-reactive protein assay when run on the TDX Analyzer. If specimens are to be stored, they should be refrigerated at 2 to 8° C. For long-term storage, the specimen should be frozen at −15° C or colder.

PROCEDURE

NOTES—Low and high positive controls should be assayed with each run.

—Start up, weekly, and monthly maintenance checks should be performed before assays are performed. See TDX System Operation Manual for maintenance procedures.

—Calibration curves should be renewed every 3 weeks or if there is a reagent pack lot number change.

—For activation procedure see System Operation Manual.

—Update CRP assay parameters as required by manufacturer.

1. Check to see if calibration is current, if needed, perform calibration prior to testing by the following procedure.

a. To calibrate, use calibration carousel.

b. Load calibration carousel with twelve cuvettes and twelve sample cartridges. Lock carousel.

c. Place 75 μL of calibrators A through F in sample cartridge. Each calibrator is run in duplicate, i.e., AA, BB, CC, etc.

d. Mix reagent pack well. Open pack and load in reagent pack position.

e. Load carousel and close cover.

f. Press RUN on keypad. The reagent pack bar code will be read, displaying the test name and calibration function. An acceptable C-reactive protein calibration curve should meet the following criteria:

a. Polarization Error (PERR) less than or equal to ±2.0 for all calibrators.

b. Root Mean Squared Error (RMSE) less than or equal to 1.0.

NOTE: Controls and/or patient samples cannot be run during a calibration because of the different sample volumes required for calibration and patient runs. It is recommended that controls be run immediately after the calibration run to verify the calibration curve.

2. To perform assay of C-reactive protein controls and patients, use a sample carousel.

3. For each patient or control, place one cuvette and one sample cartridge in carousel.

4. Add at least 50 μL of sample or control to the appropriate sample cup.

5. Load reagent pack and carousel into TDX.

6. Press RUN.

7. TDX will print:
Volumes
Repeats
Gain
Calibration date
Calibration time
Units

8. Procedure time for full carousel is approximately 17 to 20 minutes.

9. Read control values and patient values from sample concentration column.

10. Check controls to see if they fall within 2 S.D. of control value.

11. When samples contain CRP concentration higher than the calibration range, "HI" will print out instead of a result. These samples should be repeated by first making a 1:2 dilution of patient sample with saline solution.

12. Patient samples with background intensities greater than 1600 will show a "HI" printed after the BLK I readings. These samples may give questionable results. If such a sample is diluted to give a background intensity less than 1600, the diluted sample may also give a questionable result. Results from these samples should not be reported. Alternate methods should be available such as Radial Immunodiffusion for these specimens. CRP assay parameter 53.20 (MS BKG) should not be edited to a number greater than 1600.

INTERPRETATION OF RESULTS. The normal ranges[1,2] of C-reactive protein in the serum of healthy individuals using the TDX C-reactive protein assay were found to be:

$$(N = 202) \quad 95\% \leq 0.5 \text{ mg/dL}$$

$$98\% \leq 1.0 \text{ mg/dL}$$

In our laboratory the normal range has been set at less than 1.2 mg/dL. CRP values for patients in an acute phase reaction can vary over a wide range within a 24 to 48 hour time frame.

REFERENCES

1. Claus, D.R., Osmond, A.P., and Gewurz, H.: J. Lab. Clin. Med., *87*:120, 1976.

2. Shine, B., de Beer, F.C., and Pepys, M.B.: Clin. Chim. Acta, *117*:13, 1981.

ALPHA$_1$ ANTITRYPSIN

(Alpha$_1$ Proteinase Inhibitor)

Alpha$_1$ antitrypsin (AAT), or alpha$_1$ proteinase inhibitor (A$_1$PI), is the major component of the alpha$_1$ electrophoretic band in the normal serum protein electrophoresis.[8] Functionally, it is the prototypic molecule of the plasma proteinase inhibitors,[13] collectively known as "serpins":[2] a group of homologous proteins responsible for the inhibition of the serine proteases which trigger such inflammatory cascades as coagulation, kinin release, fibrinolysis, and complement activation. Other members of the serpin family include antithrombin III, ovalbumin, alpha$_1$ antichymotrypsin, and angiotensinogen. Both nucleotide[10] and amino acid[4] sequencing have been completed for AAT.

Although alpha$_1$ antitrypsin reacts more readily with leukocyte-produced elastase, it can combine with virtually all serine proteolytic enzymes, e.g. plasmin and thrombin.[1,13] Reactions are sensitive to oxidation, creating a delicate physiologic interaction among elastase, alpha$_1$ antitrypsin, and oxygen radicals released at the site of tissue damage and inflammation.[4,13]

Alpha$_1$ antitrypsin is produced primarily by hepatocytes.[2] However, monocytes and macrophages can also produce the molecule,[11] a fact which may be useful in the characterization of myeloid and monocytic leukemias.[7,9] AAT is an acute phase reactant, with a circulating half-life of approximately 6 days.[2]

Probably a single genetic locus (Pi), with multiple alleles, codes for the alpha$_1$ antitrypsin molecule.[2,13] Three allelic variants are of particular interest: M, S, and Z, although other less common alleles have also been described.[5,13] The M allele codes for normal production and secretion of the molecule; both the S and Z alleles, if present, result in a plasma deficiency.[3,4] Presence of the S and Z alleles is virtually confined to Europeans, 1:2000 of whom are homozygous ZZ or carry the SZ phenotype. Those individuals who are heterozygous MS or MZ, or homozygous SS, while they have somewhat reduced plasma alpha$_1$ antitrypsin levels, carry no significant risk of related disease, although an association with psoriasis has been described for PiMZ.[6] Persons who are SZ or ZZ phenotype have a low plasma concentration of AAT, and are predisposed to emphysema,[8] particularly if exposed to smoke or environmental pollution which appears to induce inflammation in the lungs, resulting in an influx of neutrophils and increased elastase production in the presence of oxygen radicals.[3,4] In the ZZ phenotype, liver accumulation of alpha$_1$ antitrypsin, the result of a defect in secretion, may cause severe neonatal jaundice in approximately 10% of affected individuals. Almost all ZZ adults show at least histologic evidence of liver damage.[12]

Radial immunodiffusion is used in our laboratory as a method of screening for AAT deficiencies. Nephelometric methods are also available for quantitation. AAT phenotyping is conducted at research laboratories. (See also *Acute Phase Reactants, Radial Immunodiffusion Assay*.)

REFERENCES

1. Beatty, K. et al.: J. Biol. Chem., *255*:3931, 1980.
2. Carrell, R.W.: J. Clin. Invest., *78*:1427, 1986.
3. Carrell, R.W. et al.: Nature, *298*:329, 1982.
*4. Carrell, R.W. et al.: Biochem. Soc. Symp., *49*:55, 1984.
5. Fagerhol, M.K., and Cox, D.W.: Adv. Hum. Genet., *11*:1, 1981.
6. Horne, S.L. et al.: Hum. Hered., *36*:266, 1986.
7. Krugliak, L. et al.: Am. J. Hematol., *21*:99, 1986.
8. Laurell, C.-B., and Eriksson, S.: Scand. J. Clin. Lab. Invest., *15*:132, 1963.
9. Meyer, P.R. et al.: Am. J. Clin. Pathol., *86*:461, 1986.
10. Nukiwa, T. et al.: J. Biol. Chem., *261*:15989, 1986.
11. Perlmutter, D.H. et al.: Proc. Natl. Acad. Sci. U.S.A., *82*:795, 1985.
12. Sharp, H.L.: Hosp. Pract., *6*:83, 1971.
13. Travis, J., and Salveson, G.S.: Annu. Rev. Biochem., *52*:655, 1983.

CERULOPLASMIN

Ceruloplasmin, which was first isolated by Holmberg and Laurell,[8,9] and sequenced by Takahashi et al.,[14] is the major copper-containing protein of human plasma, binding 90 to 95% of the copper found in plasma by attaching 6 to 7 cupric ions per ceruloplasmin molecule.[1] Ceruloplasmin is synthesized in the liver[11] under the control of the human ceruloplasmin gene on chromosome number 3.[17]

In addition to its role in copper homeostasis,[4] ceruloplasmin oxidizes iron from ferrous to ferric ions as part of the iron metabolism cycle,[5,6] and acts as a scavenger of superoxide anion radicals for other molecules.[5,7] It is also involved in regulation of plasma and tissue levels of biogenic amines.[5]

Metabolism of ceruloplasmin occurs through the liver,[15,16] with a circulating half-life of 2 to 3 days.[16]

As an acute phase reactant, ceruloplasmin levels are elevated with many conditions;[3] however, there has been no functional or diagnostic significance established for its role in inflammation.

Hepatolenticular degeneration, or Wilson's disease,[10,13] is a copper metabolism disorder, resulting from the inheritance of a ceruloplasmin deficiency[12] which is passed as an autosomal recessive trait. Hepatolenticular degeneration is characterized by accumulation of free copper in selected areas of the body, resulting in cirrhosis of the liver, protean central nervous system dysfunction, and formation of the Kayser-Fleischer rings, a golden-brown pigmentation encircling the cornea which hallmarks those individuals who have the disease.

Ceruloplasmin increases have been studied in patients with some types of malignant tumors, e.g. cervical cancer and Hodgkin's disease, and may be useful in monitoring clinical condition and response to therapy.[2]

Methods available for detection of ceruloplasmin are radial immunodiffusion and nephelometry. An ELISA system has also been devised.[3] (See also *Acute Phase Reactants, Radial Immunodiffusion*.)

REFERENCES

1. Calabrese, L., and Carbonaro, M.: Biochem. J., *238*:291, 1986.
2. Chakravarty, P.K. et al.: Acta Med. Okayama, *40*:103, 1986.
3. DiSilvestro, R.A., and David, E.A.: Clin. Chim. Acta, *158*:287, 1986.
4. Evans, G.W.: Physiol. Rev., *53*:535, 1973.

*5. Frieden, E., and Hsieh, H.S.: Adv. Enzymol, *44*:187, 1976.

6. Frieden, E., and Osaki, S.: Adv. Exp. Med. Biol., *48*:235, 1974.

7. Goldstein, I.M. et al.: J. Biol. Chem., *254*:4040, 1979.

8. Holmberg, C.G.: Acta Physiol. Scand., *8*:227, 1944.

9. Holmberg, C.G., and Laurell, C.-B.: Acta Chem. Scand., *2*:550, 1948.

10. Owen, C.A., *Wilson's Disease*. Park Ridge, Noyes Publications, 1981.

11. Owen, C.A., and Hazelrig, J.B.: Am. J. Physiol., *210*:1059, 1966.

12. Scheinberg, I.H., and Gitlin, D.: Science, *116*:484, 1952.

13. Scheinberg, I.H., and Sternlieb, I.: Annu. Rev. Med., *16*:119, 1965.

14. Takahashi, N. et al.: Proc. Natl. Acad. Sci. U.S.A., *81*:390, 1984.

15. Tavassoli, M.: Trans. Assoc. Am. Physicians, *98*:370, 1985.

16. Tavassoli, M. et al.: J. Cell Biol., *102*:1298, 1986.

17. Yang, F. et al.: Proc. Natl. Acad. Sci. U.S.A., *83*:3257, 1986.

HAPTOGLOBIN

Haptoglobins, originally described by Polonovski,[26] are a family of glycoproteins that migrate in the alpha$_2$ region during total protein electrophoresis.[21] Plasma concentrations under normal circumstances range from 1.0 to 2.0 mg/ml, varying with individual phenotype, and molecular weights are from 85 to 400,000 D. Haptoglobin functions by binding in a 1:1 ratio with free hemoglobin[20,23] in an irreversible, suicidal reaction, resulting in hemoglobin-haptoglobin complexes which are then removed via specific receptors[14,16,18] on Kupffer and parenchymal cells in the liver.[12,19,21] In situations where haptoglobin-binding capacity is exceeded, hemoglobin is cleared by either glomerulofiltration, followed by urinary excretion or tubular reabsorption, or by oxidation to methemoglobin and heme, which is then bound by hemopexin or albumin before being removed from circulation by hepatocytes.[12,18]

Whether removed in complex with haptoglobin or with hemopexin, iron released from the original hemoglobin is recovered and reused after digestion of the complexes.[21] Haptoglobin is important physio-logically for its role in protecting the kidneys from damage and preventing the loss of iron by urinary excretion.[9,21] Further, the rapid binding and sequestering of released hemoglobin molecules acts to limit the usefulness of hemoglobin molecules to potentially pathogenic organisms (e.g. bacteria, fungi) whose infectivity is enhanced by higher hemoglobin concentrations.[6,32,33]

Jue et al.[13] suggest a role for haptoglobin in the inhibition of prostaglandin synthesis. By restricting available heme groups, enzymatic reactions necessary early in the synthetic pathways are inhibited.

Plasma levels of haptoglobin may decrease early in inflammatory reactions, probably due not only to increased vascular permeability, but also to enhanced catabolism.[15] The behavior, then, of haptoglobin as an early acute phase protein[10] may be masked.

Haptoglobin production is apparently controlled by two loci, Hpα and Hpβ. Three common alleles are known to occur at the Hpα locus: Hpα 1F, Hpα 1S, and Hpα 2,[30,31] although rare variants occur.[5,21] Gene frequency studies within populations are available.[21]

The haptoglobin molecule is comprised of four chains, two beta chains that are common to almost all haptoglobin types,[31] and two alpha chains, which are most often α1F, α1S, or α2. Common phenotypes are designated H 1-1 (Hp 1F-1F, Hp 1F-1S, or Hp 1S-1S), H 2-1 (Hp 2-1F or Hp 2-1S), or Hp 2-2 on the basis of electrophoretic differences in alpha chains.[2,21,31]

DNA mapping[17] and amino acid sequencing[4,21] of haptoglobin have been reported.

Anhaptoglobinemia, designated "Hp O", is asymptomatic and occurs in approximately 12% of black American children, 4% of black American adults, and 32% of Nigerians.[21] Eighty to 90% of infants younger than 3 months also lack detectable haptoglobin.[8]

Haptoglobin is synthesized on membrane-bound polysomes of liver cells[27,28] as a single chain precursor molecule[1,10] that is proteolytically processed to give both alpha and beta subunits of the circulating molecule.[11] Thirty to 50% of the intravascular pool is synthesized daily.[22]

As an acute phase reactant, plasma levels increase in many acute and chronic inflammatory reactions.[24] Increased haptoglobin has been reported in stages III and IV of prostate cancer and may be useful in determining the tumor load at diagnosis and following treatment of the disease.[29] Disorders associated with significant intravascular hemolysis[3] and hemolytic transfusion reactions[7] may effect catabolism of haptoglobin, resulting in decreased serum concentrations. Chronic, low serum haptoglobin has been reported in patients with severe liver disease.[21,25]

Functional assays for haptoglobin measure the haptoglobin-binding capacity of serum or plasma,[21] often by detecting the peroxidase activity of the hemoglobin-haptoglobin complex.[10] Radial immunodiffusion or electroimmunodiffusion are often used to determine the haptoglobin levels in circulation (see also *Acute Phase Proteins*).

REFERENCES

1. Chow, V. et al.: FEBS Lett., *153*:275, 1983.
2. Connell, G.E., Dixon, G.H., and Smithies, O.: Nature, *193*:505, 1962.
3. Daniels, J.C.: In *Serum Protein Abnormalities: Diagnosis and Clinical Aspects.* Edited by S.E. Ritzmann and J.C. Daniels, Boston, Little, Brown & Co., 1975.
4. Dayhoff, M.O.: *Atlas of Protein Sequence and Structure*, Vol. 5. Suppl. 3. Washington, D.C., Natl. Biomed. Res. Found, 1979.
5. Dobryszycka, W., and Krawczyk, E.: Comp. Biochem. Physiol., *62B*:111, 1979.
6. Eaton, J.W. et al.: Science, *215*:691, 1982.
7. Fink, D.J., Petz, L.D., and Black, M.B.: JAMA, *199*:109, 1967.
8. Giblett, E.R.: Ser. Haematol., *1*:3, 1968.
9. Glaumann, H., Peters, T. Jr., and Redman, C. (eds.): *Plasma Protein Secretion by the Liver*, London, Academic Press, 1983.
10. Gordon, A.H., and Koj, A. (eds.): *The Acute Phase Response to Injury and Infection*, Amsterdam, Elsevier, 1985.
11. Haugen, T.H., Hanley, J.M., and Heath, E.C.: J. Biol. Chem., *256*:1055, 1981.
12. Hershko, C., Cook, J.D., and Finch, C.A.: J. Lab. Clin. Med., *80*:624, 1972.
13. Jue, D.M., Shim, B.S., and Kang, Y.S.: Mol. Cell Biochem., *51*:141, 1983.
14. Kino, K. et al.: J. Biol. Chem., *255*:9616, 1980.
15. Lombart, C. et al.: Rev. Fr. Etud. Clin. Biol., *13*:258, 1968.
16. Lowe, M.A., and Ashwell, G.A.: Arch. Biochem. Biophys., *216*:704, 1982.
17. Maeda, N. et al.: Nature, *309*:131, 1984.
18. Morgan, E.H., and Baker, E.: Fed. Proc., *45*:2810, 1986.
19. Murray, R.K., Connell, G.E., and Pert, J.H.: Fed. Proc., *19*:66, 1960.
20. Nagel, R.L., and Gibson, Q.H.: J. Biol. Chem., *246*:69, 1971.
21. Natelson, S., and Natelson, E.A.: *Principles of Applied Clinical Chemistry.* Vol 3. New York, Plenum Press, 1980.
22. Noyes, W.D., and Garby, L.: Scand. J. Clin. Lab. Invest., *20*:33, 1967.
23. Nyman, M.: Scand. J. Clin. Lab. Invest., *12*:121, 1960.
24. Owen, J.A. et al.: Clin. Sci., *26*:1, 1964.
25. Pintera, J.: Ser. Haematol., *4*:1, 1971.
26. Polonovski, M., and Jayle, M.F.: Compt. Rend. Soc. de Biol., *129*:457, 1938.
27. Rangei, G. et al.: Nucleic Acid Res., *11*:5811, 1983.
28. Schreiber, G. et al.: Arch. Biochem. Biophys., *212*:319, 1981.
29. Seal, U.S. et al.: Cancer, *42*:1720, 1978.
30. Smithies, O., Connell, G.E., and Dixon, G.H.: Ann. Hum. Genet., *14*:14, 1962.
31. Smithies, O., Connell, G.E., and Dixon, G.H.: Nature, *196*:232, 1962.
32. Ward, G.G., Am. J. Surg., *151*:291, 1986.
33. Weinberg, E.D.: Science, *184*:952, 1974.

Haptoglobin Latex Agglutination

PRINCIPLE. The serum specimen is mixed with antibody to haptoglobin to absorb up to 50 mg/dL haptoglobin. This mixture is then reacted with latex coated with antibody to haptoglobin. Agglutination of the latex will occur if the specimen contains > 50 mg/dL haptoglobin. A 100 mg/dL concentration can be determined by diluting the specimen 1:2 prior to absorption.

EQUIPMENT AND MATERIALS

1. Rapi/Tex-HP Test Kit (Cal.-Behring) containing:

a. Hp Antiserum—a stabilized, prediluted antiserum produced in rabbits.

b. Hp positive control serum—a stabilized human serum containing > 50 mg/dL haptoglobin.

c. Hp negative control serum—a stabilized human serum containing < 50 mg/dL haptoglobin.

d. Hp latex reagent—latex particles coated with rabbit antibody to haptoglobin.

2. Black test slide
3. Test tubes
4. Pipettes
5. Wooden applicator sticks
6. Rotator
7. Serum or plasma to be tested—markedly lipemic serum or microbial contamination may cause false positive agglutination. Store refrigerated or frozen, if not assayed immediately.

STORAGE. Store test kit reagents at 2 to 8° C. Do not freeze. Expiration date is noted on the label. All reagents contain 0.1% sodium azide as a preservative.

PRECAUTIONS. For in vitro diagnostic use. Individual blood donations for preparation of the controls were examined for hepatitis B surface antigen and for antibodies to HIV-I and were found to be nonreactive. Since no test method can ensure that infectious agents are absent, follow the usual practices recommended for handling blood and body fluids.

SPECIMEN COLLECTION AND PREPARATION. Human serum or citrated plasma may be examined. No special preparation of the specimen is required. Markedly lipemic sera or microbial contamination may cause false positive agglutination. Hemolyzed samples should not be used.

PROCEDURE
1. Bring all reagents, controls and sera to room temperature.
2. Make a 1:2 dilution in saline solution of each serum to be tested.
3. Set up 1 test tube for each control and 2 for each serum to be tested, one to be used for undiluted samples and one for the 1:2 dilution. Label each tube.
4. Place 0.2 mL Hp antiserum in each tube.
5. Add 2 μL control, serum, or 1:2 serum dilution directly into Hp antiserum.
6. Mix thoroughly and incubate for 15 minutes at room temperature.
7. Place a 35-μL drop of each test mixture on separate fields on a black slide.
8. Shake the Hp latex reagent to obtain a uniform suspension. Add 1 drop to each field containing a sample to be tested. Mix each well

with a wooden applicator stick, spreading the mixture over the field.
9. Place a rotator for 4 minutes at a speed of 145 to 160 rpm.
10. Examine immediately for agglutination.

RESULTS. The positive control should show clear agglutination; the negative control, no agglutination.

For patient specimens:

1. Agglutination in undiluted and 1:2 diluted serum fields indicates a haptoglobin concentration of > 100 mg/dL.

2. Agglutination in undiluted serum but not in diluted serum indicates a serum haptoglobin concentration of between 50 and 100 mg/dL.

3. No agglutination in either undiluted serum field or 1:2 diluted serum field indicates a haptoglobin concentration of < 50 mg/dL.

Record results on the computer sheets as > 100, 50-100, < 50.

INTERPRETATION OF RESULTS. Normal levels of haptoglobin: > 100 mg/dL.[1-3]

LIMITATIONS OF THE PROCEDURE. This test may fail to detect significant decreases in haptoglobin levels if the baseline levels were above the upper limit of the normal range, as may occur in acute phase reactions.

Reaction times longer than 4 minutes may produce false positive results.

Strength of agglutination in this test is not indicative of the amount of haptoglobin present.

REFERENCES

1. Becker, W. et al.: Meth. Clin. Chem., 1:144, 1970.
2. In lab data.
3. Ritzmann, S.E., and Daniels, J.C.: Serum Protein Abnormalities-Diagnosis and Clinical Aspects. Boston, Little Brown & Co., 1975.

CYTOKINES

Cytokines are glyco- or polypeptide molecules, produced by various cells of the body, which are active at low concentrations (10^{-10} to 10^{-15}M). They function as intracellular messengers in regulation of growth and mobility, production of secretory products, and differentiation of inflammatory leukocytes, as well as cells such as fibroblasts, osteoclasts, chondrocytes, and epithelial and endothelial cells.[82] The term *lymphokine* is commonly used to refer to those cytokines primarily produced by lymphocytes, while *monokines* are closely related cytokines principally secreted by cells of the mononuclear phagocytic system (e.g. monocytes and macrophages). Cytokines are usually identified by the presence of biologic activity in supernates of cell cultures where small quantities of a large number of cytokines may be present. Purification of individual molecules to a homologous state, or by recombinant DNA technology, presents the opportunity for more definitive characterization of molecular structure and function.

Cytokines that modulate the growth and activity of lymphocytes may be classified as *afferent*, in that their primary role appears to be in induction of immune responses (Table 7-2). The action of afferent cytokines is primarily in stimulation and control of hematopoiesis, e.g. via colony-stimulating factors (CSFs) and interleukin-3 (IL-3), and in induction and regulation of immune responses, e.g. via interleukin-1 (IL-1), interleukin-2 (IL-2), interferon (IFN), lymphocyte growth factors such as interleukin-5 (IL-5) or T cell reactive factor (TRF), B cell growth factors (BCGF) and allogeneic effect factor (AEF), and inhibitors such as immunoglobulin binding factors and soluble immune response suppressors (SIRS). *Efferent* cytokines (Table 7-2) are those that primarily effect secondary responses. They include chemotactic factors, migration inhibition factors (MIF, LIF), macrophage activating factor (MAF), lymphotoxin (tumor necrosis factor, beta), and osteoclast activating factor. Most of the cytokines described in this chapter, although usually induced by the presence of antigen, are antigen nonspecific in function and are most often genetically unrestricted.[82] Antigen specific cytokines[119] may also be produced as an integral part of immune responses.

Table 7–2. Major Human Cytokines

AFFERENT CYTOKINES
Colony-Stimulating Factors (CSFs)
Interleukin-3 (IL-3)
Interleukin-1 (IL-1)
Cachectin (TNFα)
Interleukin-2 (IL-2)
Interferons (IFN), alpha, beta and gamma
Interleukin-4 (IL-4)
Interleukin-5 (IL-5)
B Cell Stimulating Factor 2 (BSF-2, IL-6)
Allogeneic Effect Factor (AEF)
Soluble Immune Response Suppressors (SIRS)
Immunoglobulin-Binding Factors (IgBF)
DNA Synthesis Inhibitor
*IgE Differentiation Factor
*B Cell Activating Factor
*Lymphocytosis Promoting Factor

EFFERENT CYTOKINES
Macrophage Inhibition Factor (MIF)
Macrophage Activating Factor (MAF)
Leukocyte Inhibition Factor (LIF)
Lymphotoxin (LT)
Macrophage Chemotactic Factor
*PMN-activating Factor
*Eosinophil Stimulating Factor
*Fibroblast Proliferating Factor
*Fibroblast Activating Factor
*Maturation Inducing Factor
*Migration Enhancement Factor

* Recently described cytokine activities, not currently as well characterized

The characterization and nomenclature of human cytokines is ongoing.

Colony Stimulating Factors[11,76]

Differentiation and proliferation of pleuripotent hematopoietic progenitor, or stem, cells may be induced in vitro by a family of specific growth factors collectively known as colony stimulating factors or CSFs. There are four known hematopoietic CSFs: a multi-CSF known as interleukin-3 (IL-3), a granulocyte CSF (G-CSF), a macrophage CSF (M-CSF), and a factor with granulocyte-macrophage colony stimulating activity (G-M CSF).[121] Colony stimulation may be initiated via specific receptors on progenitor cells[67,103] and may involve multiple factor interaction.[11,90]

Interleukin-3[67] has multilineage hematopoietic effects. It is capable of supporting the growth and differentiation of pleuripotent stem cells, primary erythroid, lymphocytic, megakaryocytic and granuloma-crophage progenitor cells, and mast cells.[63,90,107] It is produced by activated T cells[49] and perhaps by bone marrow.[25] Synonyms that have been used for the activity of IL-3 include hematopoietic growth factor, burst-promoting activity, P-cell stimulating factor, mast cell growth factor, histamine-producing cell stimulating factor, and Thy-1 inducing activity, among others.[67] IL-3 has been purified,[49] and an IL-3 secreting clone has been produced.[25] The effects of the other colony stimulating factors are mainly restricted to a single cell lineage,[88] for example, M-CSF, also known as CSF-1,[108] specifically regulates the survival, proliferation, and differentiation of mononuclear phagocytes and their precursors.

Interleukin-1[33]

Interleukin-1, first described by Gery et al.[30] was renamed IL-1 by a group of immunologists involved in lymphokine studies.[66] Synonyms to be found in the literature include endogenous pyrogen (EP), leukocyte endogenous mediator (LEM), lymphocyte activating factor (LAF) and others.[16,66]

IL-1 is primarily produced by mononuclear phagocytes,[47,83] but also by virtually every nucleated cell type,[83] including T and B cells and natural killer cells. Although some T and B cell lines spontaneously produce IL-1,[59,83] most cells must first be induced by antigen, injury, toxins, or inflammation before IL-1 can be detected.[83] In macrophages, IL-1 can be induced intracellularly within 30 minutes, and extracellularly within 60 minutes.[17,83] There is some evidence that molecules may be released only via perforations of plasma membranes.[83]

Interleukin-1 functions as an endogenous adjuvant to T cells,[57,83] inducing activation of resting cells and production of lymphokines such as interleukin-2, and it may influence B cells at some stage of development.[31,62,83] There is evidence that it acts in combination with colony stimulating factors to promote growth of bone marrow pre-cursors.[15,17] It induces prostaglandin E_2 production,[62] which in turn causes fever via the thermoregulatory center of the brain,[15,16] and may lead to muscle wasting.[83] It causes chemotaxis and increased metabolism in neutrophils and monocytes.[83] It acts on fibroblasts, synovial cells, pancreatic cells, epithelial cells, osteoblasts, osteoclasts, natural killer cells, cells of the central nervous system, endothelial or smooth muscle cells, and chondrocytes.[16,83] Hepatocytes respond to IL-1 by decreasing the production of albumin and regulating production of several acute phase proteins;[29,67,83] thus, IL-1 is a primary mediator of acute phase reactions.

Two molecules with IL-1 activity have been cloned in humans,[4] designated IL-1α and IL-1β, which are functionally distinct.[27] Inhibitors of IL-1[83,118] have been described.

Cachectin[5]

Another factor, produced by macrophages,[9] shares many of the properties of IL-1. Termed tumor necrosis factor alpha (TNFα) or cachectin, it was first described for its hemorrhagic, necrotic effect on certain tumors.[9] It has been highly purified[1] and cloned.[87] Its primary importance may be in its ability to induce shock (e.g. in conjunction with endotoxin[9]), fever, and cachexia, the body wasting that accompanies chronic invasive diseases.[5] Like IL-1, cachectin affects many cells of the body[6] and mediates inflammation and acute phase reactions.[5]

Interleukin-2

T cell growth factor (TCGF)[69] was renamed interleukin-2 in 1979 by a group of immunologists seeking to lessen the confusion brought about by its many synonyms.[66] It is a lymphokine, produced by stimulated Ia⁻ T cells.[57] IL-2 has been cloned,[113] and its properties are fairly well defined.

Resting peripheral blood lymphocytes have no receptors for IL-2.[104] Receptors rapidly appear on T cells[58,95,104] after antigen-specific receptors on the cells complex with appropriately presented antigen[104] or with mitogen.[8] Receptors can be detected on activated B cells,[65,72,126] although they may be fewer in number and have lower affinity than those present on T cells.[72] Gamma interferon (IFNγ) can induce the appearance of IL-2 receptors on monocytes,[45] but a role for the receptor on these cells is uncertain. By contrast, the presence of IL-2 receptors on T cells is directly related to the cell's responsiveness to IL-2.[8]

Soluble IL-2 receptors (SIL-2R) are released from activated cells both in vitro and in vivo and may be useful in detection of immune cell activity in normal individuals. Elevated serum levels of SIL-2R have been described in several disease states.[56]

Probably the best described function of IL-2 is its action on T and B cells. IL-2 interaction with the IL-2 receptor on T cells results in proliferation of the cells, with subsequent amplification of immune responses.[47] B cells activated by anti-Ig or antigen develop IL-2 receptors which, in the presence of IL-2, enhance B cell activation, in conjunction with other B cell-enhancing factors (e.g. IL-4, B cell growth factor II/T cell reactive factor).[17,50,52,74,85] IL-2 may also have a role in the enhancement of gamma interferon (IFNγ) production[84] by lymphocytes.

IL-2 plays several roles in augmentation of killer cell activities.[39] First, it serves as a rapid and potent enhancer of natural killer (NK) activity,[43,114] probably via a somewhat different receptor system.[84,104] Secondly, it can act on certain normal non-T, non-B (null) cells[96] inducing a lymphokine-activated killer (LAK) population[38,71] which is capable of lysing an extensive spectrum of NK-resistant tumor cells without MHC restriction. And, IL-2 can increase the specific killing ability of cloned cytotoxic lymphocytes (CTL) in the presence of antigen.[7,42]

Normal human sera contain a factor capable of inhibiting the action of IL-2.[24]

Interferons[115]

Interferons (IFN) are a heterogeneous family of cytokines that exhibit potent immunoregulatory and antiviral activity. Named for their ability to "interfere" with viral replication in infected cells, interferons are known to exert antiproliferative, or suppressive, activity, as well as the ability to enhance certain reactions (e.g. natural killer cell activity).

Interferons are classified by their cellular origin:[109] Alpha interferon (IFNα) is produced primarily by leukocytes, beta interferon (IFNβ) by fibroblasts, and gamma interferon (IFNγ) by immune cells, predominantly stimulated lymphocytes.[115]

Interferons bind to membrane receptors, IFNα and IFNβ to a single receptor and IFNγ to another,[115] whereupon they are rapidly internalized and degraded. Synthesis of mRNA and protein ensues quickly.

Alpha and beta interferon, originally classified together as type I, or viral, interferons, are structurally related polypeptides, possessing antiproliferative and immunoregulatory, as well as antiviral, activity. IFNα can increase MHC class I molecules on lymphocytes, and can modulate antibody responses. It exerts antiproliferative effects on immune cells, but can enhance natural-killer cell activity.[44] Both IFNα and IFNβ act synergistically with IL-2 in enhancing NK cell activity.[7]

Gamma interferon, although it has less potent antiviral activity, is a good immunoregulator. It induces both Class I and Class II histocompatibility antigens on immune cells,[17,77] particularly on macrophages and dividing neoplastic B cells, but not on resting cells.[77] In the presence of IFNγ, receptors for the gamma heavy chain of immunoglobulin (FcγR) appear on myelomonocytic cells,[115] and IL-2 receptors are increased on monocytes.[45]

IFNγ may substitute for B cell growth factor II (BCGFII) in the B cell maturation sequence,[74] or may exert its enhancing effect via a role in antigen-specific differentiation and maturation of T cells.[115] The ability of IFNγ to inhibit growth of normal and neoplastic cells is documented,[106] and may occur in synergism with lymphotoxin.[115] Whether IFNγ enhances or suppresses a specific immune response is thought to be related to dosage and timing.[106]

IFNγ can also either stimulate[115] or inhibit[123,125] hematopoiesis; for example, it can induce bone marrow production of myeloid cells[115] or may suppress blood cell production by the bone marrow, as in aplastic anemia.[125] IFNγ can activate mature myelomonocytic cells (neutrophils and monocytes),[115] and is probably one of the cytokines described as macrophage activating factors[112] (see below). The effect of IFNγ on NK cell activity is weak.[7] Effects on other cells have been reported.[47]

It appears that both helper (T_H) and suppressor (T_s) cells can produce IFNγ.[115] Production may be increased during anamnestic responses, presumably as a result of memory T cells.[115] NK cells can also be potent IFNγ secretors.[114]

Gamma interferon has been cloned[36] and its structure defined.[115] Clinical trials of the molecule as a therapeutic agent are ongoing.[47]

Interleukin-4[86]

Two apparently different B cell growth factors, primarily produced by T cells, have been described: B cell growth factor I (BCGFI), also known as B stimulating factor-1 (BSF-1) and interleukin-4 (IL-4), and B cell growth factor II (BCGFII), alternately called T cell reactive factor (TRF), B cell differentiation factor (BCDF), or interleukin-5 (IL-5).

Interleukin-4 was first observed as a costimulator of B cell DNA synthesis in response to anti-IgM antibodies.[48] It is produced primarily by certain activated T cells;[86] however, B cells may also be a source.[51] Interleukin-4 has been purified[33,79] and cloned.[101,122]

Receptors for IL-4 are found on both B and T lymphocytes, where they may be enhanced by mitogen stimulation.[80] Receptors are present also on progenitor T and B cells,[103] where interaction with IL-4 probably prepares progenitor cells for response to specific growth or differentiation factors (e.g. colony stimulating factors).[88]

The effects of IL-4 are seen during several stages of B cell activation, differentiation, proliferation, and immunoglobulin secretion.[85] Within hours of contact with IL-4, resting B cells[22,77] and macrophages[13] increase their expression of the Class II histocompatibility antigens needed for immune cell interaction. Simulating antigen contact with B cells by use of antibodies to surface membrane immunoglobulins (e.g. anti-IgM, anti-Fab) results in rapid response, if cells were previously primed with IL-4.[91] Alternately, addition of IL-4 to B cells previously stimulated with anti-IgM induces progression to the S phase[86] and to proliferation.[78] T cell replacing factor (see below) and IL-2 (see above) are needed to induce immunoglobulin formation at this stage. Then, IL-4 has been shown to participate in the switch in immunoglobulin class.[85] IL-4, alone, can effect IgG and IgE production in lipopolysaccharide (LPS) stimulated B cells.[12] Whether IL-4 is primarily a B cell growth factor,[52,91] a differentiating factor,[81] or both[33] is the subject of controversy.

IL-4 promotes the growth of T helper cell lines,[22,33,70] albeit to a lesser extent than IL-2.[105] It can costimulate mast cells along with IL-3.[70] IL-4 acts on peritoneal macrophages to increase tumoricidal activity,[13] suggesting its designation as a macrophage activating factor. And, IL-4 may be a potent helper factor in generation of alloreactive cytotoxic lymphocytes (CTL) in some circumstances.[120]

Interleukin-5

Clearly distinct from interleukin-4[21] is a group of cytokines alternately known as T cell replacing factor (TRF), B cell growth factor II (BCGF II), or B cell differentiating factor (BCDF).[41] More recently, the designation interleukin-5 (IL-5) has been suggested.[55]

IL-5, as described above, acts late in humoral immune responses, effecting final maturation[53] of B cells already proliferating, and promoting immunoglobulin production and secretion.[74,85,98] IL-5 alone cannot induce proliferation of resting cells.[73]

IL-5 has been cloned,[55,101] and receptors for these cytokines have been defined on B cells.[73]

B Cell Stimulating Factor-2

An additional factor observed to participate in humoral immune responses is currently known as B cell stimulating factor-2 (BSF-2). Apparent synonyms are hybridoma plasmacytoma growth factor (HPGF),[116] hepatic stimulating factor (HSF),[29] and B$_2$ interferon (IFNB$_2$). Unlike the two lymphokines described above, BSF-2 is primarily a product of fibroblasts,[116] although epithelial cells and lymphocyte sources have been reported.[89] Receptors for BSF-2 are widely distributed in body tissues and cell lines.[111]

BSF-2 functions in the latter stages of B cell development, inducing immunoglobulin secretion[53] without clonal expansion.[28] It seems to be unique in its ability to induce increased immunoglobulin production within individual cells.[26]

BSF-2 also functions in regulation and growth of several other cells,[111] notably controlling production of many of the hepatic acute phase reactants.[29]

BSF-2 has been cloned,[46] and may soon be referred to as interleukin-6.[89]

Allogeneic Effect Factor[14]

A secreted form of T cell Ia receptor, produced by helper T cells, has been designated allogeneic effect factor. Its presence in cultures stimulates T cells to respond with lymphokine production.

Soluble Immune Response Suppressors[2]

Soluble immune response suppressors (SIRS) are immunosuppressive cytokines that are produced by T suppressor cells.[99] SIRS molecules have been cloned[3] and appear to require oxidation by H$_2$O$_2$, e.g. from macrophages, before they can suppress macrophage function[110] and, in turn, inhibit cell division and immune responses.

Immunoglobulin Binding Factors— DNA Synthesis Inhibitors

Immunoglobulin binding factors inhibit in vitro antibody production and selectively bind certain immunoglobulin molecules.[60] Best described are the human IgE-binding factors that are directly derived from cell surface IgE receptors.[75]

The suppressor lymphokines known as inhibitors to DNA synthesis arrest cell development late in G phase by binding to DNA polymerase.[61]

Both of these factors may also exert a neutralizing effect on T cell replacing factor (TRF).[60,61]

Several additional afferent activities have recently been described. *Lymphocytosis promoting factor* may increase epsilon receptors on lymphocytes,[54] and *IgE differentiation factor* may enhance production of IgE from activated B cells.[102] An additional *B cell activating factor*, shown to induce polyclonal activation of resting B cells, has also been described.[18]

Lymphotoxins[40]

Lymphotoxins, first described in 1968,[97] are efferent cytokines. They are a heterogeneous group of proteins[35] that are produced by activated T cells,[34] and appear within hours of the addition of mitogen to cell cultures.[117] Lymphotoxins are apparently distinct from cachectin (tumor necrosing factor alpha, or TNFα),[37] although they share receptors,[40] but are homologous to tumor necrosis factor beta (TNFβ)[87] and are functionally and antigenically related to differentiation-inducing factor (DIF).[40] A lymphotoxin has been cloned,[37] and two distinct molecules (alpha and beta) have been described (αLT and βLT).[117]

Lymphotoxin exerts cytostatic and cytolytic effects on transformed cells,[40] and is one of the ways immune lymphocytes cause destruction of target cells, yet it has no known effect on normal cells.[87]

Other Cytokines

Also among the cytokines classified as efferent are several which modulate macrophage function. Macrophage *migration inhibiting factor* (MIF) is the term used to describe cytokines which prevent movement of the cell. Although a single molecule with MIF activity has been purified,[23] inhibition of migration may be a consequence of metabolic activation, and thus could be induced by a large number of molecules,[32] for example, gamma interferon.[124] *Macrophage activating factors* (MAF) have the capability to enhance the bactericidal and tumoricidal functions of this naturally phagocytic cell. Gamma interferon also has properties similar to macrophage activating factor,[112] as does interleukin-4 (see above). A distinct molecule with MAF activity has been cloned.[94] Macrophage *migration enhancement factor* (MEF) has been described in rabbits,[32] apparently functioning as an antagonist to MIF. Macrophage *chemotactic factors*[72,73] are apparently a heterogenous group of cytokines sharing the characteristic of attraction for macrophages. *Maturation inducer activity*[10] is the product of a lymphokine which is capable of augmenting terminal differentiation and maturation of certain leukemic and monocytic cells.

Cytokines affecting leukocytes include *leukocyte inhibition factor*,[64] known to inhibit both random and directed migration of neutrophils, *PMN activating factor*,[19] a potent stimulator of neutrophil function, and *eosinophil activating factor*[68] which induces both chemotaxis and activation in eosinophils, as well as exerting a burst-promoting stimulation of bone marrow.

Human monocytes produce several cytokines that augment fibroblast functions, e.g. fibroblast activating factor,[20,100] leading to wound healing and fibrosis. Chemotaxins, prostaglandins, plasminogen activator, and collagenases are other examples of monocyte-derived efferent cytokines.[20]

REFERENCES

1. Aggarwal, B.B., Eessalu, T.E., and Hass, P.E.: Nature, *318*:665, 1985.
2. Aune, T.M., and Pierce, C.W.: Lymphokines, *9*:257, 1984.
3. Aune, T.M., Webb, D.R., and Pierce, C.W.: J. Immunol., *131*:2848, 1983.
4. Bell, T.V., Harley, C.B., Stetsko, D., Sauder, D.N.: J. Invest. Dermatol., *88*:375, 1987.
5. Beutler, B., and Cerami, A.: Nature, *320*:584, 1986.
6. Beutler, B., and Cerami, A.: Lymphokines, *14*:203, 1987.
7. Brooks, C.G., Holscher, M., Urdal, D.: J. Immunol., *135*:1145, 1985.
8. Cantrell, D.A., and Smith, K.A.: J. Exp. Med., *158*:1895, 1983.
9. Carswell, E.A. et al.: Proc. Natl. Acad. Sci. U.S.A., *72*:3666, 1975.
10. Chiao, J.W.: Blood Cells, *13*:111, 1987.
11. Clark, S.C., and Kamen, R.: Science, *236*:1229, 1987.
12. Coffman, R.L. et al.: J. Immunol., *136*:4538, 1986.
13. Crawford, R.M. et al.: J. Immunol., *139*:135, 1987.
14. Delovitch, T.L., Kaufman, K., and Gorczynski, R.M.: J. Exp. Med., *157*:1794, 1983.
15. Dinarello, C.A.: N. Engl. J. Med., *311*:1413, 1984.
16. Dinarello, C.A.: Rev. Infect. Dis., *6*:51, 1984.
17. Dinarello, C.A., and Mier, J.W.: N. Engl. J. Med., *317*:940, 1987.
18. Diu, A. et al.: Proc. Natl. Acad. Sci. U.S.A., *84*:9140, 1987
19. Djeu, J.Y., and Blanchard, D.K.: J. Immunol., *139*:2761, 1987.
20. Dohlman, J.G., Payan, D.G., and Goetzl, E.J.: Immunology, *52*:577, 1984.
21. Dutton, R.W., Wetzel, G.D., and Swain, S.L.: J. Immunol., *132*:2451, 1984.
22. Fernandez-Botran, R. et al.: J. Exp. Med., *164*:580, 1986.
23. Fox, R.A., and MacSween, J.M.: Immunol. Commun., *3*:375, 1974.
24. Fukushima, T. et al.: Int. Arch. Allergy Appl. Immunol., *84*:135, 1987.
25. Fung, M.C. et al.: Nature, *307*:233, 1984.
26. Gallagher, G., Taylor, N., and Willdridge, J.: J. Immunol. Methods, *105*:229, 1987.
27. Gallagher, G., Taylor, N., and Willdridge, J.: Scand. J. Immunol., *26*:295, 1987.
28. Gallagher, G. et al.: Immunology, *60*:523, 1987.

29. Gauldie, J. et al.: Proc. Natl. Acad. Sci. U.S.A., *84*:7251, 1987.

30. Gery, I., Gershon, R.K., and Waksman, B.H.: J. Exp. Med., *136*:128, 1972.

31. Gordon, J., Guy, G., and Walker, L.: Immunology, *57*:419, 1986.

32. Gordon, M.R., Chide, K., Takata, I., and Myrvik, Q.N.: J. Leukocyte Biol., *42*:197, 1987.

33. Grabstein, K. et al.: J. Exp. Med., *163*:1405, 1986.

34. Granger, G.A., and Williams, T.W.: Nature, *218*:1253, 1968.

35. Granger, G.A., Yamamoto, R.S., Fair, D.S., and Hiserodt, J.C.: Cell. Immunol., *38*:388, 1978.

36. Gray, P.W. et al.: Nature, *295*:503, 1982.

37. Gray, P.W. et al.: Nature, *312*:721, 1984.

38. Grimm, E.A., Mazumder, A., Zhang, H.Z., and Rosenberg, S.A.: J. Exp. Med., *155*:1823, 1982.

39. Grimm, E.A., and Rosenberg, S.A.: Lymphokines, *9*:279, 1984.

40. Gullberg, U. et al.: Eur. J. Haematol., *39*:241, 1987.

41. Harada, N. et al.: J. Immunol., *134*:3944, 1985.

42. Hefeneider, S.H., Conlon, P.J., Henney, C.S., and Gillis, S.: J. Immunol., *130*:222, 1983.

43. Henney, C.S., Kuribayashi, K., Kern, D.E., and Gillis, S.: Nature, *291*:335, 1981.

44. Herberman, R.B.: Semin. Oncol., *13*:195, 1986.

45. Herrmann, F., Cannistra, S.A., Levine, H., and Griffin, J.D.: J. Exp. Med., *162*:1111, 1985.

46. Hirano, T. et al.: Nature, *324*:73, 1986.

47. Horohov, D.W., and Siegel, J.P.: Drugs, *33*:289, 1987.

48. Howard, M. et al.: J. Exp. Med., *155*:914, 1982.

49. Ihle, J.N. et al.: J. Immunol., *131*:282, 1983.

50. Jelinek, D.F., and Lipsky, P.E.: J. Immunol., *139*:1005, 1987.

51. Jurgensen, C.H., Ambrus, J.L., and Fauci, A.S.: J. Immunol., *136*:4542, 1986.

52. Kehrl, J.H., Maraguchi, A., Goldsmith, P.K., and Fauci, A.S.: Cell Immunol., *96*:38, 1985.

53. Kikutani, H. et al.: J. Immunol., *134*:990, 1985.

54. Kim, K.M. et al.: Clin. Exp. Immunol., *68*:418, 1987.

55. Kinashi, T. et al.: Nature, *324*:70, 1986.

56. Kloster, B.E. et al.: Clin. Immunol. Immunopathol., *45*:440, 1987.

57. Larsson, E-L., Iscove, N.N., and Coutinho, A.: Nature, *283*:664, 1980.

58. Leonard, W.J. et al.: Nature, *300*:267, 1982.

59. Libby, P. et al.: J. Clin. Invest., *78*:1432, 1986.

60. Lowy, I. et al.: Proc. Natl. Acad. Sci. U.S.A., *80*:2323, 1983.

61. Malkowski, M. et al.: J. Immunol., *130*:785, 1983.

62. March, C. et al.: Nature, *315*:641, 1985.

63. McKearn, J.P., McCubrey, J., and Fagg, B.: Proc. Natl. Acad. Sci. U.S.A., *82*:7414, 1985.

64. Meshulam, D.H. et al.: Proc. Natl. Acad. Sci. U.S.A., *79*:601, 1982.

65. Mingari, M.C. et al.: Nature, *312*:641, 1984.

66. Mizel, S.B., and Ferrar, J.J.: Cell. Immunol., *48*:433, 1979.

67. Moore, M.A.S.: Lymphokines, *15*:219, 1988.

68. Moreau, J.F. et al.: J. Immunol., *138*:3844, 1987.

69. Morgan, D.A., Ruscetti, F.W., and Gallo, R.: Science, *193*:1007, 1976.

70. Mosmann, T.R. et al.: Proc. Natl. Acad. Sci. U.S.A., *83*:5654, 1986.

71. Mule, J.J., Smith, C.A., and Rosenberg, S.A.: J. Exp. Med., *166*:792, 1987.

72. Muraguchi, A. et al.: J. Exp. Med., *161*:181, 1985.

73. Muraguchi, A. et al.: J. Immunol., *127*:412, 1981.

74. Nakagawa, T. et al.: J. Immunol., *137*:3175, 1986.

75. Nakajima, T., Sarfati, M., and Delespesse, G.: J. Immunol., *139*:848, 1987.

76. Nicola, N.A., and Metcalf, D.: Ciba Found. Symp., *118*:7, 1986.

77. Noelle, R. et al.: Proc. Natl. Acad. Sci. U.S.A., *81*:6149, 1984.

78. O'Garra, A. et al.: Proc. Natl. Acad. Sci. U.S.A., *84*:6254, 1987.

79. Ohara, J. et al.: J. Immunol., *139*:1127, 1987.

80. Ohara, J., and Paul, W.E.: Nature, *325*:537, 1987.

81. Oliver, K.R. et al.: Proc. Natl. Acad. Sci. U.S.A., *82*:2465, 1985.

82. Oppenheim, J.J.: Methods Enzymol., *116*:357, 1985.

83. Oppenheim, J.J., Kovacs, E.J., Matsushima, K., and Durum, S.K.: Immunol. Today, *7*:45, 1986.

84. Ortaldo, J.R. et al.: J. Immunol., *133*:779, 1984.

85. Paul, W.E. et al.: Cell Immunol., *99*:7, 1986.

86. Paul, W.E., and Ohara, J.: Annu. Rev. Immunol., *5*:429, 1987.

87. Pennica, D. et al.: Nature, *312*:724, 1984.

88. Peschel, C., Paul, W.E., Ohara, J., and Green, I.: Blood, *70*:254, 1987.

89. Poupart, P. et al.: EMBO J., *6*:1219, 1987.

90. Quesenberry, P.J., Ihle, J.N., and McGrath, E.: Blood, *65*:214, 1985.

91. Rabin, E.M., Ohara, J., and Paul, W.E.: Proc. Natl. Acad. Sci. U.S.A., *82*:2935, 1985.

92. Ramb, C., Malorny, U., Feige, U., and Sorg, C.: Mol. Immunol., *20*:320, 1983.

93. Ramb, C., McEntire, J.E., and Sorg, C.: Mol. Immunol., *20*:325, 1983.

94. Ratlift, T.L. et al.: J. Reticuloendothel. Soc., *31*:393, 1982.

95. Robb, R.J., Munchk, A., and Smith, K.A.: J. Exp. Med., *154*:1455, 1981.

96. Roberts, K., Lotze, M.T., and Rosenberg, S.A.: Cancer Res., *47*:4366, 1987.

97. Ruddle, N.H., and Waksman, B.H.: J. Exp. Med., *128*:1267, 1968.

98. Schimpl, A., Hunig, T., and Wecker, E.: Lymphokines, *6*:185, 1982.

99. Schnaper, H.W., Aune, T.M., and Roby, R.K.: J. Immunol., *139*:1185, 1987.

100. Shaked, A., Sherris, D., and Mayer, L.: Curr. Surg., *44*:487, 1987.

101. Sharme, S., Mehta, S., Morgan, J., and Maizel, A.: Science, *235*:1489, 1987.

102. Sherr, E.H., Stein, L.D., and Dosch, H-M., and Saxon, A.: J. Immunol., *138*:3836, 1987.

103. Sideras, P., and Palacios, R.: Eur. J. Immunol., *17*:217, 1987.

104. Siegel, J.P., Sharon, M., Smith, P.L., and Leonard, W.J.: Science, *238*:75, 1987.

105. Smith, C.A., and Rennick, D.M.: Proc. Natl. Acad. Sci. U.S.A., *83*:1857, 1986.

106. Sonnenfeld, G., Mandel, A., and Merigan, T.C.: Cell Immunol., *40*:285, 1978.

107. Spivak, J.L., Smith, R.R.L., and Ihle, J.N.: J. Clin. Invest., *76*:1613, 1985.

108. Stanley, E.R.: Ciba Found. Symp. *118*:29, 1986.

109. Stewart, W.E., II: Nature, *286*:110, 1980.

110. Tadakuma, T., and Pierce, C.W.: J. Immunol., *117*:967, 1976.

111. Taga, T. et al.: J. Exp. Med., *166*:967, 1987.

112. Talmadge, K.W. et al.: Eur. J. Immunol., *16*:1471, 1986.

113. Taniguchi, T. et al.: Nature, *302*:305, 1983.

114. Trinchieri, G. et al.: J. Exp. Med., *160*:1147, 1984.

115. Trinchieri, G., and Perussia, B.: Immunol. Today, *6*:131, 1985.

116. vanDamme, J. et al.: J. Exp. Med., *165*:914, 1987.

117. Walker, S.M., Lee, S-C., and Lucas, Z.J.: J. Immunol., *116*:807, 1976.

118. Walsh, L.J., Lander, P.E., Seymour, G.J., and Powell, R.N.: Clin. Exp. Immunol., *68*:366, 1987.

119. Webb, D.R., Kapp, J.A., and Pierce, C.W.: Methods Enzymol., *116*:295, 1985.

120. Widmer, M.B., Acres, R.B., Sassenfeld, H.M., and Grabstein, K.H.: J. Exp. Med., *166*:1447, 1987.

121. Wong, G.C. et al.: Science, *228*:810, 1985.

122. Yokota, T. et al.: Proc. Natl. Acad. Sci. U.S.A., *83*:5894, 1986.

123. Young, N.S., Leonard, E., and Platanias, L.: Blood Cells, *13*:87, 1987.

124. Youngner, J.S., and Salvin, S.B.: J. Immunol., *111*:1914, 1973.

125. Zoumbos, N.C., Gascon, P., Djeu, J.Y., Young, N.S.: Proc. Natl. Acad. Sci. U.S.A., *82*:188, 1985.

126. Zubler, R.H. et al.: J. Exp. Med., *160*:1170, 1984.

Chapter 8

PHAGOCYTES

Phagocytosis is the process by which certain body cells, collectively known as phagocytes, ingest and remove microorganisms, effete or malignant cells, inorganic particles, and tissue debris. Although they arise from a common lineage, phagocytic cells differentiate into a heterogeneous population capable, not only of phagocytosis, but also of the secretion of molecules active in wound repair and in the modulation of inflammation, immune responses, and the phagocytic process itself. In addition, certain phagocytic cells, referred to as "accessory cells" are responsible for initiation of immune responses to virtually all antigens.

Cells comprising the phagocytic populations in man originate in the bone marrow as a pleuripotent hematopoietic stem cell, known as the colony forming unit of granulocytes and monocytes (CFU-GM). Proliferation and clonal expansion of these progenitors may be stimulated by soluble factors, e.g. granulocyte monocyte colony stimulating factor (GM-CSF), which can induce formation of both granulocytic and monocytic cell progenitors, and macrophage colony-stimulating factor (M-CSF), also referred to as colony stimulation factor 1 (CSF-1), which stimulates only the expansion of monocytic cells.[23]

Within the granulocytic cell line are two cells known to be phagocytic: the neutrophil and the eosinophil. Neutrophils are the most numerous and most mobile white cells in the blood stream; as such they are readily available, both to perform their function as phagocytes in the body and to serve as an available experimental model for study of the phagocytic process. Much less is known of the role or importance of the phagocytic properties of eosinophils.

Maturation of the neutrophil occurs in the bone marrow as a multistep process, initiated by stimulation of the hematopoietic stem cell and progressing through sequential stages of development: myeloblast, promyelocyte, myelocyte, metamyelocyte, band cells, and, finally, mature neutrophils. The average maturation time for the cell is 6 to 14 days.[6,91] Immature cells, while generally not functionally competent phagocytes, are capable of ingestion and some bactericidal activity in the latter stages of development.[6]

Under normal conditions, approximately 10^{11} mature neutrophils are released into the circulation per day.[91] There, the cells comprise 40 to 75% of the total white blood cell population. Approximately 75% of the total intravascular pool of these cells are loosely bound to blood vessel walls and are referred to as the "marginating pool." A dynamic equilibrium among attached and free cells is maintained. On the average, a cell stays in the blood stream or within the marginating pool for 6 to 10 hours,[6,91] then migrates through endothelial walls into the tissues, where it survives only another 24 to 48 hours.[6,91] Whether inside or outside of the vasculature, mature cells are available for induced migration (*chemotaxis*) to tissue sites of infection, inflammation, necrosis, or allergy.

The mononuclear phagocytic system, or the MPS, is composed of a group of cells arising from a common origin (the hematopoietic stem cell) and having similar morphology and function. Under the influence of soluble factors such as M-CSF, alone or in combination with GM-CSF, monoblasts, promonocytes, and finally mature monocytes are differentiated, a process that typically occurs within 6 days.[54] Unlike the neutrophil cell line, the cells of the MPS tend to be heterogeneous in size, cell density, morphology, and surface molecules. Only 3 to 10% of circulating leukocytes are of the MPS lineage. The average cell circulates in the vascular system for 1 to 4 days before migrating to various tissue sites, where it remains for months to years.[6] Although there is currently no data to suggest that cells are predestined for a particular tissue site,[54] they seem to adapt to their environment and differentiate further relative to their anatomic location.[5,6,61] In tissues, MPS cells may be fixed, as in the splenic sinusoids, lymph nodes, or the liver, or they may remain free, as in pleural, alveolar, or peritoneal spaces. The heterogeneous nature of tissue phases of MPS cells is evidenced by variances in cell surface receptors (see below), in functional roles, and in their responses to molecular stimuli.[15,45,57,88,91,99]

Table 8-1 lists the phagocytic cells of the body.

Mature phagocytic cells are mobile by a process known as diapedesis, a crawling movement facilitated by the forward extensions of cytoplasm known as pseudopods.

In effect, the cell forms and extends this foot-like projection, then appears to flow onto it, while maintaining contact with a cellular surface (e.g. endothelial lining of a blood vessel).

Both neutrophils and the mononuclear phagocytic system have molecular configurations on their cell walls, referred to as "receptors," which react specifically with soluble factors as a means of communicating with their environment. Certain receptors appear common to all phagocytes, whether of PMN or MPS origin,[54,84,91,95] e.g. the FcR, which reacts with the Fc portion of IgG, the CR1, reactant with the C3b, iC3b, C4b, and iC4b components of complement, and the CR3, which attaches to iC3b, C3dg and C3d. Receptors for chemotaxins (see below) such as C5a (derived from the complement system), bacterial by-products, and certain leukotrienes (produced by stimulated leukocytes) are also present on phagocytic cell membranes. Receptors for IgA have been described on neutrophils,[3] and both the neutrophil and the MPS attach to fibronectin.[17] Decay accelerating factor (DAF), described in Chapter 6, appears on stimulated neutrophils[7] and reacts with C3b and C4b. C-reactive protein (CRP) binds to neutrophils[18] either via a separate receptor or perhaps by contact with the $Fc_\gamma R$.

Certain cells of the mononuclear phagocytic system carry receptors for transferrin, alpha 2-macroglobulin and several other known molecules.[19,22] Cells of the MPS produce tumor necrosis factor-alpha (TNFα), also known as cacechtin, and may also carry the receptor for it.[29,54] Receptors for IL-2[90] and interferon (IFNγ, IFNα, and IFNβ) are available on many, if not all, cells of MPS derivation. And, some cells of this lineage have the MHC class II (Ia-like) antigens required for antigen recognition and communication with T cells in the initiation of immune responses.

Only a few of these receptors have, as yet, been studied extensively, and the phagocyte's relationship to its environment via receptors is still being investigated.

Table 8-1. Phagocytic Cells

Granulocytes	
Cell	Location
Neutrophil	Bone Marrow, Blood
Eosinophil	Bone Marrow, Blood

Mononuclear Phagocytic System	
Cell	Location
Monocyte	Blood
Macrophage	Lymph Nodes, spleen, pleural, peritoneal, and synovial spaces, other tissues
Histiocyte	Connective Tissue
Osteoclast	Bone
Pulmonary Macrophage; Alveolar Cell	Lungs
Glial/Microglial Cell	Central Nervous System
Mesangial Cell	Kidneys
Kupffer Cell	Liver
Langerhans' Cell	Skin, lymph nodes, tonsils

NOTE: Certain lymphoid organs contain dendritic cells and/or interdigitating reticulum cells that cannot phagocytize, but may function as accessory cells.

Granules are unique, membrane-bound organelles, found in phagocytic cells, which contain many of the bioactive substances associated with the functions of phagocytes. Approximately one-third of the granules in a mature neutrophil are referred to as azurophilic, or primary, granules. Contents of these granules[13,14] include lysozyme and collagenase, as well as many other molecules important in the killing and digestion of microbes.[6,95] Extracellular release of substances from the azurophilic granules may play a role in deactivation of chemotaxins, the localization of inflammation, and extracellular destruction of tissue.[39,95] The contents of azurophilic granules function optimally at an acid pH.

Secondary, or specific, granules[6,13,14,95] contain substances, e.g. cytochrome b, myeloperoxidase (MPO), and lactoferrin, which are important to the "respiratory burst" (see below). Also contained are molecules such as vitamin B_{12} binding protein, lysozyme, collagenase, chemotactic factors, the CR3 receptor molecule and complement activators.[95]

A third type of granule has been described in neutrophils but has not, as yet, been characterized.[6]

A great deal of recent study has focused on understanding the molecular basis for stimulation of phagocytic cells. At present, it appears that some molecules have broad-spectrum, potent activating ability, while others modulate specific functions. Some substances may induce the same or diverse effects on different phagocytes or on different maturational stages of a single phagocyte.[21,107] Concentration variations may affect the outcome. Often, the modulating substances are products of the phagocytes themselves.

Neutrophils are apparently stimulated not only by foreign antigenic substances, but also by C5a from the complement system, certain bioactive lipids,[85,91] bacterial byproducts, by an endogenous cationic protein,[2] and by a neutrophil activating factor (NAF) produced by cells of the MPS.[85] Certain lymphokines, retrievable from activated T cells, have been shown to be potent neutrophil activators, e.g. IFNγ enhances neutrophil activity,[59,107] as does leukocytic migration inhibition factor (LIF)[11,12] and GM-CSF.[65,67,78,116] The effects of other molecules are also under investigation.[3,18,20,42,73,86,102]

The mononuclear phagocytic system is responsive to antigen[108] and to soluble immune complexes.[112] The presence of C1q in such complexes may augment the cell's ability to respond.[10] Gamma interferon (IFNγ) is a potent enhancer of MPS activities,[9,34,35,40,41,43,76,77,89,90] while alpha and beta interferons (IFNα, IFNβ) may regulate such activities when IFNγ concentrations recede.[24,40,41,82,120] The production of complement components by the MPS system is also modulated by the presence of interferons.[43] GM-CSF,[23,55] TNFα/cachectin,[29,34] and IL-4[26] selectively enhance tumoricidal functions of the MPS cell, and may enhance other activities as well.[48,73] Leukotriene B$_4$[115] and a neutrophil-derived phagocyte activating factor[52] can stimulate metabolism, while CSF-1[114] and platelet activating factor[20] can enhance production of certain secreted molecules. Prostaglandin E$_2$ exhibits a suppressor effect on many functions of MPS cells.[74,81]

THE PHAGOCYTIC PROCESS

Although substances that stimulate the process of phagocytosis are varied, and important functional differences exist among the phagocytic cells, the process of phagocytosis is remarkably generic. Recognizable stages of phagocytosis by the neutrophil, which will serve as our model, include (1) adherence to endothelial cells or to other phagocytic cells (aggregation), (2) chemotaxis, (3) attachment, (4) ingestion, (5) degranulation, and (6) digestion.

Chemotactic factors, such as C5a and its derivative C5a des Arg, bacterially-derived factors, leukotriene B$_4$, coagulation cascade products (e.g. fibrinopeptide B), platelet products (e.g. platelet activating factor), kallikrein, and TNF[6,13,73,91] initiate phagocytosis by stimulating the cell through the first steps of the process: *adherence* and *chemotaxis*. Adherence of phagocytes to endothelial cell walls, or aggregation of cells with each other, is opposed by net electrostatic forces on the cell surfaces which induce negative surface charges.[94,113] Binding of a chemotaxin

to its receptor on the cell causes a small but significant decrease in this surface charge, thus reducing the repulsive force. Adhesive surface molecules, e.g. MAC-1, the CR3 receptor, and p150,[90,94,113] perhaps with the help of other factors,[91] can then initiate contact. Adherence of the phagocytic cell to endothelium, and maintenance of that contact, is an important criterion to its directed motion (*chemotaxis*).

Within a few seconds of contact with a chemotaxin, a complex series of metabolic and structural events occurs.[6,13,91] An increase can be noted in the transmembrane fluxes of certain ions, e.g. Ca^{++}, along with alterations in transmembrane potential. Cell shape changes coincident with an increase in membrane fluidity and deformability. The numbers of certain cell surface receptors (e.g. CR3) increase rapidly and an increase in metabolism (the respiratory burst) occurs (see below). The intracellular contractile system, which includes actin, gelsolin, myosin, and an actin binding protein, is activated, such that the microtubular cytoskeleton rearranges and the cell appears to orient itself toward the source of the chemotactic stimulant. Although the mechanism used by the cell for motility is not understood,[13,46,91,95] certain aspects such as pseudopod formation and orientation to a chemotactic gradient or impulse[111] are observable phenomena.

Attachment of phagocytes to particles may happen nonspecifically, a result of an inherent recognition, e.g. of the foreign nature of the particle, or it may be due to the presence of an opsonin and the process known as immune adherence. IgG or activated complement components (e.g. iC3b) may act as a bridge between their target molecule and a receptor-bearing phagocyte, thereby greatly increasing the efficiency of the phagocytic process.[36,70] Binding of a particle to complement receptors (CR1, CR3) or to Fc$_γ$R alone promotes optimal contact with the phagocytic cell, and may induce ingestion,[58,91,118] but attachment to both receptors often induces dramatic enhancement of the process.[36,68,91,95]

Ingestion of a particle results from extension of an advancing pseudopod over and around the particle surface, such that fusion of the pseudopod with the bulk of the cell eventually occurs. The vacuole resulting from closure of the membrane is referred to as a *phagosome*.

Degranulation of specific (secondary) granules may be triggered by soluble factors (e.g. chemotaxins, leukotrienes),[91,94] or by contact with cell receptors (e.g. Fc$_\gamma$R), or it may occur coincident with formation of a phagosome. In any case, granule contents are released within a matter of seconds into the cell, the phagosome, or into the cell's environs. An oxygen-dependent "respiratory burst" is begun that increases the oxygen consumption of the cell by several hundred fold and results in the production of cytotoxic oxygen radicals (see below). Translocation of CR3 to the cell surface occurs, presumably enhancing the cell's adherence, its chemotaxis, and its ability to attach opsonized particles.[13,84,95] Lytic molecules such as lysozyme and collagenase begin the process of digestion of susceptible cells. The contents of these granules also play a role in modulating and localizing the responses of phagocytes to inflammatory stimuli.

Degranulation of azurophilic, or primary, granules occurs when a cell has been stimulated to ingestion by Fc$_\gamma$R.[91] Granular contents are released primarily into the phagosome formed, although portions appear to escape to the cell surface and into the surrounding area,[91] where they may mediate host cell injury.

Digestion is mediated by substances released from phagocytic granules in combination with the respiratory burst they initiate and the oxygen-independent bactericidal systems.[63,95] These processes also modulate phagocytic function and the inflammatory response.[6,13,28,91,95]

"Respiratory burst"[4,28,51,91,94,96,119] refers to the enhanced oxidative metabolism initiated by the release of contents of the secondary granules. Two enzymes derived from the hexose monophosphate (HMP) shunt, designated G6PD and 6PGD, participate in the formation of NADPH oxidase, a plasma membrane-bound enzyme unique to phagocytes. NADPH oxidase, in turn, catalyzes oxygen (O_2) to superoxide (O_2^-), which is used in the production of hydrogen peroxide (H_2O_2) and certain oxidizing radicals (e.g. OH·) in the so-called MPO-independent system. Alternately, the superoxide radical may react with myeloperoxidase (MPO), an enzyme released from azurophilic or primary granules, catalyzing lipophilic amines (e.g. NH_3) into highly toxic oxidants, or inducing the oxidation of halides (e.g. Cl^-) to highly toxic ions (OCl^-). The latter, in turn, are capable of oxidizing a wide variety of biologic molecules, such as cytochromes, nucleotides, and sulfhydryl groups. Other actions of the MPO system include activation and inactivation of secreted neutrophil proteases and inactivation of toxins and other mediators of inflammation.

THE MACROPHAGE AS ACCESSORY CELL

A characteristic of the mononuclear phagocytic system that is not shared by neutrophils is the presence of class II major histocompatibility (MHC) antigens (Ia antigens) on the cell surface (see Chaps 1 and 13). A coincident characteristic is the ability of macrophages to digest, or "process," an internalized antigen in such a way that partially degraded antigen "pieces" result, which have affinity for the Class II antigens.[6,8,109,110] In combination, digestion, processing, and attachment of appropriately degraded antigen to MHC Class II antigens may be referred to as the antigen-processing or accessory cell function of macrophages.

Of the three cell lines that are required for immune responses, i.e. macrophages, T lymphocytes, and B lymphocytes, only the macrophage develops no inherent commitment to a specific antigen as it matures. The macrophage, then, is unique, in its ability to engulf virtually all foreign, effete, or undesirable cells, partially degrade them, and present them on the macrophage surface, in combination with MHC Class II antigen, for recognition by other cells.[8,109,110] While some antigens can be recognized by T and/or B lymphocytes without being processed by an accessory cell,[8] the majority of antigens cannot.

Although the requirement for accessory cell function has been well documented, the mechanism is still under investigation. It appears that some, but not all,[5,45,92] macrophages are capable of accessory cell function. (Of interest will be studies to determine which macrophages, at which sites, will be simply scavengers and which will be capable of initiating immune responses via accessory cell activity.) Organisms must be internalized before appropriate processing can occur.[109] The accessory cell must be genetically matched (MHC Class II identical) with the lymphocyte receiving the processed antigen before recognition can occur.[8] It appears that accessory cell activity is required for stimulation of both the induction of, and the suppression of, immune responses.[31,93] The relative numbers of each type of cell and the amount of antigen present, may affect the type of response which is induced.[50,93] IFNγ in the environment can increase the numbers of MHC Class II antigens, as well as the $Fc_\gamma R$, on macrophages;[35] however, the net effect of increasing the numbers of these receptors is not known. The presence of IL-1, particularly cell-bound IL-1,[50,109] may be a requirement for effective accessory cell function. Since the macrophage produces IL-1, the inhibitor to IL-1, and factors required for inhibition of the release of IL-1[50] from the cell, macrophages may have mechanisms useful in controlling their own performance of accessory functions.

The role of antigen presentation has also been attributed to B cells[87] and, under certain circumstances, to a few other types of cells.[54,110]

PHYSIOLOGIC EFFECTS OF PHAGOCYTES

Together with the ability of phagocytes to engulf and destroy undesirable substances and the function of the accessory cell population in antigen processing, phagocytes also affect other physiologic processes. Both neutrophils and the MPS, for example, produce platelet activating factor,[20] which can induce platelet aggregation and degranulation, stimulate contraction of smooth muscles, promote the chemotaxis of phagocytes, and increase vascular permeability. Oxygen metabolites from phagocytes can stimulate the synthesis of prostaglandins.[71] The term "defensins" refers to a group of azurophilic granule-related molecules which demonstrate cytotoxic properties in high concentration areas, such as those found in neutrophil-rich exudates.[39] A neutrophil-derived histamine release activating factor has also been described.[117]

Because of the potential for tissue damage from toxic products of phagocytic metabolism, the accumulation of neutrophils at sites of inflammation in the body may be an important factor in the pathogenesis of many diseases,[44,69] e.g. gout, systemic lupus erythematosus, rheumatoid arthritis, glomerulonephritis, immune vasculitis, neutrophil dermatoses, inflammatory bowel disease, myocardial infarction, emphysema, thermal injury and malignant neoplasms. A prototypic example of the role of the phagocyte may be adult respiratory distress syndrome (ARDS).[13,91] In ARDS patients, respiratory distress, hypoxia, and diffuse pulmonary infiltrates develop within 72 hours of a stimulus such as aspiration of an inducing antigen or bacterial sepsis. Vascular endothelium and alveolar epithelial cells are damaged or killed, fibrin deposition occurs, capillaries are obliterated, and fibrosis develops, presumably as a result of lung infiltration with inflammatory cells.[13,44,69] In spite of supportive therapy, more than 50% of ARDS patients die.

The mononuclear phagocytic system produces more than 100 distinct substances[79] which affect virtually every aspect of inflammation and immune responsiveness. Among the secretory products of the MPS is interleukin-1 (IL-1), known to regulate lymphocytes, induce the production of acute phase reactants, and induce fever.[54,79] The latter two functions are shared with another molecular MPS product, TNFα/cachectin.[54] The MPS has the potential to synthesize every component of the functional complement system.[43,53] Regulation of hepatic protein synthesis is a function of hepatic stimulating factor derived from the MPS.[37] Histamine-releasing factors, produced by the MPS, have a stimulatory effect on basophils and mast cells.[98] Alveolar macrophages demonstrate the ability to modulate IL-2-activated killer cells.[103] And, the MPS appears capable of regulating its own survival, growth, and differentiation via production of CSF-1 (M-CSF).[49] For further reference on the effects of the MPS, see Nathan[79] and the section on Cytokines (Chap 7).

TESTING FOR PHAGOCYTIC FUNCTION[1,91]

Efficient phagocytic function is dependent on optimal activity at each stage of the phagocytic process: chemotaxis, adherence and aggregation, attachment or opsonization, ingestion, degranulation, and digestion. Impaired phagocytic function may result from a deficiency or defective function at any step in the process. Testing for an apparent malfunction, then, may include phagocytic cell counts, tests for adherence and/or neutrophil aggregation, quantitative assays for chemotaxis, and functional testing of response to chemotaxins (e.g. Boyden test).[83] Nitroblue tetrazolium (NBT) may be used to assess the respiratory burst (see *NBT dye test* below), and bactericidal assays can demonstrate defects in opsonization and the ability to kill microbes.[30,75] Immunoglobulin and/or complement quantitation may explain impaired ability to opsonize particles.

Phagocytic assays such as those described by Stossel[104,106] may be helpful. Patient symptoms, history, and chronology of infectious agents provide important information, as does family history in many cases.

DEFECTS IN PHAGOCYTOSIS

Acquired phagocytic defects[6,13,91] occur far more frequently than primary, or congenital deficiencies. Extrinsic factors such as ethanol, hemodialysis, certain pharmacologic agents, or thermal burns can result in neutrophil dysfunction. Anti-neutrophil antibody,[97] as has been described in systemic lupus erythematosus (SLE), Felty's syndrome, rheumatoid arthritis, and drug allergies, may render a patient neutropenic. Transplacental transfer of such an antibody may confer transient effects on a newborn.[97] Neutropenia may also accompany infection, inflammation, nutritional deficiency,[25,97] chemotherapy, or radiation therapy. Defects in the locomotion or chemotaxis of neutrophils have been described in conditions including myeloblastic syndromes, Schwachman syndrome, Hodgkin's disease, juvenile periodontitis, sarcoidosis, and non-Hodgkin's lymphoma. Normal neutrophil function may be inhibited by the presence of immune complex disease, by cryoglobulins, or by bone marrow transplant. Patients with diabetes mellitus, inflammatory bowel disease, iron deficiency, or women who are pregnant, may also show evidence of phagocytic defects.

Age-related defects may impair phagocytic ability in newborns and in those of advancing age. Newborn neutrophils exhibit lowered ability to deform and to respond to chemotactic stimuli.[47,91] Deficiencies in secondary, or specific, granules of normal newborn neutrophils have been described and may appear, in part, as a lack of increase in CR3-mediated adhesion when the cell is stimulated.[91] Spontaneous resolution of these newborn abnormalities occurs with time. Macrophage function in the newborn is apparently normal.[105]

Although the ability of phagocytes to function in persons of advancing age is apparently normal,[32,66] age-related deficiency in serum-mediated ingestion is well documented,[32,66,72] and is apparently due to inability of the microenvironment to provide chemotaxins and/or opsonins. Serum from individuals over 30 years of age demonstrates diminished ability to support phagocytic activity, and the deficiency is more evident with each decade.[32]

CONGENITAL DEFECTS IN PHAGOCYTOSIS

More than 15 congenital defects in the phagocytic process have been described in the literature. These may be classified by the apparent primary defect as follows:

Neutropenia/Monocytopenia

Although primary deficiencies in neutrophils have been reported, no description of inherited monocytopenia is available in the literature.[54,99]

Disorders of Adhesion

Individuals with an inherited deficiency of the CR3 receptor,[6,13,69,91,95] and the related membrane glycoproteins LFA-1 and p150,[95] have delayed separation of the umbilical cord, recurrent infections, delayed wound healing, and the absence of pus at the site of infections. The inheritance pattern is probably autosomal recessive. The defect results in decreased peripheral blood leukocyte counts, as well as defective adherence, neutrophil aggregation, diapedesis, chemotaxis, and phagocytosis of opsonized particles. Death from overwhelming infection usually occurs without intervention in the form of bone marrow transplantation.

Disorders of Motility

Lazy leukocyte syndrome is a relatively mild disorder, where increased numbers of infections occur, but they tend to be less severe and less chronic than in other defects.[56] Lowered peripheral blood neutrophil counts reflect a tendency of the cells to stay in the bone marrow after being produced. Individuals with lazy leukocyte syndrome usually develop normally.

Disorders of Chemotaxis[13,16]

Congenital deficiencies in chemotactic factors, for example, a deficiency in the C5 component of complement, may appear as a chemotactic defect.

Primary disorders in which the phagocyte's ability to respond to chemotaxins is impaired include Chediak-Higashi syndrome, Pelger-Huet anomaly, and hyper IgE (Job's) syndrome.

Chediak-Higashi syndrome is described below (*Granular Disorders*) because of the more well known deficiencies occurring in conjunction with granular fusion.

Pelger-Huet anomaly follows a pattern of autosomal dominant inheritance.[91] Although the disorder is characterized by incomplete segmentation of neutrophil nuclei, with accompanying decrease in deformability and locomotion of cells, patients usually do not experience an abnormal number, or increased severity, of infections.

Hyper IgE (Job's) syndrome is a puzzling disorder in which patients develop relatively large concentrations of IgE (usually with specificity for *Staphylococcus aureus* and *Candida albicans*) in conjunction with decreased salivary IgA, and an increased risk for pyogenic abcesses.[64,95] Persistent eczematoid lesions and characteristic coarse facies are a corollary to this disorder. Moderate defects in chemotaxis appear to result from the presence of a potent chemotaxin inhibitor.

Granular Disorders

Genetic granular disorders have been described in which neutrophils were void of granules,[91] lacked only one of the two major types of granules (e.g. congenital specific granule deficiency), have fused granules with impaired ability to degranulate (Chediak-Higashi syndrome), or lacked only an enzyme needed for efficient respiratory burst activity (MPO deficiency; lactoferrin deficiency).

Patients with congenital specific granule deficiencies[69,95] suffer recurrent skin and deep tissue infections and impaired inflammatory responses. Peripheral white blood cell counts are usually normal; however, with Wright's staining, cells appear devoid of granules, a result of that stain's inability to demonstrate specific (secondary) granules. Peroxidase stains reveal the presence of azurophilic granules. Patient's phagocytes have impaired chemotaxis, lack lactoferrin, and are deficient in respiratory burst and certain bactericidal activities. Inherited forms of this disorder are heterozygous; different abnormalities may exist in each patient. An acquired form of this disorder is seen in some patients with thermal injuries.

Chediak-Higashi syndrome (CHS) is a rare, autosomal recessive disorder characterized by recurrent infections, partial oculocutaneous albinism, photophobia, and nystagmus.[60,91,95] Fusion of primary and secondary granules within neutrophils results in formation of the giant granules characteristic of the disease. Neutrophils in CHS patients have decreased deformability, decreased locomotive ability, and impaired degranulation.

Most patients with CHS eventually develop an "accelerated phase" of the disease, manifesting a complex of pancytopenia, fever, nonneoplastic infiltration of major organs with atypical lymphoid cells and serious infections. Death occurs as a result of infection or hemorrhage.

Myeloperoxidase (MPO) deficiency is a relatively common disorder (1/2000 individuals) which is *not* usually associated with increased susceptibility to recurrent or severe infections.[62,69,80,91,95] Although about 50% of patients have a total absence of MPO activity, and in vitro bacterial killing is demonstrably impaired within the early period after ingestion, delayed bactericidal and fungicidal killing is usually effective. In pa-

tients who also have diabetes mellitus, fungicidal activity may be insufficient.

Disorders of Oxidative Metabolism

Chronic granulomatous disease (CGD) is a rare, inherited group of disorders in which phagocytes fail to generate hydrogen peroxide (H_2O_2) and oxygen radicals upon stimulation.[13,27,28,69,95] Inheritance may be X-linked or, less commonly, autosomal recessive; thus, the majority of the > 300 known CGD-affected children have been male.

Although clinical features of the disease vary, all children with CGD share a profound impairment of oxidative metabolism and recurrent, often life-threatening infections. Pyogenic bacteria such as staphylococci and gram-negative bacilli, as well as certain fungi, e.g. aspergillus and candida are usually the cause of these infections. Organisms which produce H_2O_2 without concurrent catalase production (e.g. streptococci) are not significant pathogens. Sites of chronic infection may develop into granulomas, with obstruction of vital organs often a complication. Onset of infections is usually during the first year of life, although occasionally may not occur until adolescence or early adulthood.

The exact nature of the defect in CGD varies with each individual; however, abnormalities in cytochrome b are usually present in X-linked disease.[95,101] Decreased numbers of CR1 receptors on neutrophils of patients may also contribute to the disorder by impairing the cell's ability to ingest complement-coated particles.[38]

X-linked CGD has been associated with the absence of the Kell-related Kx antigen on leukocytes.[28]

Diagnosis of CGD,[28] and screening of individuals for carrier states of the disease, can be accomplished using the nitroblue tetrazolium (NBT) test (see below). DNA probes for the genes responsible for CGD are being developed.

Supportive therapy, e.g. prophylactic antibiotics and possibly bone marrow transplant have been the only modes of treatment for CGD. Recently, gamma interferon (IFN γ) therapy has been successful in partial correction of the phagocytic defects.[33,100]

Disorders of Oxidant Removal

Several deficiencies in the ability to remove the oxidant by-products of the respiratory burst have been described.[13] Individuals with these disorders are not usually susceptible to increased infection rates.

REFERENCES

1. Absolom, D.R.: Methods Enzymol., *132*:95, 1986.
2. Alam, M., Ranadive, N.S., and Pruzanski, W.: Inflammation, *11*:131, 1987.
3. Albrechtsen, M., Yeaman, G.R., and Kerr, M.A.: Immunology, *64*:201, 1988.
4. Babior, B.M.: Hematol. Oncol. Clin. North Am., *2*:201, 1988.
5. Becker, S. et al.: Cell. Immunol., *98*:467, 1986.
6. Bell, J.B., and Douglas, S.D.: Pediatr. Ann., *16*:379, 1987.
7. Berger, M., and Medof, M.E.: J. Clin. Invest., *79*:214, 1987.
8. Berkower, I., and Streicher, H.Z.: Pediatr. Ann., *16*:395, 1987.
9. Black, C.M., Cattarall, J.R., and Remington, J.S.: J. Immunol., *138*:491, 1987.
10. Bobak, D.A. et al.: J. Immunol., *138*:1150, 1987.
11. Borish, L., and Rocklin, R.: J. Immunol., *138*:1480, 1987.
12. Borish, L. et al.: Cell. Immunol., *113*:320, 1988.
13. Boxer, L.A., and Morganroth, M.L.: Dis. Mon., *33*:681, 1987.
14. Boxer, L.A., and Smolen, J.E.: Hematol. Oncol. Clin. North Am., *2*:101, 1988.
15. Brain, J.D.: Am. Rev. Respir. Dis., *137*:507, 1988.
16. Brown, C.C., and Gallin, J.I.: Hematol. Oncol. Clin. North Am., *2*:61, 1988.
17. Brown, E.J., and Goodwin, J.L.: J. Exp. Med., *167*:777, 1988.
18. Buchta, R., Pontet, M., and Fridkin, M.: FEBS Lett., *211*:165, 1987.
19. Buys, S.S., and Kaplan, J.: J. Cell. Physiol., *131*:442, 1987.
20. Camussi, G. et al.: J. Exp. Med., *166*:1390, 1987.
21. Carlsen, E., and Prydz, H.: Scand. J. Immunol., *27*:401, 1988.
22. Catterall, J.R. et al.: Infect. Immun., *55*:1635, 1987.
23. Chen, B.D., Clark, C.R., and Chou, T.: Blood, *71*:997, 1988.
24. Chen, B.D., and Najor, F.: Cell Immunol., *106*:343, 1987.
25. Conway, L.T. et al.: Pediatrics, *79*:728, 1987.
26. Crawford, R.M. et al.: J. Immunol., *139*:135, 1987.

27. Curnutte, J.T.: Hematol. Oncol. Clin. North Am., *2*:241, 1988.
28. Curnutte, J.T., and Babior, B.M.: Adv. Hum. Genet., *16*:229, 1987.
29. Decker, T., Lohmann-Matthes, M.-L., and Gifford, G.E.: J. Immunol., *138*:957, 1987.
30. DeWeger, R.A., Runhaar, B.A., and Denotter, W.: Methods Enzymol., *132*:458, 1986.
31. Elmasry, M.N., Fox, E.J., and Rich, R.R.: J. Immunol., *137*:2468, 1986.
32. Emanuelli, G. et al.: Gerontology, *32*:308, 1986.
33. Ezekowitz, R.A. et al.: N. Engl. J. Med. *319*:146, 1988.
34. Feinman, R. et al.: J. Immunol., *138*:635, 1987.
35. Firestein, G.A., and Zvaifler, N.J.: Cell. Immunol., *104*:343, 1987.
36. Fries, L.F. et al.: Immunology, *62*:45, 1987.
37. Fuller, G.M. et al.: Biochem. Biophys. Res. Commun., *144*:1003, 1987.
38. Gaither, T.A. et al.: Inflammation, *11*:211, 1987.
39. Ganz, T.: Infect. Immun., *55*:568, 1987.
40. Garotta, G. et al.: Biochem. Biophys. Res. Commun., *140*:948, 1986.
41. Gerrard, T.L. et al.: J. Immunol., *138*:2535, 1987.
42. Gorter, A. et al.: Immunology, *61*:303, 1987.
43. Hamilton, A.O. et al.: Biochem. J., *242*:809, 1987.
44. Harlan, J.M.: Acta. Med. Scand. (Suppl.), *715*:123, 1987.
45. Haskill, S. et al.: Cell. Immunol., *115*:100, 1988.
46. Haston, W.S., and Wilkinson, P.C.: J. Cell. Sci., *87*:373, 1987.
47. Hill, H.R. et al.: Am. J. Pathol., *128*:307, 1987.
48. Hoffman, M., and Weinberg, J.B.: J. Leukocyte Biol., *42*:704, 1987.
49. Horiguchi, J. et al.: Biochem. Biophys. Res. Commun., *141*:924, 1986.
50. Hunninglake, G.W.: Am. Rev. Respir. Dis., *136*:253, 1987.
51. Hurst, N.P.: Ann. Rheum. Dis., *46*:265, 1987.
52. Ishibashi, Y., and Yamashita, T.: Infect. Immun., *55*:1762, 1987.
53. Johnson, E., and Hetland, G.: Scand. J. Immunol., *27*:489, 1988.
54. Johnston, R.B., Jr.: N. Engl. J. Med., *318*:747, 1988.
55. Jones, M.P. et al.: Cell. Immunol., *113*:361, 1988.
56. Katzin, W.E. et al.: Cleve. Clin. Q., *53*:299, 1986.
57. Kemmerich, B., Rossing, T.H., and Pennington, J.E.: Am. Rev. Respir. Dis., *136*:266, 1987.
58. Kemp, A.S., and Turner, M.W.: Immunology, *59*:69, 1986.
59. Kowanko, I.C., and Ferrante, A.: Immunology, *62*:149, 1987.
60. Komiyama, A. et al.: Scand. J. Haematol., *37*:162, 1986.
61. Kreipe, H., Radzun, H.-J., and Parwaresch, M.R.: Histochem. J., *18*:441, 1986.
62. Lanza, F. et al.: J. Clin. Lab. Immunol., *22*:175, 1987.

63. Lehrer, R.I., Ganz, T., and Selsted, M.E.: Hematol. Oncol. Clin. North Am., 2:159, 1988.
64. Leung, D.Y.M., and Geha, R.F.: Hematol. Oncol. Clin. North Am., 2:81, 1988.
65. Lindemann, A. et al.: J. Immunol., 140:837, 1988.
66. Lipschitz, D.A., Udupa, K.B., and Boxer, L.A.: Blood, 70:1131, 1987.
67. Lopez, A.F. et al.: J. Clin. Invest., 78:1220, 1986.
68. Malbran, A., Frank, M.M., and Fries, L.F.: Immunology, 61:15, 1987.
69. Malech, H.L., and Gallin, J.I.: N. Engl. J. Med., 317:687, 1987.
70. Mantovani, B.: Exp. Cell. Res., 173:282, 1987.
71. Marshall, P.J., and Lands, W.E.M.: J. Lab. Clin. Med., 108:525, 1986.
72. Melez, K.A. et al.: Blood, 71:1726, 1988.
73. Ming, W.J., Bersani, L., and Mantovani, A.: J. Immunol., 138:1469, 1987.
74. Monick, M., Glazier, J., and Hunninghate, G.W.: Am. Rev. Respir. Dis., 135:72, 1987.
75. Moore, L.L., and Humbert, J.R.: Methods Enzymol., 132:520, 1986.
76. Murray, H.W.: Ann. Intern. Med., 108:595, 1988.
77. Murray, H.W. et al.: J. Immunol., 138:2457, 1987.
78. Naccache, P.H. et al.: J. Immunol., 140:3541, 1988.
79. Nathan, C.F.: J. Clin. Invest., 79:319, 1987.
80. Nauseef, W.M.: Hematol. Oncol. Clin. North Am., 2:135, 1988.
81. Otterness, I.G. et al.: Cell. Immunol., 114:385, 1988.
82. Pace, J.L., MacKay, R.J., and Hayes, M.P.: J. Leukocyte Biol., 41:257, 1987.
83. Pederson, M.M.: Acta. Pathol. Microbiol. Immunol. Scand, 95C:189, 1987.
84. Petty, H.R. et al.: J. Cell. Physiol., 133:235, 1987.
85. Peveri, P. et al.: J. Exp. Med., 167:1547, 1988.
86. Pichyangkul, S. et al.: Exp. Hematol., 15:1055, 1987.
87. Pierce, S.K. et al.: Immunol. Rev., 106:149, 1988.
88. Poli, G. et al.: Clin. Immunol. Immunopathol., 47:282, 1988.
89. Ralph, P., Nakoinz, I., and Rennick, D.: J. Exp. Med., 167:712, 1988.
90. Rambaldi, A. et al.: Eur. J. Immunol., 17:153, 1987.
91. Repo, H.: Ann. Clin. Res., 19:263, 1987.
92. Rich, E.A., and Ellner, J.J.: Cell. Immunol., 103:339, 1986.
93. Rich, E.A. et al.: Am. Rev. Respir. Dis., 136:258, 1987.
94. Rossi, F.: Biochem. Biophys. Acta., 853:65, 1986.
95. Rotrosen, D., and Gallin, J.I.: Ann. Rev. Immunol., 5:127, 1987.
96. Sadler, K.L., and Badwey, J.A.: Hematol. Oncol. Clin. North Am., 2:185, 1988.
97. Sakaguchi, M. et al.: Acta. Haematol. (Basel), 75:236, 1986.
98. Schulman, E.S. et al.: J. Immunol., 140:2369, 1988.
99. Seljelid, R.: Acta. Med. Scand. (Suppl.), 715:131, 1987.
100. Sechler, J.M. et al.: Proc. Natl. Acad. Sci. U.S.A., 85:4874, 1988.
101. Segal, A.W.: Hematol. Oncol. Clin. North Am., 2:213, 1988.
102. Seow, W.K. et al.: Int. Arch. Allergy Appl. Immunol., 85:63, 1988.
103. Sone, S. et al.: J. Immunol., 139:29, 1987.
104. Spangenberg, P., and Crawford, N.: Biosci. Rep., 6:715, 1986.
105. Speer, C.D. et al.: Eur. J. Pediatr., 145:418, 1986.
106. Stossel, T.P.: Methods Enzymol., 132:192, 1986.
107. Taetle, R., and Honeysett, J.M.: Blood, 71:1590, 1988.
108. Todd, R.F. 3rd, and Liu, D.Y.: Fed. Proc., 45:2829, 1986.
109. Unanue, E.R., and Allen, P.M.: Cell. Immunol., 99:3, 1986.
110. Unanue, E.R., and Allen, P.M.: Science, 236:551, 1987.
111. Vicker, M.G., Lackie, J.M., and Schill, W.: J. Cell. Sci., 84:263, 1986.
112. Vieweg, R., and Leslie, R.G.Q.: Eur. J. Immunol., 17:149, 1987.
113. Wardle, E.N.: Postgrad. Med. J., 62:997, 1986.
114. Warren, M.K., and Ralph, P.: J. Immunol., 137:2281, 1986.
115. Wasserman, J. et al.: Int. Arch. Allergy Appl. Immunol., 83:39, 1987.
116. Weisbart, R.H. et al.: Blood, 69:18, 1987.
117. White, M.V., and Kaliner, M.A.: J. Immunol., 139:1624, 1987.
118. Willis, H.E. et al.: J. Immunol., 140:234, 1988.
119. Wymann, M.P. et al.: J. Biol. Chem., 262:12048, 1987.
120. Yoshida, R., Murray, H.W., and Nathan, C.F.: J. Exp. Med., 167:1171, 1988.

NITRO BLUE TETRAZOLIUM TEST (NBT) (STIMULATED AND UNSTIMULATED)

PRINCIPLE. Fresh heparinized blood is enriched for white blood cells then incubated with NBT dye, allowing phagocytosis to occur. Following ingestion, NBT dye reacts with superoxide anions, a product of phagocyte oxygen metabolism, and is reduced to a black substance called formazan. Slides of the resultant cells are prepared, stained, and observed for the percentage of cells containing black formazan deposits. Latex particles may be added to the standard NBT test as a stimulant to phagocytosis.

EQUIPMENT AND MATERIALS

1. Bacto-latex 0.81 (Difco): Store at 2° to 8° C. DO NOT FREEZE.

2. NBT dye (Sigma): Store desiccated at 4° to 6° C.

3. Plastic microtiter plate with U-shaped wells.

4. Plastic pipets—1 ml, graduated to 0.1 ml.

5. Microscope slide 1" × 3". Use pre-cleaned slides or they may be cleaned before use by rinsing in 95% ethanol. Allow to air dry.

6. Plastic capillary pipets.

7. Commercial Wright's stain.

8. Sorenson's buffer (.067M): Add 183.4 ml of solution (a) to 66.6 ml solution (b).

Solution a: In a 1000-ml volumetric flask, add 9.08 g KH_2PO_4. QS to 1000 ml with distilled water.

Solution b: In a 1000-ml volumetric flask, add 9.475 g Na_2HPO_4. QS to 1000 ml with distilled water.

9. 0.15M phosphate buffered saline (PBS): pH 7.2. Add 266.7 ml of 0.15M KH_2PO_4 to 773.3 ml 0.15M Na_2HPO_4. Note: The PBS used for fluorescent antibody procedures is acceptable.

10. Forced air dryer.

11. Light microscope.

SPECIMEN COLLECTION AND PREPARATION.

Patient/control sample: One heparin tube per patient and control. High concentrations of heparin can block enzyme systems; thus, at least 3 ml of blood in each heparin tube is required. Blood must be used within 2 hours of extraction. NaF heparinized blood is not acceptable for NBT testing since NaF inactivates white blood cell enzymes.

PREPARATION OF REAGENTS

1. Preparation of 0.1% NBT solution: Dissolve 5 mg NBT dye in 2.5 ml 0.9% NaCl. Protect from light by wrapping tube in gauze and placing it in a plastic conical centrifuge tube. Shake until dissolved (30 to 60 minutes). Add 2.5 ml of 0.15M phosphate buffered saline (FA buffer). Label and store at 2° to 8° C. May be used up to 1 week from time of preparation.

PROCEDURE

NOTE: The NBT and the stimulated NBT are usually run in parallel. In addition, a WBC count and differential should be performed if absolute numbers are desired.

1. For each patient and control, place 0.1 ml of 0.1% NBT solution into each of 4 wells in a plastic microtiter plate; these represent stimulated and unstimulated test wells run in duplicate.

2. Add 0.1 ml of well-mixed heparinized blood to each well. Alternately, buffy coat cells may be collected after centrifugation of heparin tubes and removal of the plasma. 0.1 ml of the buffy coat is then pipetted into each of the wells. The latter procedure will increase the concentration of phagocytic cells and is strongly recommended.

3. Add 1 drop (approximately 0.05 ml) of latex to each patient and control wells labeled as stimulated assay.

4. Mix carefully with a plastic pipet.

5. Immediately place tray in moist chamber. Incubate at 37° C for 10 minutes.

6. Continue incubating at room temperature for 15 minutes.

7. Clean microscope slides in 95% ethanol and allow to dry, or use precleaned slides.

8. Mix contents of one well thoroughly with a plastic pipet, place one drop on a microscope slide and prepare blood smear. Prepare at least two blood film slides from each well. Dry immediately with a dryer.

9. Repeat for each well of all patients and controls.

10. Select one slide from each group and flood with freshly filtered Wright's stain. Stain 3½ minutes. Add an equal volume of Sorenson's buffer to each slide. Wait 10 minutes.

11. Wash with copious amounts of distilled water from a squeeze bottle. Clean backs of slides with tissue and allow to dry on a slant.

NOTE: Steps 10 and 11 can be accomplished using a slide stainer in Hematology, if desired.

12. Scan each slide under low power for the greatest concentration of leukocytes. Then, using oil immersion, count at least 50 neutrophils per slide, recording both total neutrophils and the number which contain deposits of black formazan (reduced NBT dye). Only cells containing black material larger than the granules normally appearing in neutrophils are counted. Scan and count neutrophils for latex ingestion on the stimulated slides.

RESULTS. The normal control should have >14% of the cells exhibiting reduction of NBT dye. Report the percentage of neutrophils positive for NBT reduction (i.e. positive for formazan). Stimulated NBT results are usually 2 to 3 times the normal range obtained in the NBT test. The test is reported as positive if these criteria are met. Lower percentages are reported as negative.

INTERPRETATION OF RESULTS. Normal individuals reduce NBT in greater than 14% of their neutrophils; 10% or less is considered abnormal. In some instances, the absolute number of reducing cells present may be more useful than the percentage. In these cases, a white cell count and differential should be obtained and absolute numbers calculated. NBT reduction is found impaired in individuals with chronic granulomatous disease. Patients with chronic granulomatous disease or other defects in phagocytosis or H_2O_2 production will be negative, having less than 10% of cells exhibiting NBT reduction. NBT reduction may also be used in differentiating bacterial from non-bacterial febrile disorders.[1-5]

LIMITATIONS OF PROCEDURE. Rapid performance of this procedure is necessary because white blood cells allowed to phagocytize for too long of a period may burst. This may also necessitate adjusting incubation times to slightly shorter periods. Slides should only be interpreted by personnel with extensive experience with this assay.

REFERENCES

1. Budny, J.L., Grotke, N.C., and MacGillivray, M.: N.Y. State J. Med., 76:877, 1976.
2. Feigin, R.D. et al.: J. Pediatrics, 78:230, 1971.
3. Humbert, J.R. et al.: Pediatrics, 48:259, 1971.
4. Matula, G., and Paterson, P.Y.: N. Engl. J. Med., 285:311, 1971.
5. Park, B.H., Fikrig, S.M., and Smithwick, E.M.: Lancet, 2:532, 1968.

Chapter 9

INFECTIOUS DISEASE SEROLOGY

A. Bacterial Diseases

FEBRILE AGGLUTININS

Febrile agglutinins are antibodies present in the sera of patients with certain infectious diseases characterized by the presence of persistent fever. These antibodies are demonstrable in vitro by their ability to agglutinate suspensions of bacterial antigens. Febrile agglutinin tests have been used in evaluation of infections with the following organisms:[1] (a) *Salmonella* (Widal test), (b) *Brucella*, (c) *Francisella* (*Pasteurella*), and (d) *Rickettsieae* (Weil-Felix test). Each category of diseases is discussed below.

REFERENCE

1. Insert: Febrile Antigens and Febrile Positive Control Sera, Fisher Diagnostics, Orangeburg, N.Y., 1981.

Brucellosis

Brucellosis, also known as undulant fever, Malta fever, Mediterranean fever, and Bang's disease, is caused by small gram-negative bacilli of the genus, *Brucella* (Family, *Brucellaceae*).[1,13,22] The bacteria occur as facultative intracellular parasites in mammals, and are endemic to farm animals, notably cows, pigs, and goats.[1,13,22]

Disease is transmitted to humans primarily through direct contact with infected animals or their tissues, or by ingestion of contaminated milk or milk products.[1,13] In the United States, preventative measures such as mandatory pasteurization of dairy products and vaccination and testing of domestic animals has greatly reduced the incidence of brucellosis over the last 40 years.[21] In this country, most cases occur in persons employed in occupations involving contact with livestock or dairy products, such as farming, veterinary medicine, and processing of meats and dairy goods. A smaller number of cases have occurred as a result of exposure in the laboratory or accidental self-inoculation with Brucella vaccine.[1] Evidence also suggests that airborne transmission may occur in slaughterhouses.[1,22,23]

The most common causes of human brucellosis in the United States are *Brucella abortus*, transmitted by cattle, followed by *B. suis*, transmitted by swine.[13,22] Most cases of brucellosis worldwide are due to consumption of goat dairy products contaminated with *B. melitensis*.[13,22] *B. canis* has been responsible for isolated cases resulting from contact with dogs, especially beagles,[1] and *B. rangiferi tarandi,* which occurs in reindeer, has also been reported to cause human disease.[22]

Infection with Brucella can occur through broken skin, the nasopharynx, alimentary tract, or conjunctivae.[13] The average incubation period following exposure is 10 to 14 days.[13] Subclinical infections may be recognized by serologic evidence. The clinical manifestations of Brucella infection are varied and depend on the species of the causative agent, the organ systems affected, and the stage of infection.[22] Clinical brucellosis occurs in three forms: acute, subacute, or chronic.[1,13,22,23] The symptoms of acute disease are fever which may be continuous, intermittent, or irregular, weakness, headache, sweats, vague aches and pains, cervical and/or axillary lymphadenopathy, splenomegaly, and pain over the spine, especially in the lumbar area. Some individuals exhibit hepatitis or genitourinary involvement, particularly orchitis or epididymitis. There are no distinct clinical characteristics to aid diagnosis. The organisms cause intermittent bacteremia, localize in a number of reticuloendothelial sites, and induce small granulomatous lesions in various organs. Acute disease, classified as less than 3 months' duration, may progress to the subacute form, which persists for 3 to 12 months if left untreated.[22] The majority of individuals treated with antibiotics recover completely.

Persons with chronic brucellosis may exhibit fatigue, depression, arthralgia, muscle pain, and psychoneurotic symptoms lasting 1 to several years.[1,13,22,23] Relapses of varying intensity are common. Complications of various organs and tissues may occur but rarely cause fatality. The most severe forms of human brucellosis are caused by *Brucella melitensis* and *B. suis,* while *B. abortus, B. canis,* and *B. rangiferi tarandi* usually cause mild symptoms.[22]

The diagnosis of Brucella infection is established definitively by isolation and identification of the organism, usually from cultures of blood, or sometimes from bone marrow samples, lymph node specimens, cerebral spinal fluid, or urine.[20] However, positive blood cultures are obtained in only 10 to 30% of acute cases and rarely in other forms of brucellosis.[7,22] When growth occurs, results are usually obtained in 2 to 5 days, but cultures should be held for 4 to 6 weeks before being discarded;[13] failure to do so may result in false-negative cultures.[22]

Because cultures are frequently negative or may require considerable time before results are obtained, serologic testing has been a valuable tool in the diagnosis of brucellosis. The standard method of serology has been the tube agglutination test, whereby dilutions of serum are incubated with standardized, heat-killed suspensions of Brucella organisms (usually *Brucella abortus*).[3,18] The test can detect antibodies to *B. abortus, B. suis,* or *B. melitensis* due to their antigenic cross-reactivity. Testing for *B. canis* antibody requires a specific serologic test.[11]

As in most infectious diseases, production of IgM antibody occurs early and is followed by a rise in IgG antibody, although IgM levels may remain elevated for long periods in some chronic cases.[23] Almost all acute Brucella infections induce agglutinating antibody; however, agglutination test results vary with chronic disease.[15,23] Antibody is usually detected by the end of the second week of acute illness, and peaks between the fourth and eighth weeks.[8,13,23] Presumptive evidence of infection is indicated by at least a 4-fold rise in agglutinin titer or a single titer > 80–160,[13,22,23] and should be interpreted in light of clinical symptoms, patient history, and culture results. Antibody levels decline after successful treatment with antibiotics.[13,23]

Differentiation of chronic brucellosis with low antibody titers from recovery after antibiotic therapy may be aided by addition of 2-mercaptoethanol (2ME) or dithiothreitol (DTT) to the standard agglutination test in order to remove IgM antibodies; low 2ME or DTT titers indicate a favorable response to therapy.[4,10]

Prozone reactions are not uncommon.[23] A wide range of serum dilutions should be tested, as "blocking factors," which are nonagglutinating antibodies of the IgG or IgA class, have been noted in some patients' sera, usually in low titer.[20] If suspected, these may be detected by the anti-human globulin (Coombs) test or by complement fixation.

Cross-reactions occur with antibody to *Francisella tularensis* and *Vibrio cholerae*, and may cause false-positive results in individuals who have received cholera or tuleremia vaccines.[6,9,13,16] Parallel testing of patient serum with Brucella and Francisella antigens is helpful in differentiation, since the cross-reacting antibodies are generally present in weaker titers.[9] Cross-reactions also occur between antibodies to Brucella organisms and *Yersinia enterolitica*, which contain identical O antigens; differentiation may be established by testing for H agglutinins.[20]

Slide agglutinin tests, card agglutinin tests, and microagglutination tests, which can be performed rapidly and use smaller amounts of reagents than the standard tube test, have been found to be suitable for screening purposes.[2,12,14] All sera positive in such screens should be subsequently titered with the tube test.[12] Other methods which have been developed to detect Brucella antibodies include the rose-bengal assay,[5] passive hemagglutination,[19] and ELISA.[17] Skin tests detecting delayed type hypersensitivity reactions to Brucella antigen have also been developed but have not been found to be reliable indicators of active infection.[20]

REFERENCES

1. Benenson, A.S. (Ed.): *Control of Communicable Diseases in Man.* 14th ed. Washington, DC, American Public Health Association, 1985.
2. Bettelheim, K.A., Maskill, W.J., and Pearce, J.: J. Hyg. Camb., *90*:33, 1983.
3. Buchanan, T.C. et al.: Medicine, *53*:415, 1974.
4. Buchanan, T.M., and Faber, L.C.: J. Clin. Microbiol., *11*:691, 1980.
5. Diaz, R., Maravi-Poma, E., and Rivero, A.: Bull. WHO, *53*:417, 1976.
6. Eisele, C.W., McCullough, N.B., and Beal, C.A.: Ann. Intern. Med., *28*:833, 1948.
7. Fox, M.D., and Kaufmann, A.F.: J. Infect. Dis., *136*:312, 1977.
8. Insert: Febrile Antigens, Lederle Diagnostics, Div. of Fisher Scientific, Springfield, N.J., 1973.
9. Insert: Febrile Antigens and Febrile Positive Control Sera, Fisher Diagnostics, Orangeburg, N.Y., 1981.
10. Klein, G.C., and Behan, K.A.: J. Clin. Microbiol., *14*:24, 1981.
11. Monroe, P.W. et al.: J. Clin. Microbiol., *2*:382, 1975.
12. Moyer, N.P. et al.: J. Clin. Microbiol., *25*:1969, 1987.
*13. Myrvik, Q.N., and Weiser, R.S.: *Fundamentals of Medical Bacteriology and Mycology.* 2nd ed. Philadelphia, Lea & Febiger, 1988.
14. Russell, A.O., Patton, C.M., and Kaufmann, A.F.: J. Clin. Microbiol., *7*:454, 1978.
15. Sacks, N., and van Rensburg, A.J.: S. Afr. Med. J., *50*:725, 1976.
16. Saslaw, S., and Carlisle, H.N.: Am. J. Med. Sci., *242*:166, 1961.
17. Sippel, J.E., El-Masry, N.A., and Farid, Z.: Lancet, *2*:19, 1982.
18. Spink, W.W. et al.: Am. J. Clin. Pathol., *24*:496, 1954.
19. Versilova, P.A. et al.: Bull. WHO, *51*:191, 1974.
20. Wilson, G., and Smith, G.: In *Topley and Wilson's Principles of Bacteriology, Virology, and Immunity.* Vol. 3. 7th ed. Edited by G. Wilson, A. Miles, M.T. Parker, and G.R. Smith. Baltimore, Williams & Wilkins, 1983–84.
21. Wise, R.I.: JAMA, *244*:2318, 1980.
*22. Wright, P.W.: Am. Fam. Physician, *35*:155, 1987.
23. Young, E.J.: Rev. Infect. Dis., *5*:821, 1983.

Rickettsial Diseases

Rickettsial diseases are caused by gram-negative coccobacilli of the genera, *Rickettsia, Coxiella,* and *Rochalimaea* in the family *Rickettsiaceae*. Except for *Rochalimaea quintana*, they are obligate intracellular parasites which do not grow on artificial media in vitro, but must be cultivated on live tissue.[6,7,20] In nature, they are capable of multiplying in the alimentary tract of various arthropods, and may also infect certain warm-blooded animal hosts, including humans, although the vast majority are not pathogenic to man.[19,20]

The rickettsial diseases of man are generally transmitted via an insect vector (ticks, mites, fleas, or lice), and are characterized by the presence of high fever, rash, and headache.[19,20] They may be classified into four major groups: spotted fevers, Q fever, typhus, and trench fever. In the spotted fevers, a pox-like rash appears initially on the extremities with subsequent spread to the trunk of the body. This group of infections and their causative organisms includes Rocky Mountain spotted fever (RMSF; *Rickettsia rickettsii*), Boutonneuse fever (*R. conorii*), Siberian tick typhus (*R. siberica*), Queensland tick typhus (*R. australis*), and rickettsialpox (*R. akari*). All are transmitted via tick bites except for rickettsialpox, for which mites serve as vectors. The spotted fevers that cause a significant number of cases in the United States are RMSF and rickettsialpox. RMSF is the most common rickettsial disease in the United States, occurring with increasing frequency since 1970 and causing approximately 1000 cases per year in this country.[4,6] Despite its name, the disease is not localized to western United States, but in fact, is reported in greatest frequency in the southeastern states.[4,6,19] Its cause, *R. rickettsii,* infects primarily the wood tick, *Dermacentor andersoni,* or the dog tick, *Dermacentor variabilis,* and may be found in or near wooded areas.[2] Human disease appears after a 3 to 12-day incubation period, with sudden onset of fever, headache, myalgia, nausea, and vomiting.[19,20] A characteristic macular rash erupts on the second to fifth day of illness on the palms of the hands, soles of the feet, or forehead, subsequently spreads to the trunk, and may become maculopapular, petechial, or hemorrhagic.[19,20] The disease usually lasts 2 to 3 weeks. Fatality rates vary widely and have been reported as high as 90% in some untreated cases; however, fatality can be reduced to less than 10% by treatment with antibiotics.[2,20]

Rickettsialpox is spread through the mouse mite, *Allodermanyssus sanguineus,* and is found primarily in urban residences infested with mice.[19,20] Bites from this insect leave a characteristic black hemorrhagic lesion known as an eschar, which is useful in diagnosis.[19,20] Fever and a generalized papulovesicular rash follow. The disease is self-limiting but may predispose susceptible individuals to severe secondary infections.[20]

Q fever is a disease of worldwide distribution caused by the microorganism, *Coxiella burnetti.*[6,20] Transmission among animal reservoirs such as the marsupial rat, sheep, and cattle occurs through tick vectors. Human disease is usually contracted through inhalation of contaminated barnyard dusts or handling of infected meat or milk, and occurs mainly in abbatoir workers and dairy farmers.[6,19,20] Following a 2 to 4 week incubation period, a sudden onset of fever, chills, malaise, headache, and myalgia occurs.[19] Development of pneumonitis and abnormal liver function is common. Other organ systems may also be affected. The disease is usually self-limited, lasting 1 to 3 weeks, and mortality rates are <1%.[19,20]

Epidemic typhus is caused by *Rickettsia prowazekii.* Transmission to man occurs principally through contact with contaminated feces from the body louse, *Pediculus corporis* or the head louse, *P. capitis;* usually, feces is scratched into skin wounds resulting from louse bites.[19,20] Historically, the disease has appeared primarily during periods such as war, natural disaster, or famine, when large numbers of people are living in crowded, unsanitary conditions.[6,19,20] In addition, the flying squirrel, *Glaucomys volans,* found mainly in southeastern United States and parts of Mexico, may serve as a reservoir for *Rickettsia prowazekii,* and has been associated with a few cases of human disease.[6,20,30] Clinically, the disease appears abruptly, with severe headache, high fever, chills, and myalgia following a 10- to 14-day incubation period.[19,20] Subsequently, a characteristic rash appears initially on the trunk, spreads peripherally, and darkens with time. Pneumonia, neurologic symptoms including delirium, and gangrene of various body parts may also occur. The fatality rate ranges from 5 to 50%, and varies with the age of the patient.[19] Brill-Zinsser disease, a milder form of typhus with a lower fatality rate, is due to reactivation of a latent infection in individuals who previously contracted *R. prowazekii.*[19,20] Patients with this disease may serve as a source of new typhus outbreaks under conditions of louse infestation. Brill-Zinsser disease has been found in individuals who have emigrated to the United States from endemic areas.[19,20,24]

Endemic, or murine typhus, caused by *Rickettsia typhi,* is transmitted from rats to man via the rat flea, *Xenopsylla cheopis.*[19] The disease is clinically similar to epidemic typhus, but less severe, and has a fatality of <5%.[20] The incidence of endemic typhus in the United States has decreased markedly with the advent of rat control programs, and less than 100 cases per year are reported.[6,20]

Scrub typhus, due to infection with *Rickettsia tsutsugamushi,* is found in Central Asia, the Far East, and northern Australia.[9] Transmission to man from a variety of mammals (especially rodents) and birds occurs through larvae (chiggers) of the mites of the genus, *Leptotrombidium.*[19] Bites from infected larvae result in swelling and possible ulceration at the puncture site. Other symptoms include fever, headache, rash, lymphadenopathy, conjunctivitis, pneumonitis, and deafness.[19] Fatality rates range from 1 to 60%.[19,20]

Trench fever, caused by *Rochalimaea quintana,* is transmitted from human to human through body lice.[19] The disease is found in regions of Mexico, Europe, and Africa.[8] Clinical symptoms, which follow a 2- to 4-week incubation period, are of sudden onset and include fever, chills, headache, dizziness, retroorbital pain, nystagmus, swelling of conjunctival blood vessels, back and leg pain, and an erythematous macular-papular rash on the trunk of the body.[19] Infection is mild but may last for several weeks; fatality is rare.

The diagnosis of rickettsial illnesses depends almost solely on recognition of clinical signs and examination of patient history (e.g. recent exposure to the appropriate arthropod, travel or residence in endemic areas).[8,19,31] Isolation of rickettsial organisms from blood or other body fluids/tissues is not performed routinely because of the fastidious growth requirements of the organisms[6,7,20] and the extreme danger they pose for laboratory workers,[6,12,23,34] which mandates the use of P-4 containment facilities. Demonstration of rickettsial organisms in biopsies of skin or other tissues by immunofluorescent methods may yield results by 4 to 8 days after disease onset[32,33] but also requires high level safety precautions and experienced laboratory personnel, and is not performed on a routine basis.[8]

Serologic tests often do not become positive until after treatment has begun, but are helpful in the confirmation of diagnosis.[4,8] Classically, antibodies in rickettsial diseases have been detected by the Weil-Felix test, an agglutination test based on the cross-reaction of antibody to Rickettsia with antibody to the polysaccharide (somatic "0") antigens present on the *Proteus vulgaris* strains OX-19 and OX-2, and the *Proteus mirabilis* strain OX-K.[3,9] The reactivity of sera from patients with various ricketssial diseases with the antigens used in the Weil-Felix test is summarized in Table 9–1. The Weil-Felix test may be useful in the diagnosis of RMSF, endemic typhus, epidemic typhus, scrub typhus, and occasionally Brill-Zinsser disease, with a single titer >160 or a fourfold rise in titer suggestive of disease in the presence of appropriate patient history and symptoms.[8,31] Agglutinins that cross-react with Proteus are not

Table 9–1. Rickettsial Diseases: Weil-Felix Reactions

Disease	Agent	Proteus Antigens		
		OX19	OX2	OXK
Rocky Mountain spotted fever	*R. rickettsii*	++++	+	−
Q fever	*C. burnetii*	−	−	−
Endemic typhus	*R. typhi*	++++	+	−
Brill-Zinsser	*R. prowazeki*	Usu−	−	−
Rickettsialpox	*R. akari*	−	−	−
Epidemic typhus	*R. prowazeki*	++++	+	−
Scrub typhus	*R. tsutsugamushi*	−	−	+++

found in Q fever, rickettsialpox, or most cases of Brill-Zinsser disease. Antibodies in these diseases, as well as differential diagnosis of RMSF, endemic typhus, or epidemic typhus must be accomplished with assays using rickettsia-specific antigens.[8,17,24]

The Weil-Felix test is widely available and easily performed in routine laboratories;[29] however, the diagnostic utility of the test has recently been questioned because of its low sensitivity in the early phase of disease[21,31] and its lack of specificity.[14,21,36] Because the test uses Proteus antigens, significant titers may be present in individuals with Proteus infections;[6,8,36] false-positive results have also been seen in leptospirosis, Borrelia infections, pregnancy, and hepatic disease.[6,18,31,35]

Greater specificity has been achieved with complement fixation (CF) tests using rickettsial antigens prepared from infected cell cultures or chick embryo yolk sacs.[8] However, CF, which measures primarily IgG antibodies, does not become positive for most rickettsial diseases until 2 weeks after the onset of illness;[6] its sensitivity is thus too low for use as a screening test in acute disease.[31] In addition, CF titers may be decreased significantly as a result of antibiotic treatment.[6,25] The test appears to be most useful in the distinction of recovery and chronic infection in Q fever, and in the diagnosis of Brill-Zinsser disease, where CF antibodies appear during the first week of illness.[6]

Problems with the Weil-Felix and CF tests have prompted the development of more sensitive and specific assays[6,8] such as immunofluorescence,[1,17,24,26] microagglutination,[10,25] and hemagglutination.[25,28] Of these, a microimmunofluorescence method, which allows for conservation of reagents, simultaneous testing against a panel of rickettsial antigens, and reduction in technical time, appears to possess the greatest sensitivity and specificity.[6,8] This test, which can detect antibodies by 1 week after the onset of illness,[6,8] is gaining recognition as the method of choice for rickettsial serol-

ogy.[6,21,29] Other tests which have been developed include latex agglutination[15,16] and ELISA.[5,11]

When interpreting results from rickettsia-specific tests, it is important to consider the cross-reactivity which exists between different species of rickettsiae.[13,22,24,27] Homologous and heterologous titers, though, usually differ enough to allow for correct interpretation.[8] Use of the immunofluorescence or hemagglutination methods, for which the least cross-reactivity has been observed,[8] may also be helpful. Serologic confirmation of disease is indicated by a 4-fold rise in titer or a level greater than the reference values established for the particular assay used.[6,8,31]

REFERENCES

1. Bozeman, M.F., and Elisberg, B.L.: Proc. Soc. Exp. Biol. Med., *112*:568, 1963.
2. Burgdorfer, W.: J. Med. Entomol., *12*:269, 1975.
3. Casteneda, M.R.: J. Exp. Med., *60*:119, 1934.
4. Centers for Disease Control: MMWR, *33*:188, 1984.
5. Clements, M.L. et al.: J. Infect. Dis., *148*:876, 1983.
*6. Duma, R.J.: In *Interpretive Medical Microbiology*. Edited by H.P. Dalton and H.C. Nottebart. New York, Churchill Livingstone, 1986.
7. Dyer, R.E.: JAMA, *124*:1165, 1944.
*8. Eisemann, C.S., and Osterman, J.V.: In *Manual of Clinical Laboratory Immunology*. 3rd ed. Edited by N.R. Rose, H. Friedman, and J.L. Fahey. Washington, D.C., American Society for Microbiology, 1986.
9. Felix, A.: Trans. R. Soc. Trop. Med. Hyg., *37*:321, 1944.
10. Fiset, P. et al.: Acta Virol., *13*:60, 1969.
11. Halle, S., Dasch, G.A., and Weiss, E.: J. Clin. Microbiol., *6*:101, 1977.
12. Hazard, P.B., and McCroan, J.E.: MMWR, *26*:84, 1977.
13. Hechemy, K.E.: N. Engl. J. Med. *300*:859, 1979 (letter).
14. Hechemy, K.E. et al.: J. Clin. Microbiol., *9*:292, 1979.
15. Hechemy, K.E. et al.: J. Clin. Microbiol., *12*:144, 1980.
16. Hechemy, K.E., and Rubin, B.B.: J. Clin. Microbiol., *17*:489, 1983.
17. Kenyon, R.H. et al.: J. Clin. Microbiol., *3*:513, 1976.
18. Lewthwaite, R., and Savoor, S.R.: Lancet, *1*:255, 1940.
19. Marmion, B.P.: In *Topley and Wilson's Principles of Bacteriology, Virology and Immunity*. 7th ed. Vol. 3. Baltimore, Williams & Wilkins, 1984.
20. Myrvik, Q.N., and Weiser, R.S.: *Fundamentals*

of Medical Bacteriology and Mycology. 2nd ed. Philadelphia, Lea & Febiger, 1988.
21. Newby, J.G.: JAMA, *255*:1020, 1986 (letter).
22. Newhouse, V.F. et al.: Am. J. Trop. Med. Hyg., *28*:387, 1979.
23. Oster, C.N. et al.: N. Engl. J. Med., *297*:859, 1977.
24. Philip, R.N. et al.: J. Clin. Microbiol., *3*:51, 1976.
25. Philip, R.N. et al.: Am. J. Epidemiol., *105*:56, 1977.
26. Robinson, D.M. et al.: Am. J. Trop. Med. Hyg., *25*:900, 1976.
27. Shepard, C.C. et al.: J. Clin. Microbiol., *4*:277, 1976.
28. Shirai, A., Dietel, J.W., and Osterman, J.V.: J. Clin. Microbiol., *2*:430, 1975.
29. Smith, P.W.: JAMA, *255*:1020, 1986 (letter).
30. Sonenshine, D.E. et al.: Am. J. Trop. Med. Hyg., *27*:339, 1978.
*31. Walker, D.H., Burday, M.S., and Folds, J.D.: South. Med. J., *73*:1443, 1980.
32. Walker, D.H., Cain, B.G. and Olmstead, P.M.: Am. J. Clin. Pathol., *69*:619, 1978.
33. Woodward, T.E. et al.: J. Infect. Dis., *134*:297, 1976.
34. Wright, L.J. et al.: Ann. Intern. Med., *69*:731, 1968.
35. Zarafonetis, C.J.D., Ingraham, H.S., and Berry, J.F.: J. Immunol., *52*:189, 1946.
36. Zuerlein, T.J., and Smith, P.W.: JAMA, *254*:1211, 1985.

Salmonella Infections

Bacteria of the genus *Salmonella* are members of the family, *Enterobacteriaceae* and comprise a large group of gram-negative enteric bacilli which are capable of causing disease in man. More than 1500 serotypes have been identified.[16] Transmission of *Salmonella* occurs through ingestion of food or water contaminated with feces or urine from an infected individual, or by direct contact with an infected person or animal.[4,27]

Salmonella infections clinically manifest themselves in one of three general patterns: (1) enteric fevers, (2) septicemias, and (3) gastroenteritis.[16] Enteric fevers are characterized by septicemia (bacterial invasion of the bloodstream) and enteritis (inflammation of the intestinal mucosa). The prototype of enteric fevers, called typhoid fever,[4,16] is caused by *Salmonella typhi,* although *S. paratyphi A* and *S. paratyphi B* usually induce similar symptoms, and *S. sendai* may do so occasionally. In this disease, a 1- to 3-week incubation period is typically followed by an insidious onset of headache, malaise, and anorexia, which precede the onset of fever.[4,16] Bacteremia, occurring early in the illness, seeds various organs with bacteria. Some bacteria remain in the enteric tract, where they cause abdominal distension and tenderness, usually without diarrhea. The disease lasts 3 to 5 weeks. In a small percentage of cases, perforation may occur in the gastrointestinal tract during the latter stages of disease, and peritonitis may develop. The fatality rate of 10% is primarily because of complications of intestinal hemorrhage or perforation, but may be greatly reduced by treatment with antibiotics.[4] Relapses may occur in nonfatal cases, but are usually milder and of shorter duration. Mild or clinically inapparent infection is common, particularly in endemic areas. Approximately 3 to 5% of patients become chronic carriers[16] due to survival of the organism in the biliary or urinary tracts; excretion of bacteria in the feces or urine of these individuals may continue indefinitely.

The nontyphoid enteric fevers, although clinically similar to typhoid, are usually milder and have a shorter incubation time.

Salmonella septicemias are caused most frequently by *Salmonella choleraesuis,* and occur most commonly in persons who are very young, very old, or debilitated.[16] High fevers are manifested as the organisms are transported from the intestines to the lymph nodes and bloodstream. The bacteria may then establish pyemic lesions almost anywhere in the body, although little or no enteric involvement is evident. Fatality rates are 5 to 20%.[16]

Salmonella gastroenteritis or "food poisoning," most often caused by *S. enteritidis,* is the most common of the salmonella infections.[16] A 5-fold increase in *S. enteriditis* infections associated with foods containing raw or undercooked eggs was reported from 1976 to 1985 in northeastern United States.[8,9] In a typical course of disease, ingestion of food in which there has been extensive multiplication of the bacteria is fol-

Table 9–2. Agglutinins Determined by the Use of Salmonella Group Somatic Antigens

Salmonella Antigen	Group	Organism
Salmonella Group A Antigen (Somatic 1, 2, 12)	A	*S. paratyphi* A
Salmonella Group B Antigen (Somatic 1, 4, 5, 12)	B	*S. typhimurium* *S. paratyphi* B *S. derby* *S. san diego* and others
Salmonella Groups C₁ and C₂ Antigen (Somatic 6, 7, 8)	C_1 C_2	*S. paratyphi* C *S. choleraesuis* *S. montevideo* *S. oranienburg* *S. bareilly* *S. muenchen* *S. newport* and others
Salmonella Group D Antigen (Typhoid O) (Somatic 9, 12)	D	*S. typhi* *S. enteritidis* *S. dublin* *S. panama* *S. gallinarum* *S. pullorum* and others
Salmonella Groups E₁, E₂, E₃, E₄ Antigen (Somatic 3, 10, 15)	E_1 E_2 E_3 E_4	*S. anatum* *S. meleagridis* *S. give* and others *S. newington* *S. illinois* and others *S. senftenberg* and others

lowed by a 12- to 48-hour incubation period, after which fever, headache, diarrhea, vomiting, and dehydration occur. Symptoms are usually self-limiting, lasting 1 to 5 days, and fatality is rare.

The diagnosis of salmonella infection should be suggested by clinical symptoms and confirmed by isolation and identification of the organism. In typhoid fever, positive blood cultures may be obtained during the first or second week of onset, and cultures of urine or feces generally become positive after the first week.[4,13] In septicemias, blood cultures should be set up during the first week of infection and repeated if negative.[13]

Detection of antibody to salmonella antigens has been classically performed by the Widal test,[28] whereby identification is based on the ability of antibody to agglutinate suspensions of salmonella bacteria. The antigen suspensions used in the Widal test are prepared from organisms that comprise each of five serologic groups of salmonella (A, B, C, D, and E), classified on the basis of "O" (somatic, cell wall) antigens. The antigens employed by Fisher Diagnostics are presented in Table 9–2 for reference.[14] Active infection is indicated by a fourfold rise in agglutination titer in serial serum samples.[16,21] In typhoid fever, clinically significant titers are typically reached during the second week of illness.[4,21]

The diagnostic value of the Widal test has been questioned for several reasons.[19,21,23,30] Lack of standardization in different commercial antigen preparations,[21] technical variation between laboratories,[7,23] and variation in the diagnostic criteria used for interpretation[21] have been cited as major concerns about the test. In general, "O" antigen titers are thought to be more specific and reliable indicators of infection than antibodies to "H" (flagellar) antigens,[19,23] although the value of H agglutinins remains controversial.[11,30] However, although most individuals infected with Salmonella bacteria demonstrate a rise in O antibodies, a significant percentage do not.[22,29] Treatment with antibiotics early in the course of Salmonella infection may inhibit or delay the formation of antibodies.[18,21,29] In contrast, increased levels of antibody commonly occur as a result of TAB vaccination[21,30] or exposure of asymptomatic individuals in endemic areas.[11,18,23] False-positive results may occur in individuals with immunologic disorders (e.g. rheumatoid arthritis, rheumatic fever, systemic lupus erythematosus),[23,30] and cross-reactions between typhoid and nontyphoid Salmonella antibodies have been reported.[19,21]

Antibodies to "Vi" or capsular antigens of Salmonella, are usually detectable in the sera of patients only after recovery from enteric fevers.[12] These antibodies may be useful in the detection of Salmonella carriers, but are not present in all carrier individuals;[5] tests for these antibodies are thus not recommended as a general screen for the carrier state.[21]

Because of problems with the Widal test, the intended use of the test is for presumptive evidence of infection, while definitive diagnosis should be made by isolation and identification of the organism.[14] Serial titers will provide greater confidence in the accuracy of diagnosis.[14] In developing countries lacking facilities for microbial culture, the Widal test has been of value, provided that titers are interpreted in light of reference values obtained from individuals within the geographic region of testing.[10,11,18]

Problems with the Widal test have prompted the development of other methods to detect antibody (e.g. ELISA,[3,17] RIA,[26] counterimmunoelectrophoresis (CIE),[25] passive hemagglutination[11]), as well as Salmonella antigens (e.g. coagglutination tests,[15,24] ELISA,[1,2] CIE[24]). These methods are currently being investigated to determine their clinical value.

REFERENCES

1. Araj, G.F., and Chugh, T.D.: J. Clin. Microbiol., 25:2150, 1987.
2. Barrett, T.J. et al.: J. Clin. Microbiol., 15:235, 1982.
3. Beasley, W.J., Joseph, S.W., and Weiss, E.: J. Clin. Microbiol., 13:106, 1981.
4. Benenson, A.S., Ed. Control of Communicable Diseases in Man. 14th ed. Washington, D.C., American Public Health Association, 1985.
5. Bokkenheuser, V., Suit, P., and Richardson, N.: Am. J. Public Health, 54:1507, 1964.
6. Bottone, E.J., Janda, J.M., and Motyl, M.R.: In Interpretive Medical Microbiology. Edited by H.P. Dalton and H.C. Nottebart. New York, Churchill Livingstone, 1986.
7. Carter, P.K., and Schoen, I.: Am. J. Clin. Pathol., 53:364, 1970.
8. Centers for Disease Control: MMWR, 36:10, 1987.
9. Centers for Disease Control: MMWR, 36:204, 1987.
10. Chow, C.-B.: Pediatr. Infect. Dis. J., 6:914, 1987.
11. Coovadia, Y.M., et al.: J. Clin. Pathol., 39:680, 1986.
12. Eisenberg, G.M., Palazzolo, A.J., and Flippin, H.F.: N. Engl. J. Med., 253:90, 1955.
13. Finegold, S.M., and Martin, W.J.: Bailey and Scott's Diagnostic Microbiology. 6th ed. St. Louis, C.V. Mosby Co., 1982.
14. Insert: Febrile Antigens and Febrile Positive Control Sera, Fisher Diagnostics, Orangeburg, N.Y., 1981.
15. John, T.J., Sivadasan, K., and Kurien, B.: J. Clin. Microbiol., 20:751, 1984.
*16. Myrvik, Q.N., and Weiser, R.S.: Fundamentals of Medical Bacteriology and Mycology. 2nd ed. Philadelphia, Lea & Febiger, 1988.
17. Nardiello, S. et al.: J. Clin. Microbiol., 20:718, 1984.
18. Pang, T., and Puthucheary, S.D.: J. Clin. Pathol., 36:471, 1983.
19. Reynolds, D.W., Carpenter, R.L., and Simon, W.H.: JAMA, 214:2192, 1970.
20. Rockhill, R.C. et al.: J. Clin. Microbiol., 11:213, 1980.
*21. Schroeder, S.A.: JAMA, 206:839, 1968.
22. Sen, R., and Saxena, S.N.: Indian J. Med. Res., 57:1813, 1969.
23. Senewiratne, B., Chir, B., and Senewiratne, K.: Gastroenterology, 73:233, 1977.
24. Shetty, N.P., Srinivasa, H., and Bhat, P.: Am. J. Clin. Pathol., 84:80, 1985.

25. Tsang, R.S.W., and Chau, P.Y.: Br. Med. J., *282*:1505, 1981.

26. Tsang, R.S.W. et al.: Clin. Exp. Immunol., *46*:508, 1981.

27. WHO Chron., *29*:236, 1975.

28. Widal, F.: Bull. Soc. Med. Hop. Paris, *13*:561, 1896.

29. Wilson, G.S., Mills, A.A., and Parker, M.T. (Eds.): *Topley and Wilson's Principles of Bacteriology, Virology, and Immunity.* 7th ed. Vol. 3. Baltimore, Williams & Wilkins, 1983–84.

*30. Zuerlein, T.J. and Smith, P.W.: JAMA, *254*:1211, 1985.

Tularemia

Tularemia, also known as rabbit fever, deerfly fever, and Ohara's disease, is caused by the small gram-negative bacillus, *Francisella tularensis* (previously known as *Pasteurella tularensis*). The bacterium is widespread among numerous wild birds and mammals in the northern hemisphere, particularly rodents such as the rabbit.[2,17] Transmission to man occurs via several mechanisms: (a) through direct contact of skin, conjunctivae, or oropharyngeal mucosa with blood or tissue from infected animals, (b) indirectly, through insect vectors, most notably ticks, but also deer flies, black flies, and mosquitoes, (c) via inhalation of contaminated dust from dried feces, soil, hay, or grain, or (d) by ingestion of contaminated water or insufficiently cooked rabbit meat.[2,15,17] The disease is most commonly seen in hunters, trappers, and butchers, and is also an occupational hazard for veterinarians and laboratory workers.[15]

The most common form of tularemia is the ulceroglandular type.[15,17] In this form, a 3-day incubation period is ended by abrupt onset of fever, headache, and generalized pain, followed by the appearance of a papular lesion at the site of infection and regional lymphadenopathy. The lesion develops into an ulcer and persists with fever for 2 to 3 weeks; lymphadenopathy is of longer duration and convalescence generally takes 3 to 6 months. Other forms of tularemia include the oculoglandular type, in which infection of the eyes results in ulceration of the conjunctivae and involvement of regional lymph nodes, and the glandular type, in which localized lymph nodes are affected in the absence of a primary skin lesion.[15,17] Inhalation of the organisms may lead to more severe forms: the typhoid form, a systemic infection with no localized manifestations, or the pulmonary form, which presents as pneumonia.[15,17] Prevention of tularemia may be accomplished by administration of an attenuated live vaccine in individuals at risk or by prophylactic treatment with streptomycin following a known exposure.[2,15] Streptomycin is the therapeutic drug of choice in the treatment of clinical tularemia.[7,8,17] The death rate of untreated disease is 6 to 7%.[15]

Diagnosis of tularemia is based largely on historic and clinical data. Identification of *Francisella tularensis* may be accomplished during the acute phase of disease by cultivation of discharge from lesions, blood, or sputum on special enriched media or inoculation into laboratory animals; rapid identification may be performed by fluorescent antibody staining of exudates or tissue smears.[7,8] However, isolation of the organism presents an extreme hazard to laboratory workers and should be performed only by specially equipped reference laboratories.[7,8,16]

Because of the fastidious growth requirements and biologic hazards associated with cultivating *F. tularensis,* serologic testing has been an important tool in the diagnosis of tularemia. Agglutination tests, whereby patient serum is incubated with a standardized, killed suspension of an avirulent strain of *F. tularensis,* are routinely employed in detecting antibody to the bacterium.[10,12,13,18] Agglutinins usually become positive during the second week of illness, peak at 4 to 8 weeks, and persist for years.[12,17] Titers ≤ 40 are present in apparently normal individuals; titers > 40 may be diagnostic in the presence of appropriate history and clinical data,[20] but demonstration of a fourfold rise in titer is recommended for greater confidence in the accuracy of diagnosis.[13,15]

Cross-reactions occur commonly with *Brucella abortus* antibody, and rarely with Proteus OX19.[10,13,18] The homologous titer, in this case, is virtually always higher than the heterologous one. Parallel tests using all three antigens should always be performed to detect these cross-reactions. Behan and Klein[1] have shown that cross-reactivity between *Brucella* and *Francisella* agglutinins can be reduced by addition of dithiothreitol to the test. False-positive agglutination due to heterophile antibody has also been reported.[9]

Other tests which have been developed to detect antibody include microagglutination,[3,14] ELISA,[5,19] RIA,[11] and hemagglutination.[6] A skin test to detect delayed hypersensitivity responses to *Francisella tularensis* is also available.[4]

REFERENCES

1. Behan, K.A., and Klein, G.C.: J. Clin. Microbiol., 16:756, 1982.
2. Benenson, A.S., ed.: *Control of Communicable Diseases in Man*. 14th ed. Washington, D.C., American Public Health Association, 1985.
3. Brown, S.L.: J. Clin. Microbiol., 11:146, 1980.
4. Buchanan, T.M., Brooks, G.F., and Brachman, P.S.: Ann. Intern. Med., 74:336, 1971.
5. Carlsson, H.E., et al.: J. Clin. Microbiol., 10:615, 1979.
6. Charkes, N.D.: J. Immunol., 83:213, 1959.
7. Dalton, H.P., and Nottebart, H.C. (Eds.): *Interpretive Medical Microbiology*. New York, Churchill Livingstone, 1986.
8. Finegold, S.M., and Martin, W.J.: *Diagnostic Microbiology*. St. Louis, C.V. Mosby Co., 1982.
9. Ford-Jones, L. et al.: Can. Med. Assoc. J., 127:298, 1982.
10. Francis, E., and Evans, A.C.: Public Health Rep., Wash., 41:1273, 1926.
11. Hambleton, P., and Strange, R.E.: J. Med. Microbiol., 10:151, 1977.
12. Insert: Febrile Antigens, Lederle Diagnostics, Div. of Fisher Scientific, Springfield, N.J., 1973.
13. Insert: Febrile Antigens and Febrile Positive Control Sera, Fisher Diagnostics, Orangeburg, N.Y., 1981.
14. Massey, E.D., and Mangiafico, J.A.: Appl. Microbiol., 27:25, 1974.
15. Myrvik, Q.N., and Weiser, R.S.: *Fundamentals of Medical Bacteriology and Mycology*. 2nd ed. Philadelphia, Lea & Febiger, 1988.
16. Overholt, E.L. et al.: Am. J. Med., 30:785, 1961.
*17. Smith, G., and Wilson, G.: In *Topley and Wilson's Principles of Bacteriology, Virology, and Immunity*. 7th ed. Vol. 3. Edited by G. Wilson, A. Mills, M.T. Parker, and G.R. Smith. Baltimore, Williams & Wilkins, 1984.
18. Snyder, M.J.: In *Manual of Clinical Laboratory Immunology*. 3rd ed. Edited by N.R. Rose, H. Friedman, and J.L. Fahey. Washington, D.C., American Society for Microbiology, 1986.
19. Viljanen, M.K., Nurmi, T., and Salminen, A.: J. Infect. Dis., 148:715, 1983.
20. Zuerlein, T.J., and Smith, P.W.: JAMA, 254:1211, 1985.

Febrile Agglutinins Tests[1]

(Brucella, Francisella, Proteus, and Salmonella)

PRINCIPLE. Antigenic extracts from certain bacteria are used to detect antibodies produced in a variety of febrile illnesses. Patient serum containing such an antibody will cause agglutination of the appropriate antigens

EQUIPMENT AND MATERIALS

1. Febrile antigens (Fisher Scientific), including:

   a. *Brucella abortus* antigen.

   b. *Francisella* (*Pasteurella*) *tularensis* antigen.

   c. Proteus OX19 antigen.

   d. Salmonella, group A antigen (Somatic 1, 2, 12).

   e. Salmonella, group B antigen (Somatic 1, 4, 5, 12).

   f. Salmonella, group C antigen (C_1 and C_2; Somatic 6, 7, 8).

   g. Salmonella, group D antigen (Typhoid 0; Somatic 9, 12).

   h. Salmonella, group E antigen (E_1, E_2, E_3, E_4; Somatic 3, 10, 15).

All antigens are prepared from cultures of initial isolates of specific organisms, and will give a 2+ reaction with dilutions of 1:80 or greater of standardized positive control serum to that antigen. Store at 2 to 8° C. Expiration dates are noted on the labels. Discard if gross contamination becomes evident. Contain preservative. Allow antigen to come to room temperature before use.

2. Positive control sera (rabbit; Fisher Scientific), including:

   a. *Brucella abortus* control serum.

   b. *Francisella* (*Pasteurella*) *tularensis* control serum.

   c. Proteus polyvalent control serum (OX2, OXK, OX19): Prepared for use as a positive control with OX2, OXK, or OX19 antigen.

d. Salmonella polyvalent control serum. (Somatic; groups A, B, C, D, and E): Prepared for use with Salmonella O antigen, groups A, B, C, D, and E.

Store all positive control sera at 2 to 8° C. May be used until the expiration date noted on the labels, unless gross contamination becomes evident. Contain preservative.

3. Negative control serum (Fisher Scientific): A phenolized, buffered, physiologic saline solution.

4. Agglutination slide, 30 well, each ¾ inch in diameter.

5. 0.2 ml pipets.

6. Pipette tips.

7. Wooden applicator sticks.

8. Rotator

9. 13 × 100 mm test tubes.

10. Serologic pipets, 10 ml, 5 ml, 0.5 ml and 0.1 ml.

11. 0.9% saline solution.

12. Waterbaths, set at 37° C and 48° C.

SPECIMEN COLLECTION AND PREPARATION. Serum samples may be used fresh or stored up to 24 hours at 2 to 8° C. For prolonged storage, freeze to −20° C. Do not refreeze serum. Hemolyzed or inactivated serum is not acceptable for Brucella Testing.

SCREENING PROCEDURE

NOTE: Directions are given for a slide screen test to be used for detection of any of the febrile agglutinins. If only *Salmonella* is ordered, the following is performed without *Proteus, Brucella* and *Francisella*. Or, the latter three may be done without the salmonellas.

1. Bring all antigens to be used to room temperature. Shake gently to mix.

2. Using a 0.2 ml pipet, place 0.02 ml of patient sera into 8 wells (less if fewer antigens are to be used) of an agglutination slide as indicated (see Fig. 9-1):

3. Place one drop of each positive control serum to be used into the appropriate well(s) of the slide.

4. Place one drop of negative control into each of the wells indicated.

5. Add one drop of the appropriate antigen to each well of a set (patient serum, + control, − control), making sure that all antigens react with the right controls.

6. Using wooden applicator sticks, mix the contents of each well, spreading over the entire well surface.

7. Place on a slide rotator set at approximately 180 rpm. Rotate for 3 minutes.

8. Observe immediately for agglutination, using transmitted light. All positive controls must demonstrate obvious agglutination; negative controls must be negative.

9. Any agglutination observed with patient sera must be tested further by the appropriate tube dilution test.

REPORTING. Negative results on the screening test with any antigens are reported as negative for that antigen. Any agglutination on the screening test is considered positive and *must* be confirmed with a tube test before reporting.

QUANTITATIVE PROCEDURE

1. Bring all antigens to be used to room temperature.

2. Set up ten 13 × 100 mm test tubes for each antigen to be tested. Label.

3. Add 0.9 ml saline to tube #1, 0.5 ml to tubes #2–10.

4. Pipet 0.1 ml of patient serum into tube #1. Using a 0.5 ml pipet, mix and serially dilute 0.5 ml through tube #8, discarding 0.5 ml from that tube.

5. Add one drop of the appropriate control serum to tube #9.

—For *Salmonella*, groups A, B, C, D, and E: Somatic polyvalent control serum.

—For *Proteus:* Proteus polyvalent control serum.

—For *Brucella: B. abortus* control serum.

—For *Francisella: F. tularensis* control serum.

Tube #10 will serve as a negative control.

6. Dilute the appropriate antigen(s) 1:100 with saline solution. (Prepare a sufficient amount to add 0.5 ml to each tube).

7. Add 0.5 ml of diluted antigen to each tube. Mix well. The final dilutions in each tube range from 1:20 to 1:2560.

8. Incubate in the appropriate waterbath according to the following:

Salmonella O:	48° C	18 to 24 hours
Brucella:	37° C	48 hours
Proteus:	48° C	18 to 24 hours
Francisella:	37° C	2 hours followed by:
	4° C	Overnight

9. Shake gently and observe tubes for agglutination near transmitted light according to the following code:

4+: Complete agglutination; clear supernate

3+: Nearly complete agglutination; supernate 75% clear

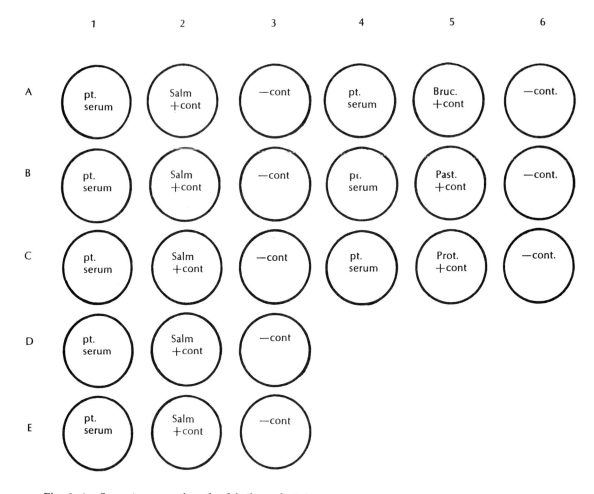

Fig. 9–1. Screening procedure for febrile agglutinins.

2+: Significant agglutination; supernate 50% clear

1+: Observable agglutination; supernate as dense as negative control

—: No agglutination; supernate as dense as negative control

10. The positive control for each antigen should be 4+; the negative control, negative. Record control results.

REPORTING. The titer is reported as the reciprocal of the highest dilution exhibiting 2+ or greater agglutination.

INTERPRETATION OF RESULTS. In no instance can the absence of febrile agglutinins be definitive evidence of the absence of disease.

Titers for all febrile agglutinins can be found in some percentage of clinically normal individuals, dependent on such factors as age, geographic location, travel, immunization, and occupation. There are no established normal ranges for these antibodies.

Blocking factors may be present in the sera of people with brucellosis. In most instances, dilution beyond 1:160 will eliminate this problem. However, if the diagnosis of brucellosis is strongly suspected, an assay for detection of blocking factor may be performed.[2]

Cross-reaction occurs with antibodies to *Brucella,* Proteus OX-2, *Francisella* and *Vibriocholera.*[1] In addition, cholera and tularemia vaccines are known to induce agglutination antibody to *Brucella.* Parallel testing of patient's serum with *Brucella, Proteus,* and *Francisella* antigens can be used if indicated to differentiate the heterologous agent.

LIMITATIONS OF THE PROCEDURE. Febrile agglutinins will not detect antibody to *Brucella canis,* nor can they be used in the diagnosis of Q fever, rickettsialpox or in most cases of Brill-Zinsser's disease.

REFERENCES

1. Insert: Febrile Antigens and Febrile Positive Control Sera, Fisher Diagnostics, Orangeburg, N.Y., 1981.

2. Meyer, M.E.: In *Manual of Clinical Laboratory Immunology.* 3rd ed. Edited by N.R. Rose, H. Friedman, and J.L. Fahey. Washington, D.C., American Society for Microbiology, 1986.

POSTSTREPTOCOCCAL DISORDERS

Streptococci of Lancefield Group A, alternately known as *Streptococcus pyogenes,* are ubiquitous human pathogens. They are a major cause of bacterial infections of the throat[52,54] (pharyngitis, tonsillitis) and of the skin (pyoderma, impetigo, wound infections) particularly, but not exclusively, in children ages 6 to 14.[19] Isolation and identification of the infecting organisms is easily accomplished in acute infections by conventional culture methods; however, the existence of a non-pathogenic "carrier" state, particularly in older children and adults, may complicate diagnosis of significant infection in the throat.[19] *S. pyogenes* appears to be spread by direct, close contact, and has been associated in the past with crowding and poor living conditions. Although the pathogenic significance of acute infection with *S. pyogenes* has long been recognized, diseases known to occur subsequent to infection i.e., *acute rheumatic fever* (ARF), *rheu-*

matic heart disease (RHD), and *post-streptococcal glomerulonephritis* (PSGN), have also been of major importance.[10]

Largely as a result of the work of Rebecca Lancefield,[36] streptococci are classified into serologic groups (e.g. A, B, C . . .) on the basis of genetically determined[11] cell wall constituents known as M proteins. Species names are independently assigned but correlate with Lancefield grouping; for example, Lancefield group A equates with *Streptococcus pyogenes.* Further, organisms belonging to *S. pyogenes,* or Lancefield group A, may be divided into more than 75 serotypes, or strains, a few of which have been cloned[49] or had their primary genetic sequence identified.[27,41,42] Resistance to streptococcal infection is serotype specific, such that cross-immunity is not evident, and recurrent *S. pyogenes* infection, albeit with different serotypes, is common. Geographic distribution of serotypes is variable, and seasonal patterns of disease are common.[55] Certain strains are associated with pharyngeal as opposed to dermal infections, and vice versa, and some serotypes are more often seen preceding rheumatic fever/rheumatic heart disease (the so-called rheumatogenic strains), while others presage renal disease (the nephritogenic strains).[33,55]

M proteins are among the major virulence factors of *S. pyogenes.* Many organisms also have hyaluronic acid capsules, which may be evidenced by the production of mucoid colonies on agar plates. Most group A streptococci, and often organisms from other groups, produce extracellular enzymes or toxins; erythrogenic toxins, streptolysins, streptokinases, hyaluronidase, desoxyribonucleases (DNAses), and nicotinamide adenine dinucleotidases (NADases) are among them. While pathogenic significance for exotoxins may be only implied, many of them are used by the clinical laboratory as aids to diagnosis (see below).

Initial infection with group A streptococci apparently requires the adherence of lipoteichoic acid (LTA) on the bacterial surface to a specific receptor, known as an adhesion factor, on human epithelial cells.[5,6] Antibody to M protein, in complex with LTA on the organism surface, may act to block primary adherence of the organism. Alternately, once attached, strongly adherent strains may be more resistant to removal by immune mechanisms or, perhaps, by therapy.[55]

Antibody to M protein initiates rapid recognition, phagocytosis, and destruction of group A streptococci, and is the only known mechanism of humoral immune destruction of highly virulent strains. An additional virulence factor is a cytoplasmic polypeptide known as endostreptosin or ESS.[37] Found only in certain strains of streptococci, notably nephritogenic strains of group A as well as a few group C and G,[4] ESS is released upon disruption of the organism in situ, and has been linked to the development of post-streptococcal glomerulonephritis.[4,37]

Lancefield groups C and G are often associated with infections of the throat in humans,[54] although usually with less symptomatic severity and are only rarely associated with post-streptococcal disease.[4,22]

Rheumatic Fever: Rheumatic Heart Disease

Acute rheumatic fever (ARF)[1] appears in some 2 to 3% of infected individuals as a consequence of group A streptococcal infection of the upper respiratory tract. It does not occur as a sequel to infections of the skin. A latent period of 10 to 35 days (average, approximately 3 weeks)[19] precedes the onset of symptoms, which usually include carditis and migratory polyarthritis, but may also involve Sydenham's chorea, erythema marginum, and/or subcutaneous nodules.[1,19,30,57,59] Although migratory polyarthritis, when present, is never disabling and responds dramatically to aspirin therapy,[19] carditis may lead to permanent disability and the condition known as *rheumatic heart disease* (RHD) in 30 to 60% of patients, depending on the severity of the inflam-

mation.[19,40] Chorea may occur as the only symptom in a small percentage of cases,[7,29] appearing as late as 6 months after the inciting streptococcal infection, and may present diagnostic difficulties. Individuals with ARF may be asymptomatic, with subclinical manifestations only. Characteristic of the disorder is a cycle of recurrences that follow subsequent streptococcal infection in 25 to 75% of cases.[19]

The current set of criteria for the diagnosis of rheumatic fever[1] is a modification of the original criteria developed by Jones.

ARF has traditionally been seasonal, appearing abruptly in the fall.[55] Only a modest number of serotypes of group A streptococci,[33,55,57] referred to as "rheumatogenic" strains, are associated with the disorder, and microepidemics of these organisms appear worldwide.[8] Genetic susceptibility to rheumatic fever, suggested by familial clustering of disease, may be linked to HLA class II antigens (e.g. DR-2, DR-4, DRw-6)[3,39,51] or B cell alloantigens, detectable by labeling with monoclonal antibody.[47] Present in the majority of individuals with rheumatic fever[47,62] and rheumatic heart disease,[60] the B cell alloantigens associated with ARF and RHD are physically distinct from, but very close to, sites on antigen-reactive B cells which actually bind to group A streptococcal membrane antigens.[60] The absence of this antigen on B cells of the tonsils of patients with rheumatic heart disease[26] may help to define individuals predisposed to the disease and may have pathogenic significance.[20]

Although the mechanisms of induction and pathogenesis are, as yet, unclear for these diseases,[61] several observations are notable. Characteristic of ARF and RHD are antibodies, reactive with streptococcal cell walls and membranes,[56] which were initially referred to as "heart reactive antibodies" (HRAs) for their ability to cross-react with skeletal and smooth muscle of vessel walls, as well as with the sarcolemmal sheath of myocardial fibers.[56] Although HRAs are present in uncomplicated streptococcal infection, their concentration is increased in ARF patients, and titers remain high for several years. HRAs have been described in diseases unrelated to streptococcal infection,[56] but cross-reactivity to streptococci is absent.

Notable among the heart reactive antibodies produced in upper respiratory streptococcal infections are those specific for the alpha helical M proteins, particularly type 5,[14,49] which appears to have at least three heart cross-reactive epitopes.[16] Myosin of both skeletal and heart muscle is at least one of the components of muscle implicated.[13,15,35]

T cell subset imbalances, e.g. decreased helper populations in combination with increased suppressor cells,[9] have been described in individuals with ARF and RHD. In addition, B cell populations characteristic of ARF and RHD, as mentioned above, may be abnormally distributed in affected individuals. Several highly purified M proteins are able to elicit cytotoxic T lymphocytes which cross-react with human target cells such as myocardial tissue.[17] And, normal T cell populations have demonstrated blastogenesis in the presence of M proteins in a macrophage-dependent reaction that shows no correlation with antibody production.[18] Lymphokine production in response to streptococcal exoenzymes can be demonstrated in patients with ARF and RHD.[50]

Rheumatic fever and rheumatic heart disease were the leading cause of death in 5- to 20-year-old individuals during the 1920s, and were second only to tuberculosis in those 20 to 30 years of age.[10] Incidence in the U.S. and economically developed countries has declined dramatically since 1945,[8,23,44] although it continues unabated in developing nations.[2,8] Widespread use of antibiotics and improved living conditions have been credited with the decline.[44,55] No corresponding decrease in the incidence of group A Streptococcal pharyngitis has been observed,[20] although its virulence may have abated.[55] Recently, unexpected localized

outbreaks of ARF have occurred in the U.S.,[12,30,45,57,59] perhaps as a result of undiagnosed or improperly treated primary infection,[20,30,32,59] and/or of the resurgence of mucoid, encapsulated rheumatogenic strains of Streptococci.[8,32,57] Notably, recent cases have not been related to crowded areas or to poor living conditions.[8,12,30]

Poststreptococcal Glomerulonephritis

Unlike rheumatic fever, poststreptococcal glomerulonephritis (PSGN) can occur as a result of either pharyngeal or skin invasion by streptococci.[46] Latent periods of 10 days and 18 to 21 days are commonly observed for the respective primary sites of infection. Clinical symptoms of the disorder include edema, hematuria, and hypertension, although asymptomatic disturbance also occurs. Nephritogenic strains of streptococci, group A[24,28,33,43] and, rarely, group C[4] have been described, which apparently share a common cytoplasmic polypeptide designated endostreptosin, or ESS,[39] as well as an exoantigenic component, nephritis strain-associated protein or NSAP,[31,58] which appears structurally and biochemically similar to streptokinase.[31] ESS is apparently liberated on disruption of certain streptococci, at the site of initial infection, then is subsequently bound to glomerular basement membrane, where it may provide a focal stimulus for the immune response. Similarly, NSAP has been suggested as a target for immune responses, initiating PSGN.[31,58] Several theories regarding the pathogenic mechanism exist, e.g. (1) that streptococcal antigens induce cross-reactive antibodies in persons with appropriate antigens,[24,43] (2) that immune complexes formed during humoral response to initial infection lodge in the glomeruli, serving as a focal point for immune-mediated damage,[37] or (3) that exotoxins such as streptokinase may deposit in the glomerulus, causing damage independent of the immune response invoked.[31,58]

Incidence of poststreptococcal glomerulonephritis has decreased in economically developed areas of the world over the past 20 years; however, the disease persists as a prototypic glomerulonephritis in the United States and worldwide.[38]

Laboratory Diagnosis of Poststreptococcal Disorders

Laboratory aids to the diagnosis of rheumatic fever fall into two categories: (1) those used to detect inflammation, e.g. the acute phase reactants such as C-reactive protein (CRP) or the erythrocyte sedimentation rate (ESR),[1] and (2) those that document a predisposing streptococcal infection, e.g. by changes in antibody titers. The laboratory contributes to diagnosis of acute glomerulonephritis by urinalysis and by demonstration of streptococcal antibody. Recommended criteria for the diagnosis of all disorders described here include documentation of recent streptococcal infection.[1] Conventional culture and identification of the inciting organism is not possible in most cases because the organism is absent by the time symptoms appear. However, documentation of prior infection may be accomplished based on historical or clinical observation, and/or on antibody tests. Assays for antibodies to streptolysin O, hyaluronidase, and DNAse B are among the most commonly used antibody tests.[21]

Streptolysin O is an oxygen-labile hemolysin produced by many strains of groups A, C, and G streptococci. The enzyme inhibition test for antibody to streptolysin O, termed the antistreptolysin O (ASO) test, is the best standardized and most widely accepted test for post-streptococcal sequelae, with 75 to 80% of ARF patients demonstrating a rise in titer 1 to 2 weeks after onset of infection. However, in the remaining 20 to 25% of individuals, and in most ARF patients with chorea as the only manifestation, the ASO titer is borderline or low.[1,29] ASO titers are not usually elevated in pyoderma or the associated glomerulonephritis.

Anti-DNAse B antibodies may appear earlier than ASO in streptococcal pharyngitis, and are more sensitive in the detection of nephritogenic skin infections. Use of the test for antibody to hyaluronidase (AHT) and/or the anti-DNAse B assay, in addition to the ASO test increases the probability of detecting evidence of recent infection.[1,19] Use of paired sera, where available, is preferable.

Antibiotic therapy,[53] e.g. with penicillin, is still universally effective against group A streptococci;[34] however, failure to eradicate the organism is not uncommon in patients with pharyngitis. Penicillin "tolerance" has been documented[25] and may be the cause of some treatment failures.[34,54] Prophylactic antibiotic therapy has been shown to prevent recurrences of streptococcal infection,[40] and, thereby, the additive effects of ARF and RHD recurrences in susceptible persons. Treatment of initial infection too early in the course of disease may significantly increase the incidence of recurrent infection.[48]

REFERENCES

1. Ad Hoc Committee to Revise the Jones Criteria (modified) of the Council on Rheumatic Fever and Rheumatic Heart Disease of the American Heart Association: Circulation, 69:204A, 1984.

2. Agarwal, B.L.: Lancet, 2:910, 1981.

3. Ayoub, E.M. et al.: J. Clin. Invest., 77:2019, 1986.

4. Barnham, M., Thornton, T.J., Lange, K.: Lancet, 1:945, 1983.

5. Beachey, E.H., and Courtney, H.S.: Rev. Infect. Dis. (9 Suppl.), 5:S475, 1987.

6. Beachey, E.H., and Ofek, I.: J. Exp. Med., 143:759, 1976.

7. Berrios, X. et al.: J. Pediatr., 107:867, 1985.

8. Bisno, A.L., Shulman, S.T., and Dajani, A.S.: JAMA, 259:728, 1988.

9. Bhatnagar, P.K., Nijhawan, R., and Prakash, K.: Immunol. Lett., 15:217, 1987.

10. Bland, E.F.: Circulation, 76:1190, 1987.

11. Caparon, M.G., and Scott, J.R.: Proc. Natl. Acad. Sci. U.S.A., 84:8677, 1987.

12. Congeni, B., Rizzo, C., Congeni, J., and Sreenivasan, V.V.: J. Pediatr., 111:176, 1987.

13. Cunningham, M.W., Hall, N.K., Krisher, K.K., and Spanier, A.M.: J. Immunol., 136:293, 1986.

14. Cunningham, M.W., Krisher, K., and Graves, D.C.: Infect. Immun., 46:34, 1984.

15. Cunningham, M.W., and Swerlick, R.A.: J. Exp. Med., 164:998, 1986.

16. Dale, J.B., and Beachey, E.H.: J. Exp. Med., 161:113, 1985.

17. Dale, J.B., and Beachey, E.H.: J. Exp. Med., 166:1825, 1987.

18. Dale, J.B., Simpson, W.A., Ofek, I., and Beachey, E.H.: J. Immunol., 126:1499, 1981.

19. Denny, F.W.: Circulation, 76:963, 1987.

20. Ferrieri, P.: Am. J. Dis. Child., 141:725, 1987.

21. Ferrieri, P., In Manual of Clinical Laboratory Immunology. 3rd ed. Edited by N.R. Rose, H. Friedman, and J.L. Fahey. Washington, D.C., American Society for Microbiology, 1986.

22. Gnann, J.W., Jr., Gray, B.M., Griffin, F.M., and Dismukes, W.E.: J. Infect. Dis., 156:411, 1987.

23. Gordis, L.: Circulation, 72:1155, 1985.

24. Goroncy-Bermes, P., Dale, J.B., and Beachey, E.H.: Infect. Immun., 55:2416, 1987.

25. Grahn, E., Holm, S.E., Roos, K.: Scand. J. Infect. Dis., 19:421, 1987.

26. Gray, E.D. et al.: J. Infect. Dis., 155:247, 1987.

27. Hollingsheal, S.K., Fischetti, V.A., and Scott, J.R.: J. Biol. Chem., 261:1677, 1986.

28. Holm, S.E., Ekedahl, C., and Bengtsson, U.: Scand. J. Infect. Dis., 5:115, 1973.

29. Hosier, D.M.: Ohio Med., 83:663, 1987.

30. Hosier, D.M., Craenen, J.M., Teske, D.W., and Wheller, J.J.: Am. J. Dis. Child., 141:730, 1987.

31. Johnston, K.H., and Zabriskie, J.B.: J. Exp. Med., 163:697, 1986.

32. Kaplan, E.L., and Hill, H.R.: J. Pediatr., 111:244, 1987.

33. Khandke, K.M., Fairwell, T., and Manjula, B.N.: J. Exp. Med., 166:151, 1987.

34. Kim, K.S., and Kaplan, E.L.: J. Pediatr., 107:681, 1985.

35. Krisher, K., and Cunningham, M.W.: Science, 227:413, 1985.

36. Lancefield, R.A.: J. Immunol., 89:307, 1962.

37. Lange, K., Ahmed, U., Kleinberger, H., and Treser, G.: Clin. Nephrol., 5:207, 1976.

38. Leung, D.T. et al.: Arch. Dis. Child., 62:1075, 1987.

39. Maharaj, B. et al.: Circulation, 76:259, 1987.

40. Majeed, H.A. et al.: J. Chron. Dis., 39:361, 1986.

41. Manjula, B.N., Trus, B.L., and Fischetti, V.A.: Proc. Natl. Acad. Sci. U.S.A., 82:1064, 1985.

42. Manjula, B.N. et al.: J. Biol. Chem., 259:3686, 1984.

43. Markowitz, A.S., and Lange, C.F., Jr.: J. Immunol., 92:565, 1964.

44. Massell, B.F., Chute, C.G., Walker, A.M., and Kurland, G.S.: N. Engl. J. Med., 318:280, 1988.

45. MMWR, 37:101, 1988.

46. Nissenson, A.R. (moderator): Ann. Intern. Med., 91:76, 1979.

47. Patarroyo, M.E. et al.: Nature, 278:173, 1979.

48. Pichichero, M.E. et al.: Pediatr. Infect. Dis. J., 6:635, 1987.

49. Poirer, T.P. et al.: Infect. Immun., 48:198, 1985.

50. Prakash, K., and Bhatnagar, P.K.: Indian J. Med. Res., 86:347, 1987.

51. Rajapakse, C.N. et al.: Br. Heart J., 58:659, 1987.

52. Roos, K.: Scand. J. Infect. Dis., 17:259, 1985.

53. Shulman, S.T. et al.: Circulation, 70:1118A, 1984.

54. Stjernquist-Desatnik, A., Prellner, K., and Christensen, P.: Acta Otolaryngol., 104:351, 1987.

55. Stollerman, B.H.: Adv. Intern. Med., 27:373, 1982.

56. vandeRijn, I., Zabriskie, J.B., and McCarty, M.: J. Exp. Med., 146:579, 1977.

57. Veasy, L.G. et al.: N. Engl. J. Med., 316:421, 1986.

58. Villarreal, H., Fischetti, V.A., vandeRijn, I., and Zabriskie, J.B.: J. Exp. Med., 149:459, 1979.

59. Wald, E.R. et al.: Pediatrics, 80:371, 1987.

60. Williams, R.C., Jr. et al.: J. Lab. Clin. Med., 105:531, 1985.

61. Zabriskie, J.B., and Friedman, J.E.: Adv. Exp. Med. Biol., 161:457, 1983.

62. Zabriskie, J.B. et al.: Arthritis Rheum., 28:1047, 1985.

Antistreptolysin O Latex Slide Test[1]

PRINCIPLE. Test serum is reacted with biologically inert latex particles coated with streptolysin O antigen. In the presence of sufficient antibody to streptolysin O (ASO) in the test serum, the latex particles will agglutinate.

EQUIPMENT AND MATERIALS

1. Rapi / Tex ASO Kit Calbiochem-Behring containing:

   a. ASO Latex Reagent

   b. ASO Positive Control

   c. ASO Negative Control

   d. Test Slide, plastic slide, six wells with black background

Store at 2 to 8° C. Do not freeze. Expiration date is specified on the label. Product instability is indicated by inappropriate reaction of the ASO Latex Reagent with the ASO controls.

2. Wooden applicator sticks

3. Test tubes

4. Pipets (50 μl, 250 μl)

5. Pipette tips

6. Normal saline solution

7. Pasteur pipets and bulbs or 40-μl pipet to place patient sample

8. Mechanical rotator (optional)

SPECIMEN COLLECTION AND PREPARATION. Serum should be examined. The specimen should be stored refrigerated or frozen if not assayed immediately. Significantly lipemic sera or those with microbial contamination may cause false-positive agglutination. Nonspecific inhibitors of hemolysis (such as cholesterol) do not interfere with the reaction.

PROCEDURE

ASO positive and negative controls should be included in each test series. Satisfactory performance is indicated by agglutination with the ASO positive control and a lack of agglutination with the ASO negative control.

Qualitative determinations: 200 IU/mL discrimination level.

1. Bring all reagents and serum samples to room temperature.

2. Prepare a 1:6 dilution of each patient serum to be tested (e.g., pipet 50 μl of sample and 250 μl of normal saline into a small test tube and mix gently).

3. Place 1 drop (≅ 40 μl) of each control and diluted patient sample on separate fields of the test slide.

4. Gently mix the ASO Latex Reagent to obtain a uniform suspension. Expel the contents of the dropper, refill and add 1 drop to each field containing a sample to be tested. Mix well with a wooden stick, spreading the mixture over most of the field. Tilt the slide through several planes for 2 minutes. A mechanical rotator may also be used (145 to 160 rpm).

5. Examine for agglutination immediately using direct light (e.g., high-intensity lamp) at a distance of approximately 10 to 15 cm from the surface of the slide. The reaction of the test serum is compared to that of the ASO positive and negative controls.

REPORTING. Agglutination of the latex particle suspension is reported as a positive result, indicating that ASO is present in the sample at a concentration of ≥ 200 IU/mL (± 15%). Lack of agglutination indicates an ASO concentration of < 200 IU/mL (⊥ 15%) and is reported as negative.

INTERPRETATION OF RESULTS. An ASO titer of 200 IU/mL is usually regarded as the upper limit of normal since less than 20% of healthy subjects yield titers of > 200 IU/mL. In newborns, the titer is usually higher than in the mother but falls sharply during the first few weeks of life as the IgG acquired from the maternal circulation is eliminated. The normal value for ASO titers of preschool children is less than 100 IU/mL. This value rises with age, peaking in school age children and decreasing in adults.

A rise in ASO titer generally takes place 1 to 4 weeks after the onset of infection with β-hemolytic streptococci, Group A. When the disease has subsided the titer gradually declines, returning to normal levels within 6 months. If the titer does not decrease, a recurrence of the infection may be indicated.

Increased ASO titers may be associated with ankylosing spondylitis (Bechterew's disease), glomerulonephritis, scarlet fever and tonsillitis. An extremely low ASO titer is observed in the nephrotic syndrome and in antibody deficiency syndromes. Elevated ASO levels are not generally found in rheumatoid arthritis except during acute attacks.[2]

LIMITATIONS OF THE PROCEDURE. Reaction times longer than 2 minutes may produce false-positive reactions. Significantly lipemic, contaminated, or plasma samples may also cause false-positive reactions. Care should be taken to keep the ASO Latex Reagent dropper vial tightly closed to prevent flocculation due to evaporation.

Strength of the agglutination reaction is not indicative of the ASO concentration.

In the qualitative test, weak reactions may occur with slightly or markedly elevated concentrations. In some cases of greatly increased ASO titer (more than 2,000 IU/mL), agglutination may be inhibited due to antibody excess (prozone). When this is suspected, it is advisable to prepare a sample dilution of 1:12 with normal saline solution and repeat the procedure.

REFERENCES

1. Insert, Rapi/Tex ASO Kit, Behring Diagnostics, Somerville, NJ, 1986.

2. Klein, G.C.: In *Manual of Clinical Immunology*. Edited by N.R. Rose and H. Friedman. American Society for Microbiology, Washington, D.C., 1976.

Antistreptolysin O[1] Tube Test

PRINCIPLE. The Anti-Streptolysin O (ASO) Tube Test is an enzyme inhibition assay. Dilutions of patient and control sera are incubated with streptolysin O reagent. Next, human red blood cells (Type O) are added to the mixture and allowed to incubate. Neutralization of the Streptolysin O reagent by Antistreptolysin O in the test serum results in inhibition of the reagent's enzymatic ability to lyse human red blood cells.

EQUIPMENT AND MATERIALS

1. 16 × 110 mm test tubes (two for each patient)

2. 13 × 100 mm test tubes (10 for each patient, 5 for the ASO positive control, 1 for the red cell control, and 1 for the streptolysin O control)

3. 37° C water bath

4. Centrifuge

5. Pipets

6. Bacto Streptolysin O Buffer (Difco) (ASO buffer): Store at room temperature before rehydration. This solution is used in diluting sera and preparing the 5% suspension of "O" cells. Pour one vial (12.4 g) of ASO buffer concentrate in a 1000-ml volumetric flask. QS to 1000 ml with distilled water. pH should be 6.6 ± 0.1. Buffer solution should then be stored at 2 to 8° C. If no concentrate is available, buffer may be prepared by dissolving 7.4 g NaCl, 3.17 g KH_2PO_4 and 1.8 g Na_2HPO_4 in 1000 ml distilled water and adjusting to pH 6.5 to 6.7 with NaOH solution. May be used indefinitely unless contamination becomes evident.

7. Anti-AB sera for typing red cells.

8. Five percent human "O" red blood cell suspension: Wash cells at least three times with 0.9% saline solution and prepare a 5% suspension of cells in ASO buffer.

9. Streptolysin O Reagent (Difco): This reagent is obtained from broth filtrates of group A Streptococci and should be stored between 2 and 8° C. Reconstitute just before using. Streptolysin O reagent is rehydrated by adding distilled water in the amount stated on the vial, and the vial is inverted several times to dissolve the reagent completely. It should be used within 20 minutes of reconstitution.

10. Antistreptolysin O Control (Difco) (ASO standard): This is a standardized gamma globulin from human plasma, to be used as a reference control for serum titrations. Store between 2 and 8° C before and after reconstitution. Reconstituted material may be used for up to 5 days when stored as directed.

11. Patient's Serum: Serum samples are used for the test. Contaminated, chylous (Streptolysin O is inhibited by cholesterol) or grossly hemolyzed sera may yield erroneous results and should not be used. Fresh or inactivated sera are equally satisfactory for the test.

PROCEDURE

1. Obtain EDTA, day old blood from Hematology. Detect type O cells as follows:

React versenated samples against anti-A,B antisera to identify tubes which do not agglutinate with the antisera. Wash and dilute as described under *Equipment and Materials,* #8.

2. Prepare the following serum dilutions in 16 × 110 tubes using Streptolysin O buffer:

a. 1:100–0.1 ml serum and 9.9 ml buffer.

b. 1:500–2 ml of 1:100 serum and 8 ml of buffer.

3. Reconstitute the Antistreptolysin O control (ASO standard) with 10 ml of distilled water to be used without further dilution as a 1:100 serum dilution.

4. Set up and label ten 13 × 100 mm tubes for each patient, 5 for the ASO positive control, 1 for the red blood control, and one for the streptolysin O control.

5. Following the table below, pipet the appropriate amounts of ASO buffer and patient serum dilutions into tubes 1 through 10 of the patient row, using the previously prepared 1:100 serum dilution in tubes 1 through 5, and the 1:500 serum dilution in tubes 6 through 10.

SERUM DILUTIONS	1:100					1:500				
TUBE #	1	2	3	4	5	6	7	8	9	10
ml serum (patient dilutions or ASO control)	1.0	0.8	0.6	0.4	0.3	1.0	0.8	0.6	0.4	0.2
ml ASO buffer	0	0.2	0.4	0.6	0.7	0	0.2	0.4	0.6	0.8

6. For the row of ASO control tubes, pipet ASO buffer and the reconstituted antistreptolysin O control in the amounts indicated in the chart above for tubes 1 through 5.

7. Shake gently to mix.

8. Pipet 1.0 ml ASO buffer into the streptolysin O control tube and 1.5 ml ASO buffer into the red cell control tube.

9. Reconstitute the streptolysin O reagent as indicated above (Equipment and Materials #9). Pipet 0.5 ml of reagent into each tube EXCEPT the red cell control tube.

10. Shake tubes gently to mix. Parafilm and incubate in 37° C waterbath for 15 minutes.

11. Remove tubes from waterbath and pipet 0.5 ml of the 5% human type O red blood cell suspension (prepared as indicated above) (Procedure Step I), into each tube.

12. Shake gently to mix. Parafilm tubes and incubate in 37° C waterbath for 45 minutes.

13. Centrifuge tubes for 3 minutes at 1500 rpm.

14. Read for the highest dilution showing complete absence of hemolysis. The ASO positive control must read ±1 tube from the titer designated on the control package insert. There should be no hemolysis in the red cell control tube and marked to complete hemolysis in the streptolysin O control tube.

REPORTING. Report patient and positive control results as the corresponding Todd unit value (TU), according to the table below.

SERUM DILUTIONS	1:100					1:500				
TUBE #	1	2	3	4	5	6	7	8	9	10
Todd Unit Value (Reciprocal of original serum dilutions)	100	125	166	250	333	500	625	833	1250	2500

NOTE: If there is no hemolysis in any of the tubes, and the control is within range, it may be necessary to titer higher than 2500 TU. If so, the following titration is suggested:

1. Place 2 ml of ASO buffer into each of six 16 × 110 tubes. To the first tube, add 2 ml of the 1:500 dilution, thus making a dilution of 1:1000. Mix and transfer 2 ml of the second tube and so on to make serial twofold dilutions through tube 6.

2. Place six 13 × 100 mm tubes in a rack. With a 1-ml pipette, place 1 ml of each of the above dilutions into their respective tubes.

3. Add 0.5 ml Streptolysin O reagent to each tube. Shake gently to mix. Incubate at 37° C for 15 minutes.

4. Add 0.5 ml 5% RBC suspension to each tube. Shake gently to mix. Incubate at 37° C for 45 minutes.

5. Following incubation, centrifuge tubes for 3 minutes at 1500 rpm and read as in #14, above. The Todd units in tubes 1–6 are now 1000, 2000, 4000, 8000, 16000, and 32000.

INTERPRETATION OF RESULTS. The normal range for ASO is generally considered to be under 200 Todd Units. However, a wide range of normal titers have been reported. A single determination of ASO should be interpreted with caution. Testing of paired sera is recommended.

Detection of < 50 TU of ASO may be due to non-specific inhibition of Streptolysin O by the lipoproteins of normal serum. Hence, titers of < 50 TU are impossible to interpret.

LIMITATIONS OF THE PROCEDURE. ASO antibody levels have often returned to normal by the onset of the pure chorea form of rheumatic fever. In addition, only 75 to 80% of streptococcal infections are associated with a rise in ASO titer. Performing more than one test for streptococcal antibody increases the probability of detecting evidence of infection.

ASO antibodies are less commonly found in pyoderma and its sequelae than are antibodies detected with Anti-DNAseB and Antihyaluronidase tests.

REFERENCE

1. Insert, Bacto-Streptolysin—O—Reagent, Difco Laboratories, Detroit, MI, 1978.

Antihyaluronidase Enzyme Inhibition[1]

PRINCIPLE. The anti-hyaluronidase test (AHT) is used as an adjunct to the antistreptolysin O (ASO) procedure for the detection of recent Group A streptococcal infection. Patient serum, if it contains antihyaluronidase, can inhibit reagent hyaluronidase added in the test. Potassium hyaluronate acts as a substrate for any hyaluronidase not neutralized by patient antibody. Finally, the addition of acetic acid indicates the presence of potassium hyaluronate by formation of a mucin clot.

EQUIPMENT AND MATERIALS

1. Bacto—AHT enzyme (Difco Laboratories)—Standardized desiccated streptococcal hyaluronidase. To rehydrate add 4 ml distilled water and rotate the vial in an end-over-end motion to effect complete solution. Do not rehydrate until ready to use. Unused portion should be discarded at the completion of the test procedure.

2. Bacto—AHT substrate (Difco Laboratories)—Standardized desiccated potassium hyaluronate. To rehydrate add 8 ml distilled water, stopper, and shake vigorously to dissolve completely. The substrate may be used up to 1 week after rehydration if it is stored at 2 to 8° C and is not allowed to become contaminated.

3. Bacto—AHT standard (Difco Laboratories)—Desiccated serum control that, when rehydrated and used in the described procedure, yields an antihyaluronidase titer of 128 units. To rehydrate add 1 ml distilled water and dissolve the contents by gentle end-over-end rotation.

4. Acetic acid 2N (prepared by adding 10 ml glacial acetic acid to 70 ml distilled water).

5. 13 × 75 mm tests tubes (seven for each serum to be tested, five for the standard, and two for reagent controls).

6. Distilled water.

7. 5 ml serologic pipettes.

8. 1 ml serologic pipettes graduated in 0.01 ml increments.

9. Waterbath at 37° C.

10. Refrigerator 2 to 8° C.

11. Interval timer.

SPECIMEN COLLECTION AND PREPARATION. Fresh or inactivated sera are equally satisfactory for the test. Store serum in the refrigerator until ready to use. Contaminated, chylous or hemoglobin-containing serum should not be used.

PROCEDURE

1. Set-up a row of chemically clean 13 × 75 mm tubes 1 through 7 for each serum to be tested. Behind this row, set up another row numbered 8 through 14. The front row is used for seven dilutions of the test serum; the first five tubes of the second row are used for five dilutions of the AHT standard; the 13th and 14th tubes are the hyaluronidase and substrate controls, respectively.

2. Serum dilutions. Add 0.25 ml distilled water to tubes 2 through 7 and 9 through 13. Add 0.6 ml distilled water to tube 14.

3. Prepare a 1:32 dilution of the patient's serum by adding 0.1 ml of serum to 3.1 ml distilled water and mixing thoroughly.

4. Add 0.25 ml of the 1:32 dilution to tubes 1 and 2.

5. Mix the contents of tube 2 by drawing the solution into a 1 ml serologic pipette (graduated in 0.01 ml) and then expelling it back into the tube. Repeat 2 more times. Transfer 0.25 ml from tube 2 to tube 3 and mix as in tube 2. Continue the dilutions through tube 7 and discard 0.25 ml from tube 7. The seven tubes will now contain 0.25 ml of 2-fold dilutions from 1:32 through 1:2048.

6. Add 0.25 ml of the rehydrated standard to tubes 8 and 9. The contents of tube 9 are mixed by drawing it into a 1-ml serologic pipette (graduated in 0.01 ml) and delivering it back into the tube. This is repeated 2 more times and then 0.25 ml is transferred to tube 10. Continue the dilutions through tube 12 and discard 0.25 ml from tube 12.

7. Add exactly 0.25 ml Bacto—AHT enzyme solution to tubes numbered 1 to 13.

8. Shake the tubes to obtain an even mixture and incubate in a waterbath at 37° C for 15 minutes.

9. Cool in the refrigerator 2 to 8° C for 10 minutes.

10. Add 0.5 ml Bacto—AHT substrate to all tubes and shake the tubes thoroughly.

11. Incubate at 37° C for 20 minutes.

12. Cool in the refrigerator at 2 to 8° C for 30 minutes.

13. Add 0.1 ml of 2 N acetic acid with a 1-ml serologic pipette to all tubes and shake the rack vigorously to obtain thorough mixing of the contents of the tubes.

14. Observe for the presence of a clot by holding each tube slightly above the eye level and shaking gently. Occasionally, the clot will adhere to the side of the tube and will be loosened by gentle shaking of the tube. The end point is also confirmed by visually comparing the turbidity in each tube containing the assay serum with the 2 control tubes; i.e., the AHT enzyme, tube 13, which should show no clot, and the AHT substrate, tube 14, which should have a definite clot. The liquid in the tubes in which a clot is present will be clear; those tubes in which no clot is present will be opalescent.

REPORTING. The antihyaluronidase titer is the reciprocal of the highest dilution having a clot (not a thread).

INTERPRETATION OF RESULTS. Quinn and Liao[2] demonstrated that normal individuals may exhibit titers up to 1:250.

LIMITATIONS OF THE PROCEDURE. Some patients with a Group A streptococcus infection do not produce a significant antihyaluronidase titer. Repeatedly negative results with this test cannot rule out a diagnosis of Group A streptococcal infection.

REFERENCES

1. Package insert, Bacto-AHT Standard, Difco Laboratories, Detroit, MI, July 1979.

2. Quinn, R.W., and Liao, S.J.: J. Clin. Invest., 29:156, 1950.

Antideoxyribonuclease-B Enzyme Inhibitor[5]

PRINCIPLE. This assay provides a means of quantitatively determining the presence of antibodies to deoxyribonuclease-B (DNase-B) by measuring enzyme inhibition. DNase-B, by its enzymatic activity, depolymerizes DNA, its substrate. However, antibodies to DNase-B can neutralize the enzyme activity and thus inhibit the depolymerization of DNA. By inclusion of a color indicator that changes from blue to pink when the DNA is depolymerized, the degree of inhibition can be determined. By testing various dilutions of a patient's serum a quantitative determination (the titer) of antibodies to DNase-B can be made by determining the highest dilution at which inhibition of the enzyme occurs.

EQUIPMENT AND MATERIALS

1. Streptonase-B kit, (Wampole Laboratories) containing:

a. Streptonase-B enzyme reagent— Streptococcal DNase-B, freeze dried. Reconstitute using 2.0 ml buffer to prepare the stock enzyme reagent. Stable for 3 months refrigerated (2 to 8° C). Do not freeze.

b. Streptonase-B substrate—calf thymus DNA with color indicator, freeze-dried. Reconstitute with 12 ml distilled water. Allow substrate to dissolve at room temperature (20 to 30° C) for 3 hours or under refrigeration (2 to 8° C) overnight.

c. Streptonase-B buffer concentrate— imidazole-calcium chloride-magnesium sulfate-gelatin. Preservative: sodium azide 0.5%. Dilute with 100 ml distilled water to prepare 125 ml of the buffer used throughout the procedure. Store refrigerated (2 to 8° C).

d. Streptonase-B positive control— anti-DNase-B serum (human), freeze-dried. Titer 1:240. Reconstitute using 0.5 ml buffer to produce a 1:10 dilution. Store refrigerated (2 to 8° C).

e. Calibrated (0.1 ml) capillary tubes and bulbs.

2. Test tubes, 10 × 75 mm disposable glass tubes

3. 37° C waterbath

4. Pipets, 0.5 ml or 1.0 ml, 2.0 ml and 10 ml, glass or plastic with 0.1 ml graduations

5. Test tube rack

SPECIMEN COLLECTION AND PREPARATION. Fresh serum, not plasma, should be used. The specimen may be stored up to 24 hours at 2 to 8° C; however, for prolonged storage (up to several years), serum should be stored frozen (−20° C). Do not thaw and refreeze more than three times. If the specimen is to be shipped at ambient temperatures, a preservative such as sodium azide 0.1% or thimerosal 0.01% should be used. Although inactivation of serum is unnecessary, inactivated serum is acceptable.

REAGENT PREPARATION

1. Streptonase-B enzyme reagent—sufficient working enzyme reagent for two titrations is prepared, immediately prior to use, by diluting 0.10 ml of stock enzyme reagent with 6.9 ml of buffer; mix well. Do not store; discard any left-over working enzyme reagent.

2. Streptonase-B substrate—1 hour before use place at room temperature (20 to 30° C). Occasionally and before use swirl gently but well. Store refrigerated (2 to 8° C). Use within 5 days. Each bottle is sufficient for two titrations.

PROCEDURE

NOTE: All reagents should be at room temperature (20 to 30° C) prior to use. The buffer concentrate must be diluted; the substrate allowed to dissolve; and the working enzyme reagent freshly prepared prior to use, as directed under Reagent Preparation. Be sure to include the serum, enzyme, and substrate controls with each testing.

1. Make a preliminary serum dilution of 1:10 for each patient (e.g. 0.1 ml and 0.9 ml buffer). The positive control is already at a 1:10 dilution when reconstituted.

2. Prepare dilutions of 1:60 and 1:85 from the 1:10 dilution as follows for each patient and the positive control:
   a. For 1:60, pipet 0.2 ml of 1:10 dilution into 1.0 ml buffer
   b. For 1:85, pipet 0.2 ml of 1:10 dilution into 1.5 ml buffer

3. Place into a test tube rack 11 test tubes for each serum and control to be tested. Also include two additional tubes, one for the enzyme control (needed for each working enzyme reagent preparation) and one for the substrate control (needed for each bottle of substrate used).

4. Prepare twofold serial dilutions from 1:60 to 1:960 and 1:85 to 1:1360 as outlined in Table 9–2 by adding 0.2 ml of buffer to each tube except tubes 1, 6, and 13; add 0.4 ml buffer to tube 13. Add 0.2 ml of the 1:60 diluted serum to tubes 1, 2, and 11, and 0.2 ml of the 1:85 dilution to tubes 6 and 7. Serially dilute by transferring 0.2 ml from tubes 2 through 5 and from tubes 7 through 10, mixing each tube thoroughly before each transfer. Discard 0.2 ml from tubes 5 and 10 so the final volume in each tube (1–10) is 0.2 ml.

5. Add 0.2 ml of working enzyme reagent to each tube except tubes 11 and 13.

6. Shake rack well to thoroughly mix tube contents and place in a 37° C waterbath for exactly 20 minutes.

7. Remove the rack from the bath after 20 minutes and add 0.4 ml of substrate to each tube.

8. Shake rack well to thoroughly mix tube contents and place in a 37° C waterbath for an additional 4 hours (4½ hours maximum) shaking the rack once after the first 15 minutes.

Table 9–2. Summary of Anti-DNase B Test Procedure

Tube No.	1	2	3	4	5	6	7	8	9	10	Serum Control 11	Enzyme Control 12	Substrate Control 13
ml of buffer	—	.02	0.2	0.2	0.2	—	0.2	0.2	0.2	0.2	0.2	0.2	0.4
ml of 1:60 serum dilution	0.2	0.2	—	—	—	—	—	—	—	—	0.2	—	—
ml of 1:85 serum dilution						0.2	0.2	—	—	—	—	—	—
ml of enzyme reagent	0.2	0.2	0.2	0.2	0.2	0.2	0.2	0.2	0.2	0.2	—	0.2	—
Shake thoroughly and incubate at 37° C for exactly 20 minutes.													
ml of substrate	0.4	0.4	0.4	0.4	0.4	0.4	0.4	0.4	0.4	0.4	0.4	0.4	0.4
Shake and incubate at 37° C for 4 hours, up to 4 1/2 hours, shaking once after the first 15 minutes.													
Titer	60	120	240	480	960	85	170	340	680	1360	—	—	—

9. Remove the rack from the bath and read results of each tube by noting change in color from blue to pink.

REPORTING. A blue or bluish-violet color indicates lack of enzymatic activity (i.e., enzyme inhibition by antibody). A pink or pinkish-violet is indicative of enzyme activity (i.e. lack of antibody inhibition).

The reciprocal of the highest dilution of serum showing inhibition (blue or bluish-violet color) is the anti-DNase-B titer of the serum. For example, if a serum produces a blue color in tubes 1, 2, 6, and 7, a bluish-violet in tube 3, a pinkish-violet in tube 8, and pink in tubes 4, 5, 9, and 10, then the titer of the serum is 240, the titer of tube 3.

The positive control should test positive to a titer of 240 within plus-or-minus one tube for a titer range of 170 to 340.

The serum control (tube 11) and the substrate control (tube 13) both must be blue and the enzyme control (tube 12) must be pink. If these results are not obtained, the test is invalid. A pink endpoint in the serum control (tube 11) can be caused by the presence of a DNase other than DNase-B in the specimen.

INTERPRETATION OF RESULTS. Expected values: The upper limit of normal (defined as the level of antibody titer exceeded by no more than 20% of a given population) for anti-DNase-B has been stated to be between 1:60 and 1:170 by Klein, et al.[14] and 1:250 by Wannamaker et al.[1] Klein et al.[4] also determined that the mean normal levels are age dependent: Preschool, 1:60, school age, 1:170, and adult, 1:85.

LIMITATION OF THE PROCEDURE. Elevated anti-DNase-B titers in streptococcal pyoderma infections with or without the sequelae of nephritis can be found in 85% of patients[2,3,6] and in over 90% of patients with acute glomerulonephritis.

Because the upper limit of normal levels of antibody titer can be expected to be exceeded by 20% of a given healthy population, a rise in the titer is more definitive evidence of a recent infection than the ab-

solute value of a single determination of anti-DNase-B titer. Ideally, serum samples should be obtained at weekly or biweekly intervals.[7]

REFERENCES

1. Ayoub, E.M., and Wannamaker, L.W.: Pediatrics, 29:527, 1962.
2. Dillon, H.C., and Reeves, M.D.: Pediatric Res., 3:362, 1969.
3. Kaplan, E.L., Anthony, B.F., Chapman, S.S., Ayoub, E.M., and Wannamaker, L.W.: J. Clin. Invest., 49:1405, 1970.
4. Klein, G.C., Baker, C.N., and Jones, W.L.: App. Microbiol., 21:999, 1971.
5. Package insert, Streptonase-B Kit, Wampole Laboratories, Cranbury, NJ, 1981.
6. Potter, E.V. et al.: J. Pediatrics, 72:871, 1968.
7. Taranta, A., and Moody, M.D.: Pediatr. Clin. North Am., 18:125, 1971.

SYPHILIS

Treponema pallidum, the causative agent of syphilis, is a thin spirochete that can be identified, in part, by its 6 to 14 corkscrew-like spirals. At 8 to 18μm in length, it is slightly longer than the diameter of an erythrocyte, but has a width of only .09 to .13μm.[49] The organism is motile, using three characteristic movements: longitudinal rotation, backward and forward migration, and flexion movements that create "waves" in the surrounding medium. Man is its only natural host; however, T. pallidum may be maintained for use in in vitro testing by injection into rabbit testis, with sacrifice of the animal and mincing of the infected testicle. More recently, the organism has been grown on cottontail rabbit epithelial cell culture.[17,43] It does not survive on artificial media. T. pallidum is composed of core structures, a sheath, and axial filaments,[13] which may contain major antigenic components for humoral immune responses. An outer envelope,[49] endoflagella,[2] and terminal nosepieces apparently used for attachment[21] are also evident. Outside a host, it is easily destroyed by heat, drying, and soap; therefore, it is almost always spread by direct contact between humans.

Three closely related treponemes have also been implicated in human disease; T.

pallidum, variant Bosnia A, causes bejel, *T. pertenue* causes yaws, and *T. carateum* is the agent known to cause pinta. The pathogenic treponemes are antigenically and structurally similar, such that differentiation is accomplished by the nature of the lesions and the clinical course of infection.

Nonpathogenic treponemes are widely distributed in nature, forming part of the normal flora of the mouth, alimentary tract, bronchi, and the urethra. Antigenically, they are similar, but not identical to the pathogenic strains.

Despite effective methods for treatment, the incidence of syphilis is still unacceptably high,[12] particularly in Florida,[37] California,[32] and New York City. Recent increases have been primarily seen in females and heterosexual males.[12] In Africa the seropositive rate is over 10% in pregnant females, suggesting that 5 to 8% of pregnancies will result in congenital infection.[51]

Acquired infection with *T. pallidum* is usually via abraded skin or mucous membrane contact with open lesions from an infected individual; thus, sexual contact is the predominant mode of acquisition. Congenital infections may be induced if primary infection or bacteremic relapse occurs during pregnancy.[16] Infection resulting from occupational exposure occurs,[63] but is extremely rare, as is transfusion-related disease.[50] Although transplanted organs have the potential to transmit the disease,[22] prophylactic treatment is an effective deterrent.

The risk of acquiring infection from sexual contact with an infected individual ranges from 5 to 30%.[8] Even when open lesions are evident on an infected person, acquired infection occurs in only about 50% of those directly exposed.[6] A transient bacteremia follows within hours of initial infection, and the organism is dispersed. It attaches to cells via one or both terminal nosepieces,[20,21] and may damage or penetrate cells,[20] particularly those in the area of initial infection. As the organisms multiply and the lesion(s) develop, hyaluronidase can be detected on the organism surface,

perhaps facilitating further dissemination.[19] A treponema-associated surface precipitate[21,52,60] has also been described.

The visible lesion in *primary syphilis,* known as a chancre, occurs at the site of contact with the organism 10 to 90 days after exposure (average: 21 days).[4,16] Usually appearing at only a single site, the chancre is a firm, painless ulcer that results probably from both the host's intense inflammatory reaction and from damage mediated by the organism.[20] Outside factors may influence the nature of lesions seen in primary and secondary syphilis,[49] e.g. the climate in the tropics encourages moister lesions, richer in treponemes. Because the chancre is painless, it may be undetected in the female. Regional lymphadenopathy accompanying the primary lesion results in painless enlargements classically known as buboes. Without therapy, the primary stage of syphilis lasts from 1 to 5 weeks, then heals spontaneously.[16]

Somewhat more than 25% of untreated syphilitics progress from primary to secondary-stage disease,[4] usually 1 to 2 months after the chancre disappears. *Secondary syphilis* manifests itself as malaise, fever, generalized lymphadenopathy, white patches on buccal mucosa, and a generalized maculopapular or pustular rash, perhaps mediated by immune complexes,[41] which frequently includes the palms and the soles of the feet. Twenty to 30% of patients develop flat genital lesions called condylomata lata, and/or exhibit pleocytosis of the cerebral spinal fluid.[16] The secondary stage can last several days to a year, but usually persists for 1 to 2 months. Relapses may occur up to 4 years after initial infection, usually during the first 2 years, and multiple relapses are not uncommon. Moist secondary papules and condylomata lata, as well as the chancre of primary syphilis, contain organisms,[49] and patients are infectious during active primary and secondary disease.

Latent syphilis is the inactive period following the secondary stage; approximately 70% of patients will remain inactive with no further signs of disease.[16] Although syphilis is considered non-infectious during this time, an asymptomatic bacteremia in infected pregnant females may pass the organism to the fetus and induce congenital infection.[2,16] The nature and location of the organism during this period in individuals with continuing infection is unclear.[49]

Late stage, or *tertiary syphilis,* may appear months to many years after secondary disease in untreated patients. Progressive inflammatory lesions of any organ or tissue may be evident, justifying the notion of syphilis as the "great imitator." Most often, the central nervous system or the cardiovascular system is involved. Benign, visceral gummas, or granulomas, can occur anywhere, but are especially noticeable on bone or skin. Perhaps the best known of tertiary syndromes, neurosyphilis may appear as acute meningitis or meningovascular involvement of any part of the central nervous system.[16] Meningovascular involvement of the spinal cord generally occurs only after prolonged incubation of more than 20 years.[16] Late-stage syphilis is not infectious, except to the fetus of an infected pregnant woman.

Transplacental transmission of *Treponema pallidum* reached an all-time low of 3 cases/100,000 births in 1980.[10] But in 1986, more cases were reported in the U.S. than for any of the previous 15 years, and the rise appears to be continuing.[23] Congenital disease has devastating effects on the infected fetus, causing fetal or perinatal death in 40% of cases,[23] usually during the second or third trimester. Twenty percent of infants will not manifest disease. Clinical symptoms in live born infants are generally absent at birth and during the first few weeks of life. The earliest findings may be nonspecific and subsequent findings so diverse that accurate and timely diagnosis may be difficult. "Early congenital disease" appears in children less than 2 years of age; "late-appearing" symptoms may not be seen until the child is 2 to 10 years old.[33] The most common observation is a maculo-papular or vesicu-

lobullous skin eruption. Condylomata lata, mucous patches, clear or hemorrhagic rhinitis, perioral fissures, painful limbs, often presenting as pseudoparalysis, generalized lymphadenopathy hepatosplenomegaly, jaundice, ascites, edema, and/or anemia are among the symptoms reported.[16,55]

The primary natural defenses against syphilis are intact skin and mucous membranes. The organism activates complement via both the classical and alternative pathways, but is not immobilized or lysed by its action.[18] Control of the organism in vivo, as suggested by experimental models,[39,52] is mediated by T cells, and effected through influx and activation of macrophages.[49] Humoral antibody may facilitate destruction by damage to organism membranes or other means.[49] Recent studies in hamsters suggest that suppressor T lymphocyte populations may be helpful in the organism's escape from total elimination by host defenses.[56]

The presence of genital ulcers in diseases such as syphilis increases the risk of transmission of the human immunodeficiency virus (HIV).[38,48] Alternatively, pre- or co-existing infection with HIV may alter the course[30,54] or the distribution of lesions[14] of syphilis. Additionally, diagnosis of syphilis may be obscured in HIV-infected persons by the absence of serologic response to *Treponema pallidum.*[27,58]

Syphilis may be diagnosed by direct identification of *T. pallidum* in specimens taken from moist lesions of primary, secondary, or congenital syphilis. Darkfield examination[40] may be performed by use of a darkfield condenser on an ordinary light microscope, allowing for illumination and characterization of floating objects by use of reflected light. Alternately, direct fluorescent antibody labeling of treponemes (DFA-TP), silver stains, or hematoxylin and eosin stains may be useful.[23] Repeated performance of direct methods is suggested[8] before negative results are accepted since a high level of expertise is needed for accurate performance and interpretation of these tests.

Serologic tests for syphilis (STS) may be used alternately or in conjunction with direct identification methods. Methods are categorized into nontreponemal (nonspecific) and treponemal (specific) tests based on the antigen used. Nontreponemal tests employ lipoidal antigens, comprised of cardiolipin, lecithin, and cholesterol to detect "reaginic" antibody, apparently formed after the interaction of T. pallidum with body tissues. Reaginic antibodies belong to the IgM and IgG classes of immunoglobulin, and are useful in screening for active, acute disease, for staging and monitoring response to therapy, and as an aid to the diagnosis of congenital infection (see below). Nontreponemal tests which are easy to perform include the Venereal Disease Research Laboratory test (VDRL), the rapid plasma reagin (RPR), the unheated serum reagin test (USR),[47] and the reagin screen test (RST). These tests are similar in performance and in their relationship to disease,[25,28,47] although the RPR may be slightly more sensitive than others.[16,28] Complement fixation tests for detection of reaginic antibody (e.g. Wasserman, cardiolipin)[44] are not generally used, as they are more labor intensive. Reaginic titers are usually elevated during symptomatic stages, but may lapse in titer during inactive phases. Sensitivity of the tests generally increases with disease progression with the exception of tertiary stage neurosyphilis, when reagin serum titers may be negative. An ELISA method for detection of reaginic antibody has been developed[45] and may facilitate differentiation between IgM and IgG classes of antibody.

Treponemal, or specific, tests for syphilis detect antibody to Treponema pallidum or its components. Included are the Treponema pallidum immobilization test (TPI), the fluorescent treponemal antibody-absorbed test (FTAabs),[15] the hemagglutination test for treponema (HATTS),[61] the microhemagglutination test (MHA-TP), and the Bio-Enza Bead Test for syphilis.[5,42] Other tests have been largely supplanted.[44] Characteristic of treponemal tests is their tendency to remain positive for the life of the individual. In general, the FTAabs test is considered more sensitive than the TPI,[1] while the HATTS test may be more sensitive than the FTAabs,[31] and microhemagglutination assays are comparable to the FTAabs once the disease is established.[1] Both the hemagglutination and the microhemagglutination tests lack sensitivity in primary stage disease.[35]

Biologic false-positives, or sera that give a reactive serologic test that is not caused by syphilis, are common among the samples testing positive, particularly in nontreponemal tests (3 to 40%).[53] They can occur in any patient,[7,35] or in normals,[46] but are more frequently seen in patients with connective tissue diseases,[26] pregnancy,[57] or other spirochetal or viral infections.[16] Transient biologic false-positives are most often associated with infection, while antibody lasting longer than 6 months may be seen with chronic disease.[36] Biologic false-positives in treponemal tests are rare.[59] Technical factors probably play an important role in many cases.[25]

Despite the high rate of biologic false-positives with nontreponemal tests, their simplicity and ease of performance render them useful for screening large populations for syphilis. Such testing is recommended as part of routine prenatal and adult care, as well as for screening units of blood for transfusion.[50] Reactive, or positive, tests are always confirmed by performance of a treponemal assay on the sample. False-negative nontreponemal tests are common early in disease and may be observed during inactive or late stages of disease. (See below.)

Diagnosis and staging of disease usually requires integration of patient history, physical findings, results of direct testing, and serology. Titers, performed primarily with nontreponemal tests, may be useful. Typical syphilis serology results are discussed below and summarized in Figure 9–2.

The first diagnostic antibody test to become reactive during the course of primary

Syphilis
Prototypic Untreated Disease and STS

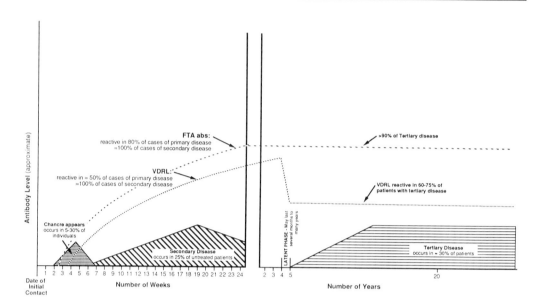

Fig. 9–2. Relative reactivity of serologic tests for syphilis during untreated disease. STS = Serologic tests for syphilis.

stage syphilis is the FTAabs. Nontreponemal tests, e.g. VDRL/RPR, become reactive sometime during this stage in most but not all cases.[28] Hemagglutination tests (HATTS, MHA-TP) lack sensitivity in detecting early disease.[28,35] Successful treatment causes the nontreponemal tests to revert to negative in about 75% of cases by 3 to 12 months, and in nearly all patients by 24 months.[3] Individuals who do not experience disease after the primary stage, without therapy, will eventually revert to negative non-treponemal tests; however, treponemal tests usually remain reactive for life, regardless of treatment.[25]

During untreated secondary stage disease, sensitivity levels approaching 100% are observed for all tests.[25] Titers of nontreponemal tests reach their highest levels (> 32) during this stage. Effective treatment returns nontreponemal titers to negative in 40% of cases during the first 12 months, and in 75% by 24 months.[3]

Nontreponemal titers gradually wane during latent disease, although treponemal antibodies will remain detectable.

In late-stage syphilis, nontreponemal tests on serum may be nonreactive in 25 to 40% of patients,[24,25] making diagnosis difficult. Treatment of late stage patients who do have reactive nontreponemal tests has little effect on antibody titer.[3] The absence of visible lesions renders direct tests useless. Treponemal tests, although they remain reactive, are not useful in establishing the diagnosis of active disease.

Testing of cerebral spinal fluid (CSF) may be helpful in diagnosis of late stage neurosyphilis. The Centers for Disease Control[9] recommend CSF examination on patients with clinical evidence of neurosyphilis, and suggest its desirability for use with asymptomatic patients with untreated disease of greater than one year duration. Others[14,62] refute their suggestion, citing large numbers of lumbar punctures ordered on patients without adequate serologic evidence of primary disease, e.g. reactive treponemal tests on serum. The reported sensitivity of VDRL testing on CSF ranges from 10 to 89% in active cases of neurosyphilis, tending to be higher in some forms than others.[14] The specificity of the test is high,[14,16] but false-negatives do occur.[3] In practice, reactive VDRL-CSFs are rare.[34] Contamination of CSF by blood, either as a result of disruption of the blood/brain barrier or a traumatic spinal tap, may induce false-positive results.[25,29] The FTAabs test is not recommended for performance on CSF.[8]

Diagnosis of congenital disease is complicated by the presence in the newborn of maternal treponemal and nontreponemal antibody of the IgG class.[33] Disease should be suspected in infants with reactive serologic tests for syphilis, regardless of the presence of symptoms, and in infants born to infected mothers.[23] Nontreponemal tests are recommended for diagnosis of congenital infections in that they detect the IgM class of antibody and can be titered. Newborns with nontreponemal titers higher than that of the mother, or in whom antibody levels do not wane over time are probably infected.[16,25] FTAabs-IgM tests are not reliable for the diagnosis of congenital infection largely because of the rheumatoid factor activity present in newborn samples.[6,23]

The effectiveness of penicillin[23] as a treatment for syphilis has remained constant since its introduction over a half century ago. Treatment is recommended for suspected infection in infants, even in the absence of definitive diagnosis. More aggressive therapy may be required to treat patients with compromised immune status.[23,58]

REFERENCES

1. Atwood, W.G., Miller, J.L., Stout, G.W., and Norins, L.C.: JAMA, 203:549, 1968.

2. Blanco, D.R., Champion, C.I., Miller, J.N., and Lovett, M.R.: Infect. Immun., 56:168, 1988.

3. Bracero, L., Wormser, G.P., and Buttone, E.J.: Mt. Sinai J. Med., 46:289, 1979.

4. Brown, W.J. et al.: *Syphilis and Other Venereal Diseases.* Cambridge, Harvard University Press, 1970.

5. Burdash, N.M., Hinds, K.K., Finnerty, J.A., and Manos, J.P.: J. Clin. Microbiol., 25:808, 1987.

6. Cannefax, G.R., Norins, L.C., and Gillespie, E.J.: Ann. Rev. Med., 18:471, 1967.

7. Catterall, R.D.: Br. J. Vener. Dis., 48:1, 1972.

8. Centers for Disease Control: *Criteria and Techniques for the Diagnosis of Early Syphilis,* 1979. (DHEW Pub. No. 98-376).

9. Centers for Disease Control, MMWR, 31:515, 1982.

10. Centers for Disease Control, MMWR, 36:173, 1987.

11. Centers for Disease Control, MMWR, 36:488, 1987.

12. Centers for Disease Control, MMWR, 37:35, 1988.

13. Cockayne, A., Bailey, M.J., and Penn, C.W.: J. Gen. Microbiol., 133:1397, 1987.

14. Dans, P.E., Cafferty, L, Otter, S.E., and Johnson R.J.: Ann. Intern. Med., 104:86, 1986.

15. Deacon, W.F., Lucas, J.B., and Price E.V.: JAMA, 198:624, 1966.

16. Feder, H.M., Jr., and Manthous, C.: Am. Fam. Physician, 37:185, 1988.

17. Fieldsteel, A.H., Cox, D.L., and Moeckli, R.A.: Infect. Immun. 35:449, 1982.

18. Fitzgerald, T.J.: Infect. Immun., 55:2066, 1987.

19. Fitzgerald, T.J., and Repesh, L.A.: Infect. Immun., 55:1023, 1987.

20. Fitzgerald, T.J., Repesh, L.A., and Oakes, S.G.: Br. J. Vener. Dis., 58:1, 1982.

21. Fitzgerald, T.J. et al.: J. Bacteriol., 130:1333, 1977.

22. Gibel, L.J., Sterling, W., Hoy, W., and Harford, A.: J. Urol., 138:1226, 1987.

23. Guidelines for the Prevention and Control of Congenital Syphilis, MMWR, 37(Suppl. 1):1, 1988.

24. Harner, R.E., Smith, J.L., and Israel, C.W.: JAMA, 203:545, 1968.

25. Hart, G.: Ann. Intern. Med., 104:368, 1986.

26. Harvey, A.M., and Shulman, L.E.: Med. Clin. North Am., 50:1271, 1966.

27. Hicks, C.B. et al.: Ann. Intern. Med., 107:492, 1987.

28. Huber, T.W. et al.: J. Clin. Microbiol., 17:405, 1983.

29. Izzat, N.N. et al.: Br. J. Vener. Dis., 47:162, 1971.

30. Johns, D.R., Tierney, M., and Felsenstein, D.: N. Engl. J. Med., 316:1569, 1987.

31. Kiraly, K., and Prerau, H.: Acta. Derm. Venereol. (Stockh), 54:303, 1974.

32. Kizer, K.W., Ault, T., and Olivas, J.M.: West. J. Med., 148:94, 1988.

33. Lane, G.K., and Oates, R.K.: Med. J. Aust., 148:171, 1988.

34. Larsen, S.A., Hambie, E.A., Wobig, E.A., and Kennedy, E.J.: In *Advances in Sexually Transmitted Diseases.* Edited by R. Morisset et al. Utrecht, VNU Science Press, 1985.

35. Larsen, S.A. et al.: J. Clin. Microbiol., 14:441, 1981.

36. Lau, R., and Forster, G.E.: Br. Med. J., 295:925, 1987.

37. Leads from the MMWR, JAMA, 257:2565, 1987.

38. Leads from MMWR, JAMA, *259*:975, 1988.

39. Lukehart, S.A., Baker-Zander, S.A., Lloyd, R.M.C., and Sell, S.: J. Immunol., *124*:461, 1980.

40. Manual of Tests for Syphilis—Atlanta: Venereal Disease Program, U.S. Communicable Disease Center, 1969. (PHS publication No. 411).

41. McNeely, M.C. et al.: J. Am. Acad. Dermatol., *14*:564, 1986.

42. Moyer, N.P., Hudson, J.D., and Hausler, W.J., Jr.: J. Clin. Microbiol., *25*:619, 1987.

43. Norris, S.J.: Infect. Immun., *36*:437, 1982.

44. Olansky, S.: Med. Clin. North. Am., *56*:1145, 1972.

45. Pederson, N.S., Orum, O., and Mouritsen, S.: J. Clin. Microbiol., *25*:1711, 1987.

46. Peter, C.R., Thompson, M.A., and Wilson, D.: J. Clin. Microbiol., *9*:369, 1979.

47. Pettit, D.E. et al.: J. Clin. Microbiol., *15*:238, 1982.

48. Potterat, J.J.: JAMA, *258*:473, 1987.

49. Paulsen, A., Kobayashi, T., Secher, L., and Weismann, K.: Acta. Derm. Venereol., (Stockh), *67*:289, 1987.

50. Puckett, A., and Pratt, G.: J. Clin. Pathol., *40*:1337, 1987.

51. Schulz, K.F., Cates, W., Jr., and O'Mara, P.R.: Genitourin. Med., *63*:320, 1987.

52. Sell, S., Baker-Zander, S., and Powece, H.C.: Lab. Invest., *46*:355, 1982.

53. Sparling, P.F.: N. Engl. J. Med., *284*:642, 1971.

54. Spence, M.R., and Abrutyn, E.: Ann. Intern. Med., *107*:587, 1987.

55. Stevens, M.C., Darbyshire, P.J., and Brown, S.M.: Arch. Dis. Child, *62*:1073, 1987.

56. Tabor, D.R., Kiel, D.P., and Jacobs, R.F.: Immunology, *62*:127, 1987.

57. Thornton, J.G. et al.: Br. Med. J., *295*:355, 1987.

58. Tramont, E.C.: N. Engl. J. Med., *316*:1600, 1987.

59. Tuffanelli, D.L., Wuepper, K.D., Bradford, L.L., and Wood, R.M.: N. Engl. J. Med., *276*:258, 1967.

60. VanderSluis, J.J., ten Kate, F.J.W., Vuzeuski, V.D., and Stolz, E.: Genitourin. Med., *63*:297, 1987.

61. Wentworth, B.B. et al.: Sex. Transm. Dis., *5*:103, 1978.

62. Whiteside-Yim, C. et al.: Ann. Intern. Med., *105*:295, 1986.

63. Williams, W.C., and Marion, E.S.: J. Fam. Pract., *25*:509, 1987.

VDRL-SERUM: QUALITATIVE AND QUANTITATIVE TESTS[4]

PRINCIPLE. A buffered saline solution suspension of cardiolipin-lecithin-cholesterol antigen is mixed with patient serum, agitated on a mechanical rotator, and examined microscopically for flocculation. This reaction occurs in the presence of reagin antibody in sera from syphilitic persons and occasionally in sera of persons with other acute and chronic conditions.

EQUIPMENT AND MATERIALS

1. VDRL Antigen (Sylvana): An alcoholic solution of 0.03% cardiolipin, 0.9% cholesterol, and sufficient purified lecithin (usually 0.21 ± 0.1%) to produce the standard reactivity. Store at room temperature in the dark. Expiration date is noted on container. Discard if precipitate forms. A new lot of antigen should be compared with antigen of known reactivity by testing against known control serum before being placed in routine use.

2. VDRL Buffered Saline Solution (Sylvana): Contains 1.0% sodium chloride, pH 6.0 ± 0.1. Store at room temperature. Check pH if an unexplained change in test reactivity occurs. Discard if pH falls out of range. Expiration date is noted on the label.

3. 0.9% saline solution.

4. Rotating machine, adjustable to 180 rpm, circumscribing a circle 1.9 cm in diameter on a horizontal plane.

5. Glass slides with ceramic rings approximately 14 mm in diameter.

6. Bottle, 30 ml, round, flat-bottomed, glass stoppered, narrow mouth.

7. Syringes (Hamilton), calibrated to deliver 1/60 ml, 1/75 ml and 1/100 ml, respectively.

8. Pipets or pipettor, capable of delivering 0.05 ml of serum.

9. Pipets: 0.1, 0.5, 1.0, and 5.0 ml.

10. Controls (Fisher): A known, titered reactive and weakly reactive serum prepared from pooled sera of rabbits immunized with floccules of VDRL antigen; diluted with stabilized bovine albumin standardized using CDC VDRL antigens. Nonreactive control serum is prepared from pooled human serum tested to be VDRL nonreactive. Store at 4° C. May be used until date noted on the label. *Do Not Freeze.*

11. Test tubes, for quantitative procedure.

12. Light microscope.

PROCEDURE
QUANTITATIVE SLIDE TEST
NOTE: Slide flocculation tests are affected by room temperature. Tests should be performed

within the temperature range 73 to 85° F (23 to 29° C).

1. Heat inactivate all sera to be tested. Examine for debris and recentrifuge those samples with evident debris. Bring all samples to room temperature.

2. Prepare antigen suspension:

a. Pipet 0.4 ml buffered saline solution onto the bottom of a 30-ml bottle. Be sure the saline solution completely covers the bottom.

b. Add 0.5 ml VDRL antigen (from lower half of a 1.0-ml pipet graduated to the tip) directly onto the saline solution while continuously, but gently, rotating the bottle on a flat surface. Add antigen drop by drop, rapidly, allowing 6 seconds for each 0.5 ml of antigen. The pipet tip should remain in the upper third of the bottle, and rotation should not be vigorous enough to splash saline solution onto the pipet. The proper speed of rotation is obtained when the center of the bottle circumscribes a 5-cm diameter circle approximately three times per second.

c. Expel the last drop of antigen out of the pipet without touching the saline solution.

d. Continue rotation of the bottle for 10 seconds.

e. Add 4.1 ml buffered saline solution, using a 5.0 ml pipet.

f. Place the top on the bottle and shake top to bottom and back approximately 30 times in 10 seconds.

g. Antigen suspension is ready for use, and may be used only during the day prepared.

h. Mix the antigen suspension gently each time it is used. *Do not* mix with the syringe, as this may cause loss of reactivity.

3. Calibrate the 1/60 ml syringe. Calibration should be performed on each Hamilton syringe before use with each run, as follows:

a. Fill the barrel of the Hamilton syringe with the fluid to be used. Place the bent needle into a 1-ml syringe that has had the needle removed and the plunger retracted to just below the 1.0 ml mark.

b. Dispense the number of drops designated for that syringe, i.e. 60 drops for the 1/60 ml syringe, 75 drops for the 1/75 ml syringe, and 100 drops for the 1/100 ml syringe.

c. Bring the plunger of the 1-ml syringe to the 1.0 ml mark. If the 1-ml syringe loses more than 2 drops, or if more than 2 drops are necessary to fill it, clean the Hamilton syringe with alcohol and repeat steps a–c. Syringes that do not deliver ± two drops from their specified number must be replaced.

5. Rotator adjustment: Using a stop watch and setting the rotator to 180 rpm, count the number of revolutions per 15 second time interval. Adjust so the machine is rotating 45 ± 1 revolutions per 15 seconds (180 rpm).

5. Pipet 0.05 ml of each of the three controls and the patient samples into the ceramic rings of a glass slide, spreading to fill the entire ring.

6. Add one drop (1/60 ml) of VDRL antigen suspension from the appropriate syringe to each ring.

7. Rotate slides for 4 minutes on the rotator (180 rpm).

8. Read microscopically immediately after rotation, using a low-power objective, at 100× magnification, as follows:

Medium and large clumps: Reactive

Small clumps: Weakly reactive

No clumps or very slight roughness: Nonreactive

REPORTING. The control sera must react appropriately to ensure accurate patient results, e.g. reactive control = reactive, etc. Record acceptable control results as required.

If controls are acceptable, record patient results as reactive, weakly reactive, or nonreactive. All sera with weakly reactive or reactive results on the qualitative slide test must be tested using the quantitative slide test. All nonreactive sera are reported as "Non-Reactive."

Record antigen lot number, control lot number, and their expiration dates.

QUANTITATIVE SLIDE TEST

Quantitative slide test to be performed on any sample demonstrating reactivity in the qualitative test.

1. Calibrate the 1/75-ml and the 1/100-ml Hamilton syringes, using the *Calibration of Syringes* procedure described in the qualitative procedure.

2. In test tubes, prepare a 1:8 dilution of each serum and the reactive control by adding 0.1 ml of the serum or control to 0.7 ml of 0.9% saline solution.

3. Mix thoroughly. Using the same pipet, transfer 0.04 ml, 0.02 ml and 0.01 ml of the 1:8 serum dilution into wells 4, 5, and 6, of a glass slide, respectively, as shown in the diagram below. Return remaining serum dilution into the dilution tube.

④   ⑤   ⑥
①   ②   ③

4. Using the same pipet, transfer 0.04 ml, 0.02 ml and 0.01 ml of the undiluted serum into wells 1, 2, and 3, respectively.

5. Add two drops (0.01 ml/drop) of 0.9%

saline solution to wells 2 and 5, using a 1/100-ml syringe.

6. Using the same syringe, add three drops of 0.9% saline solution to wells 3 and 6.

NOTE: You have prepared twofold dilutions ranging from 1:1 (well 1) to 1:32 (well 6), with a total volume in each well of 0.04 ml.

7. Rotate slide gently by hand for about 15 seconds to mix. Using a wooden applicator stick, spread the contents of each well to fill the entire ring. Start at well 6 and go back through to well 1 so that the dilutions will not be affected.

8. Using a 1/75-ml syringe, add one drop of the prepared antigen to each well.

9. Rotate slides for 4 minutes on the mechanical rotator (180 rpm).

10. Read microscopically, immediately after rotation, as in the qualitative test.

11. If all serum dilutions tested produce reactive results, prepare a 1:64 dilution of serum in saline solution by adding 0.1 ml of the 1:8 dilution to 0.7 ml saline solution. Mix and test this 1:64 dilution in three amounts as was done for the 1:8 dilution. The resulting dilutions will be 1:64, 1:128 and 1:256. Repeat until loss of reactivity is noted; then report as noted below.

REPORTING. The reactive control must be reactive (medium and large clumps) to within one dilution of the titer designated for that lot number. Record control results as required.

Record results as the greatest serum dilution that produces a reactive (not a weakly reactive) result. Sera demonstrating no more than weakly reactive flocculation are recorded as weakly reactive. Sera reactive in the quantitative test are recorded as the reciprocal of the determined dilution; e.g., a serum that is still reactive at a 1:2 dilution is reported as "reactive, titer 2."

FTA-ABS or MHA-TP testing should be performed on every sera demonstrating reactivity in the serum VDRL test.

INTERPRETATION OF RESULTS. A reactive VDRL in the presence of clinical syphilis is confirmatory evidence of the disease.

In the absence of symptoms, a reactive VDRL may be due to latent syphilis, or to a biologic false-positive.

LIMITATIONS OF THE PROCEDURE. Biologic false-positives account for 3 to 40%[6] of positive serum reagin tests; i.e., the test detects reagin that is formed in response to something other than syphilis. A wide variety of acute and chronic conditions have been associated with reagin antibody.[1-3,6]

Reagin titers may be nonreactive early in the disease or during prolonged latent periods.

Occasionally, a VDRL may be nonreactive because of a prozone phenomenon. One author estimates this may occur in 1% of secondary syphilitics.[5]

REFERENCES

1. Brown, W.J. et al.: *Syphilis and Other Venereal Diseases.* Cambridge, Harvard University Press, 1970.

2. Harvey, A.M., and Shulman, L.E.: Med. Clin. North Am., *50*:1271, 1966.

3. Krugman, S., Ward, R., and Katz, S.: *Infectious Diseases of Children.* St Louis, C.V. Mosby Co., 1977.

4. U.S. Department of Health, Education and Welfare: *Manual of Tests for Syphilis.* Public Health Service Publication #411. Washington, D.C., 1969.

5. Sparling, P.F.: N. Engl. J. Med., *284*:642, 1971.

6. Wood, R.M.: In *Manual of Clinical Immunology.* Edited by N.R. Rose and H. Friedman. Washington, D.C., American Society for Microbiology, 1976.

VDRL Spinal Fluid Procedure[3]

PRINCIPLE. Antigen from the serum VDRL tests is sensitized with 10% saline solution, then reacted with patient spinal fluid to detect the presence of reagin.

EQUIPMENT AND MATERIALS

All equipment necessary is listed under *VDRL: Serum Tests* except:

1. Boerner slides: agglutination, approximately 2" × 3", with concavities measuring 16 mm in diameter and 1.75 mm in depth.

2. 10% saline solution: Prepare by adding 10 g NaCl to a 100-ml volumetric flask. QS to 100 ml with distilled water. Store at room temperature. May be stored indefinitely.

SPECIMEN COLLECTION AND PREPARATION. Spinal fluid should be centrifuged and decanted before using. *Do not inactivate.* Spinal fluids which are visibly contaminated or grossly bloody are unsatisfactory for testing. Specimens should be stored at −20° C.

PROCEDURE

NOTE: Slide tests for syphilis are affected by room temperature. Optimum temperature of 73 to 85° F (23 to 29° C) should be maintained.

1. Thaw patient specimens if stored frozen.
2. Prepare sensitized antigen by adding one part of VDRL antigen to one part 10% saline solution. Mix by inversion and allow to stand at least 5 minutes, but not more than 2 hours, before using.
3. Calibrate the 1/100-ml syringe (labeled for CSF use), following the protocol for *Calibration of Syringes,* under VDRL Serum: Qualitative Slide Test.
4. Adjust the rotator speed to 180 rpm (45 ± 1 revolution/15 seconds), if not done previously. Procedure may be found under VDRL Serum: Qualitative Slide Test.
5. Pipet 0.05 ml of each spinal fluid sample into the concavities of a Boerner agglutination slide, spreading the sample to fill the entire surface.
6. Add one drop (0.01 ml) of sensitized antigen suspension to each spinal fluid using the 1/100-ml syringe.
7. Rotate slides for 8 minutes on a mechanical rotator at 180 rpm.
8. Read microscopically, as in the VDRL serum slide test. Record the results of the patient samples as reactive (definitive clumping), weakly reactive, or non-reactive (no clumping, or very slight roughness).
9. Those fluids reactive in the spinal fluid test are titered as follows:
   a. Using 5 or more tubes, make twofold dilutions (1:2, 1:4, 1:8, etc.) of the spinal fluid in buffered saline solution.
   b. Test the undiluted and the diluted fluids as in steps 5 through 8 above.
   c. Report the reciprocal of the greatest spinal fluid dilution that produces a reactive result.
10. Record the results as required.

REPORTING. Report nonreactive spinal fluids as "non-reactive".

Report reactive or weakly reactive spinal fluids corresponding with the titer; e.g., CSF VDRL: Reactive, titer 2.

INTERPRETATION OF RESULTS. Reactive VDRL tests on cerebral spinal fluid are virtually diagnostic of neurosyphilis; false positives are extremely rare.[1,2]

REFERENCES

1. Brown, W.J. et al.: *Syphilis and Other Venereal Diseases.* :Cambridge, Harvard University Press, 1970.
2. Jaffe, H.W.: Ann. Intern. Med., *83:*846, 1975.
3. U.S. Department of Health, Education and Welfare: *Manual of Tests for Syphilis.* Public Health Service Publication #411, Washington, D.C., 1969.

RPR Card Test[1]: Serologic Detection of Syphilis

PRINCIPLE. In the Rapid Plasma Reagin (RPR) test, the RPR card antigen suspension is a carbon particle containing cardiolipin antigen that reacts with "reagin", an antibody present in sera or plasma from many syphilitic persons, and occasionally in sera or plasma of persons with other acute or chronic conditions. When a specimen contains this antibody, flocculation occurs as a coagglutination of the carbon particles of the RPR card antigen, which appear as macroscopic black clumps against the white background of the plastic-coated card. By contrast, nonreactive specimens appear to have an even light-gray color.

EQUIPMENT AND MATERIALS

1. Macro-Vue RPR card test (BBL Microbiological Systems) containing:

   a. Antigen suspension: 0.003% cardiolipin, 0.020–0.022% lecithin, 0.09% cholesterol, 0.0125 M EDTA, 0.01 M Na_2HPO_4, 0.01 M KH_2PO_4, 0.1% thimerosal (preservative), 0.01875% charcoal, 10% choline chloride, w/v, and distilled water.

   b. Brewer diagnostic cards: Designed for use with the RPR card antigen, these are specially prepared, plastic-coated cards. In handling, care should be taken not to finger-mark the test areas on the card, as this may result in an oily deposit and improper test results. When spreading specimen within confines of test areas, avoid scratching the card with the dispenstir or stirrer. If the specimen does not spread to the outer perimeter of test area, use another test area of card.

   c. Dispenstirs and capillaries: In performing the card tests, a dispenstirs device (18 mm circle qualitative test only) or capillary may be used to transfer the specimen to the card surface. A new dispenstirs device or capillary must be used for each test specimen. When transferring from the collecting tube, the specimen must not be drawn up into the rubber bulb attached to the capillary, as this will cause incorrect readings on subsequent tests.

d. Needles: In order to maintain clear passage of the needle for accurate drop delivery, needle should be removed from the *dispensing bottle* upon completion of the tests and rinsed with distilled or deionized water. Do not wipe the needle because this will remove the silicone coating and may affect the accuracy of the drop of antigen being dispensed.

2. Controls (Fisher): A known titered reactive serum and a weakly reactive serum prepared from pooled sera of rabbits immunized with floccules of VDRL antigen; diluted with stabilized bovine albumin standardized using CDC VDRL antigens. Nonreactive control serum is prepared from pooled human serum tested to be VDRL nonreactive. Store at 4° C. May be used until date noted on the label. *Do Not Freeze.*

3. A rotator, 100 rpm, circumscribing a circle 2 cm in diameter, with automatic timer, friction drive, and a cover containing a moistened sponge or blotter.

4. Saline solution (0.9%).

5. Serum nonreactive to syphilis diluted 1:50 in 0.9% saline solution is required for diluting test specimens giving a reactive result at the 1:16 dilution.

SPECIMEN COLLECTION AND PREPARATION. To test unheated serum: Collect blood by venipuncture into a clean, dry tube without anticoagulant and allow to clot. Centrifuge the specimen at a force sufficient to sediment cellular elements and use the supernate for testing. Keep the serum in the original collecting tube.

To test plasma: Collect blood by venipuncture into a tube containing EDTA as an anticoagulant. Keep the plasma in the original collecting tube. May be stored at 2 to 8° C. Test the specimen within 24 hours of blood collection. Prior to testing, centrifuge the specimen at a force sufficient to sediment cellular elements and use the supernate for testing.

STORAGE INSTRUCTIONS. Refrigerate the RPR card antigen suspension at 2 to 8° C (35 to 45° F). All other components of the kit should be stored in a dry place at room temperature in the original kit packaging. Under refrigeration the shelf life of the antigen in the unopened ampule is 12 months from the date of manufacture.

Once the antigen has been placed in the dispensing bottle (provided in each kit) and refrigerated (2 to 8° C), the reactivity remains satisfactory for approximately three months, or until the expiration date, if it occurs sooner.

Label the dispensing bottle with the antigen lot number, expiration date, and date antigen was placed in the bottle.

PREPARATION OF REAGENTS. Preliminary preparations: When tests are to be performed, the antigen suspension should be checked with controls of graded reactivity using the particular test procedure. Only those suspensions which give the prescribed reactions should be used. Controls, RPR card antigen suspension and test specimens should be at room temperature (23 to 29° C) when used.

Prior to opening, a vigorous shaking of the ampule for 10 to 15 seconds will resuspend the antigen and dispense any carbon particles that may have become lodged in the neck of the ampule. If any carbon should remain in the neck of the ampule after this shaking, no additional effort should be made to dislodge it as this will only tend to produce a coarse antigen.

Check delivery of the needle by placing the needle firmly on a 1 mL pipet; fill the pipet with antigen suspension, and holding the pipet in a vertical position, count the number of drops delivered in 0.5 mL. The correct number of drops is given in the table that follows:

Test Method	Color of Needle Hub	Number of drops in 0.5 mL
18 mm Circle	Yellow, 20 G	30 ± 1 drop

Attach the needle to the tapered fitting on the plastic dispensing bottle. Assuring that all the antigen is below the breakline, snap the ampule neck and withdraw all of the antigen into the dispensing bottle by collapsing the bottle and using it as a suction device. Shake the card antigen dispensing bottle gently before each series of antigen droppings.

The needle and dispensing bottle should be discarded with the kit.

It is imperative that the techniques as described herein be followed in detail.

PROCEDURE

18 MM QUALITATIVE CARD TEST USING DISPENSTIRS:

1. Hold a dispenstirs device between thumb and forefinger near the stirring or sealed end. Squeeze and maintain pressure until open end is below surface of specimen, holding the specimen tube vertically to minimize stirring up of cellular elements when using original blood tube. Release finger pressure to draw up the sample.

2. Holding in a vertical position directly over the appropriate card test area (not touching card surface), squeeze dispenstirs device allowing one drop to fall onto card (approximately 0.05 mL; each dispenstirs device is designed to expel slightly in excess of 0.05 mL to compensate for small amount of specimen retained by stirring end). (If desired, sample remaining may be discharged into specimen tube from which it was drawn.)

3. Invert dispenstirs device and, with sealed stirring end, spread the specimen filling entire surface of circle. Discard dispenstirs device. Repeat procedure for number of specimens and controls to be tested.

4. Gently shake the antigen dispensing bottle before use. Holding in vertical position, dispense several drops in dispensing bottle cap to make sure the needle passage is clear. Then place one "free falling" drop (20 G, yellow hub needle) onto each test area. Do not restir; mixing of antigen suspension and specimen is accomplished during rotation. Pick up the predropped antigen from bottle cap.

5. Rotate for 8 minutes, under humidifying cover, on mechanical rotator at 100 rpm (95 to 110 rpm is acceptable). Following rotation, to help differentiate nonreactive from minimally reactive results, a brief rotating and tilting of the card by hand (three or four to-and-fro motions) must be made. Then immediately read macroscopically in the "wet" state under a high intensity incandescent lamp or strong daylight.

18 MM QUALITATIVE CARD TEST USING CAPILLARIES:

1. Using a new capillary, attach rubber bulb to capillary and remove 0.05 mL of specimen from blood collecting tube by allowing specimen to rise to measuring line on capillary, taking care not to transfer cellular elements. (If desired, a serologic pipette may be used.)

2. Place measured specimen onto circle of brewer diagnostic card, by compressing rubber bulb, while holding one finger over the hole in the bulb.

3. Using a new stirrer (broad end) for each specimen, spread to fill entire circle. Discard stirrer. Repeat procedure for number of specimens to be tested.

4. Gently shake antigen dispensing bottle before use. Holding in vertical position, dispense several drops in dispensing bottle cap to make sure the needle passage is clear. Then place one "free falling" drop (20G, yellow hub needle) onto each test area. Do not restir; mixing of antigen suspension and specimen is accomplished during rotation. Pick up the predropped antigen from bottle cap.

5. Rotate for 8 minutes under humidifying cover, on mechanical rotator at 100 rpm.

Following rotation, to help differentiate nonreactive from minimally reactive results, a brief rotation and tilting of the card by hand (three or four to-and-fro motions) must be made. Then immediately read macroscopically in the "wet" state under a high intensity incandescent lamp or strong daylight.

REPORTING. Report as: Reactive—showing characteristic clumping ranging from slight but definite (minimal-to-moderate) to marked and intense. Nonreactive—showing slight roughness or no clumping.

Note: There are only two possible reports with the card test; reactive or nonreactive, regardless of the degree of reactivity. Reactivity minimal-to-moderate (showing slight, but definite clumping) is always reported as reactive.

All reactive results should be confirmed by retesting the specimen using the quantitative procedure.

18 MM CIRCLE QUANTITATIVE CARD TEST:

1. For each specimen to be tested, place 0.05 mL of 0.9% saline solution onto circles numbered 2 to 5. A capillary (red line), or serologic pipette, 1 mL or less, may be used. *DO NOT SPREAD SALINE!*

2. Using a capillary (red line graduated at 0.05 mL, to the tip) with the rubber bulb attached, place 0.05 mL of specimen onto circle 1.

3. Refill capillary to red line with test specimen, and holding in a vertical position, deliver specimen onto circle 2. Draw mixture in and out of capillary 5 to 6 times to mix. Avoid formation of bubbles. Prepare serial twofold dilutions by mixing and transferring 0.05 mL from circle 2, to 3, to 4, to 5. Discard 0.05 mL after mixing contents in circle 5.

4. Using a new stirrer (broad end) for each specimen, start at highest dilution of serum (circle 5) and spread serum, following the entire surface of circle. Proceed to circles 4, 3, 2, and 1, and accomplish similar spreading.

5. Gently shake antigen dispensing bottle before use. Holding in vertical position, dispense several drops in dispensing bottle cap to make sure needle passage is clear. Then place one "free falling" drop onto each test area. Do not restir; mixing of antigen suspension and specimen is accomplished during rotation. Pick up the pre-dropped antigen from bottle cap.

6. Rotate for 8 minutes, under humidifying cover, on mechanical rotator at 100 rpm.

7. Following rotation, to help differentiate nonreactive from reactive minimal-to-moderate (Rm) results, a brief rotating and tilting of the card by hand (3 or 4 to-and-fro motions) must be made. Then immediately read macroscopically in the "wet" state under a high intensity incandescent lamp or strong daylight.

Unheated Serum: If the highest dilution tested (1:16) is still reactive, proceed as follows:

1. Prepare a 1:50 dilution of nonreactive serum in 0.9% saline solution. (This is to be used for making 1:32 and higher dilutions of specimens to be quantitated.)

2. Prepare a 1:16 dilution of the test specimen by adding 0.1 mL of serum to 1.5 mL of 0.9% saline solution. Mix thoroughly.

3. Place 0.05 mL of 1:50 nonreactive serum in circles 2, 3, 4 and 5.

4. Using capillary, place 0.05 mL of 1:16 dilution of test specimen in circle 1.

5. Refill capillary, make serial twofold dilutions and complete tests as described under steps 3 to 6.

Higher dilutions are prepared if necessary in 1:50 nonreactive serum.

REPORTING. Report the highest dilution giving a reactive, including those that are minimal-to-moderate reactive.

Examples:

(Und.) 1:1	1:2	1:4	1:8	1:16	Report
RM	N	N	N	N	Reactive, 1:1 dilution
R	R	R	N	N	Reactive, 1:4 dilution
R	R	R	R	N	Reactive, 1:8 dilution

LIMITATIONS OF THE PROCEDURE. The diagnosis of syphilis should not be made on a single reactive result without the support of a positive history or clinical evidence. Therefore, as with any serologic testing procedure, reactive card test specimens should be subjected to further serologic study. Serum specimens that are reactive in qualitative testing should be quantitated to establish a baseline from which changes in titer can be determined, particularly for evaluating treatment. It is also desirable to quantitate specimens that are nonreactive-rough so that an infrequent prozonal specimen may be revealed.

The RPR card tests should *not* be used for testing spinal fluids.

The Public Health Service has indicated that little reliance may be placed on a cord blood serologic test for syphilis.

Lipemia will not interfere with the card tests; however, if the degree of lipemia is so severe as to obscure the state of the antigen particles, the specimen should be considered unsatisfactory for testing.

The same criterion for testing hemolyzed samples should be used for the card tests as recommended in the Manual of Tests for Syphilis, which states, "a specimen is too hemolyzed for testing when printed matter cannot be read through it."[2]

REFERENCES

1. Insert, Macro-Vue RPR Card Test BBL Microbiology Systems, Cockeysville, MD, 1986.

2. U.S. Department of Health, Education and Welfare: *Manual of Tests for Syphilis.* Public Health Service Publication #411, Washington, D.C., 1969.

FTA-ABS (Fluorescent Treponemal Antibody Absorption Test)[1]

PRINCIPLE. The FTA-ABS is an indirect fluorescent antibody test system to aid in the confirmatory diagnosis of syphilis.

The FTA-ABS is based on the indirect fluorescent antibody procedure. Patient samples are diluted in sorbent to remove nonspecific antibodies, and the dilutions are then incubated on slides fixed with *Treponema pallidum* antigen. If specific antibodies are present in the patient's serum, stable antigen-antibody complexes are formed. The formed complexes bind fluorescein labeled antihuman gamma globulin. The resultant positive reaction is observed as apple-green fluorescence of the *T. pallidum* organisms when examined under a fluorescent microscope.

EQUIPMENT AND MATERIALS

1. FTA-ABS Fluoro-kit II (UTC) (Clinical Sciences, Inc.):

a. Substrate Slides: Each well of these slides contains fixed *Treponema pallidum* (Nichols strain) spirochetes 5 wells per slide. When stored frozen, $-20°$ C or below, these slides are stable until the labeled expiration date. Do not handle the flat surface of the slide or the envelope.

b. Fluorescent Antibody Conjugate: Lyophilized antihuman gamma globulin conjugated with fluorescein isothiocyanate (FITC). Thimerosal, 0.01% W/V, is added as a preservative. Conjugate must be titered with respect to standard controls as indicated under PROCEDURE: Titration of the conjugate. Reconstitute the conjugate with deionized water as directed by the vial label. Following reconstitution and titer verification, dilute the conjugate 1:10 with FTA PBS. Freeze 0.5 ml or greater aliquots in tightly stoppered tubes and store at $-20°$ C or below in the dark. The lyophilized conjugate is stable before reconstitution until the labeled expiration date when stored at 2 to 8° C in the dark. Frozen aliquots of diluted conjugate are stable for 90 days.

c. Conjugate Diluent: Contains 2% Tween 80 in PBS. The conjugate diluent is stable until the labeled expiration date when stored at 2 to 8° C.

d. Reactive Control Serum: Lyophilized human serum containing *T. pallidum* specific antibodies. Thimerosal, 0.01% W/V, is added as a preservative. Reconstitute with deionized water as directed by the vial label. After reconstitution, aliquot for single use and store at $-20°$ C or below. The lyophilized control serum is stable until the labeled expiration date when stored at 2 to 8° C. Frozen aliquots are stable for 90 days.

e. Nonspecific Control Serum: Lyophilized human serum from nonspecific donors. Thimerosal, 0.01% W/V, is added as a preservative. Reconstitute with deionized water as directed by the vial label. After reconstruction, aliquot for single use and store at $-20°$ C or below.

The lyophilized control serum is stable until the labeled expiration date when stored at 2 to 8° C. Frozen aliquots are stable for 90 days.

f. Sorbent: **The liquid sorbent prepared from cultures of Reiter treponemas is at optimum concentration and should not be diluted.** Thimerosal is added as a preservative. A black to grayish-white precipitate may form on standing and a small amount is acceptable. The liquid sorbent is stable until the expiration date stated on the label when stored at 2 to 8° C and sterility of the reagent is maintained. Use sterile pipettes for sorbent withdrawal.

g. PBS: Each unit contains dry powder phosphate buffered saline blend (pH 7.2 ± 0.2). Dissolve contents in deionized water as directed by the label and store at 2 to 8° C.

h. Mounting Medium: Ready to use. Contains phosphate buffered glycerol (pH 8.4 ± 0.2). Thimerosal is added as a preservative.

2. 36 to 37° C Incubator.

3. Test tubes (12 × 75 mm or comparable) and rack.

4. Pasteur and sterile pipettes.

5. Staining dish. For four slides or less, a Coplin jar will suffice; for more than four slides, use a 200-ml histologic staining dish.

6. Moist chamber. Large plastic petri dishes (bottom lined with moist paper towel) are satisfactory.

7. Volumetric flask for PBS.

8. Distilled or deionized water.

9. Forceps.

10. Properly equipped and aligned fluorescent microscope.

11. Coverslips, precleaned glass (24 × 60 mm = 1 thickness).

12. Squirt bottle.

13. 56° C ± 2° C water bath.

PRECAUTIONS

1. Do not interchange components from other sources.

2. Repeated freezing and thawing of reagent aliquots should be avoided.

SPECIMEN COLLECTION AND PREPARATION. Patient Sample: Serum specimens may be stored at 2 to 8° C if tested within 24 to 48 hours, otherwise they should be stored frozen at −20° C or below. Do not freeze and thaw sera more than once. Allow serum specimens to reach room temperature before testing. Avoid the use of sera exhibiting a high degree of lipemia, hemolysis, or microbial growth, because these characteristics may result in increased background staining/fluorescence, decrease in titers and/or unclear staining patterns.

PROCEDURE

A. Titration of Conjugate

The FTA-ABS conjugate is labeled with a working titer dilution that has been determined to give appropriate reactivity for each of the FTA-ABS control sera and the PBS nonspecific staining control. The following protocol and example of a conjugate titration is suggested to CONFIRM the titer in your laboratory with your microscope system:

1. Reconstitute the conjugate with deionized water according to the label instructions on the conjugate vial.

2. Serially dilute a 0.2-ml aliquot of the conjugate, using 2-fold dilutions in conjugate diluent, and diluting from full strength to at least three dilutions past the labeled titer on the conjugate vial.

EXAMPLE: Conjugate labeled with a titer of 1:1600. Set up test tube rack with 9 test tubes numbered 1 through 9, tube 1 containing 2.45 ml of conjugate diluent and tubes 2 through 9 containing 0.2 ml of conjugate diluent. Add 0.05 ml of reconstituted conjugate to tube 1 to make a 1:50 dilution. Mix well with a vortex mixer. Remove 0.2 ml of diluted conjugate from tube 1 and add to tube 2. Mix well, and continue serially transferring 0.2 ml through tube 9. When the series is completed, the dilutions prepared are as follows:

Tube 1 = 1:50	Tube 5 = 1:800
Tube 2 = 1:100	Tube 6 = 1:1600
Tube 3 = 1:200	Tube 7 = 1:3200
Tube 4 = 1:400	Tube 8 = 1:6400
	Tube 9 = 1:12800

3. Test each dilution of the conjugate against the following controls:

(a) PBS (nonspecific staining control).

(b) Reactive control at 1:5 in PBS (4+ control).

(c) Reactive control diluted according to

label instructions to give minimally reactive (1+ control).

4. Follow the technique instructions as outlined in the performance of FTA-ABS test section.

The working titer of the conjugate is defined as one doubling dilution less than the endpoint titer (the last conjugate dilution to give maximum (4+) fluorescence). At the working titer, the conjugate should not stain nonspecifically at three doubling dilutions below the chosen working titer, and it should give an acceptable 1+ reaction with the reactive control diluted to the minimally reactive reading standard.

The conjugate should be used at the determined titer value rather than the labeled stated value if it differs from the labeled value. When the working titer has been established, dilute the balance of the one reconstituted vial 1:10 with FTA PBS. Aliquot the diluted conjugate into 0.5 ml aliquots in labeled tubes or vials. Seal the containers and freeze immediately at −20 to −40° C. When thawing conjugate for use in this test, thaw only enough for one day's testing. Discard any unused, thawed conjugate.

B. PERFORMANCE OF FTA-ABS TEST

1. *IMPORTANT:* Heat inactivate all sera (controls and test samples) at 56° C ± 2° C for 30 minutes. Reheat previously heated sera at 56° C ± 2° C for 10 minutes on the day of testing.

2. Prepare the following control dilutions for each test run from the heat inactivated sera:

   (a) Reactive-PBS: Dilute 0.05 ml of Reactive Control in 0.2 ml PBS. Mix well.

   (b) Reactive-Sorbent: Dilute 0.05 ml of Reactive Control in 0.2 ml Sorbent. Mix well.

   (c) Nonspecific-PBS: Dilute 0.05 ml of Nonspecific Control in 0.2 ml PBS. Mix well.

   (d) Nonspecific-Sorbent: Dilute 0.05 ml of Nonspecific Control in 0.2 ml Sorbent. Mix well.

   (e) Minimally Reactive (1+) Control: The Reactive Control Serum, as reconstituted according to the vial label, is used for this control. Dilute in PBS according to the titer on the vial label. This dilution of reactive whole serum demonstrates the minimal degree of fluorescence reported as "reactive" (1+) and is used as a reading standard. Discard at the end of each run. Minimally Reactive Control should be made up fresh for each day's testing.

3. Dilute each test sample 1:5 in Sorbent. Mix well.

4. Conjugate Preparation: Remove sufficient conjugate from frozen storage for 1 day's

use and allow to equilibrate to room temperature (about 15 to 30 minutes). After equilibration, make the appropriate working titer dilution with conjugate diluent as determined in the confirmation of titer dilution procedure, taking into account the initial 1:10 dilution previously prepared.

5. Remove sufficient slides from frozen storage and allow them to equilibrate to room temperature (about 15 to 30 minutes). After equilibration, remove from foil pack and use within 1 hour.

6. Apply 0.01 ml of the following controls to individual wells on at least one slide for each test run:

   (a) Reactive control diluted 1:5 in PBS

   (b) Reactive control diluted 1:5 in sorbent

   (c) Nonspecific control diluted 1:5 in PBS

   (d) Nonspecific control diluted 1:5 in sorbent

   (e) Minimally reactive control

   (f) PBS as reconstituted

   (g) Sorbent as supplied

7. Apply 0.01 ml of test samples diluted 1:5 in sorbent to the appropriate wells of the slides.

8. Incubate the slides in a covered moist chamber at 35 to 37° C for 30 minutes.

9. Remove the slides from the moist chamber and rinse gently with deionized water using a squirt bottle. To avoid sample cross-contamination in double row slides, do not allow the rinse water to run into adjacent wells. The following technique is suggested: Direct the stream of water along the horizontal midline of the slide tilting first towards the upper row of wells followed by tilting toward the bottom row of wells.

10. Place slides into a Coplin jar or histologic staining dish filled with PBS for 5 minutes. Agitate gently.

11. Repeat step 10 using fresh PBS.

12. Rinse slides gently with deionized water for about 5 seconds. Allow slides to air dry. DO NOT BLOT.

13. Dispense 0.01 ml of the reconstituted, appropriately diluted conjugate to each well on the slide.

14. Incubate the slides in a covered moist chamber at 37° C ± 2° C for 30 minutes.

15. Remove slides from the moist chamber and rinse gently with deionized water, following procedure in step 9.

16. Place slides into a Coplin jar or histologic staining dish filled with PBS for 5 minutes. Agitate gently.

17. Repeat step 16 using fresh PBS.

18. Rinse slides gently with distilled water

for about 5 seconds. Tap off excess liquid from slide wells.

19. Apply 5 small drops of mounting medium on the mask surface between the two rows of specimen wells. Gently apply coverslip without pressure.

20. Keep slides in the dark and examine slides as soon as possible using a fluorescent microscope.

REPORTING. The controls must be examined before patient samples are read. The control results must be in the following pattern to validate procedural results. Control test results that do not give these reactions are considered unsatisfactory and patient results should not be reported. Repeat test procedure.

Control Pattern Illustration	Reaction
Reactive Control:	
a. 1:5 PBS dilution	Reactive 4+
b. 1:5 Sorbent dilution	Reactive (4+ to 3+)
Minimally Reactive (1+) Control	Reactive 1+
Nonspecific Control:	
a. 1:5 PBS dilution	Reactive (2+ to 4+)
b. 1:5 Sorbent dilution	Nonreactive
Nonspecific Serum Controls:	
a. Antigen, PBS, and Conjugate	Nonreactive
b. Antigen, Sorbent, and Congugate	Nonreactive

Using the Minimally Reactive (1+) control slide as the reading standard, record the intensity of fluorescence of the treponemas used for patient tests according to the description below.

Reading	Intensity of Fluorescence
2+ to 4+	Moderate to Strong
1+	Equivalent to Minimally Reactive (1+) Control*
± to <1+	Visible staining but less than (1+)
—	None or vaguely visible, but without distinct fluorescence

* Retest all specimens with the intensity of fluorescence of (1+).

Report patient results as follows:

Initial Test Reading	Repeat Test Reading	Report
4+, 3+, 2+		Reactive
1+	>1+	Reactive
	1+	Reactive Minimal*
	<1+	Nonreactive
<1+		Nonreactive
N− ±		Nonreactive

* In the absence of historic or clinical evidence of treponemal infection, this test result should be considered equivocal. A second specimen should be submitted for serologic testing.

INTERPRETATION OF RESULTS. The expected values in uninfected individuals are nonreactive results. Borderline results are inconclusive and cannot be interpreted as evidence of syphilis. Repeat FTA-ABS testing is recommended on all patients with borderline results.

LIMITATIONS OF THE PROCEDURE:[2]

1. The limitations of the FTA-ABS test are summarized by the following current CDC recommendations:

FTA-ABS test has never been and is not now being recommended as a routine screening test for syphilis. Its recommended uses are:

a. to confirm the reactive results of a sensitive but less specific, screening test for syphilis, such as the VDRL, or,

b. as a specific diagnostic test in patients with signs or symptoms suggestive of late syphilis.

2. Even though the FTA-ABS test is considered the most acceptable fluorescent antibody test for confirming syphilis, it is still capable of producing an occasional biological false-positive (BFP) reaction with certain conditions and/or pathologies, for example:

—Pregnancy

—Neonatal congenital syphilis

—Lupus erythematosus—*NOTE:* There seems to be some correlation between the active disease and an observable "beaded" type of fluorescence of the *Treponema pallidum.*

—Leprosy

3. Even though the FTA-ABS test has been demonstrated to be highly sensitive and specific, no absolute diagnosis should be made solely on this test or any other single laboratory procedure. The management of syphilis-suspect patients must depend on the total evaluation of each case.

4. The FTA-ABS test is not useful as an indicator of disease state, nor can it be used to assess the effects of treatment, as it remains reactive regardless of therapy.

5. The FTA-ABS test does not differentiate syphilis from the other treponematoses: pinta, yaws, or bejel.

REFERENCES

1. Insert, FTA-ABS Fluoro-Kit II, Clinical Sciences, Inc., Wippany, N.J. 1985.

2. U.S. Department of Health Education and Welfare: *Manual of Tests for Syphilis.* Public Health Service Publication #411, Washington, D.C., 1969.

Qualitative Microhemagglutination Test for Antibody to Treponema Pallidum[5]

PRINCIPLE. The Microhemagglutination *Treponema pallidum* antibody (MHA-TP) test is based on the agglutination of sensitized sheep erythrocytes by antibodies to *T. pallidum.* Prior to performing the test, the serum sample is mixed with absorbing diluent to remove most nonspecific reactants. Serum containing the specific antibody will react with the sensitized sheep cells, which are coated with *T. pallidum* antigen, to form a smooth mat of agglutinated cells in the well of the microtitration tray. Negative reactions are characterized by a compact button formed by the settling of nonagglutinated cells.

EQUIPMENT AND MATERIALS

1. SERA-TEK Treponemal Antibody Test Kit (Ames Division, Miles Laboratories):

a. Absorbing Diluent: Phosphate buffered saline solution (pH 7.2) containing soluble components of sonicated sheep red cell membranes (0.50% v/v), soluble components of sonicated bovine red cell membranes (0.25% v/v), normal rabbit testicular extract (0.1% w/w), cell components of sonicated Reiter treponeme (0.125% w/w), normal rabbit serum (1.0% v/v), and stabilizers.

b. Sensitized Cells: Lyophilized, formalinized tanned sheep erythrocytes sensitized with *T. pallidum* (Nichols strain) antigen. The rehydrated antigen is a 2.5% suspension of these cells.

c. Unsensitized Cells: Lyophilized, formalinized tanned sheep erythrocytes. The rehydrated reagent is a 2.5% suspension of these cells.

d. Reactive Control: Lyophilized human and/or rabbit serum containing antibodies to *T. pallidum*. The specific serum source is indicated on the carton.

e. Nonreactive Control: Lyophilized normal human serum.

f. Rehydrating Water: Autoclaved distilled water.

2. Microdiluters, 0.025 mL (25 μL)

3. Pipette droppers calibrated to deliver 0.025 mL (25 μL)

4. Go/No-Go delivery tester (blotter) (Dynatech Laboratories, Inc.), 0.025 mL (25 μL)

5. Disposable, clear plastic microtitration trays with roundbottom (U-shaped) cups. Trays should be free from dust and lint

6. Tray viewer

7. Pipettes

a. 20-, 25- and 50-μL automatic pipettes or 0.1-mL serologic pipettes graduated in 1/1000 mL

b. 1.0-mL serologic pipettes graduated in 1/100 mL

8. Test tubes and rack

9. Sterile distilled water

10. 0.85% saline solution

11. Bunsen burner

SPECIMEN COLLECTION AND PREPARATION. The specimen for this test must be free from particulate matter. Specimens containing particulate matter should be centrifuged prior to testing. Store sera in refrigerator at 2 to 8° C. Sera may be frozen once. Although the test is designed to use unheated serum, specimens which have been previously heated at 56° C for 30 minutes may be used.[9]

1. Set up and label one test tube for each serum to be tested and for each of the two controls.

2. Pipette 0.38 mL of Absorbing Diluent into each test tube.

3. Add 0.02 mL (20 μL) of test serum or control to labeled tubes to give a 1:20 dilution in the Absorbing Diluent.

4. Using the 20-μL pipettes, mix each diluted serum eight times. Incubate at room temperature for 30 minutes.

The absorbed 1:20 dilutions of test and control sera are now ready for testing. Quantities of absorbed sera left after withdrawal of test amounts may be stored at 2 to 8° C and retested on the same day. Absorbed sera should be at room temperature when tested.

PREPARATION OF REAGENTS. For optimal kit performance, do not interchange kit components with differing kit control numbers. Lyophilized reagents must be reconstituted with the Rehydrating Water supplied in the kit. Mix reconstituted reagents thoroughly before use to insure homogeneous suspensions or solutions. Ampules do not need to be scored prior to opening.

1. Absorbing Diluent: This reagent is ready for use and requires no reconstitution.

2. Sensitized Cells: Reconstitute each 4 × 25 test kit vial with 0.8 mL of Rehydrating Water. Reconstitute the 100 test kit vial with 2.5 mL of Rehydrating Water. Allow suspension to stand at least 1 hour prior to use.

3. Unsensitized Cells: Reconstitute each 4 × 25 test kit vial with 0.5 mL of Rehydrating Water. Reconstitute the 100 test kit vial with 1.5 mL of Rehydrating Water. Allow suspension to stand at least 1 hour prior to use.

4. Reactive Control Serum: Reconstitute with 0.5 mL of Rehydrating Water. Allow solution to stand at least 1 hour prior to use.

5. Non-Reactive Control Serum: Reconstitute with 0.5 mL of Rehydrating Water. Allow solution to stand at least 1 hour prior to use.

WORKING DILUTIONS. Prepare working dilutions of sensitized and unsensitized cells by adding one part rehydrated cell suspension to 5.5 parts absorbing diluent. Prepare only enough reagents for 1 day's testing.

Volumes of Reagents Needed: The following amounts of reagents are needed for each unknown or control to be tested:
Absorbing diluent................. 0.38 mL
Working dilution of sensitized
cells .... 0.075 mL

Working dilution of unsensitized cells .... 0.075 mL

Reactive control serum for each group of unknowns .... 0.020 mL

Nonreactive control serum for each group of unknowns .... 0.020 mL

ALL REAGENTS MUST BE AT ROOM TEMPERATURE WHEN USED.

To calculate the amount of rehydrated cell suspension needed, use the formula above (see top right column):

$$C = \frac{A \times B}{6.5}$$

Where

A = total number of tests to be run (including controls)

B = volume of working dilution per test

C = volume of rehydrated cell suspension

6.5 = total number of parts (volume) in preparing working dilution of cells (1.0 cells + 5.5 working dilution)

EXAMPLE: If running 10 tests per day:

$$C = \frac{10 \text{ tests} \times 0.075 \text{ mL Working Dilution of Sensitized Cells}}{6.5} = 0.12 \text{ mL} \begin{pmatrix} \text{Rehydrated} \\ \text{Cell} \\ \text{Suspension} \end{pmatrix}$$

0.12 mL Rehydrated Cell Suspension $\times$ 5.5 = 0.66 mL Absorbing Diluent

0.12 mL Rehydrated Cell Suspension
+ = 0.78 mL Working Dilution of Cells
0.66 mL Absorbing Diluent

Unused working dilutions of reagents must be discarded at the end of the day. This excess should be kept to a minimum to ensure that there will be sufficient reagents to run the number of tests specified by the kit.

STORAGE INSTRUCTIONS. All reagents should be stored in a refrigerator (2 to 8° C) and used prior to the expiration date. Once opened, the absorbing diluent should be stored at 2 to 8° C and used within 14 days. Reconstituted sensitized and unsensitized cells should be stored at 2 to 8° C and used within 5 days. Reconstituted control sera should be stored at 2 to 8° C and used within 5 days; alternatively, reconstituted Control Sera may be divided into aliquots of 0.1 mL or greater, frozen and stored up to 4 weeks. Working dilutions of sensitized and unsensitized cells should be stored at 2 to 8° C and used within 1 day. Reagents should be discarded if they become contaminated or do not demonstrate proper reactivity with the reactive and nonreactive controls.

PROCEDURE

1. Prepare microdiluters as follows:
   a. Clean the microdiluters by rotating in distilled water.
   b. Flame microdiluters to incandescence over a Bunsen burner; quench in distilled water to cool and blot to expel liquid.
   c. Fill each microdiluter by touching it to the surface of 0.85% saline solution. Do not wet canopy (top) of the loop.
   d. Touch the microdiluter to the marked center of one of the circles on the Go/No-Go delivery tester (blotter) and observe the dampened area within the circle.
   e. A properly prepared microdiluter will deliver all contained fluid which will be sufficient to immediately dampen the area within the circle. The solution from an improperly prepared microdiluter will not be sufficient to dampen the entire area within the circle.
2. The calibrated pipette dropper must be clean. To ensure proper delivery of fluid, gently blot excess solution from the outside of the pipette dropper with a cleansing tissue after filling. Hold the dropper in a vertical position when adding fluid to the tray cups.
3. Mark microtitration tray as shown in Figure 9-3. Thirteen wells will be required for controls. Each patient specimen will be tested in

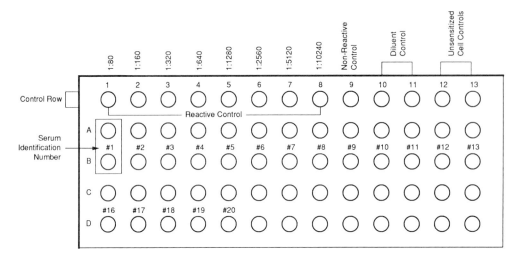

Fig. 9–3. MHA–TP microtiter plate.

duplicate. The top well will test for reactivity and the bottom well will check for nonspecific agglutination.

4. Set up control row as follows:

a. Place 0.025 mL absorbing diluent in wells 2 to 8, 10 and 11.

b. Place 0.05 mL absorbed reactive control serum (see SPECIMEN COLLECTION AND PREPARATION) in well 1 and 0.025 mL in well 12.

c. Prepare a serial dilution of the absorbed reactive control serum by placing a 0.025 mL microdiluter in well 1. Rotate for 4 seconds to fill microdiluter, remove and place in well 2 and rotate. Repeat this procedure through well 8. After mixing the contents of well 8, check the microdiluter's volume delivery on a blotter.

d. Place 0.025 mL absorbed nonreactive control serum (see SPECIMEN COLLECTION AND PREPARATION) in wells 9 and 13.

5. Place 0.025 mL of each absorbed test serum (1:20 dilution, see SPECIMEN COLLECTION AND PREPARATION) in their appropriately marked wells (Fig. 9–3).

6. Using a pipette dropper calibrated to 0.025 mL, dispense 0.075 mL working dilution of sensitized cells to wells 1 to 10 of the control row and to the top row of each specimen pair (Rows A, C, E, etc.).

7. Add 0.075 mL of the working dilution of unsensitized cells to wells 11 to 13 of the control row and to the bottom row of each specimen pair (rows B, D, F, etc.).

8. Shake all trays gently, stack and cover with an empty tray.

9. Incubate the trays, undisturbed, at 25° C ($\pm$ 5°) for at least 4 hours. The incubation period may be extended overnight with no appreciable change in pattern if assay is set up in the afternoon.

REPORTING. The reactive and nonreactive controls should be processed with each batch of tests. The reactive control serum should not vary more than plus or minus one dilution from the endpoint titer indicated on the control label, and should be nonreactive with unsensitized cells. The nonreactive control and absorbing diluent controls should be nonreactive with both sensitized and unsensitized cells.

A check of both cell suspensions should be done at the same time as the controls. Further quality control checks may be made by running characterized reactive and nonreactive sera or serum pools obtained from laboratory specimens or reference sera.

The qualitative and control titration results are obtained by reading the settling pattern of the red blood cells on the tray viewer. Readings are scored on a scale of − to 4+, using the criteria shown in the following table.

Degree of Hemagglutination	Reading	Interpretation
Smooth mat of cells covering entire bottom of cup, edges sometimes folded	4+	Reactive
Smooth mat of cells covering less area of cup	3+	Reactive
Smooth mat of cells surrounded by red circle	2+	Reactive
Smooth mat of cells surrounded by smaller red circle	1+	Reactive
Button of cells having small "hole" in center	±	Nonreactive
Definite compact button in center of cup or may have a very small "hole" in the center	−	Nonreactive

"Reactive" results are reported when a serum shows hemagglutination of 1+ or higher with the sensitized cells, and are nonreactive with the unsensitized cells.

"Nonreactive" results are reported for serum showing no hemagglutination (− or ±) with sensitized and unsensitized cells. Readings of ± may occur because of several technical factors; therefore, it is suggested that specimens giving ± readings should be retested. Repeat ± readings are reported as nonreactive.

If reactive results are seen with both sensitized and unsensitized cells, refer to section on LIMITATIONS OF PROCEDURE.

LIMITATIONS OF PROCEDURE. The SERA-TEK Treponemal Antibody Test (MHA-TP) compares favorably with the FTA-ABS in specificity, but it has been reported to be less sensitive in cases of untreated primary syphilis.[1-4,8] Treponemal tests are also recommended as diagnostic aids for patients with symptoms suggesting late syphilis regardless of reagin tests, since the reagin tests are less sensitive in such cases. Treponemal tests are not recommended for cerebrospinal fluid testing or as a screening test for syphilis.[9]

Sera from patients with infectious mononucleosis, leprosy, drug addiction, or autoimmune disease may occasionally react with the sensitized and/or unsensitized cells.[2,4,7] However, false-positive reactions because of high titer heterophile antibody can probably be resolved by determining if a serum's titer against sensitized cells is at least 4 times its titer against unsensitized control cells. When nonspecific agglutination occurs, the serum should be retested in doubling dilutions against sensitized and unsensitized cells.

1. Report "Reactive" without reference to titer if:

a. The hemagglutination titer with sensitized cells is at least 4 times that with unsensitized cells

and

b. The first dilution showing no hemagglutination with unsensitized cells has a 3+ or 4+ reaction with sensitized cells.

2. Report "inconclusive, nonspecific hemagglutination in serum control" if the hemagglutination titer with sensitized cells is no more than twice the titer with unsensitized cells.

REFERENCES

1. Coffey, E.M., Bradford, L.L., Naritomi, L.S., and Wood, R.M.: Appl. Microbiol., 24:26, 1972.
2. Cox, P.M., Logan, L.C., and Stout, G.W.: Public Health Laboratory, 29:43, 1971.
3. Dyckman, J., Storms, S., and Huber, T.: J. Clin. Microbiol., 12:629, 1980.
4. Garner, M.F., Backhouse, J.L., Daskalopoulos, G., and Walsh, J.L.: J. Clin. Pathol., 26:258, 1972.
5. Insert, Treponemal Antibody Test, Milers Inc., Elkhart, IN, 1988.
6. Jaffe, H.W., Larsen, S.A., Jones, O.G., and Dans, P.E.: Am. J. Clin. Pathol., 70:230, 1978.
7. Kaufman, R.E. et al.: Br. J. Vener. Dis., 50:350, 1974.
8. Shore, R.N.: Arch. Dermatol., 109:854, 1974.
9. U.S. Dept. of Health, Education and Welfare: Criteria and Techniques for the Diagnosis of Early Syphilis. Public Health Service, March, 1976.

B. Viral Disorders

CYTOMEGALOVIRUS INFECTION

Cytomegalovirus (CMV) is a ubiquitous virus that, depending on the population studied, has been shown to infect 50 to 100% of individuals worldwide during their lifetime.[9,39] A member of the herpes virus family, CMV consists of a double-stranded DNA genome surrounded by a protein capsid and a lipoprotein envelope. A single virion measures 180 nm in diameter and demonstrates icosahedral symmetry.[9,14,28]

CMV is highly species specific; the growth of human CMV in vitro is supported only in human cells. Fibroblasts are most effective in allowing viral replication to occur in vitro,[28,39] but growth has also been demonstrated in human endothelial cells[15] and epithelial cells[18] under special conditions. The cell types in which infection is established and maintained in vivo are uncertain, but may include epithelial cells, monocytes, and lymphocytes.[28,39] Entry of the virus into the host cell occurs through fusion of the viral envelope with the cell membrane or by phagocytosis. Interaction of CMV with its host cell may result in productive infection, latency, or oncogenic transformationn. In productive infection, the viral genome directs the replication of CMV within the host cell nucleus in a cascade-like sequence: synthesis of "immediate-early" proteins occurs first and is necessary for the synthesis of "early" proteins, which then permit DNA replication to occur; this, in turn, is followed by production of "late" proteins, which are the structural components of the virus.[9,39] The viral particles are assembled, acquire their envelope from the internal nuclear membrane and endoplasmic reticulum of the host cell,[37,41] cause lysis of the cell, and proceed to infect adjacent cells. During productive infection, a characteristic cytopathic effect (CPE)[28] becomes apparent, consisting of rounded, greatly enlarged cells (2 to 4 times normal size, hence the term, cytomegalovirus)[14] that increase in size and number over a period of several weeks. These cells often contain intranuclear inclusion bodies that bear an "owl's eye" appearance, as a result of their being eccentrically positioned and separated from the nuclear membrane by a clear halo; they are approximately 10 nm in size and stain red with hematoxylin and eosin. Occasionally, cytoplasmic inclusions may be observed. Electron microscope studies have shown that the inclusion bodies contain clusters of virions.[34,41]

Following primary infection, CMV is believed to establish a latent infection that persists for the lifetime of the host and may become reactivated in immunocompromised individuals. The site(s) of latency in humans are unknown, but epithelial cells of the salivary gland and renal tubules, skin, and lymphoid cells have all been proposed as potential candidates.[28,39]

Finally, human CMV has been shown to stimulate DNA and RNA synthesis in host cells in vitro[43] and cause in vitro transformation of human fibroblast cells, which may then exhibit malignant growth when transplanted into immunosuppressed mice.[28] The in vivo oncogenic potential of CMV in humans is unknown; reports have associated CMV infection with Kaposi's sarcoma[5] and carcinomas of the prostate, cervix, and colon,[16,23,35] but have not definitely established CMV as an etiologic agent or cofactor in these malignancies.

Transmission of CMV in nature is thought to occur orally, following close and prolonged contact with infected body secretions, sexually, by contact with infected genital secretions, and congenitally, from infected mother to fetus.[28] These modes of transmission have been supported by studies showing increased rates of seroconversion in breast-fed infants, children attending day care centers, institutionalized children, individuals of lower socioeconomic groups with poor hygiene practices, adolescents and young adults who are sexually active, and sexual contacts of infected individuals (reviewed in references 13, 28, 30). Transmission following blood transfusion or organ transplantation has also been documented.[28] Some reports indicate seroconversion in hospital employees following contact with CMV infected infants,[12,48] but medical personnel are thought not to be at significant risk as long as good personal hygiene is practiced.[1,13]

The majority of individuals who are immunologically competent will be asymptomatic after acquiring CMV infection. However, these individuals may serve as a major vector of transmisssion, as it has been estimated that at any one time, 1 to 2% of infected but asymptomatic adults are shedding CMV in their body secretions.[30]

In some previously healthy individuals, particularly young adults, a heterophile antibody-negative mononucleosis syndrome develops after CMV infection is acquired. This most frequently involves fever, myalgia, malaise, and/or headache; sore throat, splenomegaly, and lymphadenopathy occur less frequently.[14,28] Laboratory abnormalities usually include lymphocytosis, atypical lymphocytes (>10%), and abnormal liver function tests; cryoglobulins, cold agglutinins, rheumatoid factor, or antinuclear antibodies may also be present. Differential diagnosis should include testing for infection with several other viruses, particularly Epstein Barr virus (i.e. infectious mononucleosis), and for *Toxoplasma gondii*. Recovery usually occurs without complication after 6 weeks, but individuals with CMV mononucleosis continue to excrete the virus in urine, genital secretions, and saliva for months to years later.[14,28]

More serious consequences of CMV infection are observed in immunocompromised persons, most notably organ transplant recipients and patients with AIDS. CMV disease is the most frequent viral infection associated with organ transplantation, and may produce a variety of manifestations, ranging from the subclinical to the life-threatening. Symptoms include fever, malaise, myalgias, arthralgias, leukopenia, pneumonitis, hepatitis, colitis, and retinitis.[14,28] CMV has also been associated with an increased risk of superinfection with bacterial, fungal, or protozoal organisms,[26,32,46] and may contribute to decreased renal allograft function, presumably either by acting as a stimulus for graft rejection[20,25,38] or by causing an immune complex glomerulopathy.[33] The risk of CMV infection has been observed to correlate with the degree of immunosuppressive therapy the patient receives, with those receiving antilymphocyte serum having the greatest risk.[14,31] CMV infection can arise from either exposure of a CMV-seronegative recipient to an allograft from a CMV-positive donor, or from reactivation of CMV in an immunocompromised CMV-seropositive transplant recipient; clinical illness due to CMV infection, however, is more severe in the former situation.[14,47] The acquisition of donor strains of CMV by renal transplant recipients who were previously positive for a different strain of the virus has also been reported;[2,11] however, the clinical significance of this observation is unknown. Recent studies show promise of reducing the severity of CMV disease through administration of CMV-immune globulin[42] or new antiviral drugs.[6]

CMV has a high prevalence in male homosexual populations and is a common source of infection in AIDS patients.[36] Disseminated CMV infection has been well-documented in AIDS, and may involve chorioretinitis, pneumonia, hepatitis, colitis, or adrenal insufficiency.[4,36] CMV has also been implicated as a cofactor in Kaposi's sarcoma[5] and in the development of full-blown AIDS in HIV-infected individuals.[5,40]

Another group for which CMV may have serious consequences are those with congenital infection. CMV is the most common viral agent known to be transmitted congenitally, affecting 0.2 to 2.2% of live births worldwide.[44,45] In utero transmission of CMV occurs in about 30 to 40% of women who acquire primary CMV infection during pregnancy, and can also occur in those who are seropositive before the time of conception; however, congenital infections in the latter group are less likely to be clinically severe.[44] Consequences of CMV infection range from asymptomatic, in the majority of infants infected with the virus, to fulminant cytomegalic inclusion disease. The risk of severe clinical consequences to the neonate appears to be greatest when mothers acquire primary infection during the first half of gestation.[44,45] Up to 15% of congenitally-infected infants who appear well at birth may develop sequelae in the first few years of life, of which the most common is sensorineural hearing loss.[14,28,44] Mental retardation, chorioretinitis, and dental abnormalities may also develop in this group. Fulminant cytomegalic inclusion disease at birth is characterized most commonly by jaundice, petechiae, and hepatosplenomegaly; microcephaly and neuromuscular disorders are also frequently noted, and may result in irreversible mental and growth retardation and deafness in survivors.[13,14,28,45] The most frequent laboratory findings are increased serum IgM, atypical lymphocytosis, elevated hepatic transaminases, thrombocytopenia, hyperbilirubinemia, and increased cerebrospinal fluid protein.[14,28] Differential diagnosis includes toxoplasmosis, rubella, and herpes infections.

Laboratory diagnosis has traditionally involved culture of the virus from urine, saliva, or other body fluids, onto human foreskin or embryonic lung fibroblast cell lines.[14,28] The usefulness of this technique has been limited, however, as characteristic CPE generally take several days to several weeks to appear. In addition, shedding of the virus may continue long after recovery from active infection. Newer techniques for more rapid viral identification have been developed. Immunofluorescence methods employing monoclonal antibodies to the immediate early antigens of CMV have allowed detection of the virus to be accomplished 16 to 24 hours after inoculation of fibroblast lines with the clinical specimen.[3,8,19,28] Identification of the CMV genome in clinical specimens by hybridization with DNA probes has also been shown to be an effective technique for rapid viral detection.[14,21,28]

A number of serologic techniques to detect CMV antibody are available, and include complement fixation, immunofluorescence, indirect hemagglutination, latex agglutination, RIA, and ELISA.[10,14,22,28] Active CMV infection is indicated by at least a 4-fold rise in antibody titer, or the presence of IgM antibody.[28] Congenital infections are indicated by the presence of specific IgM or IgE antibodies.[28,29] In IgM-specific assays, false-positive reactions may result from the presence of rheumatoid factor, or false-negative reactions, from competition with IgG antibodies, but these may be avoided by preabsorption or fractionation of sera to remove IgG prior to testing[17] or through the use of IgM antibody capture ELISA techniques, whereby IgM in patient sera is attached to an anti-IgM antibody bound to a solid phase.[29] Active infection has also been associated with the presence of IgG antibodies to CMV early antigens,[19,24,27] while antibodies to CMV late antigens usually persist for the lifetime of the host, and are therefore unable to distinguish past from current infections.[28,29]

REFERENCES

1. Balfour, C.L., and Balfour, H.: JAMA, 256:1909, 1986.
2. Chou, S.: N. Engl. J. Med., 314:1418, 1986.
3. Chou, S., and Scott, K.M.: J. Clin. Microbiol., 26:504, 1988.
4. Collier, A.C. et al.: Am. J. Med., 82:593, 1987.
5. Drew, W.L.: Mt. Sinai J. Med., 53:622, 1986.
6. Erice, A. et al.: JAMA, 257:3082, 1987.
7. Geder, L. et al.: Science, 192:1134, 1976.
8. Gleaves, C.A. et al.: Am. J. Clin. Pathol., 88:354, 1987.
9. Griffiths, P.D., and Grundy, J.E.: Biochem. J., 241:313, 1987.
10. Grint, P.C.A. et al.: J. Clin. Pathol., 38:1059, 1985.

11. Grundy, J.E. et al.: Transplant. Proc., *19*:2126, 1987.

12. Haneberg, B., Bertnes, E., and Haukenes, G.: Acta Paediatr. Scand., *69*:407, 1980.

13. Hanshaw, J.B.: In *Infectious Diseases of the Fetus and Newborn Infant.* Edited by J.S. Remington and J.O. Klein. Philadelphia, W.B. Saunders Co., 1983.

14. Hirsch, M.S.: In *Harrison's Principles of Internal Medicine*, 11th ed. Edited by E. Braunwald, K.J. Isselbacher, R.G. Petersdorf, J.D. Wilson, J.B. Martin, and A.S. Fauci. New York, McGraw-Hill Book Co., 1987.

15. Ho, D.D. et al.: J. Infect. Dis., *150*:956, 1984.

16. Huang, E.S., and Roche, J.K.: Lancet, *1*:957, 1978.

17. Joassin, L., and Reginster, M.: J. Clin. Microbiol., *23*:576, 1986.

18. Knowles, W.A.: Arch. Virol., *50*:119, 1976.

19. Lentz, E.B. et al.: J. Clin. Microbiol., *26*:133, 1988.

20. Lopez, C. et al.: Am. J. Med., *56*:280, 1974.

21. Lurain, N.S., Thompson, K.D., and Farrand, S.K.: J. Clin. Microbiol., *24*:724, 1986.

22. McHugh, T.M. et al.: J. Clin. Microbiol., *22*:1014, 1985.

23. Melnick, J.L. et al.: Intervirology, *10*:115, 1978.

24. Middledorp, J.M. et al.: J. Clin. Microbiol., *20*:763, 1984.

25. Mourad, G. et al.: Transplant. Proc., *16*:1313, 1984.

26. Murray, H.W. et al.: Am. J. Med., *63*:574, 1977.

27. Musiani, M. et al.: Microbiologica, *1*:101, 1978.

*28. Naraqi, S.: In *Textbook of Human Virology.* Edited by R.B. Belshe. Littleton, PSG Publishing Co., 1984.

29. Nielsen, S.L. et al.: J. Clin. Microbiol., *25*:1406, 1987.

30. Onorato, I.M. et al.: Rev. Infect. Dis., *7*:479, 1985.

31. Pass, R.F. et al.: J. Infect. Dis., *143*:259, 1981.

32. Rand, K.H., Pollard, R.B., and Merigan, T.C.: N. Engl. J. Med., *298*:951, 1978.

33. Richardson, W.P. et al.: N. Engl. J. Med., *305*:57, 1981.

34. Ruebner, B.H. et al.: Am. J. Pathol., *46*:477, 1965.

35. Sanford, E.J. et al.: J. Urol., *118*:789, 1977.

36. Selwyn, P.A.: Hosp. Pract., *15* (Sep):119, 1986.

37. Severi, B. et al.: Microbiologica, *2*:265, 1979.

38. Simmons, R.L. et al.: Transplant. Proc., *2*:419, 1970.

39. Sissons, J.G.P. et al.: Immunol. Today, *7*:57, 1986.

40. Skolnik, P.R., Kosloff, B.R., and Hirsch, M.S.: J. Infect. Dis., *157*:508, 1988.

41. Smith, J.D., and DeHarven, E.: J. Virol., *12*:919, 1973.

42. Snydman, D.R. et al.: N. Engl. J. Med., *317*:1049, 1987.

43. St Jeor, S.C. et al.: J. Virol., *13*:353, 1974.

44. Stagno, S. et al.: JAMA, *256*:1904, 1986.

45. Stagno, S. and Whitley, R.J.: N. Engl. J. Med., *313*:1270, 1985.

46. Ware, A.J. et al.: Ann. Intern Med., *91*:364, 1979.

47. Weir, M.R.: Transplantation, *43*:187, 1987.

48. Yeager, A.S.: J. Clin. Microbiol., *2*:448, 1975.

Cytomegalovirus Antibody EIA Test[1]

PRINCIPLE. An enzyme immunosorbent assay (EIA) is used to detect IgG antibodies to *Cytomegalovirus (CMV).* The appropriate antigen is bound to a solid phase surface (the well in a plastic strip). Specific antibody, if present in patient's serum, binds to the attached antigen. Unbound antibody is removed by washing. Enzyme conjugated antihuman IgG is added, binding to the antibody-antigen complex. Unbound enzyme conjugate is removed by washing. Enzyme substrate is added and is hydrolyzed by the bound enzyme conjugate. After a specified time, the enzyme-substrate reaction is stopped. Spectrophotometric measurement provides an indirect measurement of specific antibody in the serum.

EQUIPMENT AND MATERIALS

CMV STAT Kit (Whittaker, M.A. Bioproducts) containing:

1. CMV antigen plate, 2 plates, 96 wells per plate, 192 tests per kit.

2. PBS-Tween 20× concentrate, phosphate buffered saline with Tween, 1 bottle, 200 mL per bottle, 0.4% sodium azide.

3. 10× conjugate, alkaline phosphatase conjugated anti-human IgG, 1 vial, 2.5 ml per vial, 0.02% sodium azide.

4. Serum diluent, 1 bottle, 50 ml per bottle, 0.1% sodium azide.

5. Conjugate diluent, 1 bottle, 25 mL per bottle, 0.1% sodium azide. Phenolphthalein monophosphate (PMP) enzyme substrate solution, 1 vial, 30 ml per vial.

6. Negative standard (human), 1 vial, 0.25 ml per vial, 0.1% sodium azide.

7. Low positive standard (human), 1 vial, 0.45 ml per vial, 0.1% sodium azide.

8. High positive standard (human), 1 vial, 0.25 ml per vial, 0.1% sodium azide.

9. Negative control (human), 1 vial, 0.25 ml per vial, 0.1% sodium azide.

10. Positive control (human), 1 vial, 0.25 ml per vial, 0.1% sodium azide.

11. Stop reagent, 1 vial, 20 gm sodium phosphate tribasic per vial.

12. Serum predilution plates, 2 plates, 96 wells each.

13. Report forms, 2 sheets.

14. Package insert, 1 sheet.

Additional Materials Required:

15. Wash bottle

16. Timer (15 minute range)

17. Calibrated precision micropipettes (200, 100 10 μl) MLA, repetman.

18. Pipettes, assorted sizes as needed.

19. Paper towels or absorbent sheets.

20. Graduate cylinders, 1 or 2 liter.

21. Disposal basin.

22. Plate shaker.

23. Spectrophotometer, plate reader.

SPECIMEN COLLECTION AND PREPARATION. Aseptically collect blood samples and prepare serum using standard techniques. If sera are stored, they should be frozen at $-70°$ C.

PRECAUTIONS

1. Use proper universal blood and body fluid precautions.

2. The CMV STAT plates are coated with inactivated virus. However, women of childbearing age should exercise caution because of the potential effect of the virus on the human fetus.

3. Reagents are intended to be used within the kit only. Do not intermix reagents. Distilled or deionized water at a neutral pH should be used where applicable. Use NaOH with care to avoid contact with skin or eyes. If contact occurs, flood with water.

4. Room temperatures of 20 to 55° C are recommended for incubation. The EIA is a sensitive technique. Care should be taken to ensure accuracy and cleanliness. Clean glassware (or disposable equipment) must be used.

REAGENT STORAGE

Kit Component	Room Temperature (20–25° C)	2–8° C
Antigen plate strips*		
Opened and resealed	8 hours	30 days
Unopened / opened in		
desiccating jar	-----	Labeled expiration
Heat resealed	-----	Labeled expiration
PBS-Tween		
20×	1 month	Labeled expiration
1×	48 hours	1 month
Conjugate		
10×	8 hours	Labeled expiration
1×	4 hours	4 hours
PMP Substrate		
1×	8 hours	Labeled expiration
Serum Diluent	8 hours	Labeled expiration
Conjugate Diluent	8 hours	Labeled expiration
Serum Controls / Standards	8 hours	Labeled expiration

*See antigen plate preparation for detailed information on storing unused strips.

PROCEDURE

Preliminary preparations: The following steps are required prior to the performance of the test. IMPORTANT: All 1× reagents must be at room temperature (20–25° C) prior to use in the assay.

1. Serum Dilution:

a. Add 10 μl of each serum to be tested to the appropriate well of the predilution plate. The kit standards and controls must be placed as shown below.

b. For each serum to be tested add 200 μl of serum diluent to a well of the predilution plate. Used portions of the plate can later be cut off and discarded.

c. Diluted sera may be stored (covered) in the predilution plates up to 24 hours prior to the test run. Plates with samples to be processed within 4 hours may be kept at room temperature; plates to be processed in 4–24 hours should be stored at 2 to 8° C. Cold plates must be allowed to equilibrate to room temperature before testing. Avoid movements which might cause the wells to splash. DO NOT place this plate on a plate shaker.

---

2. Well positions for immune status testing:

A	PC
B	LPS
C	LPS
D	LPS
E	NC
F	O
G	O
H	O

PC = Positive control
LPS = Low positive standard
NC = Negative control
O = Test sera

---

3. Well positions for quantitative, paired sera* analysis

	#1	#2
A	PC	A1
B	LPS	A1
C	LPS	C1
D	LPS	C1
E	NC	O
F	HS	O
G	NS	O
H	O	O

PC = Positive control
LPS = Low positive standard
NC = Negative control
HS = High positive standard
NS = Negative standard
A1 = Acute (or pre-vac) sample Patient #1
C1 = Convalescent (or post-vac) sample Patient #1
O = Other test sera

*Note: When evaluating paired sera (acute and convalescent) for the presence of a significant increase in CMV specific antibody each pair is tested in duplicate in adjacent (vertical, sequential) wells, as shown.

---

4. Preparing 1× reagents:

a. PBS-Tween. For each 96 well antigen plate required, dilute 100 ml of concentrated PBS-Tween to 2,000 ml with distilled or deionized water in a clean container.
If salt crystals form in the concentrate during storage, redissolve them by warming the solution to 37° C prior to diluting. Care should be taken to wash all storage vessels and dispensing tubes regularly to avoid possible contamination.

b. 10× conjugate. The 10× conjugate is diluted to a 1× working solution with conjugate diluent. Refer to the Table below to determine the volume of 10× conjugate concentrate and conjugate diluent needed to process the number of tests desired. Pipette the volumes into a clear disposable dilution tube and mix thoroughly using a vortex type laboratory mixer.

c. Stop reagent. To 20.0 gm (1 vial) of sodium phosphate tribasic add distilled or deionized water to a final volume of 1,000 ml. Mix and store in a sealed plastic container at room temperature.

Table. Conjugate volume required per number of tests.

Number of Tests	Number of Strips	10× Conjugate	Conjugate Diluent	Total 1× Conjugate
9–16	2	0.2 ml	1.8 ml	2.0 ml
17–24	3	0.3 ml	2.7 ml	3.0 ml
25–32	4	0.4 ml	3.6 ml	4.0 ml
33–40	5	0.5 ml	4.5 ml	5.0 ml
41–48	6	0.6 ml	5.4 ml	6.0 ml
49–56	7	0.6 ml	5.4 ml	6.0 ml
57–64	8	0.7 ml	6.3 ml	7.0 ml
65–72	9	0.8 ml	7.2 ml	8.0 ml
73–80	10	0.9 ml	8.1 ml	9.0 ml
81–88	11	1.0 ml	9.0 ml	10.0 ml
89–96	12	1.0 ml	9.0 ml	10.0 ml

5. Antigen plate preparation

a. Each antigen plate contains 12 strips of 8 wells coated with inactivated CMV antigen. Each test serum, standard or control will employ one of these antigen coated wells. Determine the number of wells to be used. Remove the antigen plate from the package by cutting off one end of the bag just inside the seal. Avoid contact with the base of the wells as this is the optical window for through-the-plate readers. Remove test strips not required for the immediate test run from the antigen plate and return them to the package.

b. All unused strips must be stored at 2 to 8° C. Shelf life will vary depending on how the strips are repackaged. If the strips are resealed in a package by folding the open end over twice and sealing it with tape across the entire fold, the unused strips may be used for approximately 30 days. If the sealed package is placed in a desiccating jar, the strips may be stored until the labeled expiration date. Strips may also be stored up to their labeled expiration by heat resealing the package. If the enclosed indicator card changes from blue to pink, that package of strips should not be used.

c. Number each test strip on the end tabs, if desired, and make sure the strips are firmly sealed in the antigen plate. Wash all strips carefully following the procedure below:

(1) Fill each well carefully with PBS-Tween using a wash bottle or equivalent method. Remove large air bubbles by tapping the antigen plate or by displacing them with a stream of PBS-Tween. Gently shake out PBS-Tween into a disposal basin.

(2) Repeat step 5c (1).

(3) Refill each well with PBS-Tween and antigen plate to soak for 5 minutes. Gently shake out the contents into the basin.

(4) Wrap a clean paper towel around the top and sides of the inverted antigen plate and tap the plate on the benchtop to remove residual PBS-Tween.

d. NOTE: If at any time you are interrupted during a wash step, you may allow the final soak to continue for up to ½ hour with no deleterious effect on the test. Never allow test strips to become dry during this procedure except for those few minutes as you are adding your next reagent.

6. Test

a. Serum incubation

(1) Using either a single or multiple channel 100 μl pipettor, immerse the pipette tip into a single well of the predilution plate and withdraw and expel the well contents 3–4 times to ensure proper mixing. Transfer 100 μl of the diluted sera into the appropriate wells of the CMV antigen plate.

Change tips between samples and repeat this procedure for all remaining test sera.

(2) Place the antigen plate on a plate shaker for 15 minutes at room temperature (20–25° C).

b. Conjugate incubation

(1) Shake out liquid from all wells into a disposal basin. Repeat washing steps described under antigen plate preparation, steps 5(c) through 5(d).

(2) Add 100 μl of 1× conjugate to each well.

(3) Incubate the antigen plate for 15 minutes on the plate shaker at room temperature (20–25° C).

c. Substrate incubation

(1) Shake out liquid from all wells into a disposal basin and repeat washing steps as described under antigen plate preparation, steps 5(c) through 5(d).

(2) Add 100 μl of PMP substrate to each well.

(3) Incubate the antigen plate for 15 minutes on the plate shaker at room temperature (20–25° C).

d. Stop/Read

(1) Add 200 μl stop reagent to each well.

(2) Mix the antigen plate for 2 minutes on the plate shaker.

(3) The antigen plate should be read within 1 hour of the addition of stop reagent.

CALCULATIONS

1. Immune status

a. After reading the antigen plate's absorbance, calculate the mean of the three low positive standard replicates to develop the low positive standard value (LPSV). Any single absorbance value which deviates more than 30% from the mean LPSV should not be used. The LPSV should then be recalculated from the remaining two absorbances.

Example:

	#1	#2	#3
LPS =	0.25	0.23	0.24

$$\text{LPSV} = \frac{0.25 + 0.23 + 0.24}{3} = 0.24$$

b. Test validity is checked by comparing the control sera absorbance values to that of the LPSV. The negative control absorbance must be less than the LPSV. The positive control absorbance must be greater than or equal to the LPSV.

Example:

	Absorbance	Interpretation
Negative control	.08	Valid
Positive control	.32	Valid

c. Interpretation of test samples' is performed by comparing the samples' absorbance to the LPSV. Negative test: those sera yielding absorbance values less than the LPSV; indicates no prior exposure to CMV. Positive test: those sera yielding absorbance values equal to or greater than the LPSV; indicates prior exposure to CMV.

2. Quantitative, Paired Sera Analysis. The three serum standards which are provided with a labeled index value are to be used in constructing the calibration curve.

a. Manual method: Contact technical services (800) 638-3976, for stat package insert supplement for manual calculations.

b. Calculator method: Perform a linear regression analysis of the test by entering the test absorbance values for each replicate of the three standards as the Y entries and their respective label index values as the X entries. For each control serum calculate the predicted X value (predicted index value) which corresponds to the test absorbance of the control as defined by linear regression. If the predicted index values (PIV) for the controls do not fall within the ranges stated on the vials, the test is invalid and should be repeated. Each unknown PIV is calculated in the manner as the controls.

3. Calculation of Critical Ratio

a. Calculate the mean PIV for the acute and convalescent sera.

b. To show an increase in antibody levels, the mean PIV for the acute serum should be ≤ 3.00. The mean PIV for the convalescent serum must be ≥ 1.00.

c. Calculate the critical ratio by dividing the mean PIV for the convalescent serum by the mean PIV of the acute serum.

$$\text{Critical ratio} = \frac{\text{mean PIV (convalescent)}}{\text{mean PIV (acute)}}$$

QUALITY CONTROL

1. If the r^2 value of the calibration curve is ≤ 0.95 check control values to ensure test validity.

2. The PIV's for the control sera provided must fall in their respective ranges (see vial labels). If they do not, the test is invalid and must be repeated.

3. Do not use heat inactivated sera.

4. Do not mix or interchange reagents between different kit lots.

5. Do not use reagents beyond their shelf life.

6. Do not vary incubation and reagent temperatures above or below normal room temperature ($20-25°$ C).

7. It is recommended that samples be run in duplicate until the laboratory is proficient in the assay.

INTERPRETATION OF RESULTS

1. Interpretation of immune status

PIV	Interpretation
≤ 0.79	Seronegative—absence of prior exposure to CMV
0.80–0.99	Equivocal—Sample should be retested. If retest is equivocal, the sample should be reported as equivocal, retested by an alternate method or with a new sample.
≥ 1.00	Seropositive indicates prior exposure to CMV.
1.00–2.69	Low positive
2.70–6.39	Mid positive
≥ 6.40	High positive

2. Interpretation of critical ratio

Critical Ratio	Interpretation
≤ 1.47	No significant change in antibody level. Comparable to a less than 4-fold change in antibody titer.
1.47–1.54	Lowest critical ratio which is highly suggestive of a significant rise in antibody level. Comparable in significance to a 4-fold increase in antibody titer. Results in this range suggest the possibility of active infection. It is recommended that a third sample be taken 7–14 days after sample 2. Sample 1 should then be tested with sample 3 for the critical ratio.
≥ 1.65	A critical ratio ≥ 1.65 should be interpreted as highly significant and indicative of a significant rise in CMV specific antibody level. Critical ratios ≥ 1.65 are comparable in significance to a greater than 4-fold increase in antibody titer.

a. For a critical ratio to be indicative of an increase in antibody level, PIV value for the acute serum should be ≤ 3.00 and the PIV value for the convalescent serum must be ≥ 1.00.

b. NOTE: Samples which show an increase, although negative, should be considered suspect. Example: Sample 1 = 0.20, Sample 2 = 0.80. It is recommended that a third sample be taken 7–14 days after sample 2. Sample 1 should then be compared to sample 3 for the critical ratio.

LIMITATIONS OF THE PROCEDURE

1. Icteric, lipemic, hemolyzed or heat inactivated sera may cause erroneous results and should be avoided if possible.

2. A serum obtained during the acute phase of infection when only low titers of IgM are present may be negative by this procedure.

REFERENCE

1. Insert, CMV STAT, *Cytomegalovirus* EIA Test Kit, Whittaker M.A. Bioproducts, Walkersville, Maryland, 1988.

EPSTEIN-BARR VIRUS INFECTIONS

In 1964, Epstein, Achong, and Barr[20] identified virus particles in cells from a human lymphoma endemic to certain regions of Africa.[10] Not long after, the relationship between this virus, now known as Epstein-Barr Virus or EBV, and infectious mononucleosis (IM) was described.[34] The ubiquitous nature of this virus has since caused it to be implicated in many diseases, both in immunocompromised and in apparently immunocompetent hosts.

Epstein-Barr Virus[51] is an ancient, complex virus, belonging to the gamma subgroup of the family herpesviridae. The virus is 180μ in diameter, and consists of an outer membrane envelope, with spikelike projections on its outer surface, an icosahedral nucleocapsid with 162 capsomeres, and a core of protein and linear, double stranded DNA (172,282 base pairs)[6] with single strand interruptions. Its only natural host is man. EBV demonstrates a remarkably selective tropism for B lymphocytes, oropharyngeal epithelial cells, and salivary gland cells, most often inducing "immortalization" of infected cells as a result of the effects of one or a few transforming genes (see *Burkitt's lymphoma, Nasopharyngeal carcinoma*). A few lytic forms of the virus have been observed.[1,7]

Antigens associated with the membrane of EBV-infected cells[54] include lymphocyte determined membrane antigens (LYDMA),[87] and an early membrane protein first observed on a lytic cell line.[7] Latent cells have a virus-determined membrane protein (membrane antigen, or MA)[69] which is linked to the transformation gene of the virus and may play an important role as a target for cell-mediated immune responses (see *Immune Response to EBV*).[94] Viral capsid antigens (VCA) can be demonstrated using immunofluorescence.[33] Early antigens (EA) appear in EBV-infected cells within hours of infection[31] and are considered to be a precursor to active viral production. Early antigens, as defined by immunofluorescent antibody staining,[36] may be diffuse within the nucleus and cytoplasm (EA-D) or may be restricted to cytoplasmic aggregates (EA-R). Several distinct nuclear antigens (EBNA) have been described,[81] and are expressed within the nuclei of all transformed cell lines carrying EBV DNA.

Epstein-Barr Virus asymptomatically infects virtually all people in the underdeveloped nations of the world before the age of 5 years. In industrial, "materially privileged" countries, only 25 to 50% of the population acquire the virus before the age of 18 years; 80 to 90% by 40 years.[46] EBV is a model of symbiotic viral-host interactions in most individuals;[76] however, when primary infection occurs late, in adolescence or early adulthood, clinical symptoms of infectious mononucleosis will result in approximately one-third to one-half of cases.[23] In addition, apparent or inapparent immunodeficiency (see *EBV-Associated Lymphoproliferation in Immunodeficiency*) or other defects[52] may predispose an individual to clinical disease.[73]

Epstein-Barr Virus probably infects initially via the oral route, transported by oral contact,[23] or by droplet or indirect contact.[70,85] The virus binds to receptors on oropharyngeal salivary gland epithelial cells,[80,97] and perhaps prickle epithelial cells,[29] where it penetrates and replicates.[29,80] Chronic, productive infection[46] of these oropharyngeal cells is responsible for persistent viral secretion[28,65,96] in 1 to 20% of normals, 20 to 40% of immunosuppressed or immunocompromised individuals, and up to 100% of persons with AIDS.[46] Continued recovery of EBV from saliva, the only body fluid where the virus can be demonstrated, is indicative of the lifelong infection characteristic of EBV.

Early in the course of infection, a small fraction of recirculating B lymphocytes be-

come infected with virions released from the oropharynx.[57] EBV binds via a glycoprotein in its outer membrane[88] to the $CR_2(C_{3d})$ receptor of the B cell,[24] the organism penetrates the cell, and is disseminated throughout the lymphoreticular system.[81] Inside infected cells, the genome is transported to the nucleus, where gene products are transcribed and translated, resulting in production of early antigens (EA) and nuclear antigens (EBNA), usually within 6 hours of infection. Membrane antigens, e.g. lymphocyte-determined membrane antigens (LYDMA) appear soon after EBNA and coincident with virally-induced DNA synthesis. Replication of viral DNA and synthesis of late proteins (e.g. viral capsid antigens, or VCAs) allow for assembly of progeny virions. Once a lymphocyte is transformed by the EBV genome,[94] it is immortalized, and will exhibit unlimited proliferation in cell culture. Transformed cells continue to produce EBNA, which is confined to the nucleus, but rarely are VCA or EA detectable.[46] A summary of EBV-determined antigens is available.[69]

Infectious Mononucleosis

The most common symptomatic manifestation of Epstein-Barr Virus infection is the disease known as infectious mononucleosis (IM). As previously stated, most clinical IM occurs in individuals in adolescence or young adulthood (ages 18 to 25 years) who were not previously infected. A triad of fever, pharyngitis, and diffuse lymphadenopathy is most often seen; however, malaise, fatigue, and hepatosplenomegaly are often present. Less commonly, hepatitis, cytopenias, and a range of other disorders may be seen.[46,63] Similar symptoms may be caused by cytomegalovirus (CMV), primary infection with *Toxoplasma gondii*, or with other etiologic agents.[43,81]

Not all cases of infectious mononucleosis are classic in their presentation,[12,81] and unusual forms are more frequent outside the usual age range. Although infection is most often inapparent in children, perhaps because of differences in cellular components in blood,[95] pharyngitis, fever, hyperemic throat, lymphadenopathy, and malaise may accompany infection.[4,45]

Resolution of infectious mononucleosis follows a common pattern:[64] pharyngitis disappears by 14 days after onset, fever within 21 days, and fatigue, lymphadenopathy and hepatosplenomegaly[17] by 21 to 28 days. Fatigue may, however, persist for months.

Polyclonal expansion of B cells during early stages of infectious mononucleosis is accompanied by a plethora of antibodies, many of which are autoimmune in nature. All major immunoglobulin classes increase, the earliest and highest concentration being seen in IgE.[8] During the course of IM, immunoglobulin concentrations drop to below pre-illness levels, then return to normal by 12 months after onset.

Specific antibodies reported during clinical infectious mononucleosis include heterophile antibodies (see below), cold agglutinins[42] (anti-i, others), cryoglobulins, rheumatoid factors, cytoskeletal antibodies and antibodies to ampicillin,[62] among others.[73,75,81] Rhodes, et al.[75] describe extensive epitope homology between the EBNA induced by EBV and many of the host proteins that interact with autoantibodies, e.g. heterophile antibodies and rheumatoid factors.

Early in the clinical course of IM, up to 0.05% of the peripheral blood B cells are infected with virus.[78] By the second week of illness, the number of these decreases drastically,[91] a result of the proliferation of T cells, both helper/inducers and suppressor/cytotoxic subpopulations, but a massive suppressor/cytotoxic T cell population[87,91] predominates and comprises most of the atypical lymphocytes observed hematologically during IM. These cells apparently respond, at least in part, to the LYDMA antigens previously described. EBV-specific cytotoxic T cells are detectable late in IM and reach maximum levels at 6 months post infection.[77]

Suppressor T cell populations may act nonspecifically to decrease normal immune cells and function.[48,81] Lymphocyte function tests demonstrate suppression, and significant anergy is observed.[59] Transient neutropenia, agranulocytosis, red cell aplasia, or aplastic anemia may also be seen.[73]

Lymphoid cell infiltration of several organs has been described in IM,[73] and may lead to necrosis and dysfunction.

Uninfected B cells respond to the appearance of EBV infection by the production of specific antibodies.[84] In infectious mononucleosis, IgM antibody to viral capsid antigen (VCA) appears late in the incubation period, simultaneously with anti-EA. IgM-VCA antibody converts to IgG anti-VCA, which remains detectable for years.[37] Late appearing, but also maintained lifelong, are antibodies to EBNA. Immunofluorescence and ELISA[31] have been used to detect these antibodies.

Diagnosis of infectious mononucleosis has classically been made using Hoagland's criteria,[63] based on (1) clinical features compatible with infectious mononucleosis, (2) a hematologic picture of relative and absolute lymphocytosis, with greater than 20% atypical lymphocytes (Downey cells), and (3) demonstration of heterophile antibodies. More recently, EBV-specific antibody tests have been used as an aid to diagnosis,[35] especially the VCA-IgM antibodies, which are detectable in about 97% of patients during the acute phase of illness.[40]

Heterophile antibodies are, by definition, reactant with similar antigens found in two or more unrelated species. Nearly all heterophile antibodies belong to the IgM class. Examples of heterophile antibodies, besides those defined in IM, include the ABO system, I/i system and reagin (Syphilis). The heterophile antibodies of IM, known to be directed against a "neo-antigen" on the infected B cell surface,[64] are antibodies that cross react with antigens on the surface of horse, sheep, and beef red blood cells, but not guinea pig kidney antigen. Although the antibodies can be detected using any of the

Table 9–3. Heterophile Antibodies

	Reaction With			
Source of Antibody	Sheep rbc*	Horse rbc	Beef rbc	Guinea Pig Kidney
Infectious mononucleosis	+	+	+	−
Serum sickness	+	+	+	+
Forssman-induced	+	+	−	+

*rbc = red blood cells

three red blood cell antigens, horse cells are the most sensitive,[55] and differential diagnosis (to eliminate Forssman or serum sickness antibody) may be accomplished using one of the differential slide tests currently marketed (e.g. Monospot) or the classic Davidsohn Differential slide test.[13] (Table 9–3). Heterophile antibody titer may be determined using the Paul Bunnell test. Heterophile antibodies are detectable in 90%[23,35] to 98%[81] of acute adolescent or young adult cases of infectious mononucleosis, usually remaining elevated for 8 to 12 weeks.[64] Childhood EBV infections do not commonly induce heterophile antibodies, although heterophile tests may be useful in conjunction with EBV-specific antibody panels to confirm diagnosis in children as well as in heterophile-negative adults. False-positive rapid slide tests do occur,[39,41] albeit rarely.

Treatment of infectious mononucleosis is usually conservative, limited to bed rest and symptomatic relief in most cases. Acyclovir has been shown to transiently inhibit oropharyngeal secretion of EBV[8,28] and may alleviate symptoms, but does not appear to alter the course of disease.

Fatal cases of IM do occur,[25,46,58] although rarely, and may be related to undefined defects in host response to EBV.[32]

Compelling evidence in favor of recurrent episodes of infectious mononucleosis in normal individuals does not exist.[82]

Chronic Active EBV Infection

There is currently a great deal of debate[56,77,97] about a syndrome, or group of syndromes, alternately known as chronic active EBV (CA-EBV), systemic immunodeficient EBV syndrome (SIDES),[2] chronic mononucleosis syndrome (CMS),[19] or sporadic neurasthenia.[46] Originally described by DuBois et al.,[19] Jones et al.,[47] Straus et al.,[83] and Tobi et al.,[90] the syndrome(s) has been characterized by depression,[3] mood and personality disorders, fever, anxiety, headaches,[16] chronic fatigue and/or daytime sleepiness,[30] and has often been associated with allergies.[68,81] Many authors believe in, and have attempted to prove, an association between these symptoms and chronic Epstein-Barr Virus infection.

Serologic studies using EBV-specific antigens showed that, while statistically significant differences could be detected in various antibodies to EBV antigens, e.g. anti-EA,[2,14,26] anti-EBNA,[38] and anti-VCA,[46] when compared to control groups, the use of serology in diagnosis of CA-EBV is seriously limited.[40,64] Steeper et al.[81] propose serologic grouping of CA-EBV (CMS) patients based on EBV profile, but suggest that diagnosis by this means is peremptory and must, at present, be primarily one of exclusion of all possible underlying disorders.

Lymphocytes from CA-EBV patients have been shown to suppress allogeneic, but not autologous immunoglobulin synthesis in vitro,[92] and a marked inability of mitogen to induce interleukin-2 (IL-2) and interferon production[50] by lymphocytes from these patients has been noted. The absence of antibody to a variation of the EBNA antigen, known as EBNA-K, has also been reported in CA-EBV patients.[66]

Treatment of CA-EBV diagnosed patients with gamma globulin[18] and IL-2[49] has been attempted, with some success.

Burkitt's Lymphoma

Burkitt's lymphoma (BL) is a malignant B cell lymphoproliferative disorder which is endemic to children living in the equatorial region of Africa,[10] but also may be found worldwide.[56] All cases described have demonstrated chromosomal translocations, specifically involving the myc oncogene on chromosome 8 and one of the immunoglobulin coding genes (chromosomes 2, 14, or 22).[56]

Events that induce Burkitt's lymphoma[52] probably vary somewhat in different geographic areas. In Africa, the initial event is thought to be primary exposure to EBV, which occurs by 1 to 3 years of age,[57] as the EBV genome can be detected in over 97% of Burkitt's lymphoma in that area. However, only 15% of cases outside that endemic area demonstrate EBV association.[57,73]

Environmental activators[44] are thought to reactivate the EBV genome some months before clinical detection of Burkitt's. B cells massively infected with EBV may be a target for falciparum malaria-mediated mitogenesis or for oncogene activation.[56]

Although Burkitt's lymphoma is clinically similar in various parts of the world, the absence of detectable EBV genome in some Burkitt's lymphomas suggests the virus' role is not universal.

Nasopharyngeal Carcinoma

Nasopharyngeal Carcinoma (NPC)[93] is a malignancy found predominantly in middle-aged males in southeast Asia. Unlike the situation in Burkitt's lymphoma, the association between Epstein-Barr Virus and nasopharyngeal carcinoma is strong and constant worldwide.[15] As the EBV genome is invariably identifiable within the malignant cell line, the disease is undoubtedly due to uncontrolled proliferation of EBV-carrying cells in the nasopharynx, probably reactivated by environmental factors.[44] Reacti-

vation of latent virus is associated with an increase in IgA, particularly directed against VCA and EA antigens,[44,67] an association which is useful in clinical diagnosis.

EBV-Associated Lymphoproliferation in Immunodeficiency[53,57]

Similar to other Herpes group viruses, EBV reverts to a lifelong carrier or latency state after primary infection, probably carried in both B lymphocytes and epithelial cells of the oropharynx,[76] where it is maintained in a stable host-virus balance. Individuals with a primary immunodeficiency, secondary immunodeficiency, or those who are immunosuppressed are at risk for life-threatening primary infection with EBV, or reactivation of the viral genome. Lymphoproliferative disorders in immunodeficient states range from fulminant infectious mononucleosis and invasive polyclonal B cell hyperplasia to monoclonal B cell malignancy.

Various primary immune defects, particularly those where T suppressor populations are depleted, predispose patients with immunodeficiency to EBV complications.[53,57,73,79] Probably the most studied group are those patients with X-linked lymphoproliferative syndrome,[71,72] an inherited immune defect in which development appears normal until primary EBV infection. Then, unbridled proliferation of virally-transformed B cells, fatal or chronic infectious mononucleosis, acquired hypogammaglobulinemia, or aplastic anemia develop, usually leading to death.

It is notable that Bruton's agammaglobulinemia patients, who have low or nonexistent levels of B cells but normal levels of T cells, are immune to EBV infection.

Renal transplant recipients[27,32] undergoing immunosuppression have impaired responsiveness to EBV infection or reactivation.[27] Most EBV-induced manifestations occurring in these individuals are polyclonal proliferations, either resembling infectious mononucleosis or appearing as a localized solid tumor mass.[32] Similar experience is noted with recipients of other organ transplants.[32] Notable is the observation that bone marrow transplants do not appear to predispose an individual to lymphoproliferative disorder, while thymic transplant, or simply not performing graft implant, may increase the likelihood.[73]

AIDS or ARC patients, as might be expected, frequently exhibit evidence of EBV reactivation.[74,86] T suppressor cell depletion renders patients unable to restrain polyclonal proliferation of EBV infected cells, and lymphadenopathy, or undifferentiated, EBV-associated B cell lymphomas ensue.[9,11] Hairy cell leukoplakia of the tongue, often seen in AIDS patients, can apparently result from EBV-infected prickle cells on the epithelial surface.[29]

Immune Response to EBV

Immune responsiveness to EBV infection involves humoral, cell mediated, and nonspecific elements. Humoral components include antibodies to EA, VCA, and EBNA, as described above, as well as antibodies which are apparently capable of exerting a neutralizing effect on exogenous virus. There is evidence that interferon and NK cells demonstrate enhanced activity, especially early in primary EBV infections.[46,89] EBV transformed lymphocytes are capable of alternate pathway complement activation, and the virus appears able to activate the classical pathway without the help of antibody.[60] The cell mediated immune system, however, particularly T suppressor cells in their response to the LYDMA antigen on infected cells, is most likely the protective factor.[76,91]

Development of a vaccine for Epstein-Barr Virus is in progress.[21,61]

REFERENCES

1. Alfieri, C., Ghibu, R., and Joncas, J.H.: Can. Med. Assoc. J., *131*:1249, 1984.
2. Allen, A.D., and Tilkian, S.M.: J. Clin. Psychiatry, *47*:133, 1986.
3. Amsterdam, J.D. et al.: Am. J. Psychiatry, *143*:1593, 1986.
4. Andiman, W.A.: J. Pediatr., *95*:171, 1979.
5. Andersson, J.: J. Infect. Dis., *153*:283, 1986.
6. Baer, R. et al.: Nature, *310*:207, 1984.
7. Balanchandran, N., Pittari, J., and Hutt-Fletcher, L.M.: J. Virol., *60*:369, 1986.
8. Banna, S.L., Heiner, D.C., and Horwitz, C.A.: Int. Arch. Allergy Appl. Immunol., *74*:1, 1984.
9. Birx, D.L., Redfield, R.R., and Tosato, G.: N. Engl. J. Med., *314*:874, 1986.
10. Burkitt, D.: Br. Med. J., *2*:1019, 1962.
11. Ciobanu, N., and Wiernik, P.H.: Mt. Sinai J. Med. (NY), *53*:627, 1986.
12. Copperman, S.M.: Clin. Pediatr., *16*:143, 1977.
13. Davidsohn, I.: Am. J. Clin. Pathol. (Tech. Suppl.), *2*:56, 1938.
14. DeLisi, L.E. et al.: Arch. Gen. Psychiatry, *43*:815, 1986.
15. deThé, G., and Zeng, Y.: In *The Epstein-Barr Virus: Recent Advances.* Edited by M.A. Epstein and B.G. Achong., New York, Wiley Medical, 1986.
16. Diaz-Mitoma, F., Vanast, W.J., and Tyrrell, D.L.J.: Lancet, *1*:411, 1987.
17. Dommerby, H., Stangerup, S.E., Stangerup, M., and Hancke, S.: J. Laryngol. Otol., *100*:573, 1986.
18. DuBois, R.E.: AIDS Res. (2 Suppl.), *1*:S191, 1986.
19. DuBois, R.E. et al.: South. Med. J., *77*:1376, 1984.
20. Epstein, M.A., Achong, B.G., and Barr, Y.M.: Lancet, *1*:702, 1964.
21. Epstein, M.A., and Morgan, A.J.: In *The Epstein-Barr Virus: Recent Advances.* Edited by M.A. Epstein and B.G. Achong. New York, Wiley Medical, 1986.
22. Ernberg, I., and Anderson, J.: J. Gen. Virol., *67*:2267, 1986.
23. Evans, A.S. et al.: J. Infect. Dis., *132*:546, 1975.
24. Fingeroth, J.D. et al.: Proc. Natl. Acad. Sci. U.S.A., *81*:4510, 1984.
25. Frecentese, D.F., and Cogbill, T.H.: Am. Surg., *53*:521, 1987.
26. Fudenberg, H.H., Allen, A.D., Pitts, F.N., Jr., and Allen, R.E.: Am. J. Psychiatry, *144*:1374, 1987.
27. Gaston, J.S.H., Rickinson, A.B., and Epstein, M.A.: Lancet, *1*:923, 1982.
28. Gerber, P. et al.: Lancet, *2*:988, 1972.
29. Greenspan, J.S. et al.: N. Engl. J. Med., *313*:1564, 1985.
30. Guilleminault, C., and Mondini, S.: Arch. Inter. Med., *146*:1333, 1986.
31. Halprin, J. et al.: Ann. Intern. Med., *104*:331, 1986.
32. Hanto, D.W., and Najarian, J.S.: J. Surg. Oncol., *30*:215, 1985.
33. Henle, G., and Henle, W.: J. Bacteriol., *91*:1248, 1966.
34. Henle, G., Henle, W., and Diehl, V.: Proc. Natl. Acad. Sci. U.S.A., *59*:94, 1968.
35. Henle, W., Henle, G.E., and Horwitz, C.A.: Hum. Pathol., *5*:551, 1974.
36. Henle, G., Henle, W., and Klein, G.: Int. J. Cancer, *8*:272, 1971.
37. Henle, W. et al.: J. Infect. Dis., *124*:58, 1971.
38. Henle, W. et al.: Proc. Natl. Acad. Sci. U.S.A., *84*:570, 1987.
39. Hoiby, E.A., Tjade, T., and Rotterud, O.J.: Acta. Pathol. Microbiol. Immunol. Scand., *93*:145, 1985.

40. Holmes, G.P. et al.: JAMA, 257:2297, 1987.

41. Horwitz, C.A., et al.: Am. J. Clin. Pathol., 72:807, 1979.

42. Horwitz, C.A., et al.: Blood 50:195, 1977.

43. Ho-Yen, D.O., and Martin, K.W.: J. Infect. 3:324, 1981.

44. Ito, Y.: In The Epstein-Barr Virus: Recent Advances. Edited by M.A. Barr and B.G. Achong. New York, Wiley Medical, 1986.

45. Jones, J.F.: Pediatr. Infect. Dis., 5:503, 1986.

46. Jones, J.F., and Straus, S.E.: Ann. Rev. Med., 38:195, 1987.

47. Jones, J.F. et al.: Ann. Intern. Med., 102:1, 1985.

48. Junker, A.K. et al.: Clin. Immunol. Immuno-pathol., 40:436, 1986.

49. Kawa-Ha, K. et al.: Lancet, 1:154, 1987.

50. Kibler, R. et al.: J. Clin. Immunol., 5:46, 1985.

51. Kieff, E. et al.: J. Infect. Dis., 146:506, 1982.

52. Klein, G., and Klein, E.: Nature, 315:190, 1985.

53. Klein, G., and Purtilo, D.: Cancer Res., 41:4302, 1981.

54. Klein, G. et al.: J. Natl. Cancer Inst., 39:1027, 1967.

55. Lee, C.L., Zandrew, F., and Davidsohn, I.: J. Clin. Pathol., 21:631, 1968.

56. Lenoir, G.M.: In The Epstein-Barr Virus: Recent Advances. Edited by M.A. Epstein and B.G. Achong. New York, Wiley Medical, 1986.

57. List, A.F., Greco, F.A., and Vogler, L.B.: J. Clin. Oncol., 5:1673, 1987.

58. Lukes, R.J., and Cox, F.H.: Am. J. Pathol., 34:586, 1958.

59. Mangi, R.J. et al.: N. Engl. J. Med., 291:1149, 1974.

60. Martin, H., McConnell, I., Gorick, B., and Hughes-Jones, N.C.: Clin. Exp. Immunol., 67:531, 1987.

61. Marx, J.L.: Science, 231:919, 1986.

62. McKenzie, H., Parratt, D., and White, R.G.: Clin. Exp. Immunol., 26:214, 1976.

63. McSherry, J.A.: Am. Fam. Physician, 32:129, 1985.

64. Merlin, T.L.: Hum. Pathol., 17:2, 1986.

65. Miller, G., Niederman, J.C., and Andrews, L.L.: N. Engl. J. Med., 288:229, 1973.

66. Miller, G. et al.: J. Infect. Dis., 156:26, 1987.

67. Neel, H.B., III: J. Otolaryngol., 15:137, 1986.

68. Olsen, G.B. et al.: J. Allergy Clin. Immunol., 78:308, 1986.

69. Pearson, G.R., and Luka, J.: In The Epstein-Barr Virus: Recent Advances. Edited by M.A. Epstein and B.G. Achong. New York, Wiley Medical, 1986.

70. Pochedly, C.: NY State J. Med., 87:352, 1987.

71. Purtilo, D.T. et al.: N. Engl. J. Med., 297:1077, 1977.

72. Purtilo, D.T. et al.: Am. J. Med., 73:49, 1982.

73. Purtilo, D.T. et al.: Int. Rev. Exp. Pathol., 27:113, 1985.

74. Ragona, G. et al.: Clin. Exp. Immunol., 66:17, 1986.

75. Rhodes, G. et al.: J. Exp. Med., 165:1026, 1987.

76. Rickinson, A.B., Yao, Q.Y., and Wallace, L.E.: Br. Med. Bull., 41:75, 1985.

77. Rickinson, A.B. et al.: Int. J. Cancer, 25:59, 1980.

78. Rocchi, G., deFelici, A., Ragona, G., Heinz, A.: N. Engl. J. Med., 296:132, 1977.

79. Schimke, R.N., Collins, D., and Cross, D.: Am. J. Med. Genet., 27:195, 1987.

80. Sixbey, J.W. et al.: Nature, 306:480, 1983.

81. Steeper, T.A., Horwitz, C.A., Henle, W., and Henle, G.: Ann. Allergy, 59:243, 1987.

82. Straus, S.E.: In Epstein-Barr Virus and Associated Diseases. Edited by P.H. Levine et al. Boston, Martinus Nijhoff, 1985.

83. Straus, S.E. et al.: Ann. Intern. Med., 102:7, 1985.

84. Sumaya, C.V.: Pediatr. Infect. Dis., 5:337, 1986.

85. Sumaya, C.V., and Ench, Y.: J. Infect. Dis., 154:842, 1986.

86. Sumaya, C.V. et al.: J. Infect. Dis., 154:864, 1986.

87. Svedmyr, E., and Jondal, M.: Proc. Natl. Acad. Sci. U.S.A., 72:1622, 1975.

88. Tanner, J. et al.: Cell, 50:203, 1987.

89. Thorley-Lawson, D.A.: J. Immunol., 126:829, 1981.

90. Tobi, M. et al.: Lancet, 1:61, 1982.

91. Tosaxto, G. et al.: N. Engl. J. Med., 301:1133, 1979.

92. Tosaxto, G. et al.: J. Immunol., 134:3082, 1985.

93. Trumper, A., Epstein, M.A., Giovanella, B.V., and Finerty, S.: Int. J. Cancer, 20:655, 1977.

94. Wang, D., Liebowitz, D., and Kieff, E.: Cell, 43:831, 1985.

95. Weigle, K.A., Sumaya, C.U., and Montiec, M.: J. Clin. Immunol., 3:151, 1983.

96. Yao, Q.Y., Rickinson, A.B., and Epstein, M.A.: Int. J. Cancer, 35:35, 1985.

97. Young, L.S., Sixbey, J.W., Clark, K.D., and Rickinson, A.B.: Lancet, 1:240, 1986.

Monospot[6]

PRINCIPLE. This rapid slide procedure is based on agglutination of horse red blood cells by the heterophile antibody of infectious mononucleosis (IM). Since horse red blood cells contain both Forssman and IM antigens, a differential absorption of the patient's serum is necessary to distinguish the specific heterophile antibody of IM from those of the Forssman type. This is accomplished by absorbing patient serum or plasma with both guinea pig kidney and beef erythrocyte stroma. Guinea pig kidney contains only the Forssman antigen, while beef erythrocytes contain only the antigen associated with infectious mononucleosis. Therefore, guinea pig kidney will absorb only heterophile antibodies of the Forssman type, while beef erythrocytes will absorb only the heterophile antibody of infectious mononucleosis. A positive reaction for the IM heterophile antibody is indicated by agglutination of the horse red blood cells by patient specimen absorbed with guinea pig kidney, and no agglutination (or weaker agglutination) of the horse red blood cells by patient specimen absorbed with beef erythrocyte stroma.

EQUIPMENT AND MATERIALS

1. Ortho Diagnostics, Monospot Kit containing:

a. Reagent I (guinea pig antigen): a suspension of guinea pig kidney antigen preserved with sodium azide (1%).

b. Reagent II (beef erythrocyte stroma): a suspension of beef erythrocyte stroma antigen preserved with sodium azide (1%).

c. Indicator cells (horse erythrocytes): a suspension of stabilized horse red blood cells preserved with chloramphenicol (1:3,000) and neomycin sulfate (1:10,000).

d. Positive control serum: human serum containing the heterophile antibody of infectious mononucleosis, preserved with sodium azide (0.1%).

e. Negative control serum: human serum not containing the heterophile antibody of infectious mononucleosis, preserved with sodium azide (0.1%).

f. Glass or paper slide.

g. Microcapillary pipets with rubber bulb: designed to deliver 10 lambda.

h. Wooden or plastic stirring rods.

i. Disposable plastic pipette and bulbs.

SPECIMEN COLLECTION AND PREPARATION.

Serum or plasma mixed with anticoagulants including EDTA, sodium oxalate, potassium oxalate, sodium citrate, ACD solution or heparin may be used. Inactivation of the serum is not necessary; however, inactivated serum may be used. Serum or plasma samples should be clear and particle-free.

The heterophile antibody of infectious mononucleosis is relatively stable and uncontaminated specimens of serum or plasma may be stored at 2 to 8° C for several days following collection before testing. If prolonged storage is desired, the patient specimen should be frozen.

STORAGE INSTRUCTION. When properly stored, the kit is stable through the expiration date printed on the package label. The expiration date of the kit corresponds to the shortest dated reagent. Contents of the entire kit should be discarded on the expiration date. Reagents must be stored at 2 to 8° C when not in use. Do not freeze reagents. Deterioration of indicator cells will be evidenced by hemolysis. Proper reactivity may be verified by a positive control test (see Procedure).

PROCEDURE

1. Place the slide on a flat surface under a direct light source.

2. Invert the vial of indicator cells several times to uniformly suspend the cells. Using one of the disposable microcapillary pipettes provided, deliver 10 lambda of indicator cells to one corner of both squares on the slide. To use the disposable microcapillary pipettes:

a. Insert the end of the pipette marked with a heavy black line one-quarter inch into the neck of the rubber bulb.

b. Hold the rubber bulb between the thumb and third finger.

c. Tilt the vial of indicator cells, insert the pipette, and allow the pipette to fill by capillary action to the top mark (20 lambda). Do not draw cells into the bulb.

d. To deliver 10 lambda of indicator cells to the slide, place the index finger over the hole in the top of the bulb and squeeze gently until the level of cells in the pipette returns to the first mark. Touch pipette tip to a corner of square "I" to release the cells.

e. Deliver the remaining 10 lambda of indicator cells from the pipette to a corner of square "II."

3. Place one drop of thoroughly mixed reagent I in the center of square "I."

4. Place one drop of thoroughly mixed reagent II in the center of square "II."

5. Using a disposable plastic pipette, add one drop of the serum or plasma being tested to the reagent in the center of each square on the slide.

6. Positive control serum and negative control serum are provided in each package. These control sera should be used to check the reagents upon arrival in the laboratory and daily when kit is in use.

7. Avoiding the indicator cells, mix reagent I and reagent II with the serum or plasma in each square at least ten times using a clean wooden

applicator for each square. Then using no more than ten stirring motions, blend in the indicator cells over the entire surface of each square. Start a timer upon completion of the final mixing.

8. Do not pick up or move the slide during the reaction period.

9. Observe for agglutination for no longer than 1 minute after final mixing.

REPORTING. Results are reported as positive or negative for the heterophile antibody of infectious mononucleosis.

INTERPRETATION OF RESULTS

1. Positive test: If the agglutination pattern is stronger on the left side of the slide (square I), the test is positive.

2. Negative test: If the agglutination pattern is stronger on the right side of the slide (square II), the test is negative.

3. If no agglutination appears on either square of the slide (I and II), or if agglutination is equal on both squares of the slide (I and II), the test is negative.

4. Agglutination which appears after the 1-minute reading time, or which appears when the slide is moved or rocked, is not to be interpreted as a positive result for the heterophile antibody of infectious mononucleosis.

5. A positive test result is indicative of the heterophile antibody specific for infectious mononucleosis. A titration procedure may be performed to provide quantitative indication of the level of infectious mononucleosis heterophile antibody (see *Paul-Bunnell Test*).

LIMITATIONS OF THE PROCEDURE. To obtain accurate results, only clear, particle-free serum or plasma samples should be used. False-positive results with Monospot have been reported;[5,10,11] however, because the clinical symptoms of IM are similar to many other diseases, it is often difficult to disprove the theoretical possibility of a concomitant infection.[13] The simultaneous occurrence of infectious mononucleosis and hepatitis has been reported. A result that may be interpreted as false-positive may possibly be because of residual infectious mononucleosis antibody present after clinical symptoms have subsided.[3,7]

Seronegative infectious mononucleosis has also been reported.[3] In the case of a delayed heterophile antibody response, it is possible that clinical and hematologic symptoms of IM will appear before serologic confirmation is possible.[1]

REFERENCES

1. Baehner, R.L., and Shuler, S.E.: Clin. Pediatr., 6:393, 1967.
2. Bender, C.E.: JAMA, *182*:954, 1962.
3. Carter, R.L., and Penman, H.G.: *Infectious mononucleosis.* Oxford, Blackwell Scientific Publications, 1968.
4. Hoagland, R.J.: N. Engl. J. Med., *269*:1307, 1963.
5. Horwitz, C.A. et al.: Br. Med. J., *1*:591, 1973.
6. Insert, Monospot, Ortho Diagnostics Raritan, NJ, 1983.
7. Lee, C.L., and Davidsohn, I.: Committee on Continuing Education Council on Immunohematology, ASCP, 1972.
8. Lee, C.L., and Davidsohn, I.: Joint Annual Meeting of ASCP and CAP, 1967.
9. Madhavan, T.: JAMA, *225*:314, 1973.
10. Phillips, G.M.: JAMA, *222*:585, 1972.
11. Sadoff, L., and Goldsmith, O.: JAMA, *218*:1297, 1971.
12. Starling, K.A., and Fernbach, D.J.: JAMA, *203*:810, 1968.
13. Tri, T.B., and Herbst, K.: JAMA, *225*:62, 1973.
14. Wintrobe, M.M.: In *Principles of Internal Medicine.* Edited by T.R. Harrison. Philadelphia, The Blakiston Company, 1950.

Paul-Bunnell Test (Presumptive Titer)[2]

PRINCIPLE. A suspension of sheep red blood cells is reacted with dilutions of patient serum. Agglutination indicates the presence and titer of heterophile antibodies.

EQUIPMENT AND MATERIALS

1. 0.9% saline solution.

2. Sheep erythrocytes: Prepare a 2% suspension by adding 0.5 ml of washed, packed erythrocytes to 24.5 ml 0.9% saline solution. Keep refrigerated. Diluted cells may be used up to 1 week. Discard if hemolysis occurs.

3. Positive Control (Difco): Store at 2 to 10° C. Contains 1:1000 sodium azide as a preservative. Need not be inactivated. Expiration date is noted on the label. Titer is noted on the insert. Alternatively, a positive patient sample of known titer may be ali-

quoted and stored at $-20°$ C. This control must be inactivated before use.

4. 13×100 mm test tubes (10 for each patient or control).

5. 0.1 ml, 0.5 ml and 1.0 ml pipets.

PROCEDURE

1. Perform a screening test for infectious mononucleosis to determine the presence and identity of heterophile antibody (see *Monospot*). Identification of an infectious mononucleosis antibody should precede performance of the Paul-Bunnell Test.

2. Heat-inactivate sera to be tested. Also inactivate control if necessary (see package insert-positive control).

3. Prepare a 2% sheep red blood cell suspension as described above.

4. Set up a row of 10 tubes for each serum to be tested, and a row for the positive control serum. Place 0.4 ml saline solution in the first tube of each row and 0.25 ml in each remaining tube.

5. Add 0.1 ml of control serum to tube 1 of a properly labeled row. Mix the first tube and serially transfer 0.25 ml through tube 9, discarding 0.25 ml from tube 9. The tenth tube contains no antibody and will be the negative control.

6. Repeat step 5 for each patient but continue to transfer 0.25 ml through tube 10 and discard 0.25 ml from tube 10.

7. Add 0.1 ml of the 2% cell suspension to each tube. The dilutions are now 1:7, 1:14, 1:28, etc.

8. Shake tubes to obtain an even mixture, and allow to stand at room temperature for at least 2 hours. (NOTE: Titer can be read after 15 minutes if desired, but must be allowed to incubate 2 hours before final reading is made.)

9. Shake tubes individually and observe for macroscopic agglutination. Read for the last dilution demonstrating visible agglutination. The positive control must read $\pm$ one doubling dilution from the expected value or the value printed on the package insert. Record control results.

REPORTING. Report the reciprocal of the highest dilution of serum showing visible agglutination. Always report the antibody identification (see *Monospot* test) along with the Paul-Bunnell test results.

INTERPRETATION OF RESULTS. Paul-Bunnell titers of less than or equal to 56 may be considered normal.

LIMITATIONS OF THE PROCEDURE. The Paul-Bunnell test detects heterophile antibodies of serum sickness and Forssman types, as well as those resulting from infectious mononucleosis. Therefore, this test must be used in conjunction with David-sohn-Differential[1] or the Monospot test.

REFERENCES

1. Davidsohn, I.: JAMA, *108*:289, 1937.
2. Paul, J.R., and Bunnell, W.W.: Am. J. Med. Sci., *183*:90, 1932.

Anti-EBV Capsid Antigen[3] IgM

PRINCIPLE. The EBV-M antibody test utilizes the indirect fluorescent antibody (IFA) method for the detection of IgM antibody to EBV Capsid Antigen (EB-VCA). In this procedure serum from patients suspected of having EBV Infection is layered onto EBV infected lymphoid cells which are immobilized on glass slides. Human antibody to EB-VCA will attach to the infected cells. This antibody can be detected by the reaction with a fluorescein conjugated anti-human IgM antibody and subsequent examination with a fluorescence microscope. The presence of viral related IgM antibody to EB-VCA is demonstrated by an apple-green fluorescence. Sero-negative specimens will not show this staining.

EQUIPMENT AND MATERIALS

1. EBV-M kit components: Organon Teknika, Inc.

a. EB-VCA Slides (Individually wrapped in aluminum foil packets): Five slides with 5 wells each

b. Goat Anti-Human IgM, (μ Chain Specific) Fluorescein Conjugated Containing Evans Blue Counterstain (Lyophilized): 2 plastic vials; each vial 0.5 ml after reconstitution

c. EB-VCA IgM Low Positive Control Human Serum (Lyophilized): 1 vial, 0.25 ml after reconstitution

d. EB-VCA IgM Negative Control Human Serum (Lyophilized): 1 vial, 0.25 ml

e. Phosphate Buffered Saline solution (PBS) $30\times$ Concentrate: 2 vials. The diluted PBS contains 0.15M NaCl, 0.01 M phosphate buffer, pH 7.5, with 0.01% Thimerosal

f. Mounting Fluid: 1 vial, 3 ml. Vial of mounting fluid contains:

Glycerin (reagent grade)   9 volumes
Phosphate buffered saline,
    pH 7.5   1 volume

2. Small test tubes for serum dilutions
3. Micropipets or Pasteur pipets
4. Moisture chamber for incubation of slides
5. Incubator, 37° C
6. Staining dish
7. Cover glass 24 × 50 mm. Optical glass No. 1
8. Darkfield fluorescence microscope assembly, e.g., Zeiss RA microscope or equivalent

Exciter Filter   BG-12 (3 mm) or equiva-
                  lent
Barrier Filter   OG-1 or equivalent
Light Source   HBO 200 or equivalent
Objective   24-54 × oil immersion or
                  high dry

PRECAUTIONS.   Use   proper   universal blood and body fluid precautions.

SPECIMEN COLLECTION AND PREPARATION. Obtain blood by venipuncture, removing the serum aseptically. If not used immediately, store serum at −20° C or below. The serum specimen should be obtained as soon as possible after onset of illness.

PREPARATION OF REAGENTS

1. Goat antihuman IgM, fluorescein conjugated: This preparation is a combination of Evans Blue counterstain and the fluorescein isothiocyanate (FITC) labeled specific antibody fraction of goat globulin that recognizes human IgM immunoglobulins. To reconstitute, remove the cap and dropper tip from the dispensing vial and add 0.5 ml of the diluted PBS. Replace dropper tip and cap and gently agitate until solution is complete. (Avoid vigorous shaking.)

2. EB-VCA IgM low positive control human serum: The positive control serum is prepared from human sera containing minimal IgM antibody to EB-VCA (about 2 + reactivity). Reconstitute the control serum by the addition of 0.25 ml of diluted

PBS and gently agitate until solution is complete. (Avoid vigorous shaking.) Avoid repeated freeze / thaw treatment of the control serum since this may cause loss of potency.

3. EB-VCA negative control human serum: The negative control serum is prepared from a pool of human sera that has IgG antibody to EB-VCA and undetectable (comparable to the conjugate control) IgM antibody to EB-VCA. Reconstitute the negative control serum by the addition of 0.25 ml of diluted PBS and gently agitate until solution is complete. (Avoid vigorous shaking.) Avoid repeated freeze / thaw treatment of the control serum because this may cause loss of potency.

4. Phosphate buffered saline (PBS): Each vial of buffer concentrate dilutes to 1 L with distilled water.

STORAGE INSTRUCTIONS

1. EB-VCA slides: Store at 2 to 8° C until outdated.

2. Goat anti-human IgM, fluorescein conjugated: The reconstituted preparation is stable for 4 weeks when stored at 2 to 8° C.

3. EB-VCA IgM low positive human serum: The reconstituted control serum is stable for 6 weeks when stored at 2 to 8° C.

4. EB-VCA IgM negative control human serum: The reconstituted control serum is stable for 6 weeks when stored at 2 to 8° C.

5. Phosphate buffered saline solution: Diluted PBS is stable 4 to 6 weeks at room temperature.

6. Mounting fluid: store at 2 to 8° C. Keep vial tightly capped when not in use.

PROCEDURE

1. Remove appropriate number of five-well slides from refrigerator.

NOTE: Each time the test is run, three wells are required for the controls in addition to one well for each test specimen. Allow to warm to room temperature before opening. Cut foil at indicated end, remove slide, and identify each sample by labeling the frosted area of each slide.

CAUTION: Once a packet is opened, slide should be used within 60 minutes.

2. Place each slide, well-side up, in a moisture chamber.

3. Negative control sera and conjugate control must be used each time the test is performed.

4. Prepare a 1:10 dilution of the patient serum in the PBS supplied. Dilutions may be prepared in either micro-dilution plates or tubes.

5. Place one drop (15 to 20 μl) of diluted serum or PBS into each well making certain each cell area is completely covered. *Note:* If more than 20 μl of samples are used, it may be necessary to mark between the wells on the slides with a wax pencil to prevent samples from spreading between wells. Use of a calibrated micropipet is recommended.

6. Cover moisture chamber and incubate at 37° C for 90 minutes.

Caution: Handle the chambers carefully to prevent liquid in the wells from running together while transporting them.

7. Remove slide from moisture chamber and gently rinse each slide with PBS.

8. Soak slides in two additional changes of PBS for 5 minutes each.

9. Rinse slides briefly with distilled or deionized water.

10. Allow slides to dry at room temperature.

11. Replace the slides in the moisture chamber.

12. Add one drop (15 to 20 μl) of Goat Anti-Human IgM fluorescein conjugate containing Evans Blue Counterstain to each well using the plastic dispensing vial.

13. Cover moisture chamber and incubate at 37° C for 30 minutes.

14. Remove slides from moisture chamber and gently rinse each slide with PBS. Soak in two additional changes of PBS for 5 minutes each.

15. Rinse slides with distilled or deionized water.

16. Use a tissue to wipe the water off back of slide.

17. Allow the slides to dry at room temperature.

18. Place a small drop of Mounting Fluid in each well and carefully place a cover glass to avoid trapping air bubbles.

19. Immediately examine each slide with the fluorescence microscope. (The intensity and color of fluorescent staining may vary if the filters and light source other than indicated above are used.) If the slides cannot be examined immediately, store them in a light-tight container at 2 to 8° C and examine within 24 hours.

REPORTING. Report as positive or negative for IgM Anti-EBV-VCA.

INTERPRETATION OF RESULTS

1. Conjugate Control: On occasion, a small number of cells may exhibit fluorescence. This fluorescence is insignificant in the interpretation of the EBV-M test.

2. Negative Control: The same type of cell fluorescence seen in the Conjugate Control can be expected to be seen in the Negative Control (with a slight increase in intensity).

NOTE: The 1:10 dilution used represents the amount of background seen with most patients' sera also diluted 1:10.

3. Positive Control: The positive control serum contains IgM antibody to EB-VCA at the minimally significant level.

4. Test Specimen:

a. Positive Reaction: A specimen is considered positive when it exhibits at least the amount of fluorescent staining seen in the Positive Control serum.

Periodically, a test specimen will exhibit nonspecific fluorescence over the total cell sheet. If the specimen is a "strong" positive, the reaction can be seen through the nonspecific background fluorescence. If the specimen cannot be read at a 1:10 dilution, the result is equivocal.

NOTE: It may be possible to detect a positive reaction by evaluating such a specimen at a 1:20 dilution because of decreased background staining.

b. Negative Reaction: A specimen that does not exhibit the amount of fluorescence (intensity and number of cells) observed in the positive control serum is considered as having an undetectable amount of IgM antibody to EBV-VCA.

c. Nonspecific Reaction: (1) Rheumatoid Factor: It is recognized that rheumatoid factor causes false-positive reactions in IgM test systems. *Therefore, serum determined to be positive in the EBV-M test must be tested for the presence of rheumatoid factor.* These RF(+) sera should be adsorbed with either heat-aggregated human gamma globulin or with a commercially prepared reagent.[1,2] After adsorption, sera should again be tested to confirm EB-VCA IgM fluorescence.

(2) ANA: Nonspecific staining such as that seen with Anti Nuclear Antibodies would be restricted to the nuclei of the cell.

5. Because specific IgM antibody to EB-VCA appears within 1 to 2 weeks after onset

of clinical symptoms and drops to undetectable levels within 8 to 10 weeks, the EB-VCA IgM assay is particularly helpful when only one serum specimen is available for determining the presence of current infection.

6. IgM antibody to EB-VCA as measured in the IFA tests, is demonstrable in 90% of cases of infectious mononucleosis early in illness.[2] The presence of IgM antibody is highly suggestive of acute EBV infection.

LIMITATIONS OF THE PROCEDURE

1. In some cases, human serum may contain antinuclear antibody (ANA). The distinction between ANA and antibody to VCA is based on the site of the reaction. ANA staining occurs within the nucleus of the cell whereas anti-VCA staining occurs on the cell periphery and in the cytoplasm of the cell.

2. Rheumatoid factor may cause false-positive reactions in IgM test systems.

3. A negative EB-VCA, IgM Antibody test result does not necessarily rule out current EBV infection. The specimen may have been collected before demonstrable antibody is present or after the antibody level is no longer detectable. Demonstration of elevated EB-VCA IgG titers in conjunction with specific EBV-IgM improves the specificity of serologic diagnosis.

4. In a few sera with high concentrations of IgM, a slight nonspecific fluorescence of almost all cells may be noticed. However, this fluorescence is easily distinguishable from the specific fluorescence of the cells infected by EBV.

REFERENCES

1. Gallo, D., Walen, K.H. and Riggs, J.L.: J. Clin. Microbiol., 15:243, 1982.
2. Nickoskelainen, J. and Hanninen, P.: Infect. Immunol., 11:42, 1975.
3. Package Insert, EBV-M Kit, Organon Teknika, Inc., Malvern, PA, 1986.

Anti-EBV Early Antigen[1]

PRINCIPLE. This indirect fluorescent assay (IFA) for EBV-EA is designed to detect circulating antibodies to the EBV early antigens (EA-D and EA-R) in human sera. The test system uses Raji cells that express early antigen immobilized on glass slides. The test procedure involves two steps. In the first step, human test serum is reacted with the Raji cell substrate on a glass slide. In a positive specimen, antibodies in the serum will bind to the cells and remain attached after rinsing. Fluorescein-labeled antihuman IgG added in the second step will bind to the antibodies, causing the cells to fluoresce applegreen under a fluorescent microscope. The intensity of staining is graded on a scale of 1+ to 4+ or as negative. Sera negative for EBV-EA antibody will show only red background staining of all the cells.

EQUIPMENT AND MATERIALS

1. EBV-EA kit components—Zeus Scientific

a. EBV-EA Antigen Slides: Ten 10-well substrate slides containing infected Raji cells in each well

b. Anti-Human IgG (γ) FITC-labeled conjugate: Contains 1.25% bovine albumin and Evans Blue counterstain. Two 1.5-ml vials-lyophilized

c. EBV-EA Human Positive Control Serum: Two 0.5-ml vials, lyophilized

d. EBV-EA Human Negative Control Serum: Two 0.5-ml vials, lyophilized

e. Phosphate buffered saline (PBS): Sufficient to prepare 4 L

f. Mounting fluid (buffered glycerol): 3.0 ml

g. Blotters

2. Small serologic pasteur, capillary or automatic pipettes

3. Small test tubes, 12 × 75 mm or comparable

4. Test tube racks

5. Staining dish

6. 37° C incubator

7. Moist chamber

8. Cover slips, 24 × 50 mm thickness No. 1

9. Distilled water—CAP Type 1 or equivalent

10. Wash bottle

11. Properly equipped fluorescence microscope assembly:

Exciter Filter	BG-12 (3 mm) or equivalent
Barrier Filter	OG-1 or equivalent
Light Source	HBO 200 or equivalent
Objective	24–54 × oil immersion or high dry

PRECAUTIONS

1. All sera, antisera, and buffered glycerol contain preservative; (Thimerosal, 1:10,000).

2. Use proper universal blood and body fluid precautions.

SPECIMEN COLLECTION AND PREPARATION
Only freshly drawn and properly refrigerated blood sera should be used in this assay. No anticoagulants or preservatives should be added. Avoid using hemolytic, lipemic, or bacterially contaminated sera. Sera showing bacterial contaminants may be passed through a 0.45 μ filter or centrifuged at 1000 ×g for 30 minutes before testing. Sera should be stored at 2 to 8° C for no longer than 5 days. If delay in testing is anticipated, store test sera at −20° C or lower.

PREPARATION OF REAGENTS

1. Phosphate Buffered Saline solution (PBS)—pH 7.2 ± 0.1: Empty contents of one buffer pack in 1 L of distilled water. Mix until all salts are thoroughly dissolved.

2. EBNA Human Positive and Negative Control Sera: Reconstitute with 0.5 mL of sterile distilled water (see storage instructions).

3. Anti-Human IgG (γ) FITC-Labeled Conjugate: Reconstitute with 1.5 mL of sterile distilled water. Reconstituted conjugate may be aliquoted in 0.5 ml amounts and stored at −20°C or lower in small tightly capped tubes.

NOTE: Reconstitute reagents gently but thoroughly. Reagents should be free of particulate matter. If reagents become cloudy, bacterial contamination should be suspected.

STORAGE INSTRUCTIONS

—EBV-EA Substrate Slides: −20° C or lower, stable for 2 years. 2 to 5° C, stable for 1 year.

—Anti-human IgG (γ) FITC-labeled conjugate: 2 to 5° C, stable for 90 days after reconstitution. Frozen aliquots are stable for 6 months at −20° C or lower.

—Positive and negative human EBV-EA control serum: 2 to 5° C, stable for 90 days after reconstitution. Frozen aliquots are stable for 6 months at −20° C or lower.

—Phosphate buffered saline solution: Room temperature. Store reconstituted buffer at 2 to 5° C. Stable for 30 days.

—Mounting fluid (buffered glycerol): 2 to 5° C. Stable for 1 year.

NOTE:

1. All kit components are stable until the expiration date printed on the label, provided the recommended storage conditions are strictly followed.

2. Do not freeze and thaw reagents more than once. Repeated freezing and thawing destroys antibody activity.

PROCEDURE

1. Remove substrate slide from the freezer and open the protective envelope. DO NOT APPLY PRESSURE TO FLAT SIDES OF PROTECTIVE ENVELOPE. THIS MAY DESTROY THE CELL MATRIX ON THE SLIDE. Remove slide containing the EBV-infected cells.

2. Positive, negative, and buffer controls should be run each time the test is performed.

3. Prepare 1:10, 1:20, 1:40, and 1:80 dilutions of test sera in PBS.

4. Identify each well with the appropriate patient sera and control on worksheet.

5. Spread 20 μl of test and control sera over each appropriately labeled well. Be careful not to disturb the substrate cells with the pipette tip.

6. Incubate slides in a sealed moist chamber at 37° C for 30 minutes. DO NOT ALLOW WELLS TO DRY!

7. Take slides from the moist chamber and remove excess sera from the wells by gently rinsing slides with a stream of PBS. DO NOT FLUSH THE STREAM OF PBS DIRECTLY INTO THE TEST WELLS.

8. Place slides in a staining dish and wash in PBS for two 5-minute intervals with a change of PBS. DO NOT AGITATE.

9. Remove slides one at a time from PBS. Invert slides and key wells to holes in blotters provided. Blot slides by wiping the reverse side with an absorbent wipe. POSITION THE BLOTTER AND SLIDE ON A HARD FLAT SURFACE. NOTE: BLOTTING ON BENCH PAPER OR ON PAPER TOWELS MAY DESTROY THE SLIDE MATRIX.

10. Add 20 μl of conjugate to each well.

11. Place slides in moist chamber. Incubate slides for 30 minutes at 37° C. *DO NOT ALLOW SLIDES TO DRY!*

12. Repeat steps 7, 8 and 9.

13. Add 3 to 4 drops of buffered glycerol to the mask area of each slide and coverslip. Slides should be examined immediately under a fluorescent microscope at a total magnification of 250×.

REPORTING. Report as positive or negative for Anti-EBV early antigen with titer value for positive results.

INTERPRETATION OF RESULTS

1. 1+ to 4+ applegreen fluorescence in approximately 15 to 20% of the total cell population indicates a positive reaction.

2. Positive cells express both R and D components of EA. However, the test system is not designed to differentiate between antibodies to the R and D components.

3. The red background staining due to the Evans Blue counterstain on all of the cells indicates a negative reaction.

4. All positive sera should be titered to endpoint. The endpoint is the last dilution that shows 1+ applegreen fluorescent staining.

LIMITATIONS OF THE PROCEDURE

1. A diagnosis should not be made on the basis of anti-EA titers alone. Test results for anti-EA should be interpreted in conjunction with results of antibody tests for other EBV specific antigens, i.e. VCA and EBNA.

2. Nuclear or cytoplasmic staining may be observed due to nonspecific or autoantibody reactions such as antinuclear or mitochrondrial antibodies associated with systemic lupus erythematosus and primary biliary cirrhosis respectively.

3. Nonspecific staining of all cells may be observed in some sera at low dilutions.

4. The endpoint reactions may vary due to the type of microscope employed, the light source, age of bulb, filter assembly and filter thickness.

REFERENCE

1. Package Insert, EBV-EA Kit, Zeus Scientific, Raritan, NJ, 1987.

Anti-EBV Nuclear Antigen[1]

PRINCIPLE. The test system is designed to detect circulating antibody to the Epstein Barr Virus Nuclear Antigen (EBNA) and utilizes the anti-complement immunofluorescence (ACIF) procedure. The test procedure involves three steps; in the first step, patient serum which has been heat inactivated is reacted with substrate slides containing a mixture of EBNA positive and negative cells. Antibodies to EBNA will react with the EBNA positive cell substrate and remain attached after washing. In the second step, guinea pig complement is added and reacts with the antigen-antibody complexes. Finally, fluorescein (FITC) labeled antibody to the C3 component of guinea pig complement is added and will react with the antibody-complement complexes. Serum specimens containing antibody to EBNA will show applegreen fluorescence of the cell nuclei.

EQUIPMENT AND MATERIALS

1. EBNA kit components—Zeus Scientific

a. EBNA Antigen Slides: Ten 10-well substrate slides containing EBNA positive and EBNA negative cells in each well

b. FITC labeled anti-guinea pig C3: Contains 1% bovine albumin and Evans blue counterstain. Two 1.5-ml vials, lyophilized

c. Guinea pig complement: One 0.5-ml vial, lyophilized

d. EBNA Human Positive Control Serum: Two 0.5-ml vials, lyophilized

e. EBNA Human Negative Control Serum: Two 0.5-ml vials, lyophilized

f. Complement Dilution buffer with Ca^{2+} and Mg^{2+}: One 5.0-ml vial

g. Phosphate buffered saline solution: Four packets of salts

h. Mounting fluid: (buffered glycerol) 3.0-ml vial

i. Blotters

2. Small serologic pasteur, capillary or automatic pipettes

3. Small test tubes, 12 × 75 mm or comparable

4. Test tube racks

5. Staining dish: A large staining dish with a small magnetic mixing set-up provides an ideal mechanism for washing slides between incubation steps

6. Cover slips, 24 × 50 mm thickness No. 1

7. Distilled water—CAP type or equivalent

8. Wash bottle

9. 1 L volumetric flask

10. Moist incubation chamber

11. 37° C incubator

12. 56° C water bath

13. Properly equipped fluorescence microscope assembly.

Exciter Filter	BG-12 (3 mm) or equivalent
Barrier Filter	OG-1 or equivalent
Light Source	HBO 200 or equivalent
Objective	24-54 × oil immersion or high dry

PRECAUTIONS

1. Control sera, Conjugate and Complement dilution buffers contain 0.01% thimerosal as a preservative.

2. Use proper universal blood and body fluid precautions.

SPECIMEN COLLECTION AND PREPARATION.

Only freshly drawn and properly refrigerated blood sera should be employed in this assay. No anticoagulants or preservatives should be added. Avoid using hemolytic, lipemic or bacterially contaminated sera. Sera showing bacterial contaminants may be passed through a 0.45 μ filter or centrifuged at 1000 ×g for 30 minutes before testing. Sera should be stored at 2 to 8° C for no longer than 5 days. If delay in testing is anticipated, store test sera at −20° C or lower.

PREPARATION OF REAGENTS

1. Phosphate Buffered Saline solution (PBS): Empty contents of one buffer pack in 1 L of distilled water. Mix until all salts are thoroughly dissolved.

2. EBNA Human Positive and Negative Control Sera: Reconstitute with 0.5 ml of sterile distilled water.

3. Anti-Guinea Pig C3 FITC-Labeled Conjugate: Reconstitute with 1.5 ml of sterile distilled water. Reconstituted conjugate may be aliquoted in 0.5-ml amounts and stored at −20° C or lower in small, tightly capped tubes.

4. Guinea Pig Complement: Reconstitute with 0.5-ml sterile distilled water. If not used immediately, complement should be aliquoted in 0.1-ml amounts and stored at −70° C in tightly capped tubes. To obtain an optimum working dilution of complement, take a 0.1-ml aliquot of complement and dilute to 1.0 ml with the dilution buffer provided. Do not freeze and thaw complement more than once.

NOTE: Reconstitute reagents gently but thoroughly. Reagents should be free of particulate matter. If reagents become cloudy, bacterial contamination should be suspected.

STORAGE INSTRUCTIONS

—EBNA Substrate Slides: −20° C or lower, stable for 2 years. 2 to 5° C, stable for 1 year.

—Anti-guinea pig C3 FITC-labeled conjugate: 2 to 5° C, stable for 90 days after reconstitution. Frozen aliquots are stable for 6 months at −20° C or lower.

—Positive and negative human EBNA control sera: 2 to 5° C, stable for 90 days after reconstitution. Frozen aliquots are stable for 6 months at −20° C or lower.

—Phosphate buffered saline solution: Room temperature. Store reconstituted buffer at 2 to 5° C. Stable for 30 days.

—Mounting fluid (buffered glycerol): 2 to 5° C. Stable for 1 year.

—Guinea pig complement: 2 to 5° C. Store reconstituted complement at −70° C. Stable for 6 weeks.

—Complement Dilution Buffer: 2 to 5° C. Stable for 1 year.

NOTE:

1. All kit components are stable until the expiration date printed on the label, provided the recommended storage conditions are strictly followed.

2. Do not freeze and thaw reagents more

than once. Repeated freezing and thawing destroys antibody activity.

PROCEDURE

1. Heat inactivate all sera to be tested at 56° C for 30 minutes to destroy endogenous complement.

2. Prepare 1:5, 1:10, 1:20, and 1:40 dilutions of test sera in PBS. Positive, negative, and buffer control should be run undiluted each time test is performed.

3. Remove substrate slide from the freezer, open the protective envelope, taking care not to apply pressure to the flat surfaces of the slide. Remove slide containing the cell substrate. *DO NOT APPLY PRESSURE TO FLAT SIDES OF PROTECTIVE ENVELOPE. THIS MAY DESTROY THE CELL MATRIX ON THE SLIDE.*

4. Identify each well with the appropriate patient sera and controls.

5. Spread 20 µl of test and control sera over each appropriately labeled well. Be careful not to disturb the substrate cells with the pipette tip.

6. Incubate slides in a sealed moist chamber at 37° C for 20 minutes. *DO NOT ALLOW WELLS TO DRY!*

7. Take slides from the moist chamber and remove excess sera from the wells by gently rinsing slides with a stream of PBS. *DO NOT DIRECT THE STREAM OF PBS INTO THE TEST WELLS.*

8. Place slides in a staining dish containing PBS and stir gently for 5 minutes.

9. Remove slides one at a time from PBS. Invert slides and key wells to holes in blotters provided. Blot slides by wiping the reverse side with an absorbent wipe. *POSITION THE BLOTTER AND SLIDE ON A HARD FLAT SURFACE. BLOTTING ON BENCH PAPER OR ON PAPER TOWELS MAY DESTROY THE SLIDE MATRIX.*

10. Prepare fresh guinea pig complement just before use. Add 20 µl of 1:10 diluted guinea pig complement to each well.

11. Repeat steps 6, 7, 8 and 9.

12. Add 20 µl of anti-guinea pig C3 fluorescein conjugate to each well.

13. Repeat steps 6, 7, 8 and 9.

14. Add three to four drops of buffered glycerol to the mask area of each slide and coverslip. Slides should be examined immediately under a fluorescent microscope at a total magnification of 250×.

REPORTING. Results are reported as positive or negative for anti-EBV Nuclear Antigen with titer value for positive results.

INTERPRETATION OF RESULTS

1. A positive reaction is indicated by a granular, nuclear staining pattern of apple-green fluorescence in about 25% of the cells on the EBNA slide. Only 25% of the cells should stain positive for EBNA. Nuclear staining of nearly 100% of the cells indicates the presence of antibodies to nuclear antigens (ANA) and precludes an assay for EBNA. In this case, test serum should be tested in an ANA Test System. (See *Auto antibody Tests: ANA*).

2. All positive sera should be titered to endpoint. The endpoint is the last dilution that shows 1+ applegreen fluorescent staining.

3. A negative reaction is indicated by the absence of nuclear fluorescence and a red background staining of all cells due to Evans blue counterstain. Use the reactions of the positive and negative control sera as a guide.

LIMITATIONS OF THE PROCEDURE

1. A diagnosis should not be made on the basis of anti-EBNA titers alone. Test results for anti-EBNA should be interpreted in conjunction with results of antibody tests for other EBV specific antigens, i.e. VCA and EA.

2. The endpoint reactions may vary due to the type of microscope employed, the light source, age of bulb, filter assembly and filter thickness.

REFERENCE

1. Package insert, EBNA kit, Zeus Scientific, Raritan, NJ, 1987.

VIRAL HEPATITIS[7]

The word "hepatitis" means liver inflammation. Although many agents, including radiation, chemicals, infectious organisms, and autoimmune processes, may be responsible for this inflammation, current medical practice employs the term "hepatitis" most often to describe viral hepatitis.[2] Several etiologic agents, including herpes simplex virus, Epstein Barr virus, and cytomegalovirus, are capable of inducing liver inflammation, but "hepatitis" most often refers to disease caused by viruses whose primary effect is on the liver. These viruses, and their primary modes of transmission, are listed below:

(1) Hepatitis A virus—fecal-oral route

(2) Hepatitis B virus—parenteral route (i.e. contact with blood or other body fluids)

(3) Hepatitis Delta virus—parenteral route. This virus exists only as a coinfection with Hepatitis B virus.

(4) Non A, Non B hepatitis viruses— The majority of non-A, non-B hepatitis cases in the United States are now thought to be due to a parenterally-transmitted virus termed Hepatitis C.[1,8] With the use of recombinant DNA technology, this agent has been identified as a single-stranded RNA virus.[1] An assay to detect antibodies to Hepatitis C has been developed and is being used by blood banks.[4,8] A variant form of hepatitis B called Hepatitis B-2, may also be responsible for some of the cases of post-transfusion hepatitis classified as non-A, non-B.[5] The possibility exists that other cases in this category may be attributed to an as yet unidentified agent.[8] An etiologic agent (Hepatitis E virus) transmitted by the fecal-oral route has also been included in the non-A, non-B hepatitis category.[6]

The hepatitis viruses differ in molecular structure and incubation period, but the clinical and morphologic manifestations they produce are remarkably similar.[3] (See *Hepatitis A; Hepatitis B.*)

REFERENCES

1. Choo, Q.-L, et al.: Science 244:359, 1989.
2. Fody, E.P., and Johnson, D.F.: J. Med. Technol. 4:54, 1987.
3. Hoofnagle, J.H.: *Perspectives on Viral Hepatitis—Types A and B Viral Hepatitis.* Abbott Laboratories, Diagnostics Division, North Chicago, 1981.
4. Kuo, G., et. al.: Science 244:362, 1989.
5. Lai, M.E., et al.: Blood 73:17, 1989.
6. Reyes, G.R., et. al.: Science 247:1335, 1990.
7. Vyas, G.N., et. al. (Eds.): *Viral Hepatitis.* Franklin Institute Press, Philadelphia, 1978.
*8. Waldman, A.A.: Diagnostics and Clinical Testing 27:21, 1989.

HEPATITIS A

Hepatitis A, classically referred to as infectious hepatitis, is caused by a member of the Picornaviridae family called the Hepatitis A virus (HAV). The HAV virion is a non-enveloped sphere, approximately 27 nm in diameter, consisting of a single-stranded RNA genome and a capsid containing four major structural proteins, designated VP1 through VP4.[4,8,9,11]

Transmission of the virus occurs primarily through the fecal-oral route, and is facilitated by conditions of poor personal hygiene, poor sanitation, and overcrowding.[1,4] The major mode of transmission appears to be direct person-to-person contact, but transmission by drinking from a fecally-contaminated water supply, ingesting food prepared by an infected food handler, or consuming raw shellfish containing concentrated quantities of the virus has been well-documented, and contact with infected fomites may also play a significant role in transmission.[4,6,9] Fecal contamination of food or water has resulted in a number of well-publicized common source outbreaks of Hepatitis A, but these account for only a small fraction of the total cases in the United States; most cases are acquired sporadically or endemically.[4,9] Those at high risk for contracting HAV include family members of persons with Hepatitis A, homosexual men, particularly those with oral-anal contacts, institutionalized persons (e.g. mentally retarded individuals, prisoners, military personnel), young children in day care centers, where oral behavior and lack of toilet training facilitate transmission, and contacts of these children, individuals who travel to foreign countries where sanitation is poor, and individuals who use illicit drugs.[5,9] Prevention of infection has been accomplished through the administration of immune globulin, containing antibodies to HAV, when exposure is anticipated as a result of occupation, travel, or close personal contact with an infected person, or within 2 weeks post-exposure in common source outbreaks.[9,13] A safe and effective vaccine against HAV is not yet available.[4,9,10,13] Transmission via blood transfusions or percutaneous contact has been rarely documented, most likely because the duration of viremia after infection with HAV is limited.[7,9]

The incubation period for HAV ranges from 15 to 45 days, with an average of 25 days.[2,8] During this time, the virus replicates and is shed in the stool, with peak fecal concentrations (10^8 particles/g) being reached late in the incubation period,[1,4,8] and continuing into the prodromal phase of illness. The late incubation period, when symptoms are not yet evident, is thus the period of greatest infectivity. Viremia also occurs, but is of short duration. Low concentrations of virus may be present in saliva,[8,9] but HAV has not been detected in urine, semen, or other body fluids.

Children infected with HAV at 2 years of age or younger frequently have symptoms of mild disease, including malaise, nausea, fever, diarrhea, abdominal pain, and vomiting; however, these are often not recognized as symptoms of hepatitis.[6,9] The majority of older children and adults infected with HAV, on the other hand, have symptoms of overt hepatitis A.[8,9] After the incubation period, nonspecific symptoms, including malaise, fatigue, anorexia, nausea and vomiting, and mild to moderate right upper quadrant abdominal pain, are experienced for a period lasting 2 to 15 days. These are followed by the onset of jaundice, the appearance of dark urine (due to bilirubinuria) and light-colored stool, hepatic tenderness and hepatomegaly, and occasionally, splenomegaly. Typically, hepatitis A is a self-limiting disease, with symptoms lasting from 2 weeks to 2 months. In occasional patients, symptoms may persist for 4 months or longer but eventually resolve. The fatality rate is low (0.14%).[9] Unlike hepatitis B or hepatitis non A, non B, hepatitis A has not been observed to progress to chronic liver disease or a persistent carrier state.[4,8,9]

Diagnosis of acute hepatitis A is accomplished through evaluation of clinical symptoms and patient history, demonstration of nonspecific laboratory findings associated with liver injury, and demonstration of IgM antibody to HAV. The enzymes, alanine aminotransferase (ALT, SGPT) and aspartate aminotransferase (AST, SGOT) are characteristically elevated in the sera of patients with acute viral hepatitis, reaching levels 10 to 100 fold greater than normal.[8] These enzymes become elevated during the late incubation period, reach peak levels when jaundice and other symptoms of liver injury are evident, and decline rapidly during recovery, but may remain outside of the reference range for several weeks or months after symptoms have subsided. Bilirubin is increased approximately 25-fold during periods of jaundice, while alkaline phosphatase and lactic dehydrogenase are mildly elevated.[8]

Differentiation of hepatitis A from other types of hepatitis is accomplished through demonstration of antibody to HAV. Methods of choice detect IgM antibody, which, when present in a single serum sample, indicates acute infection. IgM antibody to Hepatitis A appears about 4 to 5 weeks after exposure, reaches peak levels at 8 to 12 weeks, and becomes undetectable by 3 to 6 months.[4,9] IgG antibody rises more gradually, reaching peak levels during the convalescent phase of disease, and usually persists at detectable levels thereafter, providing life-long immunity for the individual. A fourfold rise in IgG may be used to confirm a recent infection, but is usually not observed during the acute phase of Hepatitis A.[12] Methods of choice for detecting antibody to HAV are radioimmunoassay (RIA) and enzyme linked immunosorbent assay (ELISA).[4] Methods for detecting HAV antigen in feces have also been developed,[3] but are not readily available in the clinical laboratory, and often yield negative results, as viral shedding peaks during the late incubation period of hepatitis A and is frequently absent by the time the patient presents with clinical symptoms of acute infection.[4]

REFERENCES

1. Centers for Disease Control: MMWR, *34*:313, 1985.

2. Chang, Y.-W.: Diagn. Med., p. 28, July/August 1983.

3. Chaudhary, R.K.: Am. J. Clin. Pathol., *81*:337, 1984.

*4. Coulepis, A.G., Anderson, B.N., and Gust, I.D.: Adv. Virus. Res., *32*:129, 1987.

5. Francis, D.P. et al.: Am. J. Med., *76*:69, 1984.

6. Hadler, S.C., and McFarland, L.: Rev. Infect. Dis., *8*:548, 1986.

7. Hollinger, F.B. et al.: JAMA, *250*:2313, 1983.

8. Hoofnagle, J.H.: *Perspectives on Viral Hepatitis— Types A and B Viral Hepatitis*. North Chicago, Abbott Laboratories, Diagnostics Division, 1981.

*9. Lemon, S.M.: N. Engl. J. Med., *313*:1059, 1985.

10. McLean, A.A.: Rev. Infect. Dis., *8*:591, 1986.

11. Murray, K.: Proc. R. Soc. Lond. Biol., *230*:107, 1987.

12. Perrillo, R.P.: *Perspectives on Viral Hepatitis—The Hepatitis Viruses: Differential Diagnosis*. North Chicago, Abbott Laboratories, Diagnostics Division, 1981.

13. Schiff, E.: Am. J. Gastroenterol., *82*:287, 1987.

Hepatitis A Virus Antibody-Enzyme Immunoassay for IgM (HAVAB-M EIA)

PRINCIPLE. In the HAVAB-M EIA test, a diluted serum or plasma specimen is prepared using normal saline solution then pipetted into a reaction well with diluent supplied in the kit. A bead coated with goat anti-human immunoglobulin, specific for human IgM (μ chain), is then added to the reaction well and binds any IgM in the patient's specimen during the incubation. After thorough washing, hepatitis A virus antigen (HAV Ag) is added to the reaction well and incubated with the bead. If anti-HAV IgM is present in the patient specimen, the HAV Ag binds to the bead-antibody complex. After a second wash, human anti-HAV conjugated with horseradish peroxidase (anti-HAV: HRPO) is incubated with the bead-antibody-antigen complex. Unbound enzyme conjugate is then aspirated and the beads washed. Next, o-phenylenediamine (OPD) substrate solution containing hydrogen peroxide is added to the bead and, during incubation, a yellow color develops in proportion to the amount of enzyme conjugate bound to the bead. The enzyme reaction is stopped by the addition of acid.

The absorbance values of controls and specimens are determined using a spectrophotometer with wavelength set at 492 nanometers (nm). A cutoff value and a retest range are calculated using the absorbance values of the controls. Specimens giving absorbance values equal to or greater than the cutoff are considered reactive for IgM antibody to hepatitis A virus.

Specimens that are repeatedly reactive in duplicate wells by this assay are considered positive for IgM antibody to hepatitis A virus by the criteria of the HAVAB-M EIA test. Specimens with absorbance values less than the cutoff value are considered nonreactive for IgM antibody to hepatitis A virus.

STORAGE INSTRUCTIONS

1. Store kit reagents at 2 to 8° C when received.

2. All reagents must be at 15 to 30° C (room temperature) for use, but should be returned to 2 to 8° C storage immediately after use. OPD tablets may be stored at room temperature. Caution: Do not open OPD tablet bottle until it is at room temperature.

3. Retain desiccant bags in OPD tablet bottle at all times during storage.

4. Reconstituted OPD solution MUST be held at room temperature and MUST be used within 60 minutes.

SPECIMEN COLLECTION AND PREPARATION

1. The HAVAB-M EIA test may be performed on human serum or plasma.

2. Anti-HAV IgM is stable in serum or plasma, and has been detected in stored samples after several years. If specimens are to be stored, they may be stored at 2 to 8° C for up to 5 days. However, if storage periods greater than 5 days are anticipated, the specimens must be frozen.

3. Prepare a 1:200 dilution of each specimen by adding 10 μL of specimen to 2.0 mL of 0.15M normal saline solution (NS) in test tubes and mix before use in the test procedure. (*Note:* Do not dilute controls). Use dilutions within 4 hours of preparation.

4. If specimens are to be retested, prepare new dilutions as described above.

5. Specimens containing copious amounts of precipitate may give inconsistent test results. To prevent this problem,

such specimens should be clarified by ultra centrifugation prior to testing.

EQUIPMENT AND MATERIALS

Kit contains:

1. Antibody to human IgM (goat) coated beads

2. Antibody to hepatitis A virus (human): horseradish peroxidase conjugate (Anti-HAV:HRPO)

3. Hepatitis A virus (HAV) solution (human)

4. Specimen diluent HAVAB-M EIA

5. Positive control HAVAB-M EIA (positive for anti-HAV IgM, and nonreactive for HBsAg)

6. Negative control HAVAB-M EIA (nonreactive for anti-HAV and HBsAg)

7. OPD (o-phenylenediamine 2 HCl)

8. Diluent for OPD

9. 1N sulfuric acid

10. Reaction trays

11. Cover sealers

12. Assay tubes with identifying cartons

13. Assay tube box covers

Kit *does not* include:

14. Precision pipettes with disposable tips to deliver 10 μL, 200 μL, and 300 μL

15. Device for delivery of rinse solution, such as Gorman-Rupp pump, Cornwall syringe, or equivalent

16. An aspiration device for washing coated beads such as a Pentawash® II, or Uniwash™ II cannula, or aspirator tip and a vacuum source and trap for retaining the aspirate

17. Waterbath capable of maintaining temperature at 40° C ± 1° C

18. Disposable graduated pipettes or dispenser for measuring diluent for OPD

19. Pipettes for dispensing antibody conjugate, HAV solution, and specimen diluent

20. Repipet for dispensing 1N sulfuric acid

21. Nonmetallic forceps

22. Abbott Quantum II or other spectrophotometer capable of reading absorbance at 492 nm

23. 0.15M normal saline solution for specimen dilutions

24. Single bead dispenser

PROCEDURE

This procedure may be used to test human serum or plasma. Two negative and three positive controls should be assayed with each run of specimens. Ensure that all reaction trays containing controls or specimens are subjected to the same process and incubation times. Once the assay has been started, all steps should be completed without interruption and within the time limits recommended in the procedure.

NOTE: Controls do not require dilution. Omit step 3 for controls.

CAUTION: Use a separate micropipette tip for each specimen transfer to avoid cross-contamination.

1. Bring all reagents to 15 to 30° C before beginning the assay procedure. Adjust temperature of waterbath to 40° C ± 1° C.

2. Identify the reaction tray wells for each specimen or control on data sheet. All patients are tested in duplicate.

3. To prepare 1:200 dilutions of each specimen, add 10 μl of specimens to 2.0 mL of 0.15M normal saline solution in small test tubes. Mix thoroughly. Do not dilute controls.

4. Place 10 μL of each control or diluted specimen in the bottom of the appropriate wells using a micropipette. Do not allow the controls or diluted specimens to dry in the wells.

5. Add 200 μL of specimen diluent to each well containing the specimens and controls. Tap tray to mix.

6. Remove cap from bead bottle and attach the single bead dispenser. Carefully add one bead to each well containing a control or specimen.

7. Apply cover sealer to each tray. Gently tap to ensure that each bead is covered with the reaction mixture and that any air bubbles are released. Be careful not to splash liquid onto the cover. Incubate the trays in the 40° ± 1° C water bath for 1 hour ± 5 minutes.

8. At the end of the incubation period, remove and discard the cover sealers. Aspirate the contents of the wells and wash each bead. Follow the directions under Wash Procedure Details in the kit insert. Do not allow the beads to dry out.

9. Add 200 μL of HAV solution to each well containing a bead. Apply cover sealer to each tray. Gently tap to ensure that each bead is covered with the reaction mixture and that any air bubbles are released. Be careful not to splash liquid onto the cover. Incubate the trays at room temperature (15 to 30° C) for 18 to 22 hours.

10. At the end of the incubation period, remove and discard the cover sealers. Aspirate the contents of the wells and wash each bead. Follow the directions under Wash Procedure Details in the kit insert. Do not allow the beads to dry out.

11. Add 200 μL anti-HAV:HRPO conjugate to each well containing a bead. Apply cover

sealer to each tray. Gently tap to ensure that each bead is covered with the reaction mixture and that any air bubbles are released. Be careful not to splash liquid onto the cover. Incubate the trays in the 40° C ± 1° C waterbath for 2 hours ± 5 minutes.

12. During the last 5 to 10 minutes of the incubation, prepare the OPD substrate solution by dissolving the OPD (o-Phenylenediamine-2 HCl) tablets in diluent for OPD immediately before use (as described below). The solution must not be stored longer than 60 minutes before use.

NOTE: 300 µl is required for each test specimen.

a. Using a clean pipette, deliver 5 mL of diluent for OPD for each tablet to be dissolved into a suitable clean container.

CAUTION: Use pipettes and containers known to be metal and metal ion free.

b. Transfer tablets from bottle into diluent for OPD using a nonmetallic forceps or equivalent. Return desiccant to bottle immediately (if removed to obtain tablet(s)) and close bottle tightly. Allow tablets to dissolve.

c. Swirl gently to obtain a homogeneous solution just prior to dispensing for the final incubation of the assay.

13. At the end of the incubation period, remove and discard the cover sealers. Aspirate the contents of the wells, and wash each bead as in steps 8 and 10. Do not allow the beads to dry out. Remove all excess water from top of tray by aspiration or blotting.

14. Immediately transfer beads from wells to properly identified assay tubes. Align inverted rack of oriented tubes over the reaction tray and, pressing tubes tightly over wells, invert tray and tubes together so that beads fall into corresponding tubes. Blot excess water from the top of the tube rack. Tear off the cardboard top along perforations and discard it.

15. Pipette 300 µL of the freshly prepared OPD substrate solution into each tube containing a bead and into two empty tubes to be used as substrate blanks.

NOTE: Substrate solution should be clear to pale yellow. Do not allow substrate solution to contact any metal.

16. Incubate tubes at room temperature (15 to 30° C) for 30 ± 2 minutes. To prevent foreign material from contaminating the reaction and light from affecting color development, place black plastic cover on box until incubation is complete.

17. After the 30-minute incubation, stop the enzyme reaction by adding 1.0 mL of 1N sulfuric acid to each tube containing a bead and to each of the substrate blanks. Do not allow acid solution to come into contact with any metal. Ag-

itate tubes to ensure thorough mixing. Air bubbles in the liquid or on the tube should be removed prior to reading absorbance.

Set Quantum to appropriate mode. Refer to operator's manual for detailed instructions. Read the blank using one of the two substrate blank tubes. Read the absorbance of the negative and positive controls and then read the absorbance of the unknowns.

If the above instrument is not used, set a photometer or spectrophotometer at 492 nm and zero the instrument using one of the two substrate blanks. Determine the absorbance of the controls and specimens. The cuvette should be thoroughly rinsed with distilled or deionized water following each determination of absorbance.

If there is an interruption during the reading of the samples, repeat the blank using the second substrate blank and reread the controls. Continue reading specimens. All spectrophotometric readings should be done within two hours after addition of acid.

CALCULATIONS

1. Calculation of negative control mean absorbance ($NC\bar{x}$):
Determine the mean of the negative control values.

Example:

Negative Control

Sample No.	Absorbance
1	0.060
2	0.056

$$\text{Total Absorbance} = \frac{0.116}{2} = 0.058$$

2. Calculation of positive control mean absorbance ($PC\bar{x}$):

a. Determine the mean of the positive control values.

Example:

Positive Control

Sample No.	Absorbance
1	0.885
2	0.700
3	1.190

$$\text{Total Absorbance} = \frac{2.775}{3} = 0.925$$

b. All positive control values should fall within the range of 0.7 to 1.3 times the mean. If one value is outside this range, discard this value and recalculate the mean. If two values are outside this range, the test should be repeated. If more than an occasional value falls outside this range, technique problems should be suspected.

For the example given:

$$0.7 \times 0.925 = 0.648$$
$$1.3 \times 0.925 = 1.202$$
Range: 0.648 to 1.202

In the example, no positive control sample is rejected as aberrant. The positive control mean, therefore, need not be revised.

3. Calculation of the difference between the mean positive and the mean negative control values (P-N).
Subtract the NC$\bar{x}$ from the PC$\bar{x}$.

Example:
PC$\bar{x}$ positive control mean value	0.925
$-$NC$\bar{x}$ negative control mean value	-0.058
P-N Value	0.867

The P-N value should be 0.400 or greater. If not, technique or deterioration of reagents may be suspect and the run should be repeated.

4. Calculation of the cutoff value.
Add the NC$\bar{x}$ to one-tenth of the PC$\bar{x}$.

Example:

$$NC\bar{x} + \frac{PC\bar{x}}{10} = \text{cutoff value}$$

$$0.58 + \frac{0.925}{10} = 0.150$$

0.150 is the cutoff value.

5. Calculation of the retest range.
Calculate the ± 10% retest range around the cutoff.
Example:

Cutoff value 0.150

$$0.150 \pm 10\% = 0.150 - 0.15 \text{ to } 0.150 + 0.015$$

0.135 to 0.165 is the retest range.

REPORTING. Results are reported as positive or negative for IgM antibody to Hepatitis A virus.

INTERPRETATION OF RESULTS. The presence or absence of anti-HAV IgM is determined by comparing the absorbance of the specimen to a cutoff value. The cutoff value is calculated from the negative and positive control absorbance values as explained in the Calculations section.

1. Specimens with absorbance values less than the cutoff are nonreactive for anti-HAV IgM by the criteria of the HAVAB-M EIA test.

2. Specimens with absorbance values repeatedly equal to or greater than the cutoff value are positive for anti-HAV IgM by the criteria of the HAVAB-M EIA test.

3. Specimens with absorbance values within a ± 10% range of the cutoff value should be retested to confirm the initial results.

4. While actual absorbance values for the negative and positive controls may vary, the difference of these values (P-N) is less variable. The P-N value must be greater than 0.400 to ensure the validity of each run.

LIMITATIONS OF THE PROCEDURE. The HAVAB-M EIA assay is limited to the detection of anti-HAV IgM in human serum or plasma. It can be used to determine whether a patient has, or has recently had acute or subclinical hepatitis A infection. The test cannot determine a patient's immune status to hepatitis A, since it does not measure anti-HAV IgG.

HEPATITIS B

The hepatitis B virus (HBV), the cause of Hepatitis B, is a DNA virus classified in the hepadna virus group. The intact hepatitis B virion is a 42 nm, double-shelled sphere,[13,27,31] which was first described by Dane[12] and has been subsequently referred to as the Dane particle. It contains a 27-nm nucleocapsid core, containing circular, mostly double-stranded DNA, a DNA-dependent DNA polymerase, and a polypeptide component, known as the hepatitis B core antigen (HBcAg); the core, in turn, is surrounded by an outercoat, which contains a capsid protein known as the hepatitis B surface antigen (HBsAg). HBsAg, formerly called the Australia antigen,[7] can also circulate in the sera of HBV infected patients as free particles, which are 22 nm in diameter and assume either a spherical or long filamentous shape. Four subtypes of HBsAg, adr, adw, ayw, and ayr, have been characterized and serve as useful epidemiologic markers in tracing the source of infection.[13] A third antigen, the hepatitis Be antigen (HBeAg), is thought to be associated with the core of the virus, and like HBsAg, may be detected in the sera of infected individuals.

HBV is transmitted by parenteral exposure, close, intimate contact (primarily sexual) with an infected individual, and perinatally, from infected mother to infant.[9,13,27] Hepatitis B was formerly referred to as "serum hepatitis," because percutaneous exposure to contaminated blood has long been recognized as a major mode of transmission, and cases of hepatitis B resulting from transfusion of blood or blood products, needlestick accidents among health care professionals, and sharing of contaminated needles and syringes among intravenous drug abusers have been well documented.[9,13,27] However, "serum hepatitis" has become an outmoded designation for hepatitis B since the implementation of routine screening tests for hepatitis B infection, as HBV is now responsible for only a small fraction of post-transfusion hepatitis cases (non-A, non-B hepatitis, for which there was no specific screening test, has accounted for 80 to 90% of the cases reported in the United States[20]). In addition, approximately half of the individuals with hepatitis B acquire the infection through nonparenteral routes.[13,27]

HBV has been detected in several body fluids other than blood, most notably semen and saliva.[17,23,40] The virus may thus be transmitted through sexual contact with infected persons;[9,13,29] exposure to HBV is particularly prevalent in promiscuous male homosexual populations.[9,27] Contact of broken skin or mucous membranes with secretions from infected persons has been hypothesized to result in transmission among individuals having close personal contact, e.g. household contacts or clients of institutions for the mentally retarded.[1,9,13,41] Perinatal transmission of HBV has been documented and is more likely to occur at the time of delivery than in utero.[27,36] Some cases may occur postpartum, resulting from transmission through breast milk.[37]

Following transmission, HBV undergoes an incubation period ranging from 30 to 180 days (mean, 60 days).[8,27] The outcome of hepatitis B varies considerably, causing mild or asymptomatic infection, to fulminant, potentially fatal hepatitis, or chronic forms of hepatitis. About one-quarter of those infected develop an acute viral hepatitis with symptomatology similar to that seen in hepatitis A.[9] Typically, this is a self-limiting infection involving the liver, skin, joints, intestinal mucosa, kidneys, and hematopoietic system.[27,32] The usual mode of onset involves a prodromal period, lasting 2 to 3 weeks, when the patient has malaise and digestive disturbances, such as anorexia and vomiting, and mild to moderate right upper quadrant abdominal pain. This is followed by the appearance of darkened urine, lightened feces, and/or jaundice. Symptoms generally persist for 1 to 4 weeks, and complete recovery usually follows.

In 1 to 2% of cases, however, acute hepatitis B develops into fulminant liver disease with massive hepatic necrosis. There is no effective treatment for this complication, and the fatality rate is high (60 to 90%).[22]

Approximately 6 to 10% of adults and up to 90% of infants infected with HBV become chronic carriers of the virus and serve as a major reservoir of transmission of the disease.[9,22,27] Development of a chronic carrier state may be related to the state of the host's immune defenses;[14,32] patients with chronic forms of the disease are not classically immunodeficient, but the incidence of chronicity is higher in patients undergoing immunosuppressive therapy,[32] hemodialysis,[38] or pregnancy,[32] in individuals with advanced age[32] or diseases such as leukemia or leprosy,[6] and in institutionalized persons with Down syndrome,[5] as compared to other individuals infected with the virus. About 25% of HBV carriers develop chronic active hepatitis, with hepatic inflammation and necrosis lasting at least 6 months, and often progressing to cirrhosis.[9,22,27] Furthermore, HBV carriers are at increased risk of developing primary hepatocellular carcinoma,[4,9] one of the major causes of death in the world.

Another complication that occurs in some individuals with hepatitis B is concurrent infection with the hepatitis delta virus (HDV). Discovered in 1977 by Rizzetto et al.,[35] HDV is a defective pathogen whose maturation depends on the hepatitis B virus. The HDV virion is 36 nm in size and contains an RNA genome and the delta antigen, surrounded by an outer capsid consisting of HBsAg, which is produced by HBV.[3,25] HDV is thought to be transmitted via mechanisms similar to those responsible for the spread of hepatitis B, and has an incubation period of 2 to 12 weeks.[3,25] Hepatitis delta may occur as either a coinfection with hepatitis B or as a superinfection in a chronic HBV carrier. Coinfection with both viruses is usually clinically indistinguishable from HBV infection alone, but results in a greater tendency to develop fulminant hepatitis or a biphasic relapsing hepatitis.[21,25] Resolution of hepatitis B infection results in effective termination of hepatitis delta infection. Acute HDV infection in an individual already chronically infected with HBV (i.e. HDV superinfection) almost always results in chronic HDV infection as well,[21,25] and induces clinical exacerbation and more rapid progression to cirrhosis.[16,30]

Vaccination against hepatitis B infection is recommended for individuals at high risk of exposure to HBV and also protects against hepatitis delta.[10] The vaccines available consist of inactivated HBsAg, which is prepared either by purification from plasma of HBV carriers[19] or more recently, as a recombinant product of the yeast, *Saccharomyces cerevisiae,* into which the genetic code for HBsAg has been incorporated.[39] Administration of a hepatitis B vaccine and hepatitis B immune globulin (HBIG, prepared from plasma of individuals with high titer antibodies to HBsAg) is recommended for post exposure prophylaxis of nonimmune individuals to HBV.[10]

The laboratory evaluation of hepatitis B involves quantitation of enzymes which are nonspecifically elevated as a result of liver injury, and demonstration of specific hepatitis B markers in patient sera. The most prominently elevated enzymes are alanine aminotransferase (ALT, SGPT) and aspartate aminotransferase (AST, SGOT), which may increase 10 to 100 fold during the acute stage of infection;[27] alkaline phosphatase and lactic dehydrogenase are mildly elevated.[27] In addition, significant increases in bilirubin (approximately 25-fold greater than normal) are seen during periods of jaundice.[27]

Testing for specific hepatitis B markers is performed in order to differentiate hepatitis B from other types of viral hepatitis, to monitor patients during the course of disease, to assess immunity to HBV, and to screen blood products for infectivity. A list of the hepatitis B markers that can be detected and their clinical significance follows:[9,11,24,25]

1. *HBsAg*—Hepatitis B surface antigen. This marker is the first to appear after exposure to HBV, and is an indicator of active infection, either acute or chronic. Patients with HBsAg in their sera are considered infectious.

2. *HBeAg*—Hepatitis B e antigen. This marker appears shortly after HBsAg, is present during active replication of the virus in either acute or chronic infection, and indicates a high degree of infectivity.

3. *Anti-HBc*—Antibody to hepatitis B core antigen. This antibody becomes de-

tectable shortly after the onset of symptoms. IgM antibody indicates current or recent infection, while IgG antibody appears later, persists for life, and indicates either current or past HBV infection. Hepatitis B core antigen is usually not detectable in serum unless detergent is used to expose the inner core from the surrounding HBsAg envelope.

4. *Anti-HBe*—Antibody to hepatitis Be antigen. This antibody is detectable shortly after the disappearance of HBe antigen from the serum in acutely infected individuals and indicates that the infection is being resolved. Detectable levels of this antibody persist for long periods thereafter.

5. *Anti-HBs*—Antibody to hepatitis B surface antigen. This antibody appears during the convalescent phase of hepatitis B infection, and persists long thereafter. Presence of the antibody indicates protective immunity against HBV, induced either by natural infection or vaccination.

Over the years, a number of different methodologies have been developed to detect hepatitis B markers.[26] The oldest, or first generation method, is Ouchterlony double immunodiffusion. Second generation methods include counterimmunoelectrophoresis and complement fixation, and the most current, or third generation methods, are enzyme immunoassay (ELISA), radioimmunoassay (RIA), latex agglutination, and passive hemagglutination. In the United States, blood banks screening donor blood for infectivity are required to use third generation methods for HBsAg. High sensitivity and ease of adaptability to the clinical laboratory have made ELISA the method of choice for detection of HBsAg and other HBV markers.[34] Molecular hybridization techniques for detecting HBV sequences in clinical specimens are being developed and evaluated by research laboratories.[28,33,42]

The typical sequences of hepatitis B markers during the course of acute and chronic infection[8,11,18,24,25] are illustrated in Figures 9–4A and 9-4B and are discussed below.

The first serologic marker to appear after the onset of HBV infection is HBsAg, which becomes detectable during the incubation period, 2 to 6 weeks before the onset of clinical symptoms, and reaches peak levels during the acute stage of infection, when liver enzymes are elevated.

In acute hepatitis B, the titer of HBsAg declines gradually as the patient recovers, becoming undetectable within 1 to 6 months (Fig. 9–4A). HBeAg can be detected within 1 week after the appearance of HBsAg, reaches peak titers in parallel with HBsAg, and disappears before HBsAg. Probable recovery of the patient is signaled by replacement of HBeAg with anti-HBe, which then peaks during the convalescent phase of infection and gradually declines thereafter. IgM anti-HBc appears during the acute stage of illness, 1 to 4 weeks after the appearance of HBsAg, and usually drops to undetectable levels within 6 months, while IgG anti-HBc is produced during convalescence and persists for the life of the individual. In most patients, anti-HBs does not appear until weeks to months after the disappearance of HBsAg. Anti-HBs rises during recovery and usually persists for years thereafter, providing protective immunity to the individual. The interval between the disappearance of HBsAg and the appearance of anti-HBs is often referred to as the "core window," as IgM anti-HBc may be the only indicator of recent infection detectable at that time.

The sequence of markers during a typical course of chronic hepatitis B infection is shown in Figure 9–4B, and is initially the same as in acute hepatitis B, with rises in HBsAg, HBeAg and IgM anti-HBc. In contrast to acute illness followed by recovery, however, in chronic hepatitis B, HBsAg and HBeAg persist at elevated levels for 6 months or longer (up to a lifetime in many individuals), and the patient remains infectious. As in acute infection, IgM anti-HBc levels decline after a few months and are replaced by IgG anti-HBc; however, anti-HBe and anti-HBs are not produced unless recovery eventually occurs.

Hepatitis delta infection is diagnosed by

A

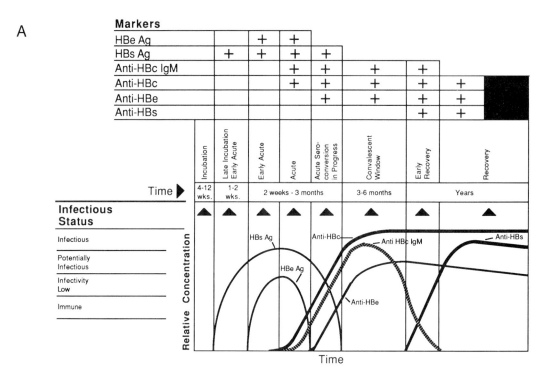

B

No Seroconversion

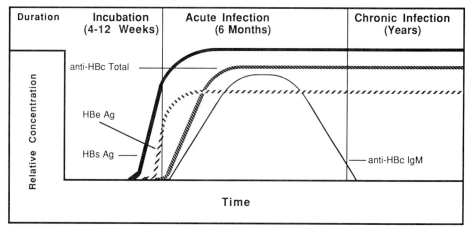

Fig. 9–4. (A) Typical sequence of HBV markers during acute hepatitis B infection; (B) Typical serologic profile in chronic hepatitis B with no recovery. (Adapted with permission from Abbott Laboratories.)

using RIA or ELISA techniques to detect anti-HDV antibodies. Acute HDV infection is characterized by the appearance of IgM anti-HDV during the acute phase of illness, followed by a decline in IgM titer and the development of IgG anti-HDV during convalescence, while in chronic hepatitis delta, both IgM and IgG anti-HDV antibodies persist.[2,15,21] Tests to detect delta antigen and molecular hybridization techniques to detect HDV RNA are also being developed.[21]

REFERENCES

1. Alter, H.J. et al.: Infect. Immun., *16*:928, 1977.

2. Aragona, M. et al.: Lancet, *1*:478, 1987.

3. Bates, H.M.: Lab. Management, p. 14, April, 1986.

4. Beasley, R.P. et al.: Lancet, *2*:1129, 1981.

5. Blumberg, B.S.: Science, *197*:17, 1977.

6. Blumberg, B.S., London, W.T., and Sutnick, A.I.: Postgrad. Med., *50*:70, 1971.

7. Blumberg, B.S. et al.: Am. J. Hum. Genet., *18*:594, 1966.

*8. Chang, Y.-W.: Diagnostic Med., p. 28, July/August, 1983.

9. Centers for Disease Control: MMWR, *34*:313, 1985.

10. Centers for Disease Control: Ann. Intern. Med., *107*:353, 1987.

11. Coslett, G.D.: *Hepatitis Learning Guide,* North Chicago, Abbott Diagnostics, 1985.

12. Dane, D.S., Cameron, C.H., and Briggs, M.: Lancet, *1*:695, 1970.

13. Dienstag, J.L., Wands, J.R., and Koff, R.S.: In *Harrison's Principles of Internal Medicine,* 11th ed. Edited by E. Braunwald et al. New York, McGraw-Hill Book Co., 1987.

14. Eddleston, A.L.W.F., and Williams, R.: Ann. Clin. Res., *8*:162, 1976.

15. Farci, P. et al.: JAMA, *255*:1443, 1986.

16. Fattovich, G. et al.: J. Infect. Dis., *155*:931, 1987.

17. Feinman, S.V. et al.: J. Lab. Clin. Med., *85*:1042, 1975.

18. Fody, E.P., and Johnson, D.F.: J. Med. Technol., *4*:54, 1987.

19. Francis, D.P.: JAMA, *256*:869, 1986.

20. Gitnick, G.: Lab. Med., *14*:721, 1983.

21. Govindarajan, S.: Lab. Management, *26*:36, 1988.

22. Gregory, D.H.: Postgrad. Med., *75*:199, 1984.

23. Heathcote, J., Cameron, C.H., and Dane, D.S.: Lancet, *1*:71, 1974.

24. Hollemweguer, E.J.: Lab. Med., *26*:30, 1988.

*25. Hollinger, F.B.: Hosp. Pract., *22*(Feb):101, 1987.

26. Hollinger, F.B., and Dressman, G.R.: In *Manual of Clinical Laboratory Immunology.* 3rd ed. Edited by N.R. Rose, H. Friedman, and J.L. Fahey. Washington, D.C., American Society for Microbiology, 1986.

*27. Hoofnagle, J.H.: Lab. Med., *14*:705, 1983.

28. Ju, L.H. et al.: J. Infect. Dis., *154*:983, 1986.

29. Koff, R.S. et al.: Gastroenterol., *72*:297, 1977.

30. Lee, S.-D., et al.: Scand. J. Infect. Dis. *19*:173, 1987.

31. Murray, K.: Proc. R. Soc. Lond. B *230*:107, 1987.

32. Neilson, J.O.: Ann. Clin. Res. *8*:151, 1976.

33. Pao, C.C., et al.: J. Clin. Microbiol. *25*:449, 1987.

34. Ratnam, S., and Tobin, A.M.: J. Clin. Microbiol. *25*:432, 1987.

35. Rizzetto, M. et al.: Gut *18*:997, 1977.

36. Schiff, E.: Am. J. Gastroenterology, *82*:287, 1987.

37. Shiraki, K. et al.: Am. J. Dis. Child, *131*:644, 1977.

38. Soulier, J.P., Junzers, P., and Zingraff, J.: Adv. Nephrol., *6*:383, 1976.

39. Stevens, C.E. et al.: JAMA, *257*:2612, 1987.

40. Ward, R. et al.: Lancet, *2*:726, 1972.

41. Wong, M.L., Lehmann, N.I., and Gust, I.D.: Med. J. Aust., *2*:52, 1976.

42. Yokota, H., Yokoo, K., and Nagata, Y.: Biochim. Biophys. Acta, *868*:45, 1986.

Hepatitis B Surface Antigen Auszyme Monoclonal Immunoassay[15]

PRINCIPLE. In the monoclonal enzyme immunoassay procedure, beads coated with mouse monoclonal antibody to hepatitis B surface antigen (anti-HBs) are incubated with serum or plasma, appropriate controls, and mouse monoclonal anti-HBs peroxidase (horseradish) conjugate (anti-HBs:HRPO). During the incubation period, any HBsAg present is bound to the solid phase antibody and simultaneously bound by the anti-HBs:HRPO. Unbound material is then aspirated and the beads washed.[2,3,5,7,10,14] Next, o-phenylenediamine (OPD) solution containing hydrogen peroxide is added to the bead and, after incubation, a yellow-orange color develops in proportion to the amount of HBsAg which is bound to the bead. The enzyme reaction is stopped by the addition of acid. The absorbance of controls and specimens is determined using a spectrophotometer with wavelength set at 492 nm. Specimens giving absorbance values equal to or greater than the absorbance value of the negative control mean plus a factor are considered reactive for HBsAg.

EQUIPMENT AND MATERIALS

1. Auszyme Monoclonal Diagnostic Kit (Abbott):

a. Anti-HBs (mouse) monoclonal coated beads; antibody to hepatitis B surface antigen (mouse monoclonal)

b. Monoclonal (mouse) conjugate; antibody to hepatitis B surface antigen (mouse monoclonal):peroxidase (horseradish). Dye: Red, No. 33

c. Positive control; human HBsAg, 9 ± 2 ng/mL in buffer with stabilizers. Dye: Bromophenol blue

d. Negative control; recalcified human plasma, nonreactive for HBsAg and anti-HBs

e. OPD (o-phenylenediamine · 2 HCl) tablets. OPD/tablet = 12.8 mg

f. Diluent for OPD; citrate-phosphate buffer containing 0.02% hydrogen peroxide

g. 1N sulfuric acid

2. Reaction trays (20 or 60 wells per tray)

3. Reaction tubes with identifying racks

4. Cover seals

5. Precision pipettes to deliver 50 μL, 200 μL, 300 μL and 1 mL

6. Disposable graduated pipettes or dispenser for measuring diluent for OPD

7. Device for delivery of rinse solution such as a Gorman-Rupp dispensing pump or equivalent

8. An aspiration device for washing beads such as a Pentawash with a vacuum source and a double trap for retaining the aspirate and maintaining adequate vacuum

9. Water bath capable of maintaining temperature ± 1° C around a set point of 39 to 40° C

10. Quantum II or spectrophotometer capable of reading absorbance at 492 nm

11. Single bead dispenser for dispensing one bead at a time from a 100 bead bottle

12. Nonmetallic forceps

13. Membrane seal puncture tool for acid bottles

14. HBsAg confirmatory assay

WARNINGS AND PRECAUTIONS

1. Handle all AUSZYME monoclonal biologic materials with universal blood and body fluid precautions. HBsAg present in the positive control may possibly be a hepatitis agent or be carried in close association with such an agent. The positive control has been heated at 60° C for at least 10 hours; nevertheless, do not assume complete inactivation. In the event of accidental exposure to HBsAg solution or positive control, consult recommendations of the Public Health Service for prophylaxis with immune serum globulin.[9]

2. Avoid contact of OPD and sulfuric acid with skin and mucous membranes. If these reagents come into contact with skin, wash thoroughly with water.

3. Avoid contact of the OPD substrate solution and 1N sulfuric acid with any oxidizing agent. Do not allow substrate solution or 1N sulfuric acid to come into contact with any metal parts.

4. Dispose of all specimens and materials used to perform the test as if they contained the infectious agents of viral hepatitis. The preferred method of disposal is autoclaving for a minimum of 1 hour at 121.5° C. Disposable materials may be incinerated. Liquid wastes not containing acid and neutralized waste may be mixed with sodium hypochlorite in volumes such that the final mixture contains 1.0% sodium hypochlorite.[11] Allow 30 minutes for decontamination to be completed.

5. Avoid splashing or forming an aerosol.

6. Spills should be wiped up thoroughly using either an iodophor disinfectant or sodium hypochlorite solution.[1,8,13]

STORAGE INSTRUCTIONS. Store kit reagents at 2 to 8° C. OPD tablets and 1N sulfuric acid may be stored at 2 to 30° C. All reagents must be brought to room temperature (15 to 30° C) for use and returned to storage conditions indicated above immediately after use. Do not open OPD tablet bottle until it is at room temperature. Retain desiccant bags in OPD tablet bottle at all times during storage. Reconstituted OPD solution MUST be stored at room temperature and MUST be used within 60 minutes. Do not expose to light.

SPECIMEN COLLECTION AND PREPARATION. Either serum or plasma may be used in the test. Remove the serum or plasma from the clot or red cells, respectively, as soon as possible to avoid hemolysis. Lipemic, icteric, or hemolyzed specimens and specimens containing precipitate may give inconsistent test results. Such specimens should be clarified by centrifugation prior to assaying. *Do not use heat-treated specimens.*

If specimens are to be stored, they should be refrigerated at 2 to 8° C. For longterm storage, the specimens should be frozen (−15° C or colder).

Because serum from heparinized patients may be incompletely coagulated, false reactive results could occur because of fibrin deposition on the bead and subsequent trapping of the HRPO conjugated antibody. To prevent this phenomenon, draw serum specimen prior to heparin therapy. Serum specimens drawn after heparin therapy may be treated with thrombin or protamine sulfate to ensure complete clotting.[6,12]

PROCEDURE

Notes

—Negative control in triplicate and positive control in duplicate should be assayed with each run of specimens. Ensure that all reaction trays are subjected to the same process and incubation times.

—Use a disposable pipette tip for each transfer to avoid cross-contamination.

—Once the assay has been started, all subsequent steps should be completed without interruption and within the recommended time limits.

—Prior to beginning the assay procedure, bring all reagents to room temperature (15 to 30° C). Adjust water bath to 38 to 41° C.

—Identify the reaction tray wells for each specimen or control on a data sheet.

—Do not splash liquid while tapping trays.

—When washing beads, follow the directions under Wash Procedure Details in the kit insert.

1. Dispense 200 μL of each specimen or control (3 negative controls and 2 positive controls [blue]) into the bottom of appropriate wells of reaction tray. All patients are run in duplicate.

2. Add 50 μL of conjugate [red] to each well containing a specimen or control.

3. Carefully add one bead to each well containing a specimen or control.

4. Apply cover seal. Gently tap tray to cover beads and remove any trapped air bubbles.

5. Perform one of the following incubations:
Procedure A: Incubate at 40° C for 3 hours
Procedure B: Incubate at room temperature for 16 hours
Procedure C: Incubate at 40° C for 75 minutes

6. During the last 5 to 10 minutes of incubation, prepare OPD substrate solution as follows:

The OPD (o-phenylenediamine · 2 HCl) tablet must be dissolved in diluent for OPD immediately before use. The solution must not be stored longer than 60 minutes before use. Three-hundred μL of OPD substrate solution is required for each test specimen as well as for two reagent blanks.

a. Using a clean pipette, transfer into a suitable container, 5 mL of diluent for OPD for each tablet to be dissolved.

b. Transfer ODP tablet(s) from bottle into container with diluent for OPD using a non-metallic forceps or equivalent. Return desiccant to bottle immediately, if removed to obtain a tablet, and close bottle tightly. Allow tablet(s) to dissolve. Do not use a tablet that is not intact.

c. Just prior to dispensing for the final incubation of the assay, swirl gently to obtain a homogeneous solution. The OPD substrate solution (OPD plus diluent for OPD) should be colorless to pale yellow. A yellow-orange color of the solution indicates that the reagent has been contaminated and must be discarded.

7. Remove and discard cover seal. Aspirate the liquid and wash each bead three times with 4 to 6 mL of distilled or deionized water.

8. Immediately transfer beads to properly identified assay tubes. When transferring beads from wells to assay tubes, align inverted rack of oriented tubes over the reaction tray. Press the tubes tightly over the wells and invert tray and tubes together so that beads fall into corresponding tubes. Blot excess water from top of tube rack.

9. Prime dispenser immediately prior to dispensing OPD substrate solution. Pipette 300 μL of freshly prepared OPD substrate solution into two empty tubes (substrate blanks) and then into each tube containing a bead.

10. Cover and incubate at room temperature for 30 minutes.

11. Add 1 mL of 1N sulfuric acid to each tube.

12. Select a wavelength of 492 nm on a spectrophotometer or use the Quantum Analyzer. Visually inspect both blanks and discard those that are contaminated (indicated by yellow-orange color). If both blanks are contaminated, the run must be repeated. Blank the instrument by using one of the two substrate blank tubes. Read negative and positive controls. Then process the test specimens. If there is an interruption during the reading of samples, repeat the blank (using the second substrate blank tube if necessary). Continue reading specimens. Determine all absorbance values within two hours after addition of acid.

REPORTING. The presence or absence of HBsAg is determined by relating the absorbance of the unknown sample to the cutoff value. The cutoff value is the absorbance of the negative control mean plus the factor 0.050 for Procedures A and B or the factor 0.025 for Procedure C.

Specimens with absorbance values greater than or equal to the cutoff value established with the negative control are to be considered reactive for HBsAg. Specimens whose absorbance values are less than the cutoff value are considered nonreactive for HBsAg.

For the run to be valid, the difference between the means of the positive and negative controls (P–N) should be 0.400 or greater for Procedures A and B, and 0.200 or greater for Procedure C. If not, technique may be suspect and the run must be repeated. If the P–N value is consistently low, deterioration of reagents may be suspect.

CALCULATIONS. *Note:* When a Quantum Analyzer is used, refer to the operations manual to determine which calculations are performed automatically. If a Quantum Analyzer is not used, perform the following calculations on the assay data.

1. Calculation of negative control mean absorbance (NC$\bar{x}$)

a. Determine the mean of the negative control values. Example:

Negative Control				
Sample No.	Absorbance			
1	0.025			
2	0.028			
3	0.028	$\dfrac{\text{Total Absorbance}}{3}$	$= \dfrac{0.081}{3} =$	0.027 (NC$\bar{x}$)
TOTAL	0.081			

b. Individual negative control values should be less than or equal to 0.100 and greater than or equal to −0.006. Negative control values should also be greater than or equal to 0.5 times NC$\bar{x}$ and less than or equal to 1.5 times NC$\bar{x}$. Where the NC$\bar{x}$ is below 0.012, the calculation of 0.5 to 1.5 times the mean may be disregarded. In such cases, all negative control values should fall within the range mean ± 0.006. If one value is outside the acceptable range, discard this value and recalculate the mean. If two values are outside the range, the test should be repeated. If more than an occasional value falls outside the range, technique problems must be corrected.

Example:		
0.5 × 0.027 = 0.014 and		
1.5 × 0.027 = 0.040	Range: 0.014 to 0.040	

In the example, no negative control sample is rejected as aberrant and the NC$\bar{x}$ need not be revised.

2. Calculation of the positive control mean absorbance (PC$\bar{x}$) Determine the positive control mean (PC$\bar{x}$). Example:

Positive Control				
Sample No.	Absorbance			
1	1.024			
2	1.030	$\dfrac{\text{Total Absorbance}}{2}$	$= \dfrac{2.054}{2} =$	1.027 (PC$\bar{x}$)
TOTAL	2.054			

3. Calculation of the P–N value
Determine the P–N value by subtracting the NCx̄ from the PCx̄. Example:

PCx̄	1.027
NCx̄	−0.027
P-N value	1.000

For the run to be valid, the P–N value must be 0.400 or greater for Procedures A and B, and 0.200 or greater for Procedure C. If not, technique or deterioration of reagents may be suspect and the run must be repeated.

4. Calculation of the cutoff value.
Determine the cutoff value by following the examples below:

a. Procedures A and B: Add the factor 0.050 to the NCx̄. Example:

NCx̄	0.027
	+0.050
Cutoff value	0.077

b. Procedure C: Add the factor 0.025 to the NCx̄. Example:

NCx̄	0.027
	+0.025
Cutoff value	0.052

INTERPRETATION OF RESULTS. Repeat testing of a specimen found reactive by the screening procedure will verify whether it is repeatedly reactive.

If repeat testing shows the specimen to be less than the cutoff, the original result may be classified as nonrepeatedly reactive. If repeats are greater than or equal to the cutoff, the specimen should be presumed reactive for HBsAg. Such results are contingent on determination of the specificity of the repeatedly reactive specimens.

False reactive results may be obtained with any diagnostic test.

Two types of false reactive results may occur with the AUSZYME monoclonal test:

1. *Nonrepeatable Reactives:* Some specimens which are reactive in the AUSZYME monoclonal screening procedure may not be reactive on repeat testing. The most common sources of such nonrepeatable reactives are:
—Improper bead washing

—Cross-contamination of nonreactive specimens caused by transfer of high titer antigen specimen[4]
—Contamination of the OPD substrate solution by oxidizing agents
—Contamination of the acid used as stopping reagent
—Contamination of reaction tray well rim with anti-HB$_s$ conjugate reagent or specimen

2. *Nonspecific Reactives:* All highly sensitive immunoassay systems have a potential for nonspecific reactions, but specificity of repeatedly reactive specimens can be confirmed by neutralization tests.

Specificity analysis must be performed prior to informing a donor or patient that he is an HBsAg carrier.

HBsAg confirmatory assay provides a method for confirmation of repeatedly reactive specimens. This enzyme immunoassay must be performed on all repeatedly reactive specimens unless they can be confirmed positive by other licensed HBsAg test systems.

A repeatedly reactive specimen, confirmed by neutralization with human anti-HBs or other licensed HBsAg tests must be considered positive for HBsAg.

LIMITATION OF THE PROCEDURE. Although the association of infectivity and the presence of HBsAg is strong, it is recognized that presently available methods for HBsAg detection are not sensitive enough to detect all potentially infectious units of blood or possible cases of hepatitis.

REFERENCES

1. Bond, W.W., Favero, M.S., Petersen, N.J., and Ebert, J.W.: J. Clin. Microbiol., 18:535, 1983.

2. David, G.S. et al.: Med. Lab. Sci., 38:341, 1981.

3. Drouet, J. et al.: In *Viral Hepatitis.* Edited by W. Szmuness, H.J. Alter, and J.E. Maynard. Philadelphia, Franklin Institute Press, 1982.

4. Epidemiologic Notes and Reports: Hepatitis B Contamination in a Clinical Laboratory - Colorado, MMWR, 29:459, 1980.

5. Goodall, A.H. et al.: Med. Lab. Sci., 38:349, 1981.

6. Grangeot-Keros, L. et al.: Vox Sang., 42:160, 1982.

7. Kennedy, R.C. et al.: Intervirology, 19:176, 1983.

8. Merck Index: Listing 4904, 1983.

9. Recommendation of the Immunization Practices Advisory Committee (ACIP): MMWR, **31**:317, 1982.

10. Shih, JW-K., Cote, P.J., Dapolito, G.M., and Gerin, J.L.: J. Virol. Methods, **1**:257, 1980.

11. Sehulster, L.M., Hollinger, F.B. Dreesman, G.R., and Melnick, J.L.: Appl. Environ. Microbiol., **42**:762, 1981.

12. *Technical Manual of the American Association of Blood Banks*, 8th Ed., Philadelphia, J.B. Lippincott Co., 1981.

13. U.S. Environmental Protection Agency, Office of Solid Waste: "Draft Manual for Infectious Waste Management," Washington, D.C., 19082. (USG PO 1982-361-082/325).

14. Wands, J.R., and Zurawski, V.R.: Gastroenterology, **80**:225, 1981.

15. Package Insert - Auszyme Monoclonal, Abbott Laboratories, North Chicago, IL, 1987.

Hepatitis B Surface Antigen Confirmation Assay[1]

PRINCIPLE. This procedure is used to confirm the presence of Hepatitis B surface antigen (HBsAg) in specimens previously determined to be repeatedly reactive for HBsAg in a screening assay. The HBsAg confirmatory assay is an enzyme-linked immunosorbent assay which uses the principle of specific antibody neutralization to confirm the presence of HBsAg. The confirmatory reagent (human antibody to hepatitis B surface antigen) is incubated with the specimen in solution. If HBsAg is present in the specimen, it will be bound by the confirmatory reagent. Beads coated with antibody to HBsAg are added later. Any neutralized HBsAg is subsequently blocked from binding to the beads. The results are visualized by subsequent addition of anti-HBsAg/peroxidase conjugate, followed by o-phenylenediamine substrate. Sulfuric acid is added to stop the reaction, which is measured spectrophotometrically. Presence of HBsAg, and subsequent neutralization, results in reduction of reaction when compared to the non-neutralized specimen in which negative control is used in place of confirmatory reagent.

By definition, a specimen is confirmed as positive if the reduction in signal of the neutralized specimen is at least 50%, and the non-neutralized control generates a signal greater than or equal to the assay cutoff.

EQUIPMENT AND MATERIALS

1. Confirmatory reagent—Antibody to hepatitis B surface antigen (human) (Solution A). Preservative: Gentamicin sulfate and thimerosal (Abbott Laboratories)

2. Negative control—Recalcified human plasma, nonreactive for HBsAg and anti-HBs (Solution B). Preservative: Gentamicin sulfate and thimerosal

3. Auszyme Monoclonal kit—for detection of HBsAg (Abbott Laboratories)

   a. Beads coated with monoclonal antibody to HBsAg (mouse)

   b. Monoclonal (mouse) conjugate; antibody to hepatitis B surface antigen (mouse monoclonal): peroxidase (horseradish)

   c. OPD (o-phenylenediamine · 2 HCl) tablets

   d. Diluent for OPD

4. 1N sulfuric acid

5. Reaction trays

6. Reaction tubes with identifying racks

7. Cover seals

8. Precision pipettes—50 μL, 200 μL, 300 μL, and 1 mL, with disposable tips

9. Waterbath (40° C ± 1° C)

PRECAUTIONS. Follow universal blood and body fluid precautions.

SPECIMEN COLLECTION AND PREPARATION. The specimens to be tested by the confirmatory neutralization test are those found to be repeatedly reactive by a screening assay.

If specimens are to be stored, they should be refrigerated at 2 to 8° C. For long-term storage, the specimens should be frozen (−15° C or colder).

STORAGE INSTRUCTIONS

1. Store reagents at 2 to 8° C.

2. All reagents should be brought to room temperature before use and returned to 2 to 8° C storage after use.

PROCEDURE

NOTES: —Depending on the procedure used to screen the specimen, the confirmatory assay may be performed by one of three procedures: A, B, or D. Confirmatory and screening procedures are identical except for the addition of duplicate controls and test specimens containing confirmatory reagents.

Screening Procedure used:*	Confirmatory Procedure to use:
Procedure A	Procedure A or B
Procedure B	Procedure B
Procedure C	Procedure A or B
Procedure D	Procedure D

* Procedures A, B, and D are described below

—If the specimen to be confirmed had an A_{492} greater than or equal to 2.000 in the screening assay, the specimen may be diluted in negative control prior to testing by the confirmatory assay.

—Negative control in triplicate and positive control in quadruplicate (two to be neutralized, two as non-neutralized controls) must be assayed with each run of unknowns. For each unknown specimen to be assayed, four samples are run (two to be neutralized, two as non-neutralized controls).

—Ensure that all reaction trays containing controls and/or unknowns are subjected to the same process and incubation times. Use a separate disposable tip for each transfer to avoid cross-contamination. Once the assay has been started, all steps should be completed without interruption.

—Prior to beginning the assay procedure, bring all reagents to room temperature (15 to 30° C). Swirl gently before using. Adjust water bath to 38 to 41° C (Procedures A and D).

—Identify the reaction tray wells for each specimen or control.

—When dispensing beads, remove cap from bead bottle, attach bead dispenser and dispense beads into wells of the reaction tray.

—Do not splash liquid while tapping trays.

—When washing beads, follow the directions in Wash Procedure Details in the AUSZYME Monoclonal package insert.

—When transferring beads from wells to assay tubes, align inverted rack of oriented tubes over the reaction tray. Press the tubes tightly over the wells and invert tray and tubes together so that beads fall into corresponding tubes. Blot excess water from top of tube rack.

—Avoid strong light during color development.

—Dispense acid in same sequence as OPD substrate solution.

—Do not allow acid solution to contact metal. If necessary, agitate tubes to ensure thorough mixing. Air bubbles should be removed prior to reading absorbance.

The following instructions are for confirmatory procedures A, B, and D:

1. Pipette 200 μL of each control into the bottom of the appropriate wells of the reaction tray (*three* wells for negative controls and *four* wells for positive controls).

2. Pipette 200 μL of serum or plasma into each of four (4) wells for each specimen being tested for confirmation.

3. Dispense 50 μL of confirmatory reagent, solution A, into two of the four wells containing positive control. Into the other two positive control wells and the three negative control wells, dispense 50 μL negative control, Solution B.

4. For each unknown specimen, dispense 50 μL confirmatory reagent, Solution A, into two of the four wells. Into the other two wells, dispense 50 μL negative control, Solution B.

5. Tap tray gently to facilitate mixing; allow neutralization reaction to proceed for 15 minutes at room temperature.

The following instructions are for procedures A and B:

6. Add 50 μL of conjugate to each well containing a specimen or control.

7. Carefully add one bead to each well containing a specimen or control.

8. Apply cover seal. Gently tap tray to cover beads and remove any trapped air bubbles.

9. Procedure A: Incubate in 40° C waterbath for 3 hours.

   B: Incubate at room temperature for 12 to 20 hours on a level surface.

10. Remove and discard cover seal. Aspirate the liquid and wash each bead three times with 4 to 6 mL of distilled or deionized water.

11. Proceed to step 15.

For procedure D:

6. Carefully add one bead to each well containing a specimen or control.

7. Apply cover seal. Gently tap the tray to cover beads and remove any trapped air bubbles.

8. Incubate in a 40° C waterbath for 2 hours.

9. Remove and discard cover seal. Aspirate the liquid and wash each bead three times with 4 to 6 mL of distilled or deionized water.

10. Pipette 200 μL of conjugate into each well containing a bead.

11. Apply new cover seal. Gently tap the tray to cover beads and remove any trapped air bubbles.

12. Incubate in a 40° C waterbath for 1 hour.

13. Remove and discard cover seal. Aspirate the liquid and wash each bead three times as in step 4.

14. Proceed to step 15.

The following instructions are for procedures A, B, and D:

15. Immediately transfer beads to properly identified assay tubes.

16. Instructions for preparation of OPD substrate solution: The OPD (o-Phenylenediamine • 2HCl) tablet must be dissolved in diluent for OPD immediately before use. The solution must not be stored longer than 60 minutes before use. During the final 5 to 10 minutes of the second incubation period, prepare the OPD substrate solution as follows:

NOTE: 300 μL is required for each test specimen.

   a. Using a clean pipette, deliver 5 mL of diluent for OPD for each tablet to be dissolved into a suitable container. CAUTION: use pipettes and containers known to be metal- and metal-ion-free.

   b. Using a nonmetallic forceps or equivalent, transfer tablet from bottle into diluent for OPD. Return desiccant to bottle immediately

if removed to obtain a tablet and close bottle tightly. Allow tablet to dissolve.

17. Pipette 300 μL of *freshly prepared OPD substrate solution* into two empty tubes (substrate blanks) and then into each tube containing a bead.

NOTE: Prime dispenser immediately prior to dispensing OPD substrate solution.

18. Cover and incubate at room temperature for 30 minutes.

19. Add 1 mL of 1 N sulfuric acid to each tube. If necessary, agitate to mix.

20. Set a wavelength of 492 nm on a spectrophotometer or use a Quantum Analyzer.

21. Visually inspect both blanks and discard those that are contaminated (indicated by yellow-orange color). If both blanks are contaminated, the run must be repeated.

22. Blank the instrument by using one of the two substrate blank tubes. Read negative and positive controls. Then read the test specimens.

23. If there is an interruption during the reading of samples, repeat the blank (using the second substrate blank tube if necessary). Continue reading specimens. Determine all absorbance values within 2 hours after addition of acid.

CALCULATIONS

1. Calculate the mean A_{492} for the three negative control values. Eliminate aberrant values as described in the AUSZYME Monoclonal package insert.

2. Determine the mean A_{492} for both the neutralized and non-neutralized positive control and each test specimen.

3. Determine the percent reduction for the positive control and for each specimen using the following equation:

$$\% \text{ Reduction} = \frac{A_{492} \text{ solution B} - A_{492} \text{ solution A}}{A_{492} \text{ solution B} - A_{492} \text{ N}\bar{x}} \times 100$$

Example:

	Mean Absorbance
Negative control (NC $\bar{x}$)	0.027
Positive control + solution B (negative control)	1.011
Positive control + solution A (confirmatory reagent)	0.019
Specimen + solution B (negative control)	0.649
Specimen + solution A (confirmatory reagent)	0.017

Positive control: $\dfrac{1.011 - 0.019}{1.011 - 0.027} = \dfrac{0.992}{0.984} \times 100 = 100.9\%$ Reduction

Specimen: $\dfrac{0.649 - 0.017}{0.649 - 0.027} = \dfrac{0.632}{0.622} \times 100 = 101.6\%$ Reduction

4. Determine the B-N value for the positive control and for each specimen using the following equation:

$$B - N = A_{492} \text{ solution } B - A_{492} \text{ NC}\bar{x}$$

Example:

Positive control: $1.011 - 0.027 = 0.984$
Specimen: $0.649 - 0.027 = 0.622$

NOTE: If a Quantum Analyzer is used for reading and an absorbance reading of greater than or equal to 2.000 is obtained for sample plus negative control, use the absorbance value of 2.000 for calculation purposes.

REPORTING. The test is valid if the B-N value for the positive control is greater than or equal to 0.400 and the positive control absorbance is reduced by at least 50% with the addition of confirmatory reagent.

A specimen is considered to be positive if both of the following criteria are met:

1. The B-N value for the specimen (or the diluted specimen) is equal to or greater than 0.025 (the assay cutoff).

2. The AUSZYME Monoclonal reactivity of the specimen (or the diluted specimen) is reduced by at least 50% by the addition of confirmatory reagent (solution A).

Any specimen yielding less than 50% neutralization should be diluted 1:500 or greater and reassayed.

A specimen that is repeatedly reactive by the AUSZYME Monoclonal test for HBsAg and is confirmed by neutralization with confirmatory reagent must be considered positive for HBsAg.

LIMITATION OF THE PROCEDURE. The association of infectivity and HBsAg is strong, although it is recognized that presently available methods for HBsAg detection are not sensitive enough to detect all potentially infectious units of blood or possible cases of hepatitis B.

REFERENCE

1. Package Insert, Confirmatory reagent, Abbott Laboratories, North Chicago, IL, 1987.

Antibody to Hepatitis B: Core Antigen Competitive EIA (Corzyme)[1]

PRINCIPLE. In the CORZYME enzyme immunoassay, beads coated with Hepatitis B core antigen (HBcAg) are incubated with serum or plasma or appropriate controls and human anti-HBc conjugated with horseradish peroxidase (anti-HBc:HRPO). After incubation, the unbound material is removed by washing the bead. Anti-HBc, if present in the specimen, will compete with anti-HBc:HRPO for a limited number of HBcAg binding sites on the bead.

Next o-phenylenediamine (OPD) solution containing hydrogen peroxide is added to the bead and, after incubation, a yellow color develops. The enzyme reaction is stopped by the addition of 1 N sulfuric acid. The absorbance of controls and specimens is determined using a spectrophotometer with wavelength set at 492 nm. Within limits, the greater the amount of anti-HBc in the specimen, the lower the absorbance. The absorbance values of unknown specimens are compared with a cutoff value to determine reactivity.

EQUIPMENT AND MATERIALS

1. CORZYME Diagnostic Kit, 100 Tests / 500 Tests (Abbott Laboratories)

   a. 100/500 Hepatitis B Core Antigen (Recombinant DNA Origin) Coated Beads

   b. 1 vial (20 mL)/1 bottle (100 mL) antibody to hepatitis B core antigen (human): Peroxidase (horseradish) conjugate. Minimum concentration: 0.2 $\mu g/$ mL. Preservative: Gentamicin sulfate, USP

c. 1 vial (3 mL)/2 vials (3 mL each) positive control. Recalcified human plasma, positive for anti-HBs and anti-HBc. Human anti-HB_c minimum titer 1:200 $\pm$ 2 log_2 dilutions. Preservative: Gentamicin sulfate, USP

d. 1 vial (4.5 mL)/2 vials (4.5 mL each) negative control. Recalcified human plasma, nonreactive for HBsAg, anti-HBs and anti-HBc. Preservative: Gentamicin sulfate, USP

e. 1 bottle (10 Tablets)/1 bottle (40 Tablets) OPD (o-Phenylenediamine · 2 HCl) Tablets. OPD/Tablet: 12.8 mg

f. 1 bottle (55 mL)/1 bottle (220 mL) Diluent for OPD (o-Phenylenediamine · 2 HCl). Citrate-phosphate buffer containing 0.02% hydrogen peroxide

An optimum combination of the following accessories is provided:

2. Reaction trays
3. Cover seals
4. Assay tubes with identifying cartons
5. 1 N sulfuric acid

Materials required but not provided:

6. Precision pipettes, EIA Pipetting Package or similar equipment with disposable tips to deliver 100 μL, 200 μL, 300 μL, and 1 mL

7. Device for delivery of rinse solution such as Gorman-Rupp dispensing pump, or equivalent

8. An aspiration device for washing beads, such as a Pentawash II with a vacuum source, such as a Gast vacuum pump or equivalent, and a double trap for retaining the aspirate and maintaining adequate vacuum

9. Water bath capable of maintaining temperature at 40° C $\pm$ 2° C

10. Quantum Analyzer or Spectrophotometer capable of reading absorbance at 492 nm

11. Single Bead Dispenser

12. Membrane Seal Puncture Tool for acid bottles

13. Nonmetallic forceps

PRECAUTIONS

1. Use proper universal blood and body fluid precautions.

2. Avoid splashing or forming an aerosol.

3. Avoid contact of OPD and sulfuric acid with skin and mucous membranes. If these reagents come into contact with skin, wash with water.

SPECIMEN COLLECTION AND PREPARATION. The CORZYME Test may be performed on human serum, or plasma. Specimens can be stored at 2 to 8° C, but if longterm storage is needed, specimens should be stored at -20° C.

PREPARATION OF REAGENTS

INSTRUCTIONS FOR PREPARATION OF OPD SUBSTRATE SOLUTION. Bring OPD Reagents to room temperature (15 to 30° C). *CAUTION:* Do not open OPD Tablet bottle until it is at room temperature.

Five to 10 minutes prior to Color Development, prepare the OPD Substrate Solution by dissolving the OPD (o-Phenylenediamine · 2 HCl) Tablet in Diluent for OPD. *DO NOT USE A TABLET THAT IS NOT INTACT.*

Using clean pipettes and metal-free containers (such as plastic ware or acid-washed and distilled water-rinsed glassware), follow the procedure below:

1. Transfer into a suitable container 5 ml of Diluent for OPD for each tablet to be dissolved.

2. Transfer appropriate number of OPD Tablets (see OPD Preparation Chart in package insert) into measured amount of Diluent for OPD using a nonmetallic forceps or equivalent. Return desiccant to bottle immediately, if removed to obtain a tablet, and close bottle tightly. Allow tablet to dissolve. Do not cap or stopper the Substrate Solution bottle while the tablets are dissolving.

NOTE: The OPD Substrate Solution must be used within 60 minutes of preparation and must not be exposed to strong light.

3. Just prior to dispensing for Color Development, swirl container gently to obtain a homogeneous solution, and remove air bubbles from tubing.

OPD Substrate Solution (OPD plus Diluent for OPD) should be colorless to pale yellow. A yellow-orange color of the Solution indicates that the reagent has been contaminated and must be discarded.

A value of less than 0.300 absorbance units for the difference between the negative and positive control means (N-P) may indicate deterioration of the kit or OPD reagents.

STORAGE INSTRUCTIONS

1. Store kit reagents at 2 to 8° C. OPD Tablets and 1 N Sulfuric Acid may be stored at 2 to 30° C.

2. Bring all reagents to room temperature (15 to 30° C) for use and return them to storage conditions indicated above immediately after use.

3. Retain desiccant bags in OPD Tablet bottle at all times during storage.

4. Reconstituted OPD Substrate Solution MUST be stored at room temperature and MUST be used within 60 minutes.

5. Replace desiccant in bead bottle, and cap bottle for storage.

HANDLING PRECAUTIONS

1. Do not use kit components beyond the expiration date.

2. Do not mix reagents from different lots.

3. Do not expose OPD reagents to strong light during storage or incubation.

4. Avoid contact of the OPD Substrate Solution with any oxidizing agent. Do not allow Substrate Solution to come in contact with any metal parts. Prior to use, rinse glassware used with OPD Solution thoroughly with 1 N acid (sulfuric or hydrochloric) using approximately 10% of the container volume followed by three washes of distilled water at the same volume.

5. Avoid microbial contamination of reagents and water used for washing. Use of disposable pipette tips is recommended.

6. Use a dedicated pipette to deliver the conjugate in order to avoid cross-contamination.

7. Adequate mixing of the Antibody conjugate and specimens is essential prior to the addition of beads. After pipetting the Conjugate solution and specimens, vigorously tap the edge of the tray several times to thoroughly mix the solution. Do not splash Antibody Conjugate Solution, specimens, or controls outside of wells or on well rims. Splashing may contaminate other wells or contaminate the beads when transferred to tubes.

8. If the desiccant obstructs the flow of beads, remove from the bead bottle prior to dispensing beads. Replace desiccant in bottle, and tightly cap bottle for storage. Do not store beads with dispenser attached to bottle.

NOTES

INCUBATION

1. Do not splash specimen or enzyme conjugate outside of well or on well rim as it will not be removed in subsequent washings and may be transferred to the tubes causing test interference.

2. When dispensing beads, remove cap from bead bottle, attach Single Bead Dispenser and dispense beads into wells of the reaction tray as directed in the Single Bead Dispenser insert.

3. Do not splash liquid while vigorously tapping trays.

COLOR DEVELOPMENT

1. When transferring beads from wells to assay tubes, align inverted rack of oriented tubes over the reaction tray. Press the tubes tightly over the wells and invert tray and tubes together so that beads fall into corresponding tubes. Blot excess water from top of tube rack.

2. Avoid strong light during color development.

3. Do not allow acid solution to contact metal. If necessary, agitate tubes to ensure thorough mixing. Air bubbles should be removed prior to reading absorbance.

PROCEDURE

1. Prior to beginning the assay procedure, bring all reagents to room temperature (15 to 30° C) and mix gently. Adjust the waterbath to 40° C ± 2°C.

2. Record the position of each specimen or control in the reaction tray for proper identification.

3. Pipette 200 μl of antibody conjugate solution into each well.

4. Pipette 100 μl of controls or specimen into appropriate wells of reaction tray. (Run the negative control in triplicate wells and the positive control in duplicate wells.) All patients are run in duplicate. Mix thoroughly by vigorously tapping the tray. Do not splash.

5. Add one bead to each well.

6. Apply cover seal. Gently tap the tray.

7. Perform incubation using either Procedure A or Procedure B:

Procedure A: Incubate trays in a 40° C ± 1° C water bath for 2 hours ± 5 minutes.

Procedure B: Incubate trays on a level surface at room temperature (15 to 30° C) for 12 to 20 hours.

8. Remove cover seal, aspirate liquid, and wash each bead 3 times with 4 to 6 mL distilled or deionized water for a total rinse volume of 12 to 18 mL.

9. Immediately transfer beads to properly labeled assay tubes.

10. Pipette 300 μL OPD solution into two empty tubes (substrate blanks) and then into each tube containing a bead. Substrate must not touch metal.

11. Cover and incubate for 30 ± 3 minutes at 15 to 30° C.

12. Add 1 mL of 1 N Sulfuric Acid to each tube.

13. Blank spectrophotometer.

14. Determine absorbance of each tube at 492 nm.

Laboratories using an instrument other than a Quantum Analyzer should read this assay as follows:

15. Read the absorbances for each Standard, Control, and specimen.

16. Rinse cuvettes thoroughly with distilled or deionized water between the reading of each specimen.

17. Refer to RESULTS section for calculations.

REPORTING. The presence or absence of anti-HBc is determined by comparing the absorbance of the specimen to a cutoff value. This cutoff value (for both Procedures A and B) is calculated from the negative control mean (NC$\bar{x}$) and positive control mean (PC$\bar{x}$) absorbance as explained in the calculations below. Unknown specimens with an absorbance value equal to, or lower than the cutoff value are considered reactive for anti-HBc. Those specimens with an absorbance value higher than the cutoff value are considered negative for anti-HBc by the criteria of the CORZYME test.

In randomly selected HBsAg positive human sera, the number of specimens found reactive for anti-HBc by CORZYME has been typically more than 90%.

Expected values for Procedure B produce a more defined separation between negative and positive populations than Procedure A.

CALCULATIONS. Laboratories using Quantum II should read this assay using Module A, Mode 1.3. If you are using a Quantumatic List No. 7523, your protocol will be automatic. If you are not, you will need to input the following information:

Name: CORZYME
C1: 0
C2: 0.4
C3: 0.6
Correct: Yes
P greater than N: No
Negative controls: 3
Minimum Negative Control: Delete
Maximum Negative Control: Delete
Negative aberrant Cutoff %: 50
Positive controls: 2
Minimum Positive Control: Delete
Maximum Positive Control: Delete
Positive Aberrant Cutoff %: 50
Minimum Control Difference: 0.300
Maximum Control Difference: Delete
Patient replicates: 1
Minimum Patient Absorbance Difference: Delete
Gray Region in %: 10
Filter 492.600: Yes

MANUAL CALCULATIONS

1. Calculation of Negative Control Mean Absorbance (NC$\bar{x}$).

   a. Determine the Mean of the Negative Control Value.

Example:

Negative Control

Sample No.	Absorbance
1	1.027
2	0.989
3	1.178

$$\frac{\text{Total Absorbance}}{3} = \frac{3.194}{3} = 1.065 \ (NC\bar{x})$$

b. All Negative Control values should fall within 0.5 to 1.5 times the Mean. If one value is outside this range, discard this value and recalculate the Mean. If two values are outside this range, the test should be repeated. If more than an occasional value falls outside this range, technique problems should be suspected.

Example: $0.5 \times 1.065 = 0.532$
$1.5 \times 1.065 = 1.597$
Range: 0.532 to 1.597

In the example above, no Negative Control sample is rejected as aberrant. The Negative Control Mean, therefore, need not be revised.

2. Calculation of Positive Control Mean Absorbance (PC$\bar{x}$).

a. Determine the Mean of the Positive Control Values.

Example:

Positive Control

Sample No.	Absorbance
1	0.051
2	0.038

$$\frac{\text{Total Absorbance}}{2} = \frac{0.089}{2} = 0.045 \ (PC\bar{x})$$

3. Determination of Cutoff Value
Calculate the Cutoff Value using the Following equation:
$0.4 \ (NC\bar{x}) + 0.6 \ (PC\bar{x}) = $ Cutoff Value
Example: $0.4 \ (1.065) + 0.6 \ (0.045) = 0.453$

Samples with absorbance values equal to or lower than the Cutoff Value are considered reactive by the criteria of the CORZYME test.

Samples with absorbance values greater than the Cutoff Value are considered negative by the criteria of the CORZYME test.

4. Determination of N-P Value
Calculate the N-P value by substracting the PC$\bar{x}$ from NC$\bar{x}$.
Example: N-P $= 1.065 - 0.045 = 1.02$

This value must be greater than 0.3. If not, technique or deterioration of reagents may be suspect and the run should be repeated.

INTERPRETATION OF RESULTS

1. Specimens with absorbance values greater than the Cutoff value are negative by the criteria of the CORZYME test.

2. Specimens with absorbance values equal to or lower than the Cutoff value are

considered reactive by the criteria of the CORZYME test.

3. Specimens with absorbance values within 10% of the Cutoff Value should be retested to confirm the initial test result. For the example given, the range for retest would be:

Cutoff Value = 0.453
Retest Range = 0.408 to 0.498

Specimens which have been found repeatedly reactive are positive for anti-HBc by the criteria of the CORZYME test.

4. To obtain semi-quantitative results, prepare and test multiple dilutions of patient specimen.

The titer of anti-HBc in a positive specimen is determined by comparing the absorbance of appropriate specimen dilution to the cutoff value.

The specimen titer is defined as that dilution of the specimen that yields an absorbance value most nearly equivalent to, but not greater than, the cutoff value.

LIMITATIONS OF THE PROCEDURE

1. Specimens containing sodium azide may give false-positive reactions and should not be tested.

2. Lipemic specimens and specimens containing precipitate may give inconsistent test results. Such specimens should be clarified by centrifugation prior to assaying.

REFERENCE

1. Package Insert—CORZYME, Abbott Laboratories, North Chicago, 1986.

Antibody to Hepatitis B Core Antigen (IgM): Corzyme-M EIA[2]

PRINCIPLE. This test is a solid phase enzyme immunoassay which uses the "sandwich principle" to measure specific anti-HBc IgM in serum or plasma. In the first incubation, antibody specific for human IgM (μ chain) coated on polystyrene beads is used to capture IgM from appropriately diluted patient samples. Hepatitis B core antigen (HBcAg) is added before the second incubation to react with IgM antibodies that are specific for HBcAg. Anti-HBc conju-

gated with horseradish peroxidase (anti-HBc:HRPO) is added before the third incubation to react with any HBcAg retained on the beads by the patient's anti-HBc IgM. Next, the beads are transferred into tubes and o-phenylenediamine (OPD) solution containing hydrogen peroxide is added to the beads. After incubation, a yellow color develops in proportion to the amount of anti-HBc:HRPO which bound to the bead during the previous incubation. The enzyme reaction is stopped by the addition of acid, and the intensity of the solution color is measured with a spectrophotometer. The absorbance at 492 nm is proportional to the quantity of anti-HBc IgM in the patients's serum. A cutoff value of 0.25 times the positive control mean ($\overline{PCx}$) plus the negative control mean ($\overline{NCx}$) is determined. Specimens giving absorbance values equal to or greater than the cutoff are considered reactive for IgM antibodies to HBcAg.

EQUIPMENT AND MATERIALS

1. Corzyme-M Diagnostic Kit (Abbott):
a. Antibody (goat), to human IgM coated on beads.
b. Antibody to hepatitis B core antigen (human):peroxidase (horseradish) conjugate. Minimum concentration 0.05 μg/mL in phosphate buffer with protein stablizers and antimicrobial agent.
c. Positive control. Recalcified human plasma positive for ant-HBc IgM (human) in specimen diluent with antimicrobial agent. Human anti-HBc IgM minimum titer 1:2.
d. Negative control. Recalcified human plasma, nonreactive for anti-HBc IgM and HBsAg in specimen diluent with antimicrobial agent.
e. Hepatitis B core antigen reagent. Human hepatitis B core antigen in phosphate buffered saline with protein stablizers and antimicrobial agent. Maximum titer 1:64.
f. Specimen diluent. Phosphate buffered saline solution with protein stablizers and antimicrobial agent.

g. OPD (o-phenylenediamine · 2 HCl) tablets. OPD/tablet: 12.8 mg.

h. Diluent for OPD (o-phenylenediamine · 2 HCl) citrate-phosphate buffer containing 0.02% hydrogen peroxide.

2. Reaction trays

3. Cover seals (tear along perforation for use)

4. Assay tubes with identifying cartons (for transfer of beads from reaction trays)

5. Assay tube box covers

6. 1N sulfuric acid

7. Precision pipettes with disposable tips to deliver 10 μL, 200 μL, 300 μL, 500 μL and 1 mL

8. Device for delivery of rinse solution, such as Gorman-Rupp Dispensing Pump or equivalent

9. An aspiration device for washing coated beads such as a Pentawash® II with a vacuum source, such as a Gast Vacuum Pump or equivalent, and a trap for retaining the aspirate

10. Water bath capable of maintaining temperature at 40° C ± 1° C

11. Disposable graduated pipettes or dispenser for measuring diluent for OPD

12. Nonmetallic forceps

13. Spectrophotometer capable of reading absorbance at 492 nm

14. Single bead dispenser

15. Test tubes and rack for dilution of specimens

16. Membrane seal puncture tool for acid bottles

STORAGE INSTRUCTIONS

1. Store all reagents at 2 to 8° C.

2. For best results, dispense reagents while cold and return to 2 to 8° C storage as soon as possible. CAUTION: Do not open OPD tablet bottle until it reaches room temperature. (Avoid unnecessary exposure to light.)

3. Retain desiccant bags in OPD tablet bottle at all times during storage.

4. Reconstituted OPD solution MUST be held at room temperature and MUST be used within 60 minutes.

SPECIMEN COLLECTION AND PREPARATION

1. Test may be performed on human serum or plasma.

2. Anti-HBc IgM is stable in serum or plasma and has been detected in stored samples (−20° C) after several years. If specimens are to be stored, they may be stored as serum or plasma at 2 to 8° C for up to 5 days. However, if storage periods greater than 5 days are anticipated, the specimens should be stored frozen.

3. Specimens containing precipitate may give inconsistent test results. Such specimens should be centrifuged prior to testing.

PROCEDURE NOTES

1. The negative control, positive control, and specimens must be run at the same time.

2. The negative and positive controls are provided in a prediluted form. They should not be diluted as specimens.

3. Handle all materials as though capable of transmitting hepatitis. In the event of accidental exposure to HBcAg solution or positive control, consult recommendations of the Public Health Service for prophylaxis with immune serum globulin.[1]

4. Do not use kit beyond the expiration date.

5. Wear disposable gloves while handling kit reagents or specimens and thoroughly wash hands afterward.

6. Avoid contact of OPD and sulfuric acid with skin and mucous membranes. If these reagents come into contact with skin, wash thoroughly with water.

7. Avoid contact of the OPD substrate solution and 1N sulfuric acid with any oxidizing agent. Do not allow substrate solution or 1N sulfuric acid to come into contact with any metal parts.

8. Dispose of all specimens and materials used to perform the test as if they contained the infectious agents of viral hepatitis. The preferred method of disposal is autoclaving for a minimum of 1 hour at 121.5° C. Disposable materials may be incinerated. Liquid wastes not containing acid and neutralized waste may be mixed with sodium hypochlorite in volumes such that the final mixture contains 1.0% sodium hypochlorite. Allow 30 minutes for decontamination to be completed.

9. Negative control in duplicate and positive control in triplicate, should be assayed with each run of specimens. Ensure that all reaction trays are subjected to the same process and incubation times.

CAUTION: Use a separate disposable pipette tip for each transfer to avoid cross-contamination.

Use a dedicated dispenser for the hepatitis B core antigen reagent to avoid accidental neutralization.

NOTE: Once the assay has been started, all subsequent steps should be completed without interruption and within the recommended time limits.

10. Prior to beginning the assay procedure, bring all reagents to room temperature (15 to 30° C). Swirl gently before using. Adjust water bath to 40° C ± 1° C.

11. Identify the reaction tray wells for each specimen or control on a data sheet.

12. When washing beads, follow the directions under Wash Procedure Details in the kit insert.

PROCEDURE

1. Prepare 1:50 dilutions of each specimen as follows: add 10 μL of specimen to a test tube and then add 0.5 mL of specimen diluent. Mix thoroughly. Do not dilute controls.

2. Pipette 200 μL of controls and 10 μL of diluted specimen into bottom of appropriate wells of reaction tray. All patients are run in duplicate.

3. Add 200 μL of specimen diluent to each well containing a specimen. Do not dilute controls. Tap trays to mix.

4. Carefully add one bead to each well containing a specimen or control.

5. Apply cover seal. Gently tap the tray to cover beads and remove any trapped air bubbles.

6. Incubate at 40° C for 1 hour ± 5 minutes.

7. Remove and discard cover seal. Aspirate the liquid and wash each bead three times with 4 to 6 mL of distilled or deionized water.

8. Pipette 200 μL of hepatitis B core antigen reagent into each reaction well containing a bead.

9. Apply new cover seal. Gently tap the tray to cover beads and remove any trapped air bubbles.

10. Incubate at room temperature (15 to 30° C) for 18 to 22 hours.

11. Remove and discard cover seal. Aspirate the liquid and wash each bead three times as in step 7.

12. Pipette 200 μL of antibody to hepatitis B core antigen (human):peroxidase (horseradish) conjugate into each reaction well containing a bead.

13. Apply new cover seal. Gently tap the tray to cover beads and remove any trapped air bubbles.

14. Incubate at 40° C for 2 hours ± 5 minutes.

15. Remove and discard cover seal. Aspirate the liquid and wash each bead three times as in step 7.

16. Remove all excess liquid from the top of the tray by aspiration or blotting.

17. Immediately transfer beads to properly identified assay tubes. When transferring beads from wells to assay tubes, align inverted rack of oriented tubes over the reaction tray. Press the tubes tightly over the wells and invert tray and tubes together so that beads fall into corresponding tubes. Blot excess water from top of tube rack.

18. The OPD (o-phenylenediamine · 2 HCl) tablet must be dissolved in diluent for OPD immediately before use. The solution must not be stored longer than 60 minutes before use.

During the last 5 to 10 minutes of the third incubation period, prepare the OPD substrate solution as follows:

NOTE: 300 μL is required for each test specimen (for each bead).

CAUTION: Use pipettes and containers known to be metal free. For example, use plastic ware or glassware washed with acid and rinsed with distilled water.

a. Using a clean pipette, transfer into a suitable container 5 mL of diluent for OPD for each tablet to be dissolved.

b. Transfer OPD tablets from bottle into container with diluent for OPD using a nonmetallic forceps or equivalent. Return desiccant to bottle immediately (if removed to obtain a tablet) and close bottle tightly. Allow tablets to dissolve. *Do not use a tablet that is not intact.*

c. Just prior to dispensing for the final incubation of the assay, swirl gently to obtain a homogeneous solution. Pipette 300 μL of OPD substrate solution into each tube containing a bead and into two empty tubes to be used as substrate blanks (substrate must not touch metal).

19. Cover and incubate at room temperature (15 to 30° C) for 30 ± 2 minutes.

20. Add 1 mL of 1N sulfuric acid to each tube. Agitate to mix.

21. Blank spectrophotometer.

22. Determine absorbance at 492 nm.

Select a wavelength of 492 nm on a spectrophotometer or use the Quantum analyzer. Visually inspect both blanks and discard those that are contaminated (indicated by yellow-orange color). If both blanks are contaminated, the run must be repeated. Blank the instrument by using one of the two substrate blank tubes. Read negative and positive controls. Then process the test specimens. If there is an interruption during the reading of samples, repeat the blank (using the second substrate blank tube if necessary). Continue reading specimens. Determine all absorbance values within two hours after addition of acid.

REPORTING. A positive or negative result for anti-HBc IgM is determined by comparing the absorbance of the specimen to a cutoff value. The cutoff value is calculated from the positive and negative control absorbance values as explained under *Calculations*. Specimens with absorbance values less than the cutoff value are considered to be nonreactive for anti-HBc IgM. Specimens with absorbance values equal to or greater than the cutoff value are considered to be reactive for anti-HBc IgM.

CALCULATIONS

1. Calculation of positive control mean absorbance ($PC\overline{x}$).

a. Determine the mean of the positive control values.

Positive Control		
Example:	Sample No.	Absorbance
	1	0.811
	2	0.902
	3	0.825
	Total	2.538

$$\frac{\text{Total Absorbance}}{3} = \frac{2.538}{3} = 0.846 \ (PC\overline{x})$$

b. All positive control values should fall within the range of 0.5 to 1.5 times the mean. If one value is outside the range, discard this value and recalculate the mean. If two values are outside this range, the test should be repeated. If more than an occasional value falls outside this range, technique should be suspect.

Example: $0.5 \times 0.846 = 0.423$
$1.5 \times 0.846 = 1.269$ Range: 0.423 to 1.269

In the example above, no positive control sample is rejected as aberrant. The positive control mean, therefore, need not be revised.

2. Calculation of negative control mean absorbance ($NC\overline{x}$). Determine the mean of the negative control values.

Negative Control		
Example:	Sample No.	Absorbance
	1	0.051
	2	0.038
	Total	0.089

$$\frac{\text{Total Absorbance}}{2} = \frac{0.089}{2} = 0.045 \ (NC\overline{x})$$

3. Calculation of the cutoff value. Cutoff value equals ($0.25 \times$ PC$\overline{x}$ absorbance value) + NC$\overline{x}$ absorbance value.

Example: ($0.25 \times$ PC$\overline{x}$) + NC$\overline{x}$ = cutoff value
(0.25×0.846) + 0.045 = 0.257 cutoff value: 0.257

4. Calculation of the retest range. Calculate the $\pm$ 10% retest range around the cutoff.

Example: cutoff value: 0.257
$0.257 \pm 10\%$ = ($0.257 - 0.026$) to ($0.257 + 0.026$)
retest range: 0.231 to 0.283

5. Calculation of the P-N value. Determine the P-N value by substracting the NC$\overline{x}$ from the PC$\overline{x}$.
Example: P-N = $0.846 - 0.045 = 0.801$

INTERPRETATION OF RESULTS

1. Specimens with absorbance values which are less than the cutoff are negative.

2. Specimens with absorbance values within $\pm$ 10% of the cutoff should be retested to confirm the initial results. If results are consistently within $\pm$ 10% of the cutoff, the borderline nature of the results should be indicated in the final report. It is recommended that patients exhibiting borderline reactive anti-HB$_c$ IgM results be closely monitored over time to distinguish rising anti-HB$_c$ IgM levels (associated with acute hepatitis B infection) from falling anti-HB$_c$ IgM levels (associated with recovery).

3. Specimens with absorbance values repeatedly equal to or greater than the cutoff value are positive.

4. The P-N value must be greater than 0.300 to ensure the validity of each run.

LIMITATIONS OF THE PROCEDURE. This assay is limited to the detection of anti-HBc IgM in human serum or plasma. In the diagnosis of acute or subclinical hepatitis B infection, supportive clinical information, including other hepatitis B markers, should be evaluated. This test cannot be used to determine a patient's immune status to hepatitis B as it does not measure anti-HBc IgG.

REFERENCES

1. Centers for Disease Control: MMWR, *31*:317, 1982.
2. Package Insert—Corzyme-M, Abbott Laboratories, North Chicago, Il, 1986.

Antibody to Hepatitis B Surface Antigen (AUSAB EIA)[3]

PRINCIPLE. The AUSAB EIA test for anti-HBs uses the "sandwich principle," a solid phase enzyme-linked immunoassay technique, to measure anti-HBs levels in serum or plasma. Polystyrene beads coated with human hepatitis B surface antigen (HBsAg) are incubated with either the patient specimen or the appropriate controls. During incubation, antibody, if present, is immunologically coupled to the solid phase antigen. After aspiration of the unbound material and washing of the bead, human antigen, tagged with biotin (B-HBsAg), and avidin, conjugated with horseradish peroxidase (A-HRPO), are incubated with the antibody—antigen complex on the bead. The biotinylated surface antigen binds to the antibody creating an antigen—antibody—antigen "sandwich." The avidin-horseradish peroxidase binds to the "sandwich" bead via phase network. Unbound conjugates are aspirated and the beads washed. Next, O-phenylenediamine (OPD) solution containing hydrogen peroxide is added to the bead and, after incubation, a yellow color develops in proportion to the amount of anti-HBs which is bound to the bead. Within limits, the greater the amount of antibody in the sample, the higher the absorbance.

The enzyme reaction is stopped by the addition of acid. The absorbance of controls and specimens is determined using a spectrophotometer with wavelength set at 492 nm. Specimens giving absorbance values equal to or greater than a designated cutoff value are considered reactive for anti-HBs.

Testing for anti-HBs can be useful for:

a. evaluating the recovery and prognosis of patients infected with hepatitis B virus (HBV)

b. screening for potential vaccine recipients, and

c. studying epidemiologic factors associated with transmission of HBV. The detection of anti-HBs is indicative of a prior immunologic exposure to the antigen or vaccine.

NOTES:

STORAGE INSTRUCTIONS

1. Store all reagents at 2 to 8° C.

2. For best results, dispense all reagents except OPD while cold and return to 2 to 8° C storage as soon as possible. CAUTION: Do not open OPD tablet bottle until it reaches room temperature. (Avoid unnecessary exposure to light.)

3. Retain desiccant bags in OPD tablet bottle at all times during storage.

4. Reconstituted OPD solution MUST be held at room temperature and MUST be used within 60 minutes.

SPECIMEN COLLECTION AND PREPARATION

1. The AUSAB EIA test may be performed on human serum, plasma, or recalcified plasma.

2. Plasma collected into ACD, CPD, or 4% citrated solution may be recalcified by the following procedure:

a. Prepare a 2.77% solution of calcium chloride in water. (Do not store solution more than 1 week.)

b. Add 0.1 mL of the calcium chloride solution to 0.9 mL of plasma and incubate at 37° C for 2 hours.

c. Recover recalcified plasma by centrifuging at 500 to 1000 × g for 15 minutes. An alternate method for recovering the recalcified plasma is to freeze the specimens following the 37° C incubation and then to thaw. This retracts the clot so that the recalcified specimen can be removed without centrifugation.

3. If specimens are to be stored, they should be refrigerated at 2 to 8° C or frozen (−15° C or colder).

4. Sodium azide to a final concentration of 0.1% w/v may be added to retard biologic growth. If specimens are to be shipped, they should be packed in compliance with applicable regulations concerning the transportation of etiologic agents.

5. Specimens containing precipitate may give inconsistent test results. To prevent this problem, such specimens should be clarified prior to assaying. (DO NOT USE HEAT-INACTIVATED SPECIMENS.)

EQUIPMENT AND MATERIALS

AUSAB EIA Test Kit (Abbott Laboratories) contains:

1. Hepatitis B surface antigen (human) (subtypes ad and ay) coated beads

2. Hepatitis B surface antigen (human):biotin conjugate

3. Avidin:peroxidase (horseradish) conjugate

4. Positive control

5. Negative control

6. OPD (o-phenylenediamine-2 HCl) tablets

7. Diluent for OPD

8. 1N sulfuric acid

Kit does not include:

9. Precision pipettes with disposable tips or similar equipment to deliver 0.1 mL, 0.2 mL, 0.3 mL and 1.0 mL

10. Disposable graduated pipettes or dispenser for measuring diluent for OPD

11. Device for delivery of rinse solution, such as Cornwall® Syringe, Gorman-Rupp Pump, or equivalent

12. An aspiration device for washing coated beads such as cannula, aspirator tip, or Pentawash® II with a vacuum source and a trap for retaining the aspirate

13. Vacuum pump for use with Penta-wash II, or equivalent

14. Water bath capable of maintaining temperature at 40°C ± 1°C

15. Repipet, for dispensing 1N sulfuric acid

16. Nonmetallic forceps

17. Spectrophotometer capable of reading absorbance at 492 nm

PROCEDURE

NOTE: Follow universal blood and body fluid precautions for all specimen, reagent handling and disposal.

1. Negative control in triplicate and positive controls in duplicate must be assayed each time the test is performed. Ensure that all reaction trays are subjected to the same conditions and incubation times.

CAUTION: Use a separate disposable pipette tip for each transfer to avoid cross-contamination.

NOTE: Once the assay has been started, all steps should be completed without interruption and within the time limits recommended by the procedure.

2. Swirl each reagent gently before using.

3. Adjust water bath to 40°C ± 1°C.

4. Identify the reaction tray wells for each specimen or control on the data sheet.

5. Pipette 200 μL of negative control into the bottom of each of three designated reaction tray wells and 200 μL of positive control into two additional wells.

6. Pipette 200 μL of each specimen to the bottom of two assigned reaction tray wells. All patient specimens are tested in duplicate.

CAUTION: Use care not to splash specimen outside of the well or high up on well rim as it will not be removed in subsequent washings and may be transferred to adjacent wells, thereby causing test interference.

7. Carefully add one hepatitis B surface antigen (human) coated bead to each well containing a control or specimen.

8. Cover the tray with an adhesive cover seal. Gently tap tray to ensure that each bead is covered with the sample and to release air bubbles. Avoid splashing liquid onto the cover.

9. Perform either Procedure A or Procedure B.

Procedure A: Incubate the tray(s) in a 40°C ± 1°C water bath for 2 hours ±5 minutes.

Procedure B: Incubate the tray(s) at room temperature on a level surface for 18 hours ±2 hours.

10. At the end of the incubation period, remove and discard cover seals. Aspirate the contents of the wells into a biohazardous waste container with a Pentawash II or equivalent system. Wash each bead three times with 4 to 5 mL of deionized or distilled water for a total rinse volume of 12 to 15 mL.

11. Calculate the amount of hepatitis B surface antigen (human):biotin conjugate (B-HBsAg) required for the number of tests to be run from the following formula:

(Number of tests required) × (0.11 mL) = Volume of B-HBsAg

12. Calculate the amount of avidin:peroxidase (horseradish) conjugate (A-HRPO) required for the number of tests to be run from the following formula:

(Number of tests) × (0.11 mL) = Volume of A-HRPO required

13. If the number of tests to be run is less than 10, each conjugate may be added individually to each reaction well in 100 μL volumes.

If the number of tests to be run is greater than 10, aliquot the appropriate volumes of B-HBsAg and A-HRPO into a clean mixing tube or beaker; mix gently and thoroughly. (Do not vortex.)

Immediately after mixing, dispense 200 μL of the conjugate mixture into each reaction well. Use a precision pipette and be careful not to splash reagent outside of well or high up on well rim as it may not be removed in subsequent washings and may be transferred to the assay tubes, thereby causing test interference.

14. Cover the reaction tray with an adhesive cover seal. Gently tap tray to ensure that each bead is covered with the conjugate and that any air bubbles are released. Avoid splashing liquid onto the cover.

15. Incubate the trays in a water bath at 40°C ± 1°C for 2 hours ±5 minutes. This applies to both Procedures A and B.

16. During the last 5 to 10 minutes of the incubation, prepare OPD substrate solution as described in the instructions.

17. At the end of the 2-hour incubation period, remove the trays from the water bath. Remove and discard the cover seals. Aspirate the contents of the well into a biohazardous waste container with a Pentawash II or equivalent system. Wash each bead three times with 4 to 5 mL of distilled or deionized water for a total rinse volume of 12 to 15 mL. Remove all excess water from top of tray by aspiration or blotting.

18. Immediately transfer beads from wells to properly identified assay tubes. Align inverted rack of oriented tubes over the reaction tray. Press tubes tightly over wells. Invert tray and tubes together so that beads fall into corresponding tubes maintaining the identity of the sample. Blot excess water from top of tube rack.

19. Instructions for preparation of OPD substrate solution: The OPD (o-Phenyl-

enediamine·2HCl) tablet must be dissolved in diluent for OPD immediately before use. The solution must not be stored longer than 60 minutes before use. During the final 5 to 10 minutes of the second incubation period, prepare the OPD substrate solution as follows: *NOTE* 300 µL is required for each test specimen.

    a. Using a clean pipette, deliver 5 mL of diluent for OPD for each tablet to be dissolved into a suitable container. CAUTION: use pipettes and containers known to be metal- and metal-ion-free.

    b. Using a nonmetallic forceps or equivalent, transfer tablet from bottle into diluent for OPD. Return desiccant to bottle immediately if removed to obtain a tablet and close bottle tightly. Allow tablet to dissolve.

    c. Immediately prior to dispensing, swirl gently to obtain a homogeneous solution.

20. Pipette 300 µL of the freshly prepared OPD substrate solution into each tube containing a bead and into two empty tubes (substrate blanks).

NOTE: Substrate solution should be clear to pale yellow. Do not allow substrate solution to contact metal.

21. Cover the carton of tubes with the black plastic lid provided. Incubate 30 minutes at room temperature.

22. After the 30 minute incubation, stop enzyme reaction by adding 1.0 mL of 1N sulfuric acid to each tube containing a bead and to each of the substrate blanks. Do not allow acid solution to contact metal. Agitate tubes to ensure thorough mixing. Air bubbles should be removed prior to measurement of absorbance.

23. When a Quantum II analyzer is used, refer to the Operations Manual for directions. Measure the blank using one of the two substrate blank tubes. Measure the absorbance of the negative and positive controls and then measure the absorbance of the test samples.

If a Quantum II analyzer is not used, set the photometer or spectrophotometer at 490 nm and zero the instrument using one of the two substrate blanks. Determine the absorbance of the controls and specimens. Thoroughly rinse cuvette with distilled or deionized water.

If there is an interruption during the measurement of samples, repeat the blank using the second substrate blank tube and remeasure the controls. Continue the measurement of specimens. The absorbance of all samples should be determined within two hours after addition of 1N sulfuric acid.

REPORTING. The presence or absence of anti-HBs is determined by comparing the net absorbance of the unknown specimen to the cutoff value.

The cutoff value is determined by adding a factor to the negative control mean as explained in the calculation section below.

Unknown specimens with absorbance values greater than or equal to the cutoff value are considered reactive for anti-HBs. Those specimens with absorbance values less than the cutoff value are considered nonreactive for anti-HBs by the test criteria.

For the run to be valid, the difference between the means of the positive and negative control (P-N) should be 0.300 or greater. If not, technique may be suspect and the test must be repeated. If the P-N value is consistently low, deterioration of reagents may be suspect.

NOTE: When a Quantum II analyzer is used, refer to Operations Manual for directions.

CALCULATIONS

1. Calculation of negative control mean (NC$\bar{\text{x}}$) absorbance.

Example:

Negative Control Sample No.	Absorbance
1	0.025
2	0.028
3	0.028
Total Absorbance	0.081

$$\frac{\text{Total Absorbance}}{3} \quad \frac{0.081}{3} = 0.027 \, (\text{NC}\bar{\text{x}})$$

Individual negative control values should be less than or equal to 0.100 and greater than or equal to −0.006. Negative control values should also be greater than or equal to 0.5 times NC$\bar{\text{x}}$ and less than or equal to 1.5 times NC$\bar{\text{x}}$. If one value is outside this range, disregard this value and recalculate the mean. If two values are outside the range, the test should be repeated. If more than an occasional value falls outside this range, technique problems must be corrected.

When the negative control mean is below 0.012, the calculation of 0.5 to 1.5 times the mean may be disregarded. In such cases, all negative control values should fall within the range: mean ± 0.006.

2. Calculation of the cutoff value

Procedure A: Add the factor 0.030 to the NC$\bar{x}$.

Example:

NC$\bar{x}$	0.027
	+0.030
Cutoff value	0.057

Procedure B: Add the factor 0.050 to the NC$\bar{x}$.

Example:

NC$\bar{x}$	0.027
	+0.050
Cutoff value	0.077

3. Calculations for determining P-N value.

a. Determine the positive control mean (PC$\bar{x}$) absorbance

Example:

Positive Control Sample No.	Absorbance
1	1.433
2	1.461

$$\frac{\text{Total Absorbance}}{2} \quad \frac{2.894}{2} = 1.447 \text{ (PC}\bar{x}\text{)}$$

b. Subtract NC$\bar{x}$ from (PC$\bar{x}$)

Example:

PC$\bar{x}$	1.447
NC$\bar{x}$	−0.027
P-N value	1.420

For the run to be valid, the P-N value should be 0.300 or greater. If not, technique or deterioration of reagents may be suspect and the run should be repeated.

4. Identification of positive specimens: Specimens with an A_{492} greater than or equal to the cutoff value are considered reactive for anti-HBs.

5. Identification of negative specimens: Specimens with an A_{492} less than the cutoff value are considered negative and, therefore, nonreactive for anti-HBs.

6. Sample retest range

Specimens with absorbance values within $\pm 10\%$ of the cutoff value should be retested.

Example:

Cutoff value: 0.077

Range: 0.069 to 0.085

Specimens which have been found repeatedly reactive are positive for anti-HBs by the criteria of the test.

INTERPRETATION OF RESULTS

1. The presence or absence of antibody to HBsAg provides useful information on the status of individuals with type B hepatitis. A positive test for anti-HBsAg can be a useful adjunct for assessing immunity or clinical recovery of the patient.

2. Repeat testing of any questionable specimen will verify whether it is repeatedly reactive for anti-HBs. Specimens whose absorbance is greater than or equal to the cutoff value are considered reactive for anti-HBs. If repeat testing shows the specimen absorbance to be less than the cutoff, the original result may be classified as nonrepeatedly reactive.

LIMITATIONS OF THE PROCEDURE. False reactive results may be obtained with any diagnostic test and usually consist of two types.

1. Nonspecific reactives

Nonspecific reactions may result from cross-reactions in the immune "sandwich" complex. Nonspecific reactions may include reactions with certain glycoproteins, such as concanavalin A,[1] which interact with HBsAg. Millman and McMichael have shown that this hepatitis B binding substance is not antibody.[2] Any highly sensitive immune system has the potential for nonspecific reaction in human serum or plasma.

2. Nonrepeatable reactives

Nonrepeatable reactive specimens, as the name implies, test nonreactive upon repeat. This phenomenon is highly dependent upon technique.

The most common sources of such nonrepeatable reactives are:

a. inadequate washing of the bead

b. cross-contamination of nonreactive

specimens caused by transfer of residual droplets of high titer, antibody-containing sera on the pipetting device

c. contamination of the OPD substrate solution by oxidizing agents

d. contamination of the acid used as a stopping reagent

e. contamination of the reaction tray well rim with conjugate reagent or specimen.

REFERENCES

1. Cawley, L.P.: Am. J. Clin. Pathol., *57*:253, 1972.

2. Millman, I., and McMichael, J.C.:, *21*:879, 1978.

3. Package Insert—AUSAB EIA, Abbott Laboratories, North Chicago, Il, 1986.

HIV INFECTION AND AIDS

First recognized in the United States in 1981[10] the Acquired Immunodeficiency Syndrome (AIDS) has rapidly emerged as a disease of pandemic proportion.[84,101] In the U.S., over 124,000 cases have been reported (as of April 1990),[9] and experts predict that the number will continue to increase throughout the 1990s.[57] An additional 1.0 to 1.5 million individuals in the U.S.[57] and 5 to 10 million persons worldwide[84] are estimated to be infected with the virus that causes AIDS (see below), but have not yet developed the disease.

In 1983–84, the virus causing AIDS was identified independently by Luc Montagnier of France[2] and Robert Gallo of the U.S.[42] and later became known as the Human Immunodeficiency Virus (HIV).[27] (Names formerly given to the virus include Human T cell Lymphotropic Virus—Type III (HTLV-III),[42] Lymphadenopathy Associated Virus (LAV),[2] and AIDS Associated Retrovirus (ARV),[78]) In 1986, a related, but genetically and antigenically distinct virus was also found to cause AIDS, primarily in patients in Western Africa.[25] This virus was termed HIV-2, while the original virus, responsible for the vast majority of AIDS cases worldwide was called HIV-1.[26] In the remainder of this discussion, the term HIV will refer to HIV-1.

HIV is a 1000 angstrom spherical particle containing two identical strands of RNA surrounded by a protein core and an outer lipid envelope.[43] Although related viruses have been discovered in other species,[34,36] human beings are the only known natural host for HIV infection. The virus has been observed to infect CD4 (+) T lymphocytes, monocytes and macrophages, B lymphocytes, microglial brain cells, intestinal cells, and bone marrow cells.[56,67,68]

Laboratory tests have shown that HIV can survive for more than a week in an aqueous environment at 23° to 37° C, but that infectivity is significantly reduced by desiccation or heating at 56° C.[112] Furthermore, in vitro inactivation of HIV is readily accomplished by treatment with a number of chemical disinfectants, including sodium hypochlorite (household bleach), ethyl alcohol, hydrogen peroxide, and nonidet-P40.[87,112]

HIV is classified as a retrovirus because it contains the enzyme activity known as reverse transcriptase, which converts the viral RNA into DNA. This DNA is acted upon by a viral integrase enzyme, and becomes integrated into the DNA of infected host cells, where it may persist as a latent provirus. Expression of the viral genes, and hence, HIV replication, may occur subsequently, and has been shown to be stimulated in vitro by activation of the infected cells with mitogens (e.g. PHA, Con A),[68,90] soluble antigens,[46,68,85] cytokines (e.g. GM-CSF),[40,70] the T cell activation protein NF-kappa B,[95] and coinfection with other viruses (e.g. herpes simplex type 1).[93]

HIV has three structural genes:[107] (1) *gag,* which encodes the core proteins of the virus, p24, p17, and p15 (p = protein; the number following = molecular weight in kilodaltons), and their precursor, p55; (2) *pol,* which codes for the enzymes, reverse transcriptase (p66/51), and endonuclease integrase (p31); and (3) *env,* which encodes a surface glycoprotein on the HIV envelope (gp 120), a transmembrane protein (gp 41), and their precursor (gp 160). Expression of these genes is controlled by a number of other genes which enhance (e.g. tat), down-regulate (e.g. nef), or have a differential effect on (e.g. rev) viral replication.[56] Following their production, HIV RNA and proteins are assembled within infected host cells and acquire an outer envelope upon budding off the surface of the cells.

HIV has been isolated from virtually every body fluid or tissue that has been investigated,[18,21,118] but epidemiologic studies have supported only blood, semen, vaginal secretions, and breast milk as vehicles of transmission.[18] Transmission of HIV, like that of Hepatitis B, has been documented to occur by three major routes: (1) sexual contact with an infected individual, (2) parenteral exposure to infected blood or its components, or transplantion of infected tissue, and (3) vertical transmission, from infected mother to infant. Sexual transmission occurs via intimate contact between homosexual or heterosexual individuals[63,86,99,108] (i.e., anal intercourse, vaginal intercourse, and possibly oral contact),[80,116] and is thought to be enhanced by the presence of open sores, such as those caused by syphilis or herpes.[53,71,103] In industrialized nations such as the U.S., transmission among homosexual/bisexual males has been predominant: approximately 70% of the AIDS cases in the U.S. have been reported among individuals in this category.[9] Heterosexual transmission, with an approximate 1:1 male:female ratio of AIDS patients, has been predominant in central, eastern, and southern Africa and some Latin American countries.[84] In the U.S., transmission via heterosexual contact has resulted in about 5% of the AIDS cases,[9] but is thought to be increasing.[84]

In industrialized countries, transmission by parenteral contact with blood has resulted primarily from the sharing of infected needles and syringes among intravenous drug users, who have comprised approximately 20% of the AIDS cases in the U.S.[9] About 2% of the AIDS cases in the U.S. have occurred in recipients of blood transfusions, and 1%, in hemophiliacs receiving coagulation factors.[9]

Far less commonly, HIV infection has been contracted by health care workers as a result of needlestick injury or mucous membrane contact with blood from infected patients or with concentrated virus in a research laboratory.[19] Numerous studies (summarized in reference 19) on thousands of health care workers with known exposures to HIV-infected blood have found that the rate of infection following exposure is very low, on the magnitude of less than 1%. This risk can be decreased even further by following recommendations issued by the Centers for Disease Control (CDC) for universal body fluid precautions.[18,21] (See also Chap 2—*Universal Precautions for Specimen Handling*). Additional precautions have been recommended for individuals working with concentrated HIV or HIV-infected animals in the laboratory.[22]

Perinatal transmission of HIV accounts for 70 to 80% of pediatric AIDS cases[9,31,129] and is thought to occur during pregnancy or delivery,[31,75,129] or during the postpartum period via breast milk feedings.[77,129,138] Studies have estimated that HIV transmission occurs in about 25 to 50% of infants born to infected mothers.[31]

No evidence has been generated in support of modes of transmission other than the three described above.[31,80] Numerous studies on household contacts of AIDS patients have indicated that casual contact does not result in transmission of HIV.[3,41,64] There is also a lack of scientific or epidemiologic evidence for transmission of the virus through insect vectors.[5,13,139] Although approximately 3% of AIDS cases reported to the CDC are classified as cause undetermined, most of these result from inability to obtain a clinical history of the patient.[9]

In the host, HIV causes a series of progressive immunologic and neurologic abnormalities, with clinical manifestations increasing in severity to eventually culminate in AIDS.[118] Following infection, a period of latency ensues for several months to several years, during which the individual is asymptomatic but may exhibit pathologic laboratory findings. The mean incubation period of HIV in adults has been estimated at 7 to 15 years.[92,111] Some patients may have an acute mononucleosis-like syndrome[29,118,128] associated with the development of HIV antibody a few days to a few weeks after infection; symptoms generally last 1 to 3 weeks, after which the patient usually becomes asymptomatic. As the virus becomes activated, chronic lymphadenopathy may develop, and increasingly severe immune abnormalities, particularly T helper cell depletion, become evident throughout the progression to AIDS. AIDS is almost universally fatal, with a mortality rate of > 90%.[9]

The resulting immunologic defects (see below) seriously impair the body's defenses against infection and malignancy. Consequently, AIDS patients are susceptible to recurrent, often life-threatening infections with any of a myriad of bacterial, viral, fungal, or parasitic organisms.[45,51,121,136] The types of infection seen vary with geographic location and risk group of the patient, and have changed in prevalence during the epidemic.[118] In the U.S., the most common life-threatening infection has been *P. carinii* pneumonia;[45,121] other infections frequently seen include toxoplasmosis, cryptococcosis, tuberculosis, *Mycobacterium avium* and *intracellulare,* cytomegalovirus, herpes simplex, candidiasis, *Streptococcus pneumoniae,* and *Haemophilus influenzae.*[45]

Malignancies commonly seen in AIDS are Kaposi's sarcoma[61,115] (observed predominantly in homosexual males), non-Hodgkin's lymphoma, and primary lymphoma of the brain;[1,118] other malignancies may also occur secondary to HIV infection.[118]

Neurologic symptoms, thought to result from HIV infection of the brain, may become evident in some patients early in the course of infection and resolve, but often progress to more severe manifestations with time.[104] Neurologic syndromes associated with HIV include vacuolar myelopathy, subacute encephalitis, aseptic meningitis, and peripheral neuropathy, and may be evidenced by symptoms such as dementia, motor dysfunction, behavioral changes, and parasthesias.[104,118]

Classification systems defining stages along the broad clinical spectrum of HIV infection have been developed by the Walter Reed Army Institute of Research[110] and the CDC[12] on the basis of clinical symptoms and laboratory findings. An updated surveillance definition of AIDS has also been published by the CDC.[17]

Pediatric AIDS, which constitutes approximately 1% of AIDS cases in the U.S.,[9] is described by a separate CDC classification system.[14] In infants, AIDS is predominantly characterized by failure to thrive, persistent oral candidiasis, chronic pulmonary infiltrates, hepatosplenomegaly, lymphadenopathy, diarrhea, and recurrent bacterial infections, although other symptoms may also occur.[119]

The profound decrease in disease resistance seen in AIDS patients is a consequence of the numerous complex effects of HIV on the immune system.[7,73,120] The most pronounced effect of the virus is that exerted on the T helper (CD4+) lymphocytes. HIV is thought to infect these cells through binding of the viral envelope protein gp120 to the CD4 receptor,[32,66,91,117] and causes massive depletion and profound functional abnormalities in this cell population. Destruction of the T helper cells is thought to result in part, from replication of the virus within the cell and cytotoxic immune responses to viral proteins on the surface of infected cells.[68,109] Because molecular studies have detected HIV in only 1 out of every 10,000 to 100,000 lymphocytes,[54] other mechanisms[68,109] are also thought to contribute to cell death, including (1) destruction by cytotoxic T cells or antibodies directed against soluble gp120 passively attached to uninfected T helper cells,[123] (2) fusion of T cells to form giant syncytia through interaction of surface CD4 and gp120,[81] and (3) alteration of cytokine production in different cell types, with deleterious effects on the T helper cells.[114] Whatever the mechanism(s) of cell death, the decrease in CD4 cells is progressive throughout the course of HIV infection[73,109] and is a hallmark characteristic of AIDS. Peripheral blood CD4 numbers < 400/mm^3 are evident beginning at the Walter Reed WR3 stage of HIV infection,[109,110] and strongly predict a poor prognosis with subsequent development of AIDS.[37,48,102,125]

Functional abnormalities observed in the T helper lymphocytes include decreased in vitro proliferation in response to mitogens and antigens, decreased delayed type hypersensitivity response to skin recall antigens, and decreased production of interleukin-2 in response to antigen stimulation.[7,73,120]

The CD8 lymphocyte population (i.e. cytotoxic/suppressor T cells) increases significantly at the time of HIV antibody seroconversion,[44,74] possibly reflecting an early defensive immune response.[44,133] Thereafter, CD8 counts rise slowly and remain elevated until 6 to 12 months prior to development of AIDS, when they start to decrease.[74] The early elevation of CD8 cells, coupled with the decrease in CD4 cells, generates a decreased CD4/CD8 ratio below the normal value of 1.0.

HIV is capable of infecting cells of the monocyte/macrophage lineage,[59,79,96] possibly via nonspecific phagocytosis, binding to their surface CD4 receptors, or ingestion of immune complexes containing HIV through Fc or complement receptors.[127] Because HIV can replicate in monocytes and macrophages, but does not cause their death, these cells may serve as important reservoirs for HIV, facilitating persistence and dissemination of the virus within the host.[59,127] Functional abnormalities have been observed in monocytes from AIDS patients, including decreased chemotaxis, decreased in vitro killing of microorganisms, and altered monokine production.[7,59,73]

Functional abnormalities of B lymphocytes, most notably polyclonal B cell activation with resulting elevation in total serum immunoglobulins, and unresponsiveness to stimulation with B cell mitogens or antigens, are common in HIV-infected individuals.[7,73,120] These defects may be due to direct infection of the B cells with HIV, abnormal regulation by T cells, or co-infection with viruses such as EBV or CMV.[58,73] Decreased cytotoxicity against virus-infected cells or tumor cells by cytotoxic T lymphocytes or natural killer cells have also been noted in association with HIV infection.[7,30,73] Other abnormalities in immune function include the presence of circulating immune complexes, autoimmune phenomena (e.g. anti-lymphocyte antibodies), production of suppressor factors, serum elevations[7,73,120] in beta-2-microglobulin, acid labile alpha interferon, alpha-1-thymosin, and soluble interleukin-2 receptors,[69,122] and a decrease in serum thymulin.[7,73,120]

In addition to the laboratory abnormalities discussed above, leukopenia, lymphopenia, thrombocytopenia, and anemia are frequently observed in individuals with HIV infection.[118]

Specific laboratory tests for HIV infection are used to screen donated blood products for infectivity, to diagnose and monitor patients, to determine the prevalence of infection in different populations, and to perform investigations in research laboratories. The majority of these tests detect antibody to HIV.

The most widely used antibody test is the ELISA method for HIV-1 antibody,[126] which became available in 1985.[100] (See also *HIV Antibody EIA; Enzyme Immunoassay and Enzyme Linked Immunosorbent Assay*). Specific tests for HIV-2 antibody have also been developed.[26,47] Because the ELISA is highly sensitive, highly specific, and readily adaptable in the clinical laboratory, it is routinely employed as a screening test for HIV antibody.

Federally licensed ELISA procedures are available through a number or commercial manufacturers, and have sensitivity and specificity values > 98–99%.[16,126,131] False values may be obtained as a result of procedural, technical, or test kit errors,[135] but can be reduced by repeat testing of initially reactive specimens. False-negative results may be obtained if the test specimen is collected too early in the course of infection; on the average, individuals develop HIV antibody 6 to 12 weeks after exposure to the virus,[16] but periods as long as 3 years preceding seroconversion have been reported.[55,62,106] Seronegative results may also be obtained from HIV infected neonates with severely depressed immunity.[6,60] False-positive results may occur in the presence of autoantibodies or HLA antibodies directed toward solid phase bound antigens derived from the cell line used to grow HIV;[72,126,135] nonspecific binding may also occur in association with certain disease states (e.g. some viral infections, autoimmune diseases, and hematologic malignancies).[126] Presence of passively transferred HIV-specific maternal antibody (IgG) may complicate results in infants.[60]

To reduce the incidence of false-positive results, it is essential that a confirmatory test be performed on repeatedly reactive ELISA specimens. The need for confirmation is particularly evident in populations with a low prevalence of HIV infection, where the predictive value of a positive antibody result by ELISA alone is low, but increases to almost 100% when followed by a confirmatory procedure.[18]

The most commonly employed confirmatory test is the Western blot (WB) procedure,[98,126,132] which detects antibodies to individual HIV antigens. Technically labor intensive, it is performed primarily by specialized reference or research laboratories. In the WB method, HIV antigens are obtained after detergent treatment of the virus, separated by electrophoresis on a polyacrylamide gel, and immobilized by transfer onto nitrocellulose paper. Incubation of patient serum with the paper allows any HIV antibodies present to bind to their corresponding antigens. Presence of these antibodies is detected by addition of an anti-human immunoglobulin-peroxidase conjugate, followed by substrate, producing

bands at the electrophoretic positions of the corresponding HIV antigens. Variances in banding patterns appear during the course of HIV infection and are useful in monitoring patients.[126] Antibodies to gp160, gp120, p24, and p17 are the first to appear, while bands representing antibodies to p66/51, p31, and gp41 become evident a few weeks later. Over the next few months, titers increase, as seen by a thickening of the bands, then plateau, until progression to AIDS, when antibodies to p24, and to a lesser extent, p31, decline or disappear. This latter development signifies a poor prognosis.[35,130]

Interpretation of the WB has been complicated by a lack of standardization of the procedure and criteria for positivity.[28] In an attempt to resolve discrepancies among different laboratories, the national Public Health Service organized a consultation group in 1988 and summarized various interpretative criteria as follows:[28] (1) positive = presence of bands p24, p31, and gp41 or gp120/160, (2) negative = no bands present; other patterns were classified as (3) probably positive, or (4) indeterminate. All patients in the latter two categories should be followed clinically and retested at a later time to reevaluate their antibody status.

Although the WB is a more specific test than the ELISA, false-positive results may occur for some of the same reasons as discussed for ELISA.[98] Combination of a repeatedly reactive ELISA with a positive WB yields an estimated false positive rate of 1 to 5 per 100,000 samples tested when rigid quality assurance measures are followed.[8,16]

Confirmatory tests other than WB include immunofluorescence[78,132] and radioimmunoprecipitation;[132,135] however, the former cannot detect antibodies to individual HIV antigens, while the latter is too labor intensive to perform outside of the research laboratory.

Efforts are ongoing to improve the sensitivity, specificity, and ease of performance of the serologic tests available. ELISA and WB methods using recombinant HIV antigens have been introduced by a number of sources,[4] and reportedly have excellent performance,[33,94] but have not yet been licensed in the U.S. Rapid screening procedures (e.g. latex agglutination)[105,124] have also been developed, and will be particularly useful in developing nations lacking sophisticated laboratory equipment and personnel and in clinics where immediate counseling of clients is desirable.

In addition to serologic techniques, HIV can be cultured from peripheral blood cells or other clinical specimens from the patient by in vitro infection of activated lymphocytes or permissive T cell lines;[50,135] however, because of the low number of lymphocytes infected, cultures are frequently negative or require several weeks before results are obtained. A reverse transcriptase assay[50] may be performed as an indication of presence of HIV, but is most suited to the research laboratory setting.

Other techniques have been developed to allow more rapid detection of the virus, including an ELISA test for p24 antigen.[49,130] By this method, antigen is detectable in the early acute phase of infection, disappears concurrent with the development of HIV antibody, and then reappears again late in the course of infection.[49,65,130] This reappearance of antigen signifies reactivation of the virus, and predicts a poor prognosis with progression to AIDS.[35,49]

Because of the small number of HIV-infected lymphocytes in patients, molecular hybridization techniques to detect the HIV genome in peripheral blood lymphocytes were extremely difficult prior to the development of the polymerase chain reaction (PCR).[97] By this method, the desired DNA is amplified a number of times upon reaction with specific primer sequences and DNA polymerase; the amplified DNA can then be more easily detected by Southern blot or dot blot analysis. This technique can detect as few as 1 to 10 copies of viral DNA / 1 million cells,[88] and has been a valuable research tool for detecting HIV infection in individuals with negative or equivocal antibody results.[38,76,82]

Although there have been improvements in laboratory detection, HIV infection continues to spread in the absence of an effective treatment or vaccine. Development of a vaccine has been hampered by properties of the virus, lack of a good animal model, and ethical problems.[89] Attempts to reconstitute the immune system in patients with AIDS have been largely unsuccessful.[52] A number of antiviral drugs have been developed and are undergoing clinical trials.[137] Notably, 3'-azido-3'-deoxythymidine (AZT) has been observed to reduce the level of p24 antigenemia and prolong the lifespan of AIDS patients;[24,39] however, AZT is not a cure for AIDS. Treatment of AIDS is therefore largely experimental, in addition to the supportive treatments used to control individual infections and malignancies.[45]

At present, the key to combating this disease is prevention. Massive educational efforts for the public have been aimed at modification of sexual behaviors and habits of intravenous drug users.[11,20] Efforts put forth by individuals to follow these precautions will definitely have an impact on the future course of this pandemic.

REFERENCES

1. Ahmed, T.: In *AIDS and Other Manifestations of HIV Infection.* Edited by G.P. Wormser, R.E. Stahl, and E.J. Bottone. Park Ridge, Noyes Publications, 1987.
2. Barre-Sinoussi, F. et al.: Science, *220*:868, 1983.
3. Berthier, A. et al.: Lancet, *2*:598, 1986.
4. Bianco, C.: Lab. Management, *27*:37, 1989.
5. Booth, W.: Science, *237*:355, 1987.
6. Borkowsky, W. et al.: Lancet, *1*:1168, 1987.
7. Bowen, D.L., Lane, H.C., and Fauci, A.S.: Ann. Intern. Med., *103*:704, 1985.
8. Burke, D.S. et al.: N. Engl. J. Med., *319*:961, 1988.
9. Centers for Disease Control: HIV / AIDS Surveillance Report, April, 1990.
10. Centers for Disease Control: MMWR, *30*:250, 1981.
11. Centers for Disease Control: MMWR, *35*:152, 1986.
12. Centers for Disease Control: MMWR, *35*:334, 1986.
13. Centers for Disease Control: MMWR, *35*:609, 1986.
14. Centers for Disease Control: MMWR, *36*:225, 1987.
15. Centers for Disease Control: MMWR, *36*:285, 1987.

16. Centers for Disease Control: MMWR, *36*:509, 1987.

17. Centers for Disease Control: MMWR, *36*(Suppl. 1S):3s, 1987.

*18. Centers for Disease Control: MMWR, *36*(Suppl. 2s):1s, 1987.

*19. Centers for Disease Control: MMWR, *37*:229, 1988.

20. Centers for Disease Control: MMWR, *37*:261, 1988.

21. Centers for Disease Control: MMWR, *37*:377, 1988.

22. Centers for Disease Control: MMWR, *37*(Suppl. S4):1, 1988.

23. Centers for Disease Control: MMWR, *38*:165, 1989.

24. Chaisson, R.E. et al.: Arch. Intern. Med., *148*:2151, 1988.

25. Clavel, F. et al.: Science, *233*:343, 1986.

26. Clavel, F. et al.: N. Engl. J. Med., *316*:1180, 1987.

27. Coffin, J. et al.: Science, *232*:697, 1986 (letter).

*28. Consortium for Retrovirus Serology Standardization: JAMA, *260*:674, 1988.

29. Cooper, D.A. et al.: Lancet, *1*:537, 1985.

30. Cunningham-Rundles, S. et al.: Adv. Exp. Med. Biol., *187*:97, 1985.

*31. Curran, J.W. et al.: Science, *239*:10, 1988.

32. Dagleish, A.G. et al.: Nature, *312*:763, 1984.

33. Dawson, G.J. et al.: J. Infect. Dis., *157*:149, 1988.

34. Desrosiers, R.C., and Letvin, N.L.: Rev. Infect. Dis., *9*:438, 1987.

35. DeWolf, F. et al.: J. Infect. Dis., *158*:615, 1988.

36. Essex, M., and Kanki, P.J.: Sci. Am., *259*:64, 1988.

37. Fahey, J.L. et al.: Mt. Sinai J. Med., *53*:657, 1986.

38. Farzadegan, H. et al.: Ann. Intern. Med., *108*:785, 1988.

39. Fischl, M.A.: N. Engl. J. Med., *317*:185, 1987.

40. Folks, T.M. et al.: Science, *238*:800, 1987.

41. Friedland, G.H. et al.: N. Engl. J. Med., *314*:344, 1986.

42. Gallo, R.C. et al.: Science, *224*:500, 1984.

43. Gallo, R.C., and Montagnier, L.: Sci. Am., *259*:41, 1988.

44. Giorgi, J.V. et al.: J. Clin. Immunol., *7*:140, 1987.

*45. Glatt, A.E., Chirgwin, K., and Landesman, S.H.: N. Engl. J. Med., *318*:1439, 1988.

46. Gluckman, J.C., Klatzmann, D., and Montagnier, L.: Ann. Rev. Immunol., *4*:97, 1986.

47. Gnann, J.W.: Science, *237*:1346, 1987.

48. Goedert, J.J. et al.: JAMA, *257*:331, 1987.

49. Goudsmit, J. et al.: Lancet, *2*:177, 1986.

50. Griffith, B.P.: Yale J. Biol. Med., *60*:575, 1987.

51. Groopman, J.E.: Prog. Allergy, *37*:182, 1986.

52. Gupta, S., and Gottlieb, M.S.: J. Clin. Immunol., *6*:183, 1986.

53. Handsfield, H.H. et al.: Third International Conference on AIDS, Washington, DC, June 1987.

54. Harper, M.E. et al.: Proc. Natl. Acad. Sci. U.S.A., *83*:772, 1986.

55. Haseltine, W.A.: N. Engl. J. Med., *320*:1487, 1989.

*56. Haseltine, W.A., and Wong-Staal, F.: Sci. Am., *259*:52, 1988.

57. Heyward, W.L., and Curran, J.W.: Sci. Am., *259*:72, 1988.

58. Ho, D.D., Pomerantz, R.J., and Kaplan, J.C.: N. Engl. J. Med., *317*:278, 1987.

59. Ho, D.D., Rota, T.R., and Hirsch, M.S.: J. Clin. Invest., *77*:1712, 1986.

60. Ho Pyun, K. et al.: N. Engl. J. Med., *317*:611, 1987.

61. Hymes, K.B.: In *AIDS and Other Manifestations of HIV Infection*. Edited by G.P. Wormser, R.E. Stahl, and E.J. Bottone. Park Ridge, Noyes Publications, 1987.

62. Imagawa, D.T. et al.: N. Engl. J. Med., *320*:1458, 1989.

63. Jaffe, H.W. et al.: Ann. Intern. Med., *99*:145, 1983.

64. Jason, J.M. et al.: JAMA, *255*:212, 1986.

65. Kessler, H.A. et al.: JAMA, *258*:1196, 1987.

66. Klatzmann, D. et al.: Nature, *312*:767, 1984.

67. Klatzmann, D. et al.: Science *225*:59, 1984.

*68. Klatzmann, D., and Gluckman, J.C.: Immunol. Today, *7*:291, 1986.

69. Kloster, B.E. et al.: Clin. Immunol. Immunopathol., *45*:440, 1987.

70. Koyanagi, Y.: Science, *241*:1673, 1988.

71. Kreiss, J.K. et al.: N. Engl. J. Med., *314*:414, 1986.

72. Kuhnl, P., Seidl, S., and Holzberger, G.: Lancet, *1*:1222, 1985.

*73. Lane, H.C., and Fauci, A.S.: Ann. Rev. Immunol., *3*:477, 1985.

74. Lang, W. et al.: J. AIDS, *2*:63, 1989.

75. Lapointe, M. et al.: N. Engl. J. Med., *312*:1325, 1985 (letter).

76. Laure, F. et al.: Lancet, *1*:538, 1988.

77. LePage, P. et al.: Lancet, *2*:400, 1987.

78. Levy, J.A. et al.: Science, *225*:840, 1984.

79. Levy, J.A. et al.: Virology, *147*:441, 1985.

*80. Lifson, A.: JAMA, *259*:1353, 1988.

81. Lifson, J.D. et al.: Science, *232*:1123, 1986.

82. Loche, M., and Mach, B.: Lancet, *2*:418, 1988.

83. Mann, J.M. et al.: JAMA *256*:721, 1986.

84. Mann, J.M. et al.: Sci. Am., *259*:82, 1988.

85. Margolick, J.B. et al.: J. Immunol., *138*:1719, 1987.

86. Marmor, M. et al.: Ann. Intern. Med., *105*:969, 1986 (letter).

87. Martin, L.S., McDougal, J.S., and Loskoski, S.L.: J. Infect. Dis., *152*:400, 1985.

88. Marx, J.L.: Science, *240*:1408, 1988.

89. Matthews, T.J., and Bolognesi, D.P.: Sci. Am., *259*:120, 1988.

90. McDougal, J.S. et al.: J. Immunol., *135*:3151, 1985.

91. McDougal, J.S. et al.: Science, *231*:382, 1986.

92. Medley, G.F. et al.: Nature, *328*:719, 1987.

93. Mosca, J.D. et al.: Nature, *325*:67, 1987.

94. Motz, M., et al.: Lancet, *2*:1093, 1987 (letter).

95. Nabel, G., and Baltimore, D.: Nature, *326*:711, 1987.

96. Nicholson, J.K.A. et al.: J. Immunol., *137*:323, 1986.

97. Ou, C.-Y. et al.: Science, *239*:295, 1988.

98. Package Insert: HIV Western Blot Kit, Biotech

Research Laboratories, Inc., and Du Pont de Nemours and Co., Inc., Wilmington, DE, 1987.

99. Padian, N. et al.: JAMA, 258:788, 1987.

100. Petricciani, J.C.: Ann. Intern. Med. , 103:726, 1985.

101. Piot, P. et al.: Science, 239:576, 1988.

102. Polk, B.F. et al.: N. Engl. J. Med., 316:61, 1987.

103. Potterat, J.J.: JAMA, 258:473, 1987 (letter).

104. Price, R.W. et al.: Science, 239:586, 1988.

105. Quinn, T.C. et al.: JAMA, 260:510, 1988.

106. Ranki, A., et al.: Lancet, 2:589, 1987.

107. Ratner, L. et al.: Nature, 313:277, 1985.

108. Redfield, R.R. et al.: JAMA, 254:2094, 1985.

*109. Redfield, R., and Burke, D.S.: Sci. Am., 259:90, 1988.

110. Redfield, R.R., Wright, D.C., and Tramont, E.C.: N. Engl. J. Med., 314:131, 1986.

111. Rees, M.: Nature, 326:343, 1987.

112. Resnick, L. et al.: JAMA, 255:1887, 1986.

113. Richman, D.D.: N. Engl. J. Med., 317:192, 1987.

114. Ruddle, N.H.: Immunol. Today, 7:8, 1986.

115. Safai, B. et al.: Ann. Intern. Med., 103:744, 1985.

116. Salahuddin, S.Z. et al.: Lancet, 2:1418, 1984.

117. Sattenau, Q.J. et al.: Science, 234:1120, 1986.

*118. Schupbach, J. (ed.): Current Topics in Microbiology and Immunology. Vol. 142. Berlin, Springer Verlag, 1989.

119. Scott, G.B. et al.: N. Engl. J. Med., 310:76, 1984.

120. Seligmann, M. et al.: N. Engl. J. Med., 311:1286, 1984.

121. Selwyn, P.A.: Hosp. Pract., 21(Sept):119, 1986.

122. Sethi, K.K., and Naher, H.: Immunol. Letters, 13:179, 1986.

123. Siliciano, R.F. et al.: Cell, 54:561, 1988.

124. Spielberg, F. et al.: Lancet, 1:580, 1989.

125. Spira, T.J. et al.: J. Clin. Immunol., 9:132, 1989.

*126. Steckelberg, J.M., and Cockerill, F.R.: Mayo Clin. Proc., 63:373, 1988.

127. Takeda, A., Tuazon, C.U., and Ennis, F.A.: Science, 242:580, 1988.

128. Tucker, J. et al.: Lancet, 1:585, 1985.

129. van der Graaf, M., and Diepersloot, R.J.A.: Infection, 14:203, 1986.

130. von Sydow, M. et al.: Br. Med. J., 296:238, 1988.

131. Waldman, A.A., and Calmann, M.: Lab. Management, August, 1986, p. 31.

132. Waldman, A.A., and Olesko, W.R.: Lab. Management, September, 1986, p. 45.

133. Walker, C.M. et al.: Science, 234:1563, 1986.

134. Weber, J.N. et al.: Lancet, 1:119, 1987.

135. Weiss, S.H.: In AIDS and Other Manifestations of HIV Infection. Edited by G.P. Wormser, R.E. Stahl, and E.J. Bottone. Park Ridge, Noyes Publications, 1987.

136. Wormser, G.P., Stahl, R.E., and Bottone, E.J. (Eds.): AIDS and Other Manifestations of HIV Infection. Park Ridge, Noyes Publications, 1987.

137. Yarchoan, R., Mitsuya, H., and Broder, S.: Sci. Am., 259:110, 1988.

138. Ziegler, J.B. et al.: Lancet, 1:896, 1985.

139. Zuckerman, A.J.: Br. Med. J., 292:1094, 1986.

HIV Antibody EIA[6]

PRINCIPLE. Human Immunodeficiency Virus (HIV) coated beads are incubated with a specimen diluent and human serum or plasma and appropriate controls. Any antibody to HIV is bound to the HIV antigens on the solid phase. After aspiration of the unbound material and washing of the bead, goat antibody to human IgG, conjugated with horseradish peroxidase, is incubated with the bead-antigen-antibody complex. Unbound enzyme conjugate is then aspirated and the beads washed. Next, o-phenylenediamine (OPD) substrate solution containing hydrogen peroxide is added to the bead and, after incubation, a yellow-orange color develops in proportion to the amount of antibody to HIV which is bound to the bead.

EQUIPMENT AND MATERIALS

1. Abbott HIV EIA Diagnostic Kit including:

a. HIV antigen coated beads (Inactivated)

b. One vial (20 mL) or two vials (100 mL each) antihuman conjugate (goat). Antihuman IgG (goat): Peroxidase (horseradish)

Minimum concentration: 0.01 μg/mL in HEPES buffer. Preservatives: antimicrobial agents

c. One vial (0.45 mL) or two vials (0.45 mL each) positive control

Inactivated human plasma positive for antibody to HIV. Minimum titer: 1:2. Preservatives: Antimicrobial agents and 0.1% sodium azide

d. One vial (0.3 mL) or two vials (0.3 mL each) negative control. Human plasma negative for antibody to HIV. Preservatives: Antimicrobial agents and 0.1% sodium azide

e. Two vials (20 mL each) or four vials (100 mL each) specimen diluent containing bovine and goat sera. Preservative: 0.1% sodium azide

f. One bottle (10 tablets) or two bottles (40 tablets each) OPD (o-Phenylenediamine-2 HCl) Tablets. OPD/tablet: 12.8 mg

g. One bottle (55 mL) or two bottles (220 mL each) diluent for OPD (o-Phenylenediamine-2 HCl). Citrate-phosphate buffer containing 0.02% hydrogen peroxide.

   h. 1N sulfuric acid

2. Abbott Quantum II analyzer

3. Waterbath at 40° C

4. Abbott Pentawash II bead washing system or equivalent

5. Distilled or deionized water

6. Disposable pipets

7. Precision pipettes to deliver 200 μL, 300 μL, and 10 μL, with tips

8. Nonmetallic forceps

PRECAUTIONS

1. Handle all Abbott HIV EIA biologic materials as though capable of transmitting infection.[1] HIV antigen coated on beads has been inactivated by detergent and sonication prior to coating. Positive Control has been inactivated by heat treatment.

2. The negative and positive controls are provided in prediluted form. They should not be diluted as specimens. Each run should also include a known positive and a known negative patient control that is treated the same as the test specimens.

3. Do not mix reagents from different lots. Any OPD tablet, diluent for OPD, or sulfuric acid lot, however, may be used with any Abbott HIV kit lot.

4. Do not use kit beyond expiration date.

5. Avoid microbial contamination of reagents when removing aliquots from the reagent vials. Use of disposable pipette tips is recommended.

6. Water for washing should be stored in clean containers to prevent contamination of water with HRPO inactivating substance.

7. Use a clean dedicated dispenser for the conjugate solution to avoid neutralization.

8. Do not expose OPD reagents to strong light during incubation or storage.

9. Avoid contact of OPD and sulfuric acid with skin and mucous membranes. If these reagents come into contact with skin, wash thoroughly with water.

10. Avoid contact of the OPD substrate solution and 1N sulfuric acid with any oxidizing agent. Do not allow substrate solution or 1N sulfuric acid to come into contact with any metal parts. Prior to use, thoroughly rinse glassware used for OPD solution with 1N sulfuric acid using approximately 10% of the container volume. Follow with three washes of distilled water at the same volume.

11. For cleanup of spills[2,5,7] see package insert.

STORAGE INSTRUCTIONS

1. Store kit reagents at 2 to 8° C. OPD Tablets and 1 N Sulfuric Acid may be stored at 2 to 30° C.

2. Bring all reagents to room temperature (15 to 30° C) before use (approximately 30 minutes) and return to storage conditions indicated above immediately after use.

SPECIMEN COLLECTION AND PREPARATION

1. If specimens are to be stored, they should be refrigerated at 2 to 8° C or frozen. Avoid multiple freeze-thaw procedures. If specimens are to be shipped, they should be packed in compliance with Federal regulations covering the transportation of etiologic agents.

2. Either serum or plasma may be used in the test. Remove the serum or plasma from the clot or red cells as soon as possible to avoid hemolysis. When possible, clear, nonhemolyzed specimens should be used. Specimens containing precipitate may give inconsistent test results. Such specimens should be clarified by ultracentrifugation prior to assaying.

PROCEDURE

1. Commercial negative control in duplicate and commercial positive control in triplicate should be assayed with each run of specimens. Do not dilute the controls from the kit.

2. Identify the reaction tray wells for each specimen or control on a data sheet.

3. Prepare patient/patient control dilutions by dispensing 10 μL of each specimen or patient control into bottom of appropriately labeled test tube. Add 200 μL of specimen diluent to each tube. Mix thoroughly.

4. Dispense 10 μL of each control or diluted specimen (from Step 3) into bottom of appropriate wells of reaction tray.

5. Dispense 200 μL of specimen diluent to each well containing a control or diluted specimen.

6. Carefully add one bead to each well containing a control or diluted specimen.

7. Apply cover seal. Gently tap the tray to cover beads and remove any trapped air bubbles.

8. Incubate at 40° C for 1 hour ± 5 minutes.

9. Remove and discard cover seal. Aspirate the liquid and wash each bead three times with 4 to 6 mL of distilled or deionized water.

10. Pipette 200 μL of conjugate into each well containing a bead.

11. Apply new cover seal. Gently tap the tray to cover beads and remove any trapped air bubbles.

12. Incubate at 40° C for 2 hours ± 10 minutes.

13. Remove and discard cover seal. Aspirate the liquid and wash each bead three times as in first incubation.

14. Instructions for preparation of OPD substrate solution: The OPD (o-Phenylenediamine · 2 HCl) tablet must be dissolved in diluent for OPD immediately before use. The solution must not be stored longer than 60 minutes before use. Five to 10 minutes prior to end of incubation, prepare the OPD substrate solution as follows:

NOTE: 300 μL of OPD substrate solution is required for each test specimen as well as for each of two reagent blanks.

CAUTION: Use pipettes and containers known to be metal free such as plastic ware or acid washed/distilled water rinsed glassware.

a. Using a clean pipette, transfer into a suitable container 5 mL of diluent for OPD for each tablet to be dissolved.

b. Transfer OPD tablet(s) from bottle into container with diluent using a nonmetallic forceps or equivalent. Return desiccant to bottle immediately, if removed to obtain a tablet, and close bottle tightly. Allow tablet(s) to dissolve. *Do not use a tablet that is not intact.*

c. Just prior to dispensing for the final incubation of the assay, swirl gently to obtain a homogeneous solution.

15. Immediately transfer beads to properly identified assay tubes.

NOTE: When transferring beads from wells to assay tubes, align inverted rack of oriented tubes over the reaction tray. Press the tubes tightly over the wells and invert tray and tubes together so that beads fall into corresponding tubes. Blot excess water from top of tube rack.

16. Prime dispenser immediately prior to dispensing OPD substrate solution. Pipette 300 μL of freshly prepared OPD substrate solution into each tube.

17. Cover and incubate at room temperature for 30 ± 2 minutes.

18. Add 1 mL of 1 N sulfuric acid to each tube.

19. Blank spectrophotometer with a substrate blank at 492 nm.

20. Determine absorbance of controls and specimens at 492 nm. When a Quantum Analyzer is used, refer to the Operator's Manual to determine which calculations are performed automatically. If a Quantum Analyzer is not used, perform manual calculations.

CALCULATIONS. The presence or absence of antibody to HIV is determined by relating the absorbance of the specimen to the cutoff value. The cutoff value is the absorbance of the negative control mean plus 0.1 times the positive control mean. For the run to be valid, the difference between the means of the positive and negative controls (P-N) should be 0.400 or greater. If not, technique may be suspect and the run must be repeated. If the P-N value is consistently low, deterioration of reagents may be suspect.

1. Calculate the mean of the negative control absorbance values ($NC\bar{x}$).

Example: Negative Control		
Sample No.	Absorbance	
1	0.060	
2	0.056	$\dfrac{\text{Total Absorbance}}{2} = \dfrac{0.116}{2} = 0.058 \ (NC\bar{x})$
Total	0.116	

Individual negative control values must be less than or equal to 0.100 and greater than or equal to 0.010.

Individual negative control values must be within the range 0.5 to 1.5 times the negative control mean. If one value is outside this range, the test must be repeated. If more than an occasional value falls outside this range, technique problems should be investigated.

2. Calculate the mean of the positive control absorbance values (PCx̄).

Example: Positive Control

Sample No.	Absorbance
1	0.835
2	0.925
3	1.015
Total	2.775

$$\frac{\text{Total Absorbance}}{3} = \frac{2.775}{3} = 0.925 \text{ (PCx)}$$

Individual positive control values must be less than or equal to 1.999 or greater than or equal to 0.400.

Individual positive control values must be within the range 0.5 to 1.5 times the positive control mean. If one value is outside the acceptable range, discard this value and recalculate the mean. If two values are outside the range, the test should be repeated.

3. Calculation of the cutoff value

Cutoff Value = NCx̄ + (0.1 × PCx̄)

Example:

NCx̄ = 0.058

PCx̄ = 0.925

Cutoff Value = 0.058 + (0.1 × 0.925) = 0.151

4. Calculations for Determining P-N

Example:

NCx̄ = 0.058

PCx̄ = 0.925

P-N = (0.925-0.058) = 0.867

For the run to be valid, the P-N value should be 0.400 or greater. If not, technique or deterioration of reagents may be suspect and the run should be repeated.

REPORTING. Results are reported as positive or negative for HIV antibody.

INTERPRETATION OF RESULTS

1. Specimens with absorbance values less than the cutoff value are not reactive by the criteria of Abbott HIV EIA and may be considered negative for the antibody.

2. Specimens with absorbance values greater than or equal to the cutoff value are considered reactive by the criteria of Abbott HIV EIA and should also be retested before interpretation using the original sample source. If the results from the second run do not agree with the first, a third run must be performed.

3. Initially reactive specimens that do not react in either of the duplicate repeat tests are considered negative for antibodies to HIV.

4. Specimens which have been found repeatedly reactive are interpreted to be positive for antibody to HIV by the criteria of Abbott HIV EIA.

5. Initially reactive specimens that are nonreactive upon repeat testing should be retested using the original sample source.

LIMITATIONS OF THE PROCEDURE. Because the HIV EIA was designed to test individual units of blood or plasma, most data regarding its interpretation were derived from testing individual samples. Insufficient data are available to interpret tests performed on other body specimens, pooled blood, or processed plasma, and products made from such pools; testing of these specimens is not recommended.

ABBOTT HIV EIA detects antibodies to HIV in blood and thus is useful in screening blood and plasma donated for transfusion and further manufacture, in evaluating patients with signs or symptoms of AIDS, and in establishing prior infection with HIV. Clinical studies continue to clarify and refine the interpretation and medical significance of the presence of antibodies to HIV.[9] For most uses, it is recommended that repeatedly reactive specimens be investigated by an additional more specific, or supplemental, test. A person who has antibodies to HIV is presumed to be infected with the virus and appropriate counseling and medical evaluation should be offered. Such an evaluation should be considered an important part of HIV antibody testing and should include test result confirmation on a freshly drawn sample.

AIDS and AIDS-related conditions are clinical syndromes and their diagnosis can only be established clinically.[4] EIA testing alone cannot be used to diagnose AIDS, even if the recommended investigation of reactive specimens suggests a high probability that the antibody to HIV is present (see *HIV Infection and AIDS*). A negative test result at any point in the investigation of individual subjects does not preclude the possibility of exposure to or infection with HIV. The risk of an asymptomatic person with a repeatedly reactive serum developing AIDS or an AIDS-related condition is not known.[8]

Data obtained from testing persons both at increased and at low risk for HIV infection suggest that repeatedly reactive specimens with high absorbance on EIA are more likely to demonstrate the presence of the HIV antibodies by additional more specific, or supplemental, testing.[3] Reactivity at or only slightly above the cutoff value is more frequently nonspecific, especially in samples obtained from persons at low risk for HIV infection; however, the presence of antibodies in some of these specimens can be demonstrated by additional more specific, or supplemental, testing.

REFERENCES

1. Centers for Disease Control: MMWR, *31*:577, 1982.

2. Bond, W.W., Favero, M.S., Petersen, N.J., and Ebert, J.W.: J. Clin. Microbiol., *18*:535, 1983.

3. Carlson, J.R., Bryant, M.L., Hinrichs, S.H. et al.: JAMA, *253*:3405, 1985.

4. Centers for Disease Control: MMWR, *31*:507, 1982.

5. Merck Index, Listing 4904, 1983.

6. Package Insert, HIV EIA, Abbott Laboratories, Diagnostic Division, North Chicago, IL., 1987.

7. U.S. Environmental Protection Agency, Office of Solid Waste: "Draft Manual for Infectious Waste Management," Washington, D.C., 1982. (USG PO 1982-361-082/325).

8. Taylor, J.M., Schwartz, K., and Detels, R.: J. Infect. Dis., *154*:694, 1986.

9. Weber, J.N. et al.: Lancet, *1*:119, 1987.

RUBELLA (GERMAN MEASLES)

Rubella, the causative agent of German measles, is a member of the viral family Togaviridae, and the only known virus in the genus Ribivirus, It is a single-stranded, spherical RNA virus, enveloped, and approximately 60nm in diameter.[8,28]

Signs and symptoms of acute rubella infection vary from subclinical cases, which are common, to a relatively benign clinical disease characterized by low fever, lymphadenopathy, arthralgia, a transient erythematous rash, and occasionally conjunctivitis, coryza, or headache.[21,31] Central nervous system involvement or thrombocytopenia are rare complications,[21] as is a benign, self-limiting and late occurring arthritis.[45] The disease is classically most common in school-age children (5 to 14 years) and in young adults. The prognosis is almost uniformly excellent; rubella is one of the most benign of all acquired diseases.

The viremia characteristic of acute rubella infection may involve the placenta and fetus of a woman who is pregnant during the illness. Gestational age at the time of infection correlates with fetal infection rates; few, if any, escape damage if less than 7 weeks gestation have elapsed. The majority of those exposed at less than 16 weeks gestation will have defects,[24,35,40] while the risk of "serious morbidity" after 16 weeks gestation is small.[24] Congenital rubella syndrome, or CRS, may be characterized by abortion or stillbirth, or by defects in the central nervous system, heart, eyes, or ears of liveborn infants, either at birth or later in childhood. Persistent T cell abnormalities[30] and growth retardation[41] have also been described. The Centers for Disease Control (CDC) has developed criteria for aiding in the diagnosis of congenital rubella syndrome.[22]

Infection in utero is usually accompanied by substantial fetal IgM production, usually detectable in cord blood and in fetal circulation at birth. Conversion of IgM to IgG occurs during the first year of life, and is then maintained, in most cases, for years.

Since 1969, when the first vaccine for rubella was licensed, greater than a 99% decline has occurred in the number of cases reported.[31] A combined approach to vaccination was adopted in 1981[21] such that susceptible adolescents and young adults are immunized, as well as pre-school children.[2] The MMR, or measles, mumps and rubella combination vaccine is currently in use,[3] administered at the recommended age of 15 months.[27,37] Continued diligence of vaccination at both age levels is recommended.[25]

Vaccination during pregnancy remains contraindicated, a result of theoretical risk to the fetus; interruption of pregnancy in the case of inadvertent vaccination is not recommended.[16]

Both natural infection and immunization usually result in life long immunity to rubella, detectable by the demonstration of serum antibody.[7] Reinfections do occur, more often in vaccinated individuals, but are uncommon, usually subclinical, and accompany waning antibody levels (titer <1:8).

Hemagglutination inhibition[6,38] (HI or HAI) and hemagglutination inhibition testing for IgM,[42] have long been accepted as the standard for rubella antibody testing. Immunofluorescence,[4] ELISA,[14,43,44] complement fixation, passive hemagglutination, latex agglutination, and radioimmunoassay[20] have been extensively compared,[9,10,23,37] in general exhibiting greater sensitivity than HI testing. Most recently, a disperse-dye immunoassay,[32] a single radial hemolysis,[1,15,26] and a capture ELISA[13] for detecting virus-specific IgM have been introduced. Extensive evaluation of commercial kits for detection of rubella antibody is available in the literature.[5,11,12,17,19,29,33,36,39,46]

Recommendations for the standardization of rubella antibody testing have been developed by the National Committee for Clinical Laboratory Standards (NCCLS).[34]

(See also *Rubella Antibody Test: Latex Agglutination*)

REFERENCES

1. Balfour, H.H., Jr. et al.: Lancet, 2:1284, 1981.
2. Bart, K.J., Orenstein, W.A., and Hinman, A.R.: Dev. Biol. Stand., 65:45, 1986.
3. Böttinger, M.: Dev. Biol. Stand., 65:37, 1986.
4. Brown, G.C. et al.: Science, 145:943, 1964.
5. Castellano, G.A. et al.: J. Infect. Dis., 143:578, 1981.
6. Centers for Disease Control: A Procedural Guide to the Performance of Standardized Rubella Hemagglutination Inhibition Tests. Atlanta, 1970.
7. Chantler, J.R., and Davies, M.A.: J. Gen. Virol., 68:1277, 1987.
8. Clarke, D.M. et al.: Nucleic Acids Res., 15:3041, 1987.
9. Cleary, T.J. et al.: Res. Commun. Chem. Pathol. Pharmacol., 19:281, 1978.
10. Cremer, N.E., Hagens, S.J., and Cossen, C.: J. Clin. Microbiol., 11:746, 1980.
11. Fayram, S.L. et al.: J. Clin. Microbiol., 25:178, 1987.
12. Freeman, S., Clark, L., and Dumas, M.: J. Clin. Microbiol., 18:197, 1983.
13. Gerna, G. et al.: J. Clin. Microbiol., 25:1033, 1987.
14. Hancock, E.J. et al: J. Infect. Dis., 154:1031, 1986.
15. Hedman, K. et al.: J. Infect. Dis., 154:1018, 1986.
16. JAMA, 258:753, 1987.
17. Kleeman, K.T., Kiefer, D.J., and Halbert, S.P.: J. Clin. Microbiol., 18:1131, 1983.
18. Madsen, R.D. et al.: Am. J. Clin. Pathol., 79:206, 1983.
19. Meegan, J.M., Evans, B.K., and Horstmann, D.M.: J. Clin. Microbiol., 16:644, 1982.
20. Meurman, O.H., Viljanen, M.K., and Granfors, K.: J. Clin. Microbiol., 5:257, 1977.
21. MMWR, 30:37, 1981.
22. MMWR, 35:770, 1986.
23. Morgan-Capner, P. et al.: J. Clin. Pathol., 32:542, 1979.
24. Munro, N.D. et al.: Lancet, 2:201, 1987.
25. Nokes, D.J., and Anderson, R.M.: Lancet, 1:1441, 1987.
26. Nommensen, F.E.: J. Clin. Microbiol., 25:22, 1987.
27. Orenstein, W.A. et al.: Dev. Biol. Stand., 65:13, 1986.
28. Porterfield, J.S. et al.: Intervirology, 9:129, 1978.
29. Pruneda, R.C., and Dover, J.C.: Am. J. Clin. Pathol., 86:768, 1986.
30. Rabinowe, S.L. et al.: Am. J. Med., 81:779, 1986.
31. Robertson, S.E. et al.: Am. J. Pub. Health, 77:1347, 1987.
32. Rothe, U. et al.: Bio. Biochim. Acta, 45:1325, 1986.
33. Sever, J.L. et al.: J. Clin. Microbiol., 17:52, 1983.

34. Skendzel, L.P.: Lab. Med., *18*:461, 1987.

35. Skinner, C.W.: Am. J. Dis. Child, *101*:78, 1961.

36. Steece, R.S. et al.: J. Clin. Microbiol., *19*:923, 1984.

37. Steece, R.S. et al.: J. Clin. Microbiol., *21*:140, 1985.

38. Stewart, G.C. et al.: New Engl. J. Med., *276*:554, 1967.

39. Storch, G.A. and Myers, N.: J. Infect. Dis., *149*:459, 1984.

40. Tartakow, I.J.: J. Pediatr., *66*:380, 1965.

41. Tokugawa, K. et al.: Rev. Infect. Dis., *8*:874, 1986.

42. Vesikari, T. and Vaheri, A.: Br. Med. J., *1*:221, 1968.

43. Voller, A., and Bidwell, D.E.: Br. J. Exp. Pathol., *56*:338, 1975.

44. Voller, A., and Bidwell, D.E.: Br. J. Exp. Pathol., *57*:243, 1976.

45. Yaneg, J.E. et al.: Ann. Intern. Med., *64*:772, 1966.

46. Zartarjan, M.V. et al.: J. Clin. Microbiol., *14*:640, 1981.

Rubella Antibody Test[2]: Latex Agglutination

PRINCIPLE. The Rubascan card test is based upon the principles of passive latex agglutination. Latex is sensitized using solubilized rubella virus antigens from disrupted virions. When mixed with serum containing rubella antibodies on a card surface, this latex reagent will agglutinate, forming visible clumps. In the absence of antibody, or if the concentration is sufficient to react, the latex will remain smooth and evenly dispersed.

EQUIPMENT AND MATERIALS

1. Rubascan Kit (Becton Dickinson) containing:

   a. Rubascan Latex antigen with 0.02% gentamicin and 0.2% sodium azide (preservatives)

   b. Rubascan high reactive control (human serum), with 0.1% sodium azide (preservative)

   c. Rubascan low reactive control (human serum), with 0.1% sodium azide (preservative)

   d. Rubascan nonreactive control (human serum), with 0.1% sodium azide (preservative)

   e. Rubascan card dilution buffer, phosphate buffered saline solution, containing bovine serum albumin, with 0.02% sodium azide (preservative)

   f. Rubascan test cards, qualitative

   g. Plastic stirrers

   h. Dispensing needle, 21 guage, green hub

2. Centrifuge

3. Rotator

4. Humidifying cover

5. High intensity incandescent lamp

6. Micropipettors, 100 and 25 μl delivery

7. Pipettor tips

PRECAUTIONS. Reagents: Do not use beyond the expiration date. Upon removal from the refrigerator, allow the reagents to warm to room temperature (23 to 29° C) before use. Do not mix reagents from different kit lot numbers. To assure proper drop delivery when dispensing Rubascan latex antigen, the dispensing bottle must be held vertically. The Rubascan latex antigen has been prepared from disrupted vaccine strain virus which has been judged to be inactivated by bioassay procedures. Reagents contain sodium azide which may react with lead and copper plumbing to form highly explosive metal azides. On disposal, flush with a large volume of water to prevent azide build-up.

SPECIMEN COLLECTION AND PREPARATION. The manner of serum collection varies with testing objectives. Single-serum specimens are required for qualitative antibody level determinations. In suspected clinical infections or exposure, two serial serum specimens for quantitative testing should be obtained. The first should be collected within 3 days of the onset of rash, or at the time of exposure, and tested upon arrival at the laboratory. This specimen should then be subsequently stored frozen until the second specimen is collected 7 to 21 days after the onset of rash, or at least 30 days after exposure if no clinical symptoms occur. Both specimens should then be tested simultaneously for antibodies to rubella.

Whole blood is collected and the serum is

separated. Specimens may be stored up to 48 hours at 2 to 8° C. Specimens should be frozen if longer storage is required. Do not heat inactivate the serum. The presence of particulate matter, lipemia, or hemolysis does not affect the test.

STORAGE INSTRUCTIONS. Refrigerate at 2 to 8° C. DO NOT FREEZE. Reagents should be returned to refrigeration when not in use.

PROCEDURE

Test cards: Cards must be flat for proper reactions. If necessary, flatten cards by bowing back in a direction opposite to that of the curl. Care should be taken not to finger-mark the test areas, since this may result in an oily deposit and improper tests results. Use each card once and discard. Store cards in the original package in a dry area at room temperature prior to use.

Dispensing needle: Upon completion of daily tests, remove the needle from the dispensing bottle and recap the bottle. Rinse the needle with distilled water to maintain clear passage and accurate drop delivery. Do not wipe the dispensing needle because it is silicone-coated.

PERFORMANCE OF QUALITATIVE TESTING

1. Remove the cap from the Rubascan latex antigen bottle and attach the green hub needle to the tapered fitting.
2. Mark the card to identify the low reactive and non reactive controls and all samples being tested.

With Undiluted Specimens:

3. With a micropipettor, place 25 µl of low reactive control onto the appropriate circle.
4. With the same micropipettor and a new tip each time, repeat the procedure in step 3, using the nonreactive control and each sample being tested.

With 1:10 Specimen Dilutions:

3. With a micropipettor, add 100 µl of card dilution buffer to the appropriate squares for each control and sample being tested.

With a micropipettor, add 25 µL of card dilution buffer to the appropriate circles for each control and sample being tested.

4. Using the same micropipettor with a new tip, place 25 µl of low reactive control directly into the buffer in the appropriate square and mix the serum and buffer by drawing up-and-down with the micropipettor 12 times. Avoid the formation of bubbles. The serum in this square is now a 1:5 dilution.

Using the same micropipettor and tip, transfer 25 µl of the 1:5 dilution from the square and place directly into the buffer in the correspondingly numbered circle. Mix by drawing up-and-

down the micropipettor six times. Withdraw 25 µl from the circle and discard. The serum in the circle is now a 1:10 dilution.

Repeat the procedures in step 4 for the nonreactive control and for each sample being tested. *With 1:10 dilutions and undiluted specimens:*

5. Using a new plastic stirrer for each circle, spread the serum to fill the entire circle.
6. While holding the bottle cap over the tip of the needle, gently invert the dispensing bottle several times to thoroughly mix the Rubascan latex antigen.
7. Holding the bottle in a vertical position, dispense several drops of antigen into the bottle cap until a drop of uniform size has been formed. Dispense one free-falling drop of antigen (approximately 15 µl) onto each circle containing the serum. Recover the predropped antigen from the bottle cap.
8. Place the card on a rotator and rotate for 8 minutes at 100 rpm under a moistened humidifying cover.
9. Immediately following mechanical rotation, read the card macroscopically in the wet state under a high intensity incandescent lamp. Gently tilt the card (three or four back-and-forth motions) to help differentiate weak agglutination from no agglutination.

REPORTING

1. The reactive control should show agglutination, while the nonreactive control should show no agglutination.

2. Report as positive: Reactive—showing any agglutination of the Rubascan latex antigen.

3. Report as negative: Nonreactive—showing no agglutination of the Rubascan latex antigen.

In undiluted samples, strong reactivity may cause the center of the test circle to appear clear, because agglutinated latex has migrated to the periphery. Furthermore, reduction in the degree of agglutination has been reported with rare high titered specimens when Rubascan testing is performed undiluted. Optimal sensitivity has been ensured by screening all serum samples undiluted and repeating negative samples at a 1:10 dilution.

INTERPRETATION OF RESULTS. The presence of antibodies is an indication of previous exposure to the virus, and a single specimen can be used to estimate the immune status of the individual. Because it is the opinion of the Immunization Practice Advisory Committee that any detectable antibody is indicative of immunity and protection against subsequent viral infection, the sensitive test configuration using undiluted specimens may be preferred. An alternative procedure using specimens diluted 1:10 is provided for use when it is desired to collect data at a sensitivity level approximating that expected with hemagglutination inhibition methods. However, this protocol method using 1:10 dilutions will fail to detect low level antibody specimens that would be reactive undiluted.

PERFORMANCE OF QUANTITATIVE TESTING (SERA DILUTED 1:15 THROUGH 1:160)

1. Remove the cap from the Rubascan latex antigen bottle and attach the green hub needle to the tapered fitting.

2. Mark squares and circles on the card to identify high reactive, low reactive and nonreactive controls, and all samples being tested.

3. Dilution of high reactive control:

   a. With a micropipettor, add 100 μl of card dilution buffer to the appropriate square in the row marked "High Reactive".

   b. With a micropipettor, add 25 μl of card dilution buffer to circles 1 through 6.

   c. With a micropipettor, place 25 μl of high reactive control directly into the buffer in the appropriate square and mix the serum and buffer by drawing up-and-down with the micropipettor 12 times. Avoid the formation of bubbles. The serum in the square is now a 1:5 dilution.

   d. Using the same micropipettor and tip, transfer 25 μl of the 1:5 dilution from the square, and place directly into the buffer in circle 1. Mix by drawing up-and-down with the micropipettor six times. The serum in circle 1 is now a 1:10 dilution.

   e. Using the same micropipettor and tip, transfer 25 μl of the 1:10 dilution directly into the buffer in circle 2, mix as before, and continue this preparation of serial twofold dilutions through circle 6. Withdraw 25 μl from circle 6 and discard. The resulting serum dilutions are twofold starting at a 1:10 dilution.

4. Dilution of low reactive control: Repeat step 3, except that serial dilutions only go through circle 4, and 25 μl diluted serum is discarded from circle 4.

5. Nonreactive control: With a micropipettor add 25 μl of nonreactive

control to circle 1 in the row marked "Nonreactive Control."

6. Dilution of test samples:

   a. Using a new micropipettor tip for each sample being tested, repeat the procedures in step 3.

   b. If further dilutions are required, continue the procedures described in step 3 through the next row of circles.

7. Using a new plastic stirrer for each control and test sample, start at the highest numbered circle and spread the serum dilution to fill the entire circle. Using a separate stirrer for each row, proceed to the next lower circle and spread the serum dilution in a similar manner. Repeat this procedure until the contents of all circles are spread.

8. While holding the bottle cap over the tip of the needle, gently invert the dispensing bottle several times to thoroughly mix the antigen.

9. Holding in a vertical position, dispense several drops of antigen into the bottle cap until a drop of uniform size has been formed. Dispense one free-falling drop of antigen (approximately 15 μl) onto each circle containing the serum dilutions. Recover the pre-dropped antigen from the bottle cap.

10. Place the card on a rotator and rotate for 8 minutes at 100 rpm under a moistened humidifying cover.

11. Immediately following mechanical rotation, read the card macroscopically in the wet state under a high intensity incandescent lamp. Gently tilt the card (three or four back-and-forth motions), to help differentiate weak agglutination from no agglutination.

REPORTING. Report reactivity in terms of the highest dilution showing any agglutination of the Rubascan latex reagent. Specimens showing no agglutination at any dilution are reported as nonreactive.

The reactive controls are formulated to produce agglutination within the labeled dilutions. The nonreactive control should show no agglutination.

INTERPRETATION OF RESULTS. Demonstration of seroconversion or a fourfold or greater rise in antibody titer on properly collected paired specimens, indicates recent exposure to rubella virus with the Rubascan test system. Seroconversion may also be indicated by a positive test result of 1:5 or greater after an initial nonreactive result of less than 1:5. In rare instances, a low titered sample will exhibit equivocal results (borderline agglutination) even upon repeat testing. In such cases, testing of additional samples or the use of an alternative test procedure may be helpful.

LIMITATIONS OF THE PROCEDURE. The Rubascan qualitative card test has been designed to detect the presence of rubella antibody. At a single dilution the qualitative protocol will perform satisfactorily with both acute phase and convalescent phase antibodies. In cases when the presence or absence of a fourfold titer rise in paired specimens must be demonstrated, the quantitative protocol is required.

The quantitative protocol should be used with properly paired specimens to determine recent infection. Care must be used in the timing of sample collection. If the first (acute phase) sample is taken too late or the second (convalescent phase) sample is taken too soon, the seroconversion or fourfold rise in titer characteristic of recent infection may not be seen. The acute phase specimen should be collected as nearly as possible to the time of exposure and no later than 3 days after the onset of rash. The convalescent phase specimen should be taken 7 to 21 days after the onset of the rash or at least 30 days after exposure, if no clinical symptoms appear (possible inapparent infection). *BOTH SPECIMENS SHOULD BE TESTED SIMULTANEOUSLY.* The absence of a fourfold titer rise does not necessarily rule out the possibility of exposure and infection.

Serum specimens with obvious microbial contamination should not be assayed with this method.

The use of plasma in the Rubascan quantitative card test has not been established.

REFERENCES

1. Centers for Disease Control: MMWR, *30*:37, 1981.

2. Insert, Rubascan, Becton Dickinson Microbiology Systems, Cockeysville, MD, 1988.

C. Fungal Infections

ASPERGILLOSIS

The genus Aspergillus is comprised of a group of saprophytic molds which are ubiquitous in nature and capable of inducing disease in man. *Aspergillus fumigatus* is the species most commonly linked to disease; however, *A. flavus, A. niger,* and several other species have also been implicated as human pathogens.[1,4,16]

Most cases of aspergillosis involve the respiratory system. Inhaled spores, or allergens, from the mold, may induce a variety of clinical manifestations, depending on the immunologic status of the host (atopic, nonatopic, or immunosuppressed).[8,9]

Atopic individuals, or those prone to type I hypersensitivity responses,[6] may develop extrinsic asthma, with reaginic activity directed against Aspergillus antigens, and affecting primarily the bronchial tree. In some individuals, typically young to middle-aged adults with a history of recurrent, corticosteroid-dependent asthma, colonization of the respiratory tract with Aspergillus may occur, resulting in Allergic Bronchopulmonary Aspergillosis (ABPA).[3,8,11] Clinical manifestations of ABPA include chest pain, wheezing, fever, general flu-like symptoms, and eosinophilia of both sputum and blood. Pulmonary infiltrates are seen, and expectoration of brown sputum plugs containing eosinophils and mycelia may occur. Bronchial wall damage may result from deposition of immune complexes containing IgG, IgM, or IgA antibodies and complement (i.e. Gell and Coombs Type III hypersensitivity reaction),[6] or cell-mediated hypersensitivity (Type IV hypersensitivity reaction).[6] Early recognition and treatment of the disease is essential in preventing progression to end-stage ABPA, characterized by irreversible bronchiectasis and pulmonary fibrosis.[3,11]

Infection of nonatopic individuals who are not immunosuppressed may result in the development of hypersensitivity pneumonitis or noninvasive pulmonary aspergilloma. Hypersensitivity pneumonitis, or extrinsic allergic alveolitis (EAA), may be induced by inhalation of Aspergillus spores and subsequent formation of immune complexes in the bronchi and lungs. Asthma and eosinophilia are not usually associated with this condition, whose symptoms are described elsewhere (see *Hypersensitivity Pneumonitis*). Pulmonary aspergilloma is the formation of a fungus ball, or a gummous mass containing thousands of tangled hyphae, resulting from colonization by Aspergillus of pre-existing cavities of the lung due to complications of other pulmonary disorders, such as tuberculosis, sarcoidosis, lung cancer, cystic fibrosis, or ABPA.[11] In most cases of aspergilloma, the colony is noninvasive and non-atopic, although about one-fourth of the cases may eventually exhibit atopy.

Invasive or disseminated aspergillosis is a serious condition affecting immunocompromised patients, most commonly, individuals with acute leukemia, lymphoma, or organ transplantation, and profound granulocytopenia.[1,8] The disease is usually fatal, and generally presents as an acute pneumonia that disseminates to the gastrointestinal tract, brain, liver, kidneys, heart, and skin.

Bronchial infection or colonization with Aspergillus is suggested by repeated isolation of the organism from sputum cultures or demonstration of hyphae in sputum or bronchial brushings. However, a significant number of patients with bronchopulmonary aspergillosis or aspergilloma yield negative results, even on repeat culture.[16] Antibody tests are useful in detecting aspergillosis and frequently provide the earliest evidence of ABPA and aspergilloma.[7] The most widely used method for detecting Aspergillus antibody is Ouchterlony double immunodiffusion.[12] Other commonly used techniques are counterimmunoelectrophoresis, which reportedly has a comparable sensitivity to that of Ouchterlony, and immunofluorescence, which appears to have greater sensitivity but less specificity than the diffusion methods.[7]

The antibodies detected are usually of the IgG class, but IgM and IgA have also been implicated. Using broth filtrates or whole cell homogenates as antigen, precipitins have been detected in greater than 90% of patients with aspergilloma and 70% of patients with ABPA,[4,15] while the incidence of precipitins in normal subjects has reportedly ranged from 0 to 11%.[4,10] Multiple precipitin bands (≤ 15–20) may be observed, and attest to the number of antigen-antibody systems present in the disease.[16] One to four precipitin bands are usually noted: one to two bands indicate strong exposure to Aspergillus, and three to four bands indicate aspergilloma or invasive aspergillosis.[17] The number of precipitin bands correlated well with high titers in one study, and removal of the patient from exposure to Aspergillus antigen resulted in seroconversion to negative.[5] An additional precipitin band may be caused by the reaction of C-substance, often found in antigen extracts of Aspergillus,[14] with C-reactive protein in patient sera. However, since this reaction is Ca^{++}-dependent, formation of the precipitin can be prevented by incorporating EDTA into the agarose of the immunodiffusion plates,[14] or the precipitate can be solubilized by treatment with sodium citrate.[16]

Although immunoprecipitation methods are often helpful in diagnosing aspergillosis in the immunocompetent individual, they often fail to detect invasive disease in the patient who is immunocompromised.[13] Diagnosis of disseminated aspergillosis is confounded by the fact that cultures in these patients are almost uniformly negative in blood and sputum,[1,8] and may be negative even when invasive techniques such as bronchoscopy and open lung biopsy are used to obtain the specimen.[18] These shortcomings have prompted the search for a more sensitive method of detecting invasive infection. Studies suggest that the more sensitive methods of RIA and ELISA may detect Aspergillus antibody in a significant number of patients with invasive disease, as well as noninvasive infections,[12,13] but these have not yet received widespread application. RIA and ELISA technology has also been applied to the detection of Aspergillus antigen, but has had only limited success;[7,13,18] however, these methods may improve as more highly purified reagents are developed.[2,14]

Other tests that are useful in the detection of Aspergillus infections include skin tests and quantitation of serum IgE. The latter is useful in the diagnosis of ABPA, since IgE levels are markedly elevated in virtually all patients with this condition.[8]

Skin tests, either via prick test or intradermal injections, are also helpful. With atopy (eg. asthma or ABPA), immediate reactions are noted. In the absence of atopy, "delayed" or Arthus reactions become visible within 3 to 4 hours. Skin tests are diagnostic for allergic bronchopulmonary disease when both immediate and "delayed" reactions are noted.[16] With the other manifestations of the disease, skin tests provide evidence of the presence of antibody, but are not diagnostic.

In our laboratory, we detect serum precipitins to Aspergillus by double immunodiffusion. (See also *Hypersensitivity Pneumonitis, Ouchterlony Technique: Double Immunodiffusion.*)

REFERENCES

1. Bennett, J.E.: In *Harrison's Principles of Internal Medicine.* 11th ed. Edited by E. Braunwald et al. New York, McGraw-Hill Book Co., 1987.
2. Bennett, J.E.: Rev. Infect. Dis., *9*:398, 1987.
3. Brown, G.P., and Hunninghake, G.W.: In *Basic and Clinical Immunology.* 6th ed. Edited by D.P. Stites, J.D. Stobo, and J.V. Wells, Norwalk, Appleton and Lange, 1987.
4. Campbell, M.J., and Clayton, Y.M.: Am. Rev. Respir. Dis., *89*:186, 1964.
5. Coleman, R.M., and Kaufman, L.: Appl. Microbiol., *23*:301, 1972.
6. Coombs, R.R.A., and Gell, P.G.H.: In *Clinical Aspects of Immunology.* Edited by P.G.H. Gell, R.R.A.

Coombs, and P.J. Lachmann. Oxford, Blackwell Scientific, 1975.
*7. deRepentigny, L., and Reiss, E.: Rev. Infect. Dis., *6*:301, 1984.
*8. Doyle, T., Symon, H., and Sutherland, P.: Med. J. Aust., *145*:466, 1986.
9. Fink, J.N., and Sosman, A.J.: Med. Clin. North Am., *58*:157, 1974.
10. Galant, S.P. et al.: Am. Rev. Respir. Dis., *114*:325, 1976.
11. Greenberger, P.A., and Patterson, R.: Ann. Allergy, *56*:444, 1986.
12. Harvey, C., Shaw, R.J., and Longbottom, J.L.: J. Allergy Clin. Immunol., *79*:324, 1987.
13. Hopwood, V., and Warnock, D.W.: Eur. J. Clin. Microbiol., *5*:379, 1986.
14. Jones, J.M.: Lab. Management, March, 1985, p.53.
15. Kaufman, L.: In *Rapid Methods and Automation in Microbiology.* Edited by R.C. Tilton. Washington, D.C., American Society for Microbiology, 1981.
*16. Rosenberg, M. et al.: Ann. Intern. Med., *86*:405, 1977.
17. Schwartz, R.H. et al.: Am. J. Dis. Child., *120*:432, 1970.
18. Talbot, G.H. et al.: J. Infect. Dis., *155*:12, 1987.

CANDIDIASIS

The genus, Candida, contains a group of ubiquitous fungi that are commonly found among the normal flora of the human mouth, vagina, and intestinal tract.[2,4,10,11] *Candida albicans* is the species of yeast most frequently isolated from the human body and is primary cause of Candidiasis. Other species of Candida, such as *Candida tropicalis* and *Candida parapsilosis,* have been implicated in a smaller number of cases of the disease.

Candidiasis can present itself in one of two basic forms: (1) Superficial Candidiasis, or minor, self-limiting infections of mucocutaneous surfaces commonly seen in healthy individuals; these infections include vulvovaginal candidiasis, oral candidiasis (thrush), and cutaneous candidiasis; and (2) Invasive Candidiasis, or potentially life-threatening, systemic infections that occur in immunocompromised hosts, including individuals with AIDS, Chronic Mucocutaneous Candidiasis, severe diabetes mellitus, extensive burns, organ transplants in conjunction with immunosuppressive therapy, or hematologic malignancies. Invasive candidiasis has been described as the most common serious fungal infection in hospitalized patients,[9] increasing in incidence in recent years with increased usage of invasive procedures such as central venous catheterization and total parenteral nutrition, and therapeutic regimens such as antitumor chemotherapy or therapy with large doses of broad-spectrum antibiotics.[5,8,10]

Superficial Candida infections are best diagnosed by demonstration of pseudohyphae on wet smears prepared from scrapings of skin, nails, and oral or vaginal mucosa, and confirmation by culture.[2] Invasive candidiasis poses a difficult diagnostic problem, as it is not associated with a single typical clinical picture,[10,15] and the diagnosis of deep or systemic infections involves the preparation of histologic sections of biopsy specimens or culture of blood, cerebral spinal fluid, synovial fluid, or surgical specimens.[2] However, culture of Candida from areas of the body not externally exposed is not easily accomplished, and surgical or needle biopsies pose a threat of further infection in the compromised host. Conversely, the significance of cultures from areas of the body with external access (for example, the urinary or digestive tracts) is often difficult to determine, as these might be easily contaminated during collection of the specimen through contact of sites normally colonized by Candida. Repeatedly positive cultures from normally sterile body fluids (blood, cerebral spinal fluid, synovial fluid) usually signify infection, but are demonstrable in less than 40% of patients with invasive Candidiasis.[5,15]

Thus, much effort has been directed toward developing a serologic assay which, ideally, would be capable of detecting invasive candidiasis in the early stages of disease, so that treatment may be initiated promptly, while at the same time, differentiating systemic disease from superficial infection. Detection of antibody to *Candida albicans* has been performed using a variety of test systems, of which the most widely used are double immunodiffusion (Ouchterlony), counter-immunoelectrophoresis, and latex agglutination.[1,5,8,13,16] Methods of whole cell agglutination, immunofluores-

cence, RIA, and ELISA have also been developed. Although numerous studies have been published on these tests, differences in patient populations studied, lack of antigen standardization, and variances in test techniques have resulted in findings which lack in agreement and are difficult to compare.[5,16] Collaborative studies using the most common methods of counterimmunoelectrophoresis, Ouchterlony, and latex agglutination, have found these tests to have sensitivity and specificity levels >80% when used on a patient population with a largely intact immune response.[5,12,14] However, false-positive results may be encountered, as up to 100% of the normal population may have low titers of antibody to *C. albicans,* which tend to rise in association with hospitalization.[1,16] Therefore, serologic tests on these patients should be performed quantitatively on serial specimens in order to yield the most accurate results.

Unfortunately, a high percentage of false-negative results have been encountered when these tests are performed on immunocompromised patients with invasive candidiasis, and may be caused by impaired ability of the host to produce an antibody response or by an excess of circulating antigens.[1,5] Numerous attempts have been made to increase the sensitivity and predictive value of serologic tests in this group of patients, and to more accurately discriminate between superficial and invasive candidiasis. Some of the more recent advances include the production of monoclonal antibodies to fungal antigens, increased characterization and purification of Candida antigens, and the development of more sensitive assay systems, such as RIA and ELISA.[5]

Another approach undertaken by laboratories in order to detect infection in immunosuppressed patients who do not produce a measurable antibody response has been to investigate the detection of circulating Candida antigens.[1,3,7,9] At least two different antigens are present in the blood of infected patients: (1) a soluble, heat-stable antigen, thought to be mannan, the major cell wall polysaccharide of Candida, which must be dissociated from immune complexes prior to detection, and (2) a heat-labile cytoplasmic protein antigen.[3] Because these antigens, however, are present in low concentrations (in the range of ng/ml), and antigenemia appears to occur only transiently during the infection, a suitable assay system for detection of Candida antigens in the routine clinical laboratory is not yet available.[1,7] Serum quantitation of the Candidal metabolites, arabinotol, and mannose, by gas liquid chromatography has also been investigated and shows some promise, but requires considerable technical expertise and is not suitable for routine testing.[5,7]

Despite the problems encountered with serologic test systems for Candida, these assays have demonstrated an acceptable level of accuracy in patients with a largely intact immune system, and have been useful as an adjunct to other laboratory and clinical findings in immunocompromised patients. Some laboratories have found that the predictive values of these tests increased when combinations of different test systems were used in diagnosis.[6,15] Their value is also increased when tests are performed on serial specimens, as levels of antigen and antibody will fluctuate during the course of infection.

Our laboratory employs a double immunodiffusion method to detect antibody, using *Candida albicans,* Strain B35, type A, as the antigen (see also *Ouchterlony Technique: Double Immunodiffusion*).

REFERENCES

1. Anonymous: Lancet, *2*:1373, 1986.
2. Bennett, J.E.: In *Harrison's Principles of Internal Medicine,* 11th ed. Edited by E. Braunwald et al. New York, McGraw-Hill Book Co., 1987.
3. Bennett, J.E.: Rev. Infect. Dis., *9*:398, 1987.
4. Bodey, G.P., and Fainstein, V. (Eds.): *Candidiasis,* New York, Raven Press, 1985.
*5. deRepentigny, L., and Reiss, E.: Rev. Infect Dis., *6*:301, 1984.
6. Fisher, J.F., Trincher, R.C., and Agel, J.F.: Am. J. Med. Sci., *290*:135, 1985.
7. Hopwood, V., and Warnock, D.W.: Eur. J. Clin. Microbiol., *5*:379, 1986.
8. Jones, J.M.: Lab. Management, March 1985, p.53.
9. Kahn, F.W., and Jones, J.M.: J. Infect. Dis., *153*:579, 1986.
*10. Kauffman, C.A., and Jones, P.G.: Postgrad. Med., *80*:129, 1986.
11. Kirkpatrick, C.H., Rich, R.R., and Bennett, J.E.: Ann. Intern. Med., *74*:955, 1971.
12. Kozinn, P.J. et al.: Am. J. Clin. Pathol., *70*:893, 1978.
13. Kozinn, P.J., and Taschdjian, C.L.: In *Candidiasis.* Edited by G.P. Bodey and V. Fainstein, New York, Raven Press, 1985.
14. Merz, W.G. et al.: J. Clin. Microbiol., *5*:596, 1977.
15. Platenkamp, G.-J. et al.: J. Clin. Pathol., *40*:1162, 1987.
16. Smith, J.M.B., Mason, A.B., and Meech, R.J.: N.Z. Med. J., *97*:155, 1984.

HYPERSENSITIVITY PNEUMONITIS

Hypersensitivity pneumonitis (HP), also known as *extrinsic allergic alveolitis,* is an immunologically induced disorder of the peripheral airways (bronchioles, alveoli) and interstitial tissues of the lung which develops as a result of intense and often prolonged exposure to certain inhaled particles. The disorder is related to, but must be differentiated from immunologically related asthma,[16,19] and from such fibrotic lung diseases as asbestosis and berylliosis, which are not proven to be immunologically induced.[16]

Hypersensitivity pneumonitis may occur in subacute, acute, or chronic form.[14] Subacute, or asymptomatic pneumonitis, is characterized by the presence of certain immunologic factors, e.g. precipitating antibodies to the antigen involved, but without clinical manifestation. Acute attacks involve breathlessness, cough, fever, chills, and aching, which follow exposure by 4 to 6 hours and subside within 24 to 48 hours. Chronic illness is most commonly insidious, involving cough, increasing breathlessness, weight loss and generalized malaise. Chronic disease may appear with or without previous acute attacks. In either acute or chronic forms, continued exposure may lead to irreversible fibrotic lung disease. Even after acute attacks, impairment of pulmonary function can persist.[21]

Pathologic observations[23,40,41] of these diseases include interstitial alveolar infiltrate in all cases, granuloma formation and, as a later development, interstitial fibrosis in many. There are activated macrophages, increased lymphocyte populations and plasma cells, and mast cell infiltrates.

Many hypersensitivity pneumonitis patients are occupationally exposed to the inducing antigens. Farmer's lung disease, the first of these to be described[8,10,15,52] is a hazard to farmers, a result of exposure to thermophilic actinomycetes in moldy hay. Pigeon breeder's disease,[3] or bird fancier's disease[20,39] is induced by exposure to proteins associated with birds, e.g. pigeon droppings, bird feathers of both domestic and exotic varieties.[7] More recently, chemical exposures such as anhydrides[59] (e.g. trimellitic anhydride or TMA)[16,58] and isocyanates[5] (e.g. toluene diisocyanate) have been implicated in disease. Although federal recommendations[33] and standards have been developed to protect against occupational exposure, these primarily focus on levels of toxicity and exposure limits. However, it should be noted that recommended levels of exposure may still allow for sensitization and development of symptoms in certain workers.[16]

Potential antigens that could cause hypersensitivity pneumonitis may be infinite when the number and variety of inhalable substances is considered.[43] Particles with a diameter of $<10\mu m$ are capable of reaching deeper regions of the lungs on inhalation. A listing of known and suspected causes of hypersensitivity pneumonitis to date can be found in Table 9–4.

Diagnosis of hypersensitivity pneumonitis has classically been based on characteristic symptoms, physical findings, radiologic studies, pulmonary function testing, and demonstration of precipitating antibodies, usually IgG, against likely antigens. Pulmonary or dermal antigenic challenge may help with diagnosis.[16] Avoidance of exposure to the inciting antigen, with subsequent remission of symptoms, may also be useful.

Precipitating antibodies, long thought to be important in the pathogenesis of hypersensitivity pneumonitis (see below) are demonstrable in serum[38] and in bronchial alveolar lavage (BAL)[51] of patients. Demonstration of antibody to an agent known to induce HP does not correlate with clinical disease;[11,14,35] indeed, in a study of farmers,[31] 50% of those with precipitating antibodies had no history of disease. This observation was also noted in pigeon breeder's disease.[11] Although antibody can be found in asymptomatic as well as symptomatic individuals, higher levels of antibody are most often associated with symptoms.[30,35] Not all patients with clinical evidence of hypersensitivity pneumonitis have demonstrable antibody. In addition to the original double immunodiffusion precipitin test,[38] complement fixation,[35] immunofluorescence,[37] counterimmunoelectrophoresis, radioimmunoassay, and enzyme immunoassay[29] have been developed to detect appropriate antibodies. All of the latter procedures are more sensitive than double immunodiffusion, and are sensitive enough to detect antibody in most, if not all, patients and in many exposed persons as well.[44] Antibody levels appear to decrease with time after the last acute exposure[18] and may be useful in following the course of illness.[30]

Hypersensitivity pneumonitis apparently results from a complex series of interactions between the inhaled substances and the cells and proteins of the patient's body. Some antigens, specifically the thermophilic actinomycetes known to cause Farmer's Lung, have an adjuvant effect, demonstrable with both antibody producing and cell-mediated reaction inducing cells.[6,44] Antibody may play a role, via the Arthus or immune complex mechanisms described as Type III hypersensitivity reactions by Coombs and Gell,[9] although serum transfer probably does not confer the disease.[46] There is evidence that certain inhalants can activate complement via the alternative pathway without antibody involvement,[12] although the clinical significance of this is not known.

Lesions in hypersensitivity pneumonitis demonstrate mononuclear infiltrates,

Table 9–4. Examples of Hypersensitivity Pneumonitis*

Disorder	Exposure	Inducing Agent(s)
Farmer's Lung	Moldy hay, crops	Thermophilic Actinomycetes *Micropolyspora faeni* *Thermoactinomyces vulgaris* Others[56]
Bird Fancier's Diseases	Avian dust, products, or feathers	Avian Proteins
Pigeon Breeder's Disease Turkey Handler's Disease Duck Fever Feather Plucker's Disease Others[2,7,57]		
Bagassosis	Moldy sugarcane	Thermophilic Actinomycetes *Thermoactinomyces sacchari* *Thermoactinomyces vulgaris*
Mushroom Worker's Disease	Mushroom compost	Thermophilic Actinomycetes *Micropolyspora faeni, Thermoactinomyces vulgaris*
Malt Worker's Lung	Moldy barley	*Aspergillus clavatus*
Wood Worker's Diseases	Moldy wood, sawdust	
Sequoiosis		*Cryptostroma corticale, Graphium*
Maple Bark-Stripper's Disease		*Cryptostroma corticale*
Wood Pulp Worker's Disease		*Alternaria*
Wood Trimmer's Disease		*Rhizopus, Mucor*
Sawmill-Related Alveolitis[4]		Rhizopus
Familial Hypersensitivity Pneumonitis		*Bacillus subtilis*
Suberosis	Moldy cork dust	Penicillium species
Humidifier Disease[22,42]	Contaminated humidifiers, air conditioners	Thermophilic Actinomycetes *(T. vulgaris, T. candidus)* Penicillium, Cephalosporium, amoeba
Chemical-Related Diseases	Reactive chemicals	
TDI Hypersensitivity Pneumonitis		Toluene diisocyanate (TDI)
TMA Hypersensitivity Pneumonitis		Trimellitic anhydride (TMA)
MDI Hypersensitivity Pneumonitis		Diphenyl methane diisocyanate (MDI)
Epoxy Resin Lung		Heated epoxy resin
Drug-Related Disease	Therapeutic drugs	Gold Salts[32] Methotrexate[28] Nadolol[27] Sulfasalazine[53]
Metal-Related Disease	Pearl Oyster Shells[55] Diamond[54]	Cobalt
Cheese Washer's Disease	Cheese casings	Penicillium species
Summer-Type Hypersensitivity Pneumonitis[24] Others[44]	Infected hair	*Trichosporon cutaneum*

* Adopted from Salvaggio,[44] Grammer and Patterson,[16] and others.

comprised of significantly activated macrophages[1,50] and many T cells,[36,51] large increases in mast cell populations,[49] some neutrophils,[21] and plasma cells.[40]

Studies[1] of the macrophages in bronchial alveolar lavage (BAL) demonstrated the presence of DR and DRQ antigens, as well as an increase in HLA Class I antigen positive cells, suggesting that these cells are structurally ready to encourage antigen recognition by T cells. Interleukin-1 production by the activated macrophages may act to encourage the monoclonal proliferation of lymphocytes.[51] In several studies[26,48] the majority of the T cells recovered from bronchioalveolar lavage carried CD_8 markers, signifying their role as suppressor cells. In another study,[25] the CD_8/CD_4 ratios in bronchioalveolar lavage from symptomatic and asymptomatic individuals were approximately the same; however, the authors found suppressive activity predominating in functional assays using only cells from symptomatic individuals. An increase in T_{AC}, or clonal expansion markers, can be demonstrated on T suppressor and T cytotoxic cell populations,[48] suggesting active in situ proliferation of those cell lines.[13] T suppressor and cytotoxic T cell proliferations and production of suppressive lymphokines almost never happen in asymptomatic persons[16] or in other diseases.[1] Together, these observations suggest an immunoregulatory imbalance. Schuyler, et al.,[46] were able to induce hypersensitivity pneumonitis in guinea pigs by transfer of mitogen- or antigen- activated patient T cells, followed by challenge to the animal with the specific antigen.

Marked increases in the mast cell populations[21,49] in the bronchioalveolar lavage of patients with hypersensitivity pneumonitis suggest a role for mast cell degranulation in pathogenesis, e.g. that symptoms may result from a late phase reaction induced by mast cell degranulation.[49]

Thorough reviews of what is known of the pathogenic mechanisms in hypersensitivity pneumonitis are available.[44,45]

Treatment for individuals with hypersensitivity pneumonitis centers on avoidance of the antigen. Pharmacologic management is rarely helpful.[16]

REFERENCES

1. Agostini, C. et al.: J. Clin. Immunol., 7:64, 1987.

2. Balasubramaniam, S.K. et al.: Clin. Pediatr., 26:174, 1987.

3. Barboriak, J.J., Sosman, A.J., and Reed, C.E.: J. Lab. Clin. Med., 65:600, 1965.

4. Belin, L.: Int. Arch. Allergy Appl. Immunol., 82:440, 1987.

5. Bernstein, I.L.: J. Allergy Clin. Immunol., 70:24, 1982.

6. Bice, D., McKarron, K. Hoffman, E.O., and Salvaggio, J.E.: Int. Arch. Allergy Appl. Immunol., 55:267, 1975.

7. Burdon, J.G., and Stone, C.: Am. Rev. Respir. Dis., 134:1319, 1986.

8. Campbell, J.M.: Br. Med. J., 2:1143, 1932.

9. Coombs, R.R.A., and Gell, P.G.H.: In Clinical Aspects of Immunology. Edited by P.G.H. Gell and R.R.A. Coombs. Oxford, Blackwell Scientific Publications, 1968.

10. Dickie, H.A., and Rankin, J.: JAMA, 167:1069, 1958.

11. doPico, G.A. et al: Am. Rev. Respir. Dis., 113:451, 1976.

12. Edwards, J.H., Baker, J.T., and Davies, B.H.: Clin. Allergy, 4:379, 1974.

13. Fink, J.N.: J. Lab. Clin. Med., 109:619, 1987 (Editorial).

14. Fink, J.N. et al.: Ann. Intern. Med., 68:1205, 1968.

15. Frank, R.C.: AJR., 79:189, 1958.

16. Grammer, L.C., and Patterson, R.: Ann. Allergy, 58:151, 1987.

17. Hansen, P.J., and Penny, R.: Int. Arch. Allergy Appl. Immunol., 47:498, 1974.

18. Hapke, E.J. et al.: Thorax, 23:451, 1968.

19. Hargreave, F.E., and Pepys, J.: J. Allergy Clin. Immunol., 50:157, 1972.

20. Hargreave, F.E., Pepys, J., Longbottom, J.L., and Wraith, D.G.: Lancet, 1:445, 1966.

21. Haslam, P.L. et al.: Am. Rev. Respir. Dis., 135:35, 1987.

22. Hodgson, M.J. et al.: Am. J. Epidemiol., 125:631, 1987.

23. Kawanami, O. et al.: Am. J. Pathol., 110:275, 1983.

24. Kawane, H., and Soejima, R.: Chest, 92:577, 1987.

25. Keller, R.H. et al.: Am. Rev. Respir. Dis., 130:766, 1984.

26. Leatherman, J.W., Michael, A.F., Schwartz, B.A., and Hoidal, J.R.: Ann. Intern. Med., 100:390, 1984.

27. Levy, M.B., Fink, J.N., and Guzzetta, P.A.: Ann. Intern. Med., 105:806, 1986.

28. Louie, S., and Lillington, G.A.: Thorax, 41:703, 1986.

29. Marx, J.J., and Gray, R.L.: J. Allergy Clin. Immunol., 80:109, 1982.

30. Marx, J.J. Jr., Motszko, C., and Wenzel, F.J.: J. Clin. Microbiol., 1:480, 1975.

31. Marx, J.J. Jr. et al.: J. Allergy Clin. Immunol., 62:185, 1978.

32. McCormick, J. et al.: Am. Rev. Respir. Dis., 122:145, 1980.

33. MMWR, 32(Suppl 3S), 1983.

34. Moira Chan-Yeung, M.B.: J. Allergy Clin. Immunol., 70:32, 1982.

35. Moore, V.L., and Fink, J.N.: J. Lab. Clin. Med., 85:540, 1975.

36. Moore, V.L., Pederson, G.M., Hauser, W.C., and Fink, J.N.: J. Allergy Clin. Immunol., 65:365, 1980.

37. Parratt, D., and Peel, J.A.: J. Clin. Pathol., 25:846, 1972.

38. Pepys, J., and Jenkins, P.A.: Thorax, 20:21, 1965.

39. Reed, C.E., Sosman, A., and Barbee, R.A.: JAMA, 193:81, 1965.

40. Reijula, K., and Sutinen, S.: Pathol. Res. Pract., 181:418, 1986.

41. Reyes, C.N., Wenzel, F.J., Lawton, B.R., and Emanuel, D.A.: Chest, 81:142, 1982.

42. Robertson, A.S., Burge, P.S., Wieland, G.A., and Carmalt, M.H.B.: Thorax, 42:32, 1987.

43. Salvaggio, J.E.: J. Allergy Clin. Immunol., 70:5, 1982.

44. Salvaggio, J.E.: Int. Arch. Allergy Appl. Immunol., 82:424, 1987.

45. Salvaggio, J.E.: J. Allergy Clin. Immunol., 79:558, 1987.

46. Schuyler, M., Subramanyan, S., and Hassan, M.D.: J. Lab. Clin. Med., 109:623, 1987.

47. Selman, M. et al.: Clin. Immunol. Immunopathol., 44:63, 1987.

48. Semenzato, G. et al.: J. Immunol., 137:1164, 1986.

49. Soler, P. et al.: Thorax, 42:565, 1987.

50. Stankus, R.P., Cashner, R., and Salvaggio, J.E.: J. Immunol., 120:685, 1978.

51. Teles De Araujo, A., Alfarroba, E., and Freitas E. Costa, M.: Eur. J. Respir. Dis. (Suppl.), 146:203, 1986.

52. Totten, R.S., Reid, D.H.S., Davies, H.O., and Moran, T.J.: Am. J. Med., 25:803, 1958.

53. Valcke, Y., Pauwels, R., and Van Der Straeten, M.: Chest, 92:572, 1987.

54. VanCutsem, E.J., Cueppens, J.L., Lacquet, L.M., and Demedts, M.: Eur. J. Respir. Dis., 70:54, 1987.

55. Weiss, W., and Baur, X.: Chest, 91:146, 1987.

56. Wenzel, F.J., Gray, R.L., Roberts, R.C., and Emanuel, D.A.: Am. Rev. Respir. Dis., 109:464, 1974.

57. Wolf, S.J., Stillerman, A., Weinberger, M. and Smith, W.: Pediatrics, 79:1027, 1987.

58. Zeiss, C.R. et al.: Ann. Intern. Med., 98:8, 1983.

59. Zeiss, C.R. et al: J. Allergy Clin. Immunol., 70:15, 1982.

Ouchterlony Technique: Double Immunodiffusion

PRINCIPLE. Sera suspected of containing specific antibody are diluted and placed in wells concentric to a well to which antigen is added. Precipitin bands are formed if antibody is present.

EQUIPMENT AND MATERIALS

1. Agar gel double immunodiffusion plates (Ouchterlony; Cooperbiomedical): Contains 0.1% sodium azide. Store at 2 to 8° C. May be used until the expiration date noted on the label.

2. Antigen as follows:

a. *Thermoactinomyces vulgaris* #1 (broth antigen; Greer Laboratories): Prepared from broth filtrate by the procedure of Edwards.[1] The lyophilized extract was reconstituted at 20 mg/mL using normal saline containing 0.1% sodium azide and Tris buffer.

b. *Micropolyspora faeni* (broth antigen; Greer Laboratories): Prepared from broth filtrate as described above.

c. *Aspergillus fumigatus* (culture filtrate; Meridian Diagnostics)

d. Pigeon serum (Greer Laboratories): Diluted 1:10 in normal saline.

e. *Candida albicans* (Meridian Diagnostics): Strain B35, type A.

NOTE: All antigens are stored at 2 to 8° C. Expiration dates are noted on the vial labels.

3. Positive control sera:

Anti-*Aspergillus fumigatus*—(Meridian Diagnostics)

Anti-*Candida albicans*—(Meridian Diagnostics)

Anti-*Micropolyspora faeni*—(Greer labs)

Anti-Pigeon serum—(Greer labs)

Anti-*Thermoactinomyces vulgaris*—(Greer labs)

The control serum was produced by immunizing goats or rabbits with the antigen. Serum from the animal was tested to detect the presence of specific precipitin bands and to determine the concentration of the precipitating antibody by the relative position of the precipitin bands. The control serum is supplied lyophilized and is reconstituted with distilled water

4. Capillary pipets

5. Tubes and pipets or microtiter system (0.05 ml) for preparing serum dilutions

6. Moist chamber for incubation

7. 7.5% acetic acid: To prepare, add 7.5 ml of glacial acetic acid to 92.5 ml of distilled water. Store at room temperature. May be used indefinitely

8. 5% sodium citrate: Add 5 g sodium citrate to 100 ml distilled water. Store at room temperature. May be used indefinitely or until cloudiness occurs

9. 0.9% saline solution.

10. Patient serum: Use fresh or freeze at −20° C until ready to use

PROCEDURE

1. Prepare the following dilutions of patient

serum and positive controls in saline-1:1 (undiluted), 1:2, 1:4, 1:8, and 1:16.

NOTE: The dilutions of control/sera may be covered with parafilm or corked and stored at 2 to 8° C for subsequent use. Discard if contamination occurs.

2. Using the Ouchterlony worksheet provided (Fig. 9–5), indicate:
   a. Patient information and dates.
   b. Plate number.
   c. Dilutions of patient serum or control to be placed in the five concentric wells of each group.
   d. Antigen to be used.
3. Using a capillary pipet, fill all wells with the appropriate patient/control dilution or antigen (wells will hold approximately 5 μl).
4. Cover the plate and place in a moist chamber.
5. Incubate 72 hours, observing daily, using transmitted light. Sketch the precipitin bands on the template sheet, and record the highest dilution exhibiting precipitate under "results."
6. For *Pigeon Serum, Candida, Thermoactinomyces vulgaris, Micropolyspora faeni:* After 72 hours, observe for precipitate, sketch and record. Cover each group of wells with 7.5% acetic acid and allow to stain for about 5 minutes; rinse gently with a stream of tap water. Again observe for precipitate, sketch and record the maximum dilution with precipitate.
7. For *Aspergillus* only: Overlay with 5% sodium citrate and allow to react for 45 minutes. Rinse in a gentle stream of tap water. Overlay with 7.5% acetic acid and allow to react for 5 minutes. Rinse in a gentle stream of tap water. Again observe for precipitin lines. Report only those lines that are not dissolved by reaction with sodium citrate.
8. All positive controls must exhibit precipitin bands ± one doubling dilution from the designated titer for that control.
9. Report the highest dilution exhibiting precipitate.

INTERPRETATION OF RESULTS. In the presence of clinical symptoms, detectable levels of precipitating antibody may be considered significant.[2]

Plate #

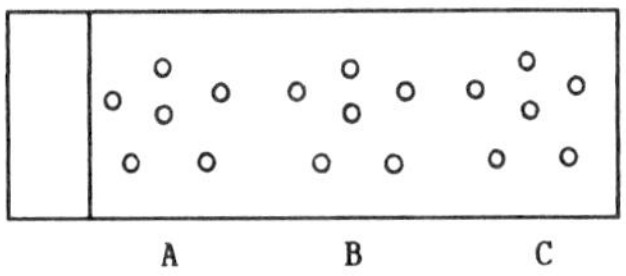

	Pt. Name:	________	Date Rec'd:	________	Antigen:
A	Hosp. No.:	________	Date Begun:	________	________
	Floor/Dr:	________	Date CRC'd:	________	
	Pt. Name:	________	Date Rec'd:	________	Antigen:
B	Hosp. No.:	________	Date Begun:	________	________
	Floor/Dr:	________	Date CRC'd:	________	
	Pt. Name:	________	Date Rec'd:	________	Antigen:
C	Hosp. No.:	________	Date Begun:	________	________
	Floor/Dr:	________	Date CRC'd:	________	

Results:

Interpretation:

	24h	48h	72h	stain
A				
B				
C				

Fig. 9–5. Ouchterlony Worksheet

REFERENCES

1. Edwards, J.H.: J. Lab. Clin. Med., 79:683, 1972.
2. In lab data—Establishment of normal ranges.

CRYPTOCOCCOSIS

Organisms of the genus Cryptococcus are ubiquitous, normally saprophytic organisms which are capable of causing the opportunistic human infections collectively known as cryptococcoses. Of the seven species of Cryptococci which have been described,[36] only one, *Cryptococcus neoformans,* grows well at 37° C[7] and is a common medical isolate. Rarely is one of the other species implicated in human disease.[16]

Cryptococcus neoformans exists in nature and in human infection in its asexual, yeast-like budding form, incapable of the production of hyphae, chlamydospores or germ tubes. It is found worldwide in pigeon droppings and soil.[37] Of the known serogroups of *C. neoformans,* only serogroup pair A/D has been isolated from pigeons,[7] where it apparently lives as a commensal, causing no known avian disease. All natural and human isolates are capable of forming large heteropolysaccharide capsules.[7] These may be absent in free living forms but are readily produced once the organism infects tissues,[7] especially in individuals where some immune responsiveness is evident (see below).

Several sexual, or perfect, forms of *Cryptococcus neoformans* have been described in nature and have been given the genus name Filobasidiella.[7,36]

Man probably acquires Cryptococcus by inhalation of aerosolized organisms from his environment.[33] Communicable transfer from human to human has not been documented.[7]

Prior to the advent of AIDS, Cryptococcus was the second most commonly significant fungal isolate;[11] however, the estimated risk to the general population was low, approximately 0.15% per year.[14] Predisposing illnesses are many, including lymphoreticular disorders, hepatitis, diabetes mellitus, systemic lupus erythematosus, chronic lung diseases, alcoholism, sarcoidosis, and renal failure and transplant. All immunosuppressive therapies apparently predispose patients to Cryptococcus; indeed, the incidence of the disease has increased with iatrogenic intervention in host responsiveness.[32] Fungal infections are among the most frequent causes of death in non-AIDS immunocompromised patients, with Candida, Aspergillus and Cryptococci accounting for the majority.[13]

Cryptococcoses also occur in apparently healthy people,[41] although subtle defects in the immune responses of these individuals may antedate infection (see below).

Asymptomatic, nonprogressive colonization of the respiratory tract occurs in some individuals and may be difficult to differentiate from clinical infection,[11,13] especially when it is found coincident with underlying pulmonary disease. Pulmonary cryptococcosis[24] in its localized form is characterized by rather non-specific symptoms, e.g. cough, chest pain, and/or increased sputum production. As such, it may spontaneously resolve or, more often in patients with predisposing disorders, may spread to the meninges or elsewhere.

Cryptococcal meningitis, when it occurs in apparently healthy individuals,[41] may be difficult to diagnose, but treatment is usually successful. Headache, fever, nausea, unconsciousness, and increased meningeal signs and pathologic reflexes are common symptoms. Immunocompromised patients are much more prone to treatment failure[10] or to dissemination.[24]

Disseminated cryptococcosis is defined as spread of the organism, presumably via hematogenous or lymphatic routes, to involve two or more non-contiguous organs, excluding the central nervous system.[13] The vast majority of disseminated disease is seen in patients with predisposing illness.[11] Dykstra et al.[12] studied the relationship between capsule size and an organisms's propensity to disseminate. They suggest that poorly encapsulated cryptococci may spread earlier and easier than those with large capsules. Data from AIDS patients[4] (see below) suggests that immune responsiveness on the part of the host may be a primary factor in capsule formation, i.e. encapsulation may occur almost solely as a result of selective pressure from the host, and, lacking that pressure, the organism may remain smaller and, therefore, more easily disseminated. It is of interest to note that Cryptococcemia[32] may occur in the presence of a known primary pulmonary infection, or without an observable focal infection.

Dissemination most often involves the bone or the skin. Cutaneous disease comprises 10 to 15% of cryptococcal disseminations.[21] Cellulitis,[5,21] perhaps the most dangerous of these, is seen only in markedly immunocompromised patients.

Rarely, disseminated cryptococcosis can involve the peritoneum, spleen, thyroid, parathyroid, adrenals, prostate, pituitary, heart, liver, eyes, lymph nodes, kidney, pancreas, ovaries, skeletal muscle, urinary tract, or gastrointestinal system.

Certain individuals may be more susceptible to clinical infection with cryptococcus as a result of selective immune deficiencies. Subtle deficiencies in cell mediated immunity[17,18,28,38] may predispose to illness; for example, lymphocyte transformation responses to the organism may be defective.[9] Hypogammaglobulinemia may allow the organism to invade successfully.[19] And, NK (natural killer) cells may play a role in early resistance, but not in patient survival.[27]

Studies of patients with Cryptococcal disease suggest that lymphocytes,[29] K (killer) cells,[30] monocytes[8] and/or antibody[10,22] may be instrumental in recovery.

Cryptococcus is the fifth most common infection seen in AIDS patients, eclipsed only by cytomegalovirus, Candida, *Pneumocystis carinii,* and *Mycobacterium avium-intracellulare.*[15] It ranks fourth among those organisms capable of threatening life.[25] Between 6 and 7%[14,45] of AIDS patients develop this infection.

Poorly encapsulated strains of Cryptococcus can and do cause infection in AIDS patients.[4] It is probable that organisms may simply not encapsulate in immune-deprived

atmospheres, since unencapsulated strains, recovered from AIDS patients, can apparently form capsules readily in immunocompetent mice.[4]

The presentation and progression of cryptococcosis in AIDS patients differs considerably from that seen in others with cryptococcal infection. Brain or meningeal disease is a more common occurrence,[45] and disseminated infection is often the initial observation.[31,34,44]

Pulmonary disease, when it occurs, is almost always clinical in AIDS patients[43] and disseminates more readily, despite therapy.[14,43] Much higher levels of antigen persist in serum, even though the organism may have been killed by therapy.[14] The organism may disseminate to unlikely sites, such as the mediastinum,[44] the pleural cavity,[31] or the joints.[34] The first case of oral cryptococcosis has also been described.[28]

Recent studies[3,35,39] suggest that serogroup pair A/D has been exclusively identified worldwide in AIDS patients.

Diagnosis of cryptococcosis is often difficult. Pulmonary infection may be demonstrated by sputum culture or lung biopsy[26] or by latex agglutination test[1] for antigen in serum. None of these tests are particularly reliable[13,26] as indicators of pulmonary infection, as they lack sensitivity. Cryptococcal meningitis is often first diagnosed via India ink prep or Nigrosin stain,[13] where the presence of a wide capsule on a morphologically identifiable yeast is considered a positive test. However, antigen latex agglutination from serum or cerebral spinal fluid is a more sensitive indicator of meningeal infection.[13] Kaufman and Reiss[23] discuss immunofluorescence, enzyme immunoassay, and tube agglutination procedures for detection of antibody, and enzyme immunoassay and latex agglutination tests for antigen. They suggest that an effective serologic battery of tests includes latex agglutination for detection of antigen and tube agglutination and immunofluorescence for detection of antibody.

Latex agglutination tests for antigen are sensitive and specific,[2] although false-positives and false-negatives[20] occur. False positives may be caused by rheumatoid factors in patient samples binding to the immunoglobulin-coated latex beads, but may be removed by a simple pronase procedure.[40] Latex agglutination for cryptococcal antigen is used (1) to detect cryptococcal infections not detected by India ink, (2) to confirm the presence of cryptococcal infections first detected by other tests (India ink, culture), and (3) to quantitate antigen titer over time, to monitor the course of infection.

Damsker and Bottone[6] suggest the culture of buffy coats from AIDS patients may help with early diagnosis of *Mycobacterium tuberculosis, Mycobacterium avium-intracellulare,* and *Cryptococcus.* Walsh et al.[42] suggest differentiation of suspected fungal infection by the use of several observable factors; for example, they noted that Cryptococcus was almost always community acquired, while Aspergillus and Candida were nosocomial.

REFERENCES

1. Bloomfield, N., Gordon, M.A., Elmendorf, D.F. Jr.: Proc. Soc. Exp. Biol. Med., *114*:64, 1963.
2. Boom, W.H. et al.: J. Clin. Microbiol., *22*:856, 1985.
3. Bottone, E.J., Salkin, I.F., Hurd, N.J., and Wormser, G.P.: J. Infect. Dis., *156*:242, 1987.
4. Bottone, E.J., and Wormser, G.P.: AIDS Res., *2*:219, 1986.
5. Carlson, K.C. et al.: J. Am. Acad. Dermatol., *17*:469, 1987.
6. Damsker, B., and Bottone, E.J.: AIDS Res., *2*:343, 1986.
7. Davis, C.E.: In *Infectious Diseases and Medical Microbiology.* 2nd ed. Edited by A.I. Braude, C.E. Davis, and J. Fierer. Philadelphia, W. B. Saunders Co., 1986.
8. Diamond, R.D., and Allison, A.C.: Infect. Immun., *14*:714, 1976.
9. Diamond, R.D., and Bennett, J.E.: J. Infect. Dis., *127*:694, 1973.
10. Diamond, R.D., and Bennett, J.E.: Ann. Intern. Med., *80*:176, 1974.
11. Duperval, R., Hermans, P.E., Brewer, N.S., and Roberts, G.D.: Chest, *72*:13, 1977.
12. Dykstra, M.A., Friedman, L., and Murphy, J.W.: Infect. Immun., *16*:129, 1977.
13. Edson, R.S., Fernandez-Guerrero, M.L., Roberts, G.D., and VanScoy, R.E.: Minn. Med., *70*:337, 1987.
14. Eng, R.H., Bishburg, E., and Smith, S.M.: Am. J. Med., *81*:19, 1986.
15. Fauci, A.S.: Ann. Intern. Med., *100*:92, 1984.
16. Gluck, J.L., Myers, J.P., and Pass, L.M.: South Med. J., *80*:511, 1987.
17. Graybill, J.R., and Alford, R.H.: Cell Immunol., *14*:12, 1974.
18. Graybill, J.R., and Taylor, R.L.: Arch. Allergy Appl. Immunol., *57*:101, 1978.
19. Gupta, S. et al.: Am. J. Med., *82*:129, 1987.
20. Haldane, D.J. et al.: Ann. Neurol., *19*:412, 1986.
21. Hall, J.C. et al.: J. Am. Acad. Dermatol., *17*:329, 1987.
22. Henderson, D.K., Kan, V.L., and Bennett, J.E.: Clin. Exp. Immunol., *65*:639, 1986.
23. Kaufman, L., and Reiss, E.: In *Manual of Clinical Laboratory Immunology.* 3rd ed. Edited by N.R. Rose, H. Friedman, and J.L. Fahey. Washington, D.C., American Society for Microbiology, 1986.
24. Kerkering, T.M., and Duma, R.J., and Shadomy, S.: Ann. Intern. Med., *94*:611, 1981.
25. Kovacs, J.A. et al.: Ann. Intern. Med., *103*:533, 1985.
26. Lewis, J.L., and Rabinovich, S.: Am. J. Med., *53*:315, 1972.
27. Lipscomb, M.F.: Amer. J. Pathol., *128*:354, 1987.
28. Lynch, D.P., and Naftolin, L.Z.: Oral Surg. Oral Med. Oral Pathol., *64*:449, 1987.
29. Miller, G.P., and Puck, J.: J. Immunol., *133*:166, 1984.
30. Nabavi, N.: Infect. Immun., *51*:556, 1986.
31. Newman, T.G., Soni, A., Acaron, S., and Huang, C.T.: Chest, *91*:459, 1987.
32. Perfect, J.R., Durack, D.T., and Gallis, H.A.: Medicine, *62*:98, 1983.
33. Poblete, R.B., and Kirby, B.D.: Am. J. Med., *82*:665, 1987.
34. Ricciardi, D.D. et al.: J. Rheumatol., *13*:455, 1986.
35. Rinaldi, M.G. et al.: J. Infect. Dis., *153*:642, 1986.
36. Rippon, J.W., *The Pathogenic Fungi and the Pathogenic Actinomycetes,* 2nd ed. Philadelphia, W. B. Saunders Co., 1982.
37. Ruiz, A., Fromtling, R.A., and Bulmer, G.S.: Infect. Immun., *31*:560, 1981.
38. Schimpff, S.C., and Bennett, J.E.: J. Allergy Clin. Immunol., *55*:430, 1975.
39. Shimizu, R.Y., Howard, D.H., and Clancy, M.N.: J. Infect. Dis., *154*:1042, 1986.
40. Stockman, L., and Roberts, G.D.: J. Clin. Microbiol., *17*:945, 1983.
41. Tjia, T.L., Yeow, Y.K., and Tan, C.B.: J. Neurol. Neurosurg. Psychiatry, *48*:853, 1985.
42. Walsh, T.J., Hier, D.B., and Caplan, L.R.: Neurology, *35*:1654, 1985.
43. Wasser, L., and Talavera, W.: Chest, *92*:692, 1987.
44. Witt, D. et al.: Am. J. Med., *82*:149, 1987.
45. Zugir, A. et al.: Ann. Intern. Med., *104*:234, 1986.

Cryptococcal Antigen[7] Latex Agglutination Test: Qualitative / Quantitative Procedures

PRINCIPLE. Latex particles coated with antibody to cryptococcal antigen are reacted with patient sample. Capsular polysaccharide antigen, if present in the sample, will cause agglutination of the particles.

EQUIPMENT AND MATERIALS

1. Latex Agglutination Test for *Cryptococcus neoformans* Antigen International Biological Laboratories, Inc. (IBL), including:

a. Latex coated with anti-cryptococcal globulin (rabbit) in glycine buffered saline solution, pH 9.0

b. Latex coated with normal globulin (rabbit), in glycine buffered saline solution, pH 9.0

c. Positive control: 0.25 μg/ml concentration of capsular polysaccharide antigen from *Cryptococcus neoformans*

d. Negative control: Rabbit serum known to be negative for cryptococcal antigen

e. Diluent: Glycine buffered saline solution, pH 9.0, with 0.1% bovine serum albumin

NOTE: All of the above reagents contain 1:10,000 Merthiolate. Store at 2 to 8° C. Do not freeze. Expiration dates are noted. Do not mix reagents between lot numbers of kits.

2. Patient sample: CSF, urine or serum samples may be tested using this method. Remove all cellular material before testing. Specimens must be heat inactivated before testing. Repeated freezing and thawing will not impair specimen reactivity.

3. Boerner slides
4. 1 ml pipets, with bulb
5. Pasteur pipets
6. Test tubes
7. Rotator set at 160 rpm
8. Wooden applicator sticks
9. 56° C waterbath
10. Transmitted light source

PROCEDURE (QUALITATIVE)

1. Inactivate patient sample(s) to be tested by heating specimen in 56° C waterbath for 30 minutes.

2. Set rotator speed at approximately 160 rpm.

3. Perform positive control as follows:

a. Set up five test tubes in a rack. Add 0.2 ml of diluent to each tube.

b. Add 0.2 ml of the positive control to tube 1, mix and transfer 0.2 ml through tube 5. The dilutions are 1:2 through 1:32.

c. Using pasteur pipets, add a drop from tube 1 to well 1 of Rows A and B of a Boerner slide, as shown below:

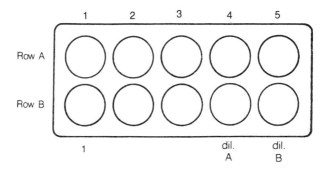

d. Add a drop from each of tubes 2 to 5 to wells 2 to 5 of Row A, respectively.

e. Place one drop of diluent into wells 4 and 5 of Row B.

f. Gently resuspend the anticryptococcal globulin-latex suspension. Place one drop into each of the wells in Row A, and into well 4 of Row B.

h. Gently resuspend the latex beads coated with normal globulin. Place one drop into wells 1 and 5 of Row B.

i. Mix the contents of each well using separate wooden applicator sticks, spreading the contents of each well over its entire surface.

j. Rotate at 160 rpm for 10 minutes.

k. Observe immediately using transmitted light.

l. Read for 2+ to 4+ agglutination. Slight agglutination is considered negative. The positive control should be reactive to at least a titer of 4 (well 2). No agglutination should occur in well 1 of row B, nor in the diluent control wells (4 and 5). If any of the controls do not react properly, discard the kit.

4. On a clean Boerner slide and using pasteur pipets, place one drop of each patient sample to be tested into one well of Row A and into the corresponding well of Row B as indicated:

Patient Number

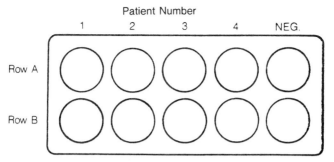

5. Again using a pasteur pipet, place a drop of negative control in one well of Row A and into the corresponding well of Row B, as indicated in the diagram.

6. Gently resuspend the anticryptococcal globulin-latex reagent, and place one drop into each well of row A.

7. Resuspend the normal globulin sensitized-latex and place one drop into each well of row B.

8. Mix the contents of each well using separate applicator sticks, spreading the contents to fill the entire well surface.

9. Place on the slide rotator and rotate at 160 rpm for 10 minutes.

10. Observe immediately for agglutination using transmitted light. A positive reaction is one with 2+ to 4+ agglutination. Less than 2+ agglutination in patient sample wells is considered negative.

11. Contents of both wells in which globulin-latex reagents are reacted with negative control serum should not be agglutinated. If either of the negative control serum wells are agglutinated, discard the kit and repeat the test (and the positive control run) with a new kit.

REPORTING (QUALITATIVE). Samples are reported as negative for cryptococcal antigen if both wells (Rows A & B) containing the sample have 1+ or less agglutination and all controls are properly reactive.

If >1+ agglutination is observed in Row A only, the specimen should be titered using the quantitative procedure for cryptococcal antigen.

If >1+ agglutination occurs in both Rows A and B of a sample, the presence of rheumatoid factor in the sample is indicated. The sample should be titered using both latex globulin reagents following the quantitative procedure guidelines.

PROCEDURE (QUANTITATIVE)

1. If longer than 4 hours has elapsed since the specimen(s) were inactivated, repeat inactivation by heating at 56° C for 10 minutes.

2. Ensure that the slide rotator is set at approximately 160 rpm.

3. Prepare 2-fold dilutions of the specimen to be tested by placing 0.1 ml of glycine diluent into each of several test tubes, adding 0.1 ml of sample to the first tube, mixing and serially transferring 0.1 ml through the last tube.

NOTE: Begin with 5 tubes, enough for one row of a Boerner slide and continue if the titer needs to be extended.

4. If the specimen was *agglutinated only by the anticryptococcal globulin-latex* in the qualitative test:

a. Transfer a drop from each of the specimen dilutions to a corresponding well on a clean Boerner slide.

b. Add a drop of the anticryptococcal globulin-latex to each well.

c. Mix well, using separate applicator sticks for each well and spreading the contents to fill the entire well.

d. Place on the slide rotator and rotate for 10 minutes at 160 rpm.

e. Observe immediately using transmitted light. The reciprocal of the last dilution with at least 2+ agglutination is the titer to be reported.

5. If the specimen was *agglutinated by both the anticryptococcal globulin-latex and the normal globulin-latex reagents:*

a. Place one drop from each tube into each of two wells, one in row A and one in the corresponding well of row B of a clean Boerner slide.

b. Place one drop of the anticryptococcal globulin-latex reagent into the wells of Row A.

c. Place one drop of the normal globulin-latex reagent into each well in Row B.

d. Mix well using wooden applicator sticks and spreading the contents to fill the entire well.

e. Rotate on the slide rotator at 160 rpm for 10 minutes.

f. Observe for agglutination using transmitted light. *For each row of wells,* determine the last well that has at least 2+ agglutination.

6. If the endpoint has not been reached, return to the last tube of the tube dilution(s) and

prepare further twofold dilutions by mixing and transferring 0.1 ml of sample dilution through tubes containing 0.1 ml of glycine diluent. Repeat steps a–f.

7. Report the reciprocal of the last dilution with at least 2+ agglutination.

REPORTING (QUANTITATIVE)

If agglutination of patient sample was observed only with anticryptococcal globulin-latex reagent, the sample is reported as positive for cryptococcal antigen to the titer observed.

If agglutination was observed with both reagents, the titer observed with each is reported, e.g.,

Anticryptococcal latex reagent: Titer 16
Normal latex globulin reagent: Titer 4

INTERPRETATION OF RESULTS.

Those specimens yielding negative results in the latex agglutination assay should not be assumed negative for *Cryptococcus neoformans.*

Any titer observed with anticryptococcal globulin reagent alone should be considered presumptive evidence of clinical infection with *C. neoformans.*[4]

Samples that exhibit rheumatoid factor activity must be considered equivocal and untestable using the latex agglutination assay, *unless* a fourfold or greater increase in titer is noted using the anticryptococcal globulin reagent, as compared with the normal globulin-sensitized latex reagent.

LIMITATIONS OF THE PROCEDURE.

Interference by rheumatoid factor activity occurs in up to 10% of samples tested for cryptococcal antigen.[1,2]

Although the latex agglutination test is highly specific,[2,5,6] it does not detect all cases of Cryptococcosis.[3,5,6]

REFERENCES

1. Bennett, J.E., and Bailey, J.W.: Am. J. Clin. Pathol., *56*:360, 1971.
2. Dolan, C.F.: Am. J. Clin. Pathol., *58*:358, 1972.
3. Duperval, R. et al.: Chest, *72*:13, 1977.
4. Goodman, J.S., Kaufman, L., and Koenig, M.G.: N. Engl. J. Med., *285*:434, 1971.
5. Gordon, M.S., and Vedder, D.K.: JAMA, *197*:961, 1966.
6. Kaufman, L., and Blumer, S.: Appl. Microbiol., *16*:1907, 1968.
7. Package Insert, Cryptococcal Antigen Latex Agglutination Test, International Biological Laboratories, Inc., Cranbury, N.J., 1985. Reprinted with permission of Wampole Laboratories Division, Carter-Wallace, Inc., Cranbury, NJ 08512.

D. Protozoal Infections

TOXOPLASMOSIS

Toxoplasmosis is a disease caused by the ubiquitous, protozoan parasite, *Toxoplasma gondii.*[8,12,17] Although the definitive hosts for this parasite are confined to the cat family, a wide spectrum of other mammals and birds may serve as secondary hosts.

Toxoplasma gondii exists naturally in three forms: (1) the *tachyzoite*, or proliferative form (also known as endozoite or trophozoite), (2) the *tissue cyst* (also known as *bradyzoite* or *cystozoite*), and (3) the *oocyst.*[8,12,17]

Tachyzoites are crescent or oval-shaped forms, with one rounded end and one pointed end. They are approximately 3 by 7µm in size and stain well with either Wright or Giemsa stain. In this form, *Toxoplasma gondii* is easily destroyed by freezing and thawing, heat, desiccation, and gastric juice. Tachyzoites are present during the acute stage of infection, during which they are capable of invading all mammalian cells except non-nucleated erythrocytes. The tachyzoites proliferate within vacuoles in the cytoplasm of the cells, ultimately causing the cells to burst and release the tachyzoites, which may then invade surrounding cells or become phagocytized by cells of the reticuloendothelial system.

After continued multiplication of the organism, tissue cysts form within the vacuoles of infected host cells. The cysts range from 10 to 200µm in size and may contain thousands of organisms. Any body cell may be host to cyst formation; however, the brain, skeletal, and heart muscle are the most common sites. Cysts have a spherical shape in the brain, but assume an elongated shape in muscle, where they conform to the shape of the muscle fiber. They can be visualized by staining with periodic acid Schiff stain. The cysts may be destroyed by desiccation, freezing at $-20°$ C for 18 to 24 hours, or heating above 66° C. Once formed, tissue cysts persist for the life of the host, and are thought to be responsible for recurrent episodes of disease in immunocompromised individuals.[10,14]

Oocysts are formed and excreted only by members of the cat family. Following ingestion of Toxoplasma in prey, tachyzoites invade the intestinal mucosa of the cat, and undergo a typical coccidian sexual cycle, which ultimately results in the formation of oocysts. Oocysts appear in cat feces after a latent period of 3 to 24 days, are shed in massive amounts (up to 10 million in a single day), and are excreted for 7 to 20 days. Oocysts are highly resistant to desiccation and may remain viable for more than a year under appropriate soil and weather conditions, during which they may be transported by insect or earthworm vectors.

Transmission of Toxoplasma in nature occurs through (1) ingestion of tissue cysts in raw or partly cooked meat (especially pork and lamb, and to a lesser extent, beef),[4] (2) ingestion of oocysts on food or hands in contact with cat feces or soil contaminated with cat feces, and (3) congenitally, by transplacental transfer from infected mother to infant.[8,11,12,17] Transmission may also occur through blood transfusion, organ transplantation, and handling of infected animals or contaminated glassware in the laboratory.[12,17]

After entering the body, usually through the intestine, Toxoplasma tachyzoites are released from cysts or oocysts and invade host cells directly or through phagocytosis. Parasitemia develops, and the organisms spread throughout the body.[18] As the host's immune system becomes active, encystment occurs, as described above, and the tachy-zoites are probably cleared.[2,17] A chronic or latent state ensues with encysted organisms apparently living in symbiosis with the host. Some evidence infers that encysted organisms are occasionally freed,[13,17] possibly explaining the persistence of high antibody titers after acute disease subsides.

Toxoplasma has a worldwide distribution. In the United States, serologic evidence of infection with Toxoplasma gondii has been observed in 5 to 30% of children and young adult populations and up to 70% of older adults.[12] The majority of individuals with acquired toxoplasmosis are asymptomatic. Symptomatic infections in the immunologically normal host are self-limiting and most frequently involve local (usually cervical) or generalized lymphadenopathy; malaise, fever, hepatosplenomegaly, myalgias, arthralgias, sore throat, headache or maculopapular rash may also be present.[12] These clinical features, along with the atypical lymphocytes and lymphocytosis which may occur, closely resemble those seen in infectious mononucleosis; however, heterophile antibody tests are negative.

Toxoplasma gondii infection in the immunodeficient or immunosuppressed host poses a much more difficult problem, often resulting in disseminated disease.[12,19] This most frequently involves the central nervous system, producing diffuse encephalopathy, meningoencephalitis, or cerebral mass lesions. Resulting clinical symptoms include changes in mental status, headache, focal neurologic abnormalities, and seizures. Hepatitis, pneumonitis, and acute necrotizing myocarditis have also been noted, the latter sometimes mimicking rejection of a cardiac transplant.[12,19] Prior to the advent of AIDS, disseminated toxoplasmosis predominantly affected individuals with neoplasia (especially hematologic malignancies), organ transplants, or collagen vascular disorders,[12,19] but was a relatively rare disease even in these immunocompromised patients.[10,11] By contrast, toxoplasmic encephalitis is the most common opportunistic infection of the central nervous system in

AIDS patients, reportedly occurring in up to 40% of these patients.[10,11] Early diagnosis and treatment are essential in preventing a fatal outcome.

Another group of patients in which *Toxoplasma gondii* causes significant morbidity and mortality are those who have contracted the infection congenitally. From available data, the incidence of congenital toxoplasmosis in the United States has been estimated at 1:1000 to 1:8000 live births.[11] Transmission of infection to the fetus results in one-third to one-half of women who become infected with *T. gondii* during pregnancy,[11,12] and may cause clinical abnormalities at birth or later in life, premature delivery, stillbirth, or spontaneous abortion. Congenital transfer of organisms occurs only if acute maternal infection is acquired during pregnancy, but may result whether or not symptoms of infection are evident in the mother.[11,12,17] The risk to the fetus is related to the gestational age at the time of infection. When maternal infection is acquired during the third trimester, the likelihood of fetal infection is greatest, but the disease is most often subclinical; when maternal infection is acquired during the first trimester, the likelihood of fetal infection is lowest, but the disease is clinically more severe.[11,12,17] Clinical trials in France, where the incidence of Toxoplasma infection is high, suggest that prenatal screening of mothers and fetuses, and subsequent treatment of infected mothers during pregnancy or infected infants after birth reduces the severity of disease.[5]

Most infants with congenital toxoplasmosis appear normal at birth, and the disease often goes unrecognized at that time.[17] However, symptoms may develop at any time from early infancy to adulthood, and are most often ocular, although neurologic manifestations may also occur.[3,16,17,22] When recognized in the neonate, congenital toxoplasmosis is usually severe, classically occurring as a triad of bilateral chorioretinitis, cerebral calcification, and micro- or hydroencephaly, although one or more of these symptoms may be absent.[1,3,9] Death, if it occurs, is related to micro- or hydroencephaly, or to severe mental and motor retardation.[9]

The diagnosis of toxoplasmosis requires sophistication, both for the congenital and the disseminated forms, as clinical symptoms may mimic those seen in other infections, or in the infant, may be absent at birth. Diagnosis of acute toxoplasmosis is established by demonstration of tachyzoites in tissue sections or smears, demonstration of characteristic lymph node histology, serologic testing, and rarely, isolation of *Toxoplasma gondii* from clinical specimens by inoculation into mice.[12] Serologic testing plays an important role in diagnosis, as isolation of the organisms is a lengthy process not practically performed by most laboratories, and appropriate tissue specimens for histologic study are often difficult to obtain.[7] Seroconversion to an antibody-positive status, a detectable fourfold rise in titer, or the demonstration of high levels of IgM antibody to Toxoplasma by a reliable method is usually diagnostic (see below);[4,7] in the absence of these, a single high titer of antibody is presumptive evidence of acute or recent infection, but it must be noted that high titers may persist for long periods in some individuals.[4]

The diagnosis of congenital toxoplasmosis involves demonstrating elevated cerebral spinal fluid protein, isolating trophozoites in fluids or tissue, and/or demonstrating nonmaternal antibody through serologic techniques.[17]

Patients with AIDS pose a special problem for diagnosis. Unlike other groups of immunocompromised patients with toxoplasmosis,[19] AIDS patients rarely produce IgM antibody to *Toxoplasma gondii* or demonstrate a rise in serum IgG antibody, likely as a result of their inability to mount a normal antibody response.[10,14] The absence of IgG antibody, however, indicates that the patient has not been exposed to the organism in the past, and may therefore be used to exclude a diagnosis of Toxoplasma reactivation.[14] In some patients, a rise in cerebral spinal fluid antibody has been demonstrated, even though serum titers are not elevated.[10] In the absence of IgM antibody or rising titers of IgG antibody, demonstration of the organism in sedimented cerebral spinal fluid, brain aspirate, or in some cases, brain biopsy, is necessary for definitive diagnosis.[10,14] Often, a presumptive diagnosis based on clinical and radiologic evidence is used.

The methylene blue dye test (MBDT),[6] developed by Sabin and Feldman,[20] is the definitive test for antibody to *Toxoplasma gondii*.[8] Exquisitely sensitive and specific for antibody to the organism, the test involves the reaction of live Toxoplasma with dilutions of patient serum in the presence of normal human serum as a source of complement.[21] After the addition of methylene blue, the organisms are observed microscopically. In the absence of specific antibody, the organisms appear stained. In the presence of antibody to Toxoplasma, the organisms are lysed and lose their ability to incorporate the dye.

The indirect fluorescent antibody test (IFA) has been the most widely used serologic assay for Toxoplasma antibody. IgG titers parallel those of the MBDT, appearing 1 to 2 weeks after infection, peaking at 6 to 8 weeks, and gradually declining thereafter, with low titers often persisting for life.[12] A single IFA titer ≥ 80 or an MBDT titer ≥ 1000 are considered presumptive evidence of recent Toxoplasma infection.[12,17] The IgM IFA is a technically simple and reliable method for detecting acute acquired infection or congenital infection. However, false-positive results may occur in patients who have high levels of rheumatoid factor (RF) or antinuclear antibodies (ANA), and false-negatives may occur because of competitive inhibition by specific IgG antibodies.[7,8] Many of these false results may be eliminated by absorption of the test serum with heat-aggregated IgG (to remove RF) or a Staphylococcus/Streptococcus preparation (to remove IgG and IgA), or separation of IgM by gel filtration prior to testing.[7,8]

IgG and IgM ELISA tests have also been developed to detect antibody to *Toxoplasma gondii*. These are more sensitive than IFA, but like IFA, may yield false-positive results if pre-absorption steps are not performed.[7] Use of a double-sandwich ELISA, whereby anti-human IgM antibodies adsorbed to a solid substrate bind IgM in the test serum, has also been shown to prevent false positive results caused by RF or ANA.[15,23] Complement fixation and indirect hemagglutination tests have been developed, but detect different antibodies than the other serologic methods, with titers rising several weeks or months later, and persisting at high levels for long periods of time;[8,12] these methods are thus less useful in establishing diagnosis, but may be helpful in assessing the stage of infection when used in conjunction with other methods. (See also *Toxoplasma gondii IFA*.)

REFERENCES

1. Alford, C.A., Stagno, S., and Reynolds, D.W.: Bull. N.Y. Acad. Med., *50*:160, 1974.
2. Anderson, S.E., Bautista, S.C., and Remington, J.S.: Clin. Exp. Immunol., *26*:375, 1976.
3. Anderson, S.E., and Remington, J.S.: South Med. J., *68*:1433, 1975.
4. Carter, A.D., and Frank, J.W.: Can. Med. Assoc. J., *135*:618, 1986.
5. Daffos, F. et al.: N. Engl. J. Med., *318*:271, 1988.
6. Endo, T., and Kobayashi, A.: Exp. Parasitol., *40*:170, 1976.
7. Fuccillo, D.A. et al.: Diagn. Clin. Immunol., *5*:8, 1987.
8. Hughes, H.P.A.: Clin. Top. Microbiol. Immunol., *120*:105, 1985.
9. Krogstad, D.J., Juranek, D.D., and Walls, K.W.: Ann. Intern. Med., *77*:773, 1972.
10. Luft, B.J., and Remington, J.S.: J. Infect. Dis., *157*:1, 1988.
11. McCabe, R., and Remington, J.S.: N. Engl. J. Med., *318*:313, 1988.
*12. McLeod, R., and Remington, J.S.: In *Harrison's Principles of Internal Medicine.* 11th ed. Edited by E. Braunwald et al. New York, McGraw-Hill Book Co., 1987.
13. Miller, M.J., Aronson, W.J., and Remington, J.S.: Ann. Intern. Med., *71*:139, 1969.
14. Mills, J.: Rev. Infect. Dis., *8*:1001, 1986.
15. Naot, Y., and Remington, J.S.: J. Infect. Dis., *142*:757, 1980.
16. O'Connor, G.R.: Bull. N.Y. Acad. Med., *50*:192, 1974.

*17. Remington, J.S., and Desmonts, G.: In *Infectious Diseases of the Fetus and Newborn Infant.* 2nd ed. Edited by J.S. Remington and J.O. Klein. Philadelphia, W.B. Saunders Co., 1983.

18. Remington, J.S., and Gentry, L.O.: Ann. N.Y. Acad. Sci., *174*:1006, 1970.

19. Ruskin, J., and Remington, J.S.: Ann. Intern. Med., *84*:193, 1976.

20. Sabin, A.B., and Feldman, H.A.: Science, *108*:660, 1948.

21. Schreiber, R.D., and Feldman, H.A.: J. Infect. Dis., *141*:366, 1980.

22. Stagno, S. et al.: Pediatrics, *59*:669, 1977.

23. Tomasi, J.-P., Schlit, A.-F., and Stadtbaeder, S.: J. Clin. Microbiol., *24*:849, 1986.

Toxoplasma Gondii—IFA[3]

PRINCIPLE. *Toxoplasma gondii* antibodies are detected in serum by a standardized kit that employs *Toxoplasma gondii* substrate affixed to substrate slides. Patient sera is reacted with the substrate. The second incubation is the interaction of FITC labeled anti-human globulin with *T. gondii* antibodies attached to the *T. gondii* substrate. Presence of antibody is indicated by apple green fluorescence of the organism.

EQUIPMENT AND MATERIALS. Indirect fluorescent antibody toxoplasma test system kit, Zeus Scientific, Inc., Consisting of:

1. Rabbit antihuman globulin polyvalent (lyophilized) labeled with fluorescein isothiocyanate (FITC); contains phosphate buffered saline (PBS), pH 7.6 ± 0.1 in 1.25% bovine albumin and Evans blue counterstain

2. Fifteen eight-well substrate slides; each well contains formalin-fixed *Toxoplasma gondii* organisms (RH strain) harvested from mouse peritoneal fluid and purified. Each well contains 50 to 100 organisms per high power field (400 ×) for optimum reactivity and readability

3. Human negative control serum (lyophilized) for *T. gondii* antibody at a 1:16 working dilution when reconstituted with 1.0 mL sterile distilled water

4. Human low titer positive control serum (lyophilized) for *T. gondii* at a 1:16 working dilution when reconstituted with 1.0 mL sterile distilled water. End point titer is 1:32 to 1:128.

5. Human high titer positive control serum (lyophilized) for *T. gondii* antibody at a 1:16 working dilution when reconstituted with 1.0 mL sterile distilled water. The approximate end point titer is 1:512 to 1:2048

6. Phosphate buffered saline (PBS), pH 7.6 ± 0.1, sufficient to make 5 liters. Buffered glycerol, 3.0 mL, pH 9.0 ± 0.1

7. All sera, antisera and buffered glycerol contain preservative; thimerosal, mercury derivative 1:10,000

ADDITIONAL MATERIALS REQUIRED (BUT NOT PROVIDED)

1. Test tubes, 13 × 100, test tube racks or microtitration system equipment

2. Small serologic, pasteur or automatic pipettes

3. Staining dish: Large staining dish with a small magnetic mixing set-up provides an ideal mechanism for washing slides between incubation steps

4. Moist chamber

5. Cover slip, 24 × 50 mm thickness No. 1

6. Distilled water—CAP type 1 or equivalent

7. Properly equipped fluorescence microscope assembly

STORAGE INSTRUCTIONS

1. *Toxoplasma gondii* substrate slides—store at −20° C or lower. Stable for 2 years. Do not refreeze thawed slides.

2. Rabbit anti-human globulin—reconstitute with 3.0 mL sterile distilled water. Store in small aliquots at −20° C or lower. Frozen aliquots are stable for 6 months. Thawed aliquots are stable for 90 days at 2 to 5° C. Do not refreeze.

3. Human negative control serum: Reconstitute with 1.0 mL sterile distilled water. Store in small aliquots at −20° C or lower. Frozen aliquots are stable for 6 months. Thawed aliquots are stable for 90 days at 2 to 5° C. Do not refreeze.

4. Human high titer positive control serum: Reconstitute with 1.0 ml of sterile distilled water. Store in small aliquots at −20° C. Frozen aliquots are stable for 6

months. Thawed aliquots are stable for 90 days at 2 to 5° C. Do not refreeze.

5. Human low titer positive control serum: Reconstitute with 1.0 mL of sterile distilled water. Store in small aliquots at −20° C. Frozen aliquots are stable for 6 months. Thawed aliquots are stable for 90 days at 2 to 5° C. Do not refreeze.

6. Buffered glycerol: Stable for 2 years at 2 to 5° C.

7. Phosphate buffered saline solution (PBS): Store packets at room temperature or 2 to 8° C once rehydrated. Packets are stable until expiration date. Rehydrated PBS is stable for 30 days.

SPECIMEN COLLECTION AND PREPARATION. Only fresh or properly refrigerated serum should be used. Specimens can be stored at −20° C until tested. Hemolyzed or contaminated specimens should not be tested.

PRECAUTIONS

1. Use universal blood and body fluids precautions.

2. Do not freeze and thaw reagents more than once. Repeated freezing and thawing destroys antibody reactivity.

3. Do not apply pressure to the slide envelope. This may damage substrate organisms.

4. The components of this kit are matched for optimum sensitivity and reproducibility. Reagents from other kits or sources should not be interchanged. Follow kit procedures carefully.

5. Reconstitute reagents gently but thoroughly. Reagents should be free of particulate matter. If reagents become cloudy, bacterial contamination should be suspected.

6. Reagents that appear bacterially contaminated should be discarded.

7. Always run controls with each batch of tests.

PROCEDURE
Reagent Preparation:

1. Phosphate buffered saline solution (PBS) pH 7.6 ± 1.0: Empty contents of each buffer pack in one liter of distilled water. Mix until all salts are thoroughly dissolved.

2. Human negative control serum: Reconsti-

tute with 1.0 mL of sterile distilled water. This represents a 1:16 dilution.

3. Human low titer positive control serum—reconstitute with 1.0 mL sterile distilled water. This represents a 1:16 dilution.

4. Human high titer positive control serum—reconstitute with 1.0 mL sterile distilled water. This represents a 1:16 dilution.

5. Rabbit anti-human globulin: Reconstitute with 2.0 mL sterile distilled water. Use as reconstituted. Do not dilute.

TEST PROCEDURE

1. Prepare serial twofold dilutions of patient sera in PBS. Two dilutions of each patient's serum should be tested at 1:16 and 1:64.

2. Remove the appropriate number of substrate slides from the freezer and allow slides to reach room temperature before opening packets.

3. Open packets, remove slides and identify patient and control wells.

4. Add one drop (approx. 0.01 mL) of test and control sera to each appropriately identified well. Include positive, negative, and buffer controls.

5. Place slides in a moist chamber and incubate at 25°C for 30 minutes.

6. Rinse slides briefly in a gentle stream of distilled or deionized water.

7. Wash slides in a staining dish containing PBS for 10 minutes with two changes of buffer.

8. Rinse slides briefly with distilled or deionized water, and air dry slides. Do not disturb.

9. Add one drop, approx. 0.01 mL, of conjugate to each well and incubate in a moist chamber at 25°C for 30 minutes.

10. Repeat steps 6 through 8.

11. Place a small amount (4 to 5 drops) of mounting media between the two rows of wells, and coverslip.

12. Examine slides in the dark with a properly assembled fluorescence microscope. Slides should be examined immediately or stored at 2 to 5° C in the dark for no longer than 24 hours before reading. Stored slides should not be mounted.

13. If patient sera is positive at a titer of 1:64, further dilution of the specimen is required. Prepare serial 2-fold dilutions of patient serum in PBS. Test dilutions of 1:64, 1:128, 1:256, 1:512 and 1:1024. If patient is positive at 1:1024, report as > 1024.

14. For endpoint control, titer the human high titer positive control serum. Use the manufacturer's assayed values as a guide, making serial dilutions which will give a definitive endpoint titer. Remember the human high titer positive control serum is stored at a working dilution of 1:16.

REPORTING. Examine the slide for the relative staining intensity of the *Toxoplasma gondii* substrate organisms. A negative reaction is one that demonstrates no staining along the periphery of the substrate organisms or one that shows only polar staining of the substrate organisms. Positive reactions are observed as staining 1+ to 4+ along the periphery of the substrate organisms. A 1+ reaction is one that shows weak but distinct applegreen peripheral staining and represents the end point reaction in a titration. A 4+ reaction is one that shows strong applegreen staining at the periphery of the substrate organisms.

INTERPRETATION OF RESULTS	
Negative	Nondiagnostic
1:16–1:64	Usually reflects only some past exposure or may represent early disease with a rising titer.
1:256	Usually indicates relatively recent exposure or current involvement.
1:1024 or higher	Very significant. The clinician should be advised to consider toxoplasmosis and to further attempt to identify the disease.

EXPECTED VALUES. The expected value in the normal population is negative. However, healthy individuals may contain toxoplasma antibodies at low titers and occasionally at high titers.

LIMITATIONS OF THE PROCEDURE

1. False positive reactions may occur with sera from patients with high titer rheumatoid factor[2] and antinuclear antibodies.[1]

2. A single test by itself is not diagnostic. The results of this test system should be interpreted in the light of the patient's history, physical examination, and clinical symptoms by a medical authority.

REFERENCES

1. Araujo, F.G. et al.: Appl. Microbiol., 22:270, 1971.

2. Hyde, B. et al.: J. Clin. Pathol., 148:42, 1975.

3. Package Insert—Indirect fluorescent antibody Toxoplasma test system. Zeus Scientific, Inc., Raritan, New Jersey, 1987.

Chapter 10

ALLERGY

This chapter will concentrate on those allergies that are acute, adverse inflammatory reactions to antigenic stimuli, and are commonly characterized by release of chemical mediators (e.g. histamine) from basophils and mast cells. Depending in part on the stimulus and the mode of entry into the body, allergies can result in a wide variety of symptoms, including skin rashes, respiratory pruritus, sneezing, coughing, wheezing, congestion, dypsnea, difficulty breathing, laryngo- and/or bronchospasm, abdominal pain, vomiting, diarrhea, rhinorrhea, eye irritation, angioedema, hypotension, cardiovascular collapse, and shock. Allergic reactions may be generalized (systemic), involving multiple organ systems, or localized such that only a single organ or closely associated organs are affected. The term *anaphylaxis* refers to those severe, systemic allergic reactions that result when the organs involved are primarily blood vessels and smooth muscles of the circulatory system.[108]

ALLERGY AND IgE

The role of IgE in allergic reactions was first established by Ishizaka, Ishizaka, and Lee,[47] who demonstrated that structural changes in the Fc portion of IgE could result in release of the chemical mediators responsible for allergic reactions. The mechanism by which IgE acts as an immunologic trigger for allergic reactions in vivo, referred to as *immediate hypersensitivity,* was defined as Type I immunopathology by Coombs and Gell[17] (see below and Chap. 1). Classic immediate hypersensitivity reactions occur within 20 to 30 minutes of exposure to an antigen referred to in this situation as an *allergen.* Symptoms resolve, usually within an hour, if the allergen is removed from the environment. Continued exposure to allergen over time results in chronic forms of immediate hypersensitivity characterized by maintenance of high levels of chemical mediators at target sites. In practice, allergies may result from sporadic, seasonal, or continuous exposure to an allergen.

Although most allergic reactions are immunologic, i.e. are mediated by IgE, identical symptoms may result from non-immunologic stimuli. The latter are referred to as *anaphylactoid* or *pseudoallergic* reactions (see below).

IgE is one of the five classes of human immunoglobulins. Although present in small quantities in normal sera, IgE concentration is elevated in persons with parasitic infections,[31,66,87] in some normal individuals,[79] and in the 10 to 20% of the general population worldwide who develop allergies during their lifetimes.[32,79] Proclivity for IgE production in response to allergens appears to be a function of the nature of exposure (repetitive, small amounts are more effective) in those individuals who are genetically prone to allergic responses (atopic individuals). Two genetic loci appear to be involved: a specific immune response (Ir) gene associated with the Major Histocompatibility Complex (MHC) on chromosome 6 allows for immune recognition of specific allergens, while a separate non-MHC locus probably determines regulation of IgE production.[7] Both atopic and non-atopic individuals have resting B cells capable of IgE production as well as T cell populations which can promote IgE synthesis[89] and regulation.[32,89] Speculation that defective immunoregulation is responsible for atopy in affected individuals remains to be proven.[28,32] It is intriguing, however, to note relationships between certain cell-mediated immune deficiency states and elevated IgE levels, with or without associated allergic syndromes.[3,33]

Modulation of IgE production by B cells appears to be a function of T lymphocytes[18,32,89] although the mechanisms are yet to be elucidated. The cytokine interleukin-4 (IL-4), however, is apparently essential for IgE synthesis.[4,19,63,80,81,97,98] The pleiotrophic effects of this molecule include enhancement of the growth of B cells, T cells, and NK cells[80] and induction of an antigen referred to as CD23 (BLAST-2; B cell-derived B cell growth factor)[37,38,80] on B cells, which probably functions as the IgE receptor on those cells.[38] CD23 released from B cells may play a regulatory role in IL-4-induced IgE synthesis.[80] Ishizaka[46] describes IgE binding factors (IgEBF) in serum that may be breakdown products of the IgE receptor and that serve to selectively regulate IgE responses.[73] Gamma interferon (IFNγ) appears to act as an inhibitor to the secretion of IgE by B cells.[26,63]

In general, serum concentrations of IgE increase in response to an allergenic stimulus, then wane with time. Seasonal pollen allergies, for example, are associated with regular increases and decreases of serum IgE related to levels of pollen inhalation.[34] Salivary immunoglobulin levels correspond with those of serum.[39] Immunotherapy can be effective in suppressing seasonal rises in antibody,[34,106] but does not affect postseasonal levels, which tend to remain elevated despite the absence of stimulus.[107] While serum IgE is catabolized at higher fractional rates than other immunoglobulins in normals, catabolism is significantly less in atopic people[23] and undoubtedly contributes to maintenance of higher concentrations in atopics.

The amino acid sequence, domains, and functional relationships of IgE have been defined.[20] Although extensive structural heterogeneity of the molecule has not been described, functional heterogeneity has been reported by several authors[56,59,60] who describe a functionally active IgE (IgE+), found only in atopic individuals, which is associated with increased responsiveness to allergens.

The mechanism by which IgE triggers allergic responses involves tissue mast cells and basophils as effector cells. The two cell lines are distinct and functionally similar, but their derivations and mechanisms of response differ greatly.[62,96]

Mast cells[29,45] are derived from precursor cells in the bone marrow, which migrate to specific tissue sites to mature.[96] They are found distributed throughout the body,[29,45,50] but principally in loose connective tissue of serosa and in mucosa and submucosa of the skin, alimentary and respiratory tracts. The thymus, lymph nodes, synovium, myometrium, heart and blood vessels, bone marrow, and nervous system are heavily populated. Most abundant concentrations of mast cells are found near small blood vessels, nerves, and the basement membrane of airways. Up to a million mast cells may be found in a gram of tissue in some situations.[111] Mast cells are present from birth and are maintained in stable concentrations throughout life, although a regulation mechanism has not been described.[96]

Two types of mast cells are present in humans, differing from one another by their content of specific proteases. Tryptase- and chymase-containing cells predominate in skin, while cells with only tryptase are prevalent in the lung.[96]

Basophils[85,96] derive from the bone marrow, then remain in the peripheral blood where they comprise approximately 1% of the circulating leukocytes. With an average half life of only 3 days, they are rarely found extravascularly. Basophils respond to chemotactic stimuli, as do other polymorphonuclear leukocytes, and will accumulate in many inflammatory reactions.[96] The numbers of circulating basophils in atopic individuals are significantly increased over nonatopics, and there is evidence that relative numbers are stable over time.[85]

Mast cells and basophils have high affinity IgE receptors (Fc_ER)[23,67] on their surfaces which are unique to these cells. Comprised of an alpha, a beta, and two gamma subunits,[54,58] they bind to a 76 amino acid sequence at the $C_E{}^2/C_E{}^3$ junction of the Fc portion of IgE.[43] IgE dissociates slowly from the receptor, once bound, with a half life of 8 to 14 days.[22] Basophils carry approximately twice the number of IgE receptors as mast cells.[96]

Low affinity IgE receptors ("Fc_ERII")[37,49,96] differ significantly from those described above, and may be found on eosinophils, macrophages, platelets, and B cells. Although these may be triggered by similar mechanisms, they do not appear to play a significant role in initiation of immediate hypersensitivity reactions. Gordon and Guy[37] speculate that the Fc_ERII may be the CD23 antigen of B cells, described above.

Binding of IgE to the high affinity of IgE receptor primes mast cells and basophils for subsequent activity; however, the cells remain quiescent even when IgE is attached. An entirely different picture emerges when cross-linkage of adjacent IgE molecules, by allergen or by anti-IgE, occurs. When dimeric[22,61] allergens of a size greater than 200Å[51] cross-link at least 10% of the cell's receptors,[22,61,83] explosive activation and degranulation results. Evidence suggests an orderly set of intracellular events,[48,96] probably requiring both Ca^{2+}[48] and IL-2,[68] facilitate degranulation and subsequent activity.

Among a heterogeneous group of molecules collectively referred to as *histamine releasing factors* (HRF: see below),[40,41,56,60] some work via IgE-dependent reactions and may be responsible for the altered IgE(IgE+) described above.[56,60]

Some of the chemical mediators of allergic reactions are preformed by mast cells and basophils and stored in granules within the cells' cytoplasm. Of these, several are released into the environment upon activation of the cell (1° preformed mediators), while others remain associated with the granule after discharge (1° preformed granule-associated mediators). After activation of the cell occurs, synthesis of a separate group of mediators is initiated (1° generated mediators), which are subsequently released from the cell over time. Table 10–1 lists selected primary mediators.

Secondary mediators contribute to allergic reactions but are produced by cells other than basophils and mast cells. In general terms, these serve either to enhance inflammation or to inactivate substances already released. Table 10–1 lists several secondary mediators with their cellular sources.

Histamine, the predominant preformed mediator, is produced by both basophils and mast cells, comprising about 10% of the granular contents in resting cells. Working through specific receptors, designated H_1 and H_2, histamine has both pro-inflammatory and anti-inflammatory effects.[96,111] Interaction with H_1 receptors effects bronchoconstriction, increased vascular permeability and smooth muscle contraction while H_2 receptor stimulation is responsible for increased gastric acid, pepsin and mucous secretions.[111] Collective actions of histamine release also include urticaria, angioedema, headache, flushing, and the

Table 10–1. Chemical Mediators of Allergy[50,75,96,99,111]

1° Preformed Mediators	Cellular Source
Histamine	Mast cells, basophils
Eosinophil Chemotactic Factor	Mast cells
Neutrophil Chemotactic Factor	Mast cells, basophils
Proteolytic Enzymes (e.g.	
kininogenase, arylsulfatase A)	Mast cells, basophils
1° Preformed Granule-Associated Mediators	
Heparin	Mast cells
Chymotrypsin	
Arylsulfatase B	
1° Generated Mediators	
Leukotrienes (LTB$_4$, LTC$_4$, LTD$_4$, LTE$_4$)	Mast cells
Prostaglandin D$_2$	Mast cells
Platelet-Activating Factor	Mast cells, basophils
Others[50]	
2° Mediators	
Arylsulfatase B	Eosinophils
Histaminase	Eosinophils
Major Basic Protein	Eosinophils
Leukotrienes	Neutrophils
Plasmin	Eosinophils
Phospholipase D	Eosinophils
Prostaglandins	Eosinophils, neutrophils
Serotonin	Platelets
Platelet-Activating Factor	Neutrophils, eosinophils
Others[96]	Macrophages

wheal (swelling) and flare (redness) reactions that characterize positive skin reactions.[96,111]

Among the *proteolytic enzymes* are molecules that can generate kinins, initiate intravascular coagulation, and effect complement activation. Beyond its anticoagulant function, *heparin* has primarily anti-inflammatory effects, e.g. it can bind histamine and inhibit complement sequences. *Leukotrienes* are potent bronchoconstriction mediators. Leukotriene B$_4$ (LTB$_4$) is an active neutrophil chemotactic factor. LTC$_4$ induces bronchoconstriction and increases vascular permeability. LTD$_4$ effects coronary vasoconstriction. Originally, LTC$_4$, LTD$_4$, and LTE$_4$ were referred to collectively as slow-reacting substance of anaphylaxis (SRS-A). Among the *prostaglandins,* prostaglandin D$_2$ (PGD$_2$) constricts bronchi and effects systemic vasodilation, increased vascular permeability and pulmonary hypertension. It is a potent hypotensive. PGE$_2$ induces bronchodilation and blocks histamine release from mast cells and ba-

sophils. PGF$_2$ is an effective vasoconstrictor, as is PGI$_2$. *Platelet-activating factor* aggregates and induces degranulation of platelets. Its presence attracts neutrophils and eosinophils, increases vasopermeability, and causes bronchoconstriction.

In vivo, mediators are probably released multiply from cells after appropriate activation,[77] e.g. initial mast cell/basophil activation induces the release of 1° preformed and preformed granule-associated mediators. 1° generated mediators subsequently are formed by the activated cells and released over a period of time. Accumulation of cells in response to chemotaxins may facilitate release and/or generation of 2° mediators.

In most cases, the initial response to isolated allergen exposure spontaneously resolves within about an hour. In up to 28% of cases,[99] however, *protracted* reactions lasting 5 to 32 hours occur, despite adequate treatment. An additional 20% of patients may experience a second wave, or *biphasic* reaction within 8 hours after the apparent remission of the initial event.[99,101] Evidence suggests that both biphasic and protracted anaphylaxis are mediated solely by Type I, IgE-mediated responses,[76,96] although they are generally unresponsive to conventional treatments. Collectively, these reactions are referred to as *late phase reactions* (LPR).

Although the mechanism of late phase reactions remains to be elucidated, the central role of mast cell degranulation in the reaction is generally accepted.[21] LPR are characterized by infiltrations of eosinophils and neutrophils (2 to 8 hours), deposition of fibrin, and, subsequently macrophage and fibroblast influx (<24 hours).[27,50,96] There is evidence of protracted elevations of histamine[93] and other mediators.[71] Late phase reactions are most likely provoked by inflammatory mediators and chemotaxins generated during initial reactions, then maintained by complex interactions of secondary cells and mediators.[23,56,96]

Elevations of IgE in atopic individuals may appear in response to many different types of stimuli[99] with resultant symptomology. Atopic individuals may react to foods,[1,36,42,74,96] especially milk, egg whites, fish, legumes, nuts, shell fish, citrus fruits, grains, and chocolate. Prevalence of food allergies is probably low;[96] 4 to 6% in infants, 1 to 2% in young children, and less than 1% in adults. Food intolerance, it should be noted, often occurs as a result of factors other than IgE-mediated hypersensitivity.[96]

Inhaled allergens (e.g. ragweed pollen) may elicit allergic rhinitis[16,114] (hay fever); they and other inhalants[6,82,100,105] such as house dust, house dust mites, cockroach residue, molds, animal or human dander, or pollens may also induce development of allergic (extrinsic) asthma[14,104] in sensitive individuals. Environmental pollutants,[2] cigarette smoke,[53] and/or viral infection probably act synergistically to facilitate asthma and contribute to more severe disease. Exposure to inhaled allergens in occupational settings may elicit either allergic rhinitis or occupational asthma.[11,12,24]

Classically, asthma is a disease of inflamed, hyperirritable airways[44] which manifests as reversible airway obstruction associated with bronchospasm, mucosal edema, cellular infiltrates, and increased secretions.[50,84] Circumstantial evidence clearly implicates the mast cell in the initiation of allergen-induced bronchospasm[30,95] and the eosinophil in its pathogenesis.[35,70,110] Approximately 50% of IgE-mediated asthmatic responses are followed by secondary, late responses (late asthmatic responses or LAR)[50,76,111] analogous to the late phase response described above.

Atopic dermatitis[8,90] is a skin disorder associated primarily with inhaled allergens or foods.[78,90] The disorder is usually seen in patients with a personal or family history of atopy, and 90% of individuals demonstrate increased levels of IgE to a variety of allergens.[9] Patch tests and observation of skin lesions implicate IgE hypersensitivity in combination with evidence of type IV (delayed hypersensitivity) reactions.[3,8]

Protein drugs such as insulin or other hormones,[99,113] antibiotics (e.g. penicillin, tetracycline, nitrofurantoin, streptomycin, sulfonimides), and vitamins (folic acid, thiamine) can induce IgE-mediated-reactions, as can exposure to seminal or vaginal fluids.[5,99,116] Vaccines grown in egg embryo, or foreign proteins used in therapy (tetanus antitoxin, gammaglobulin) can also cause IgE-mediated allergy. Insect venoms[25,65,117] (e.g. fire ants, honeybees, and wasps) elicit IgE-mediated hypersensitivity in 0.5 to 5% of the population,[108] but not all insect induced anaphylactic reactions are IgE-mediated[59] (see below). Most individuals allergic to insect stings lose sensitization over time.[91,117]

Anaphylactic reactions in which histamine is released may be caused by a variety of stimuli (*histamine releasing factors,* or HRF) in reactions which are not dependent on IgE. The reactions elicited are clinically similar to IgE-mediated responses and are treated identically, but differ from one another in the nature of specific mediators.[48] Collectively, they are referred to as *anaphylactoid,* or *pseudoallergic responses.* The list of inducing agents is long,[29,99] and includes certain cytokines (e.g. IL-1),[40,103] components of complement activation,[72] coagulation and fibrinolysis,[99] protein kinase C,[69] and neuropeptides such as substance P and ATP.[111] Environmental exposure to insect stings,[86] heterologous seminal fluid,[99] or food may elicit responses.[99] Drugs[92,99,115] including opiates, curare, polymixin B, desferal, aspirin, and steroidal antiinflammatory drugs may be responsible. Sterilizers used in hemodialysis[99] or radio-contrast medias used for radiographic examination may cause responses. Recently, non-IgE anaphylactic reactions have been described during exercise[94] or upon exposure to sulfiting agents in foods.[102]

Preparation of reliable allergens for use in diagnosis and immunotherapy of IgE-induced hypersensitivity has been a chronic problem. Not only are difficulties encountered in recognition and purification of allergenic substances, but identification of cross reactions,[112] concentration and storage conditions have not been standardized.[88] Monoclonal antibodies[13] have been helpful in recent standardization[15,100] and development of a nomenclature system[64] for allergenic extracts.

Diagnosis of IgE-mediated hypersensitivity is most often made by careful physical examination and history, and by skin testing.[88] Because IgE is attached to mast cells in skin, a prick or scratch of skin with allergen, or its intradermal injection, will result in a characteristic reaction (wheal and flare) that appears within 15 to 30 minutes and usually resolves within an hour. Although skin testing is subjective in reading and interpretation, and reliable antigens are not yet available,[88] it remains a tool for diagnosis and evaluation of therapy. Performance of peripheral blood eosinophil counts, and radioimmunoassay assays used for detection of total IgE (Radioimmunosorbent Test, or RIST) or allergen-specific IgE (Radioallergosorbent Test, or RAST) may be helpful. A recent study[109] of discrepancies between skin testing and RAST indicates 18% discordant results, usually the result of reactive skin tests that did not correlate with positive RAST. It is likely that enhanced sensitivity and specificity of the allergens used in testing will improve in vitro testing results. Micro RAST tests, an adaptation that reportedly enhances sensitivity and speed,[52] and enzyme immunoassay (EIA) techniques[57] have recently been developed.

REFERENCES

1. Anderson, J.A., and Sogn, D.D. (eds.): *Adverse Reactions to Foods.* NIH Publication No. 84-2442, July, 1984.
2. Andrae, S. et al.: Arch. Dis. Child., *63*:473, 1988.
3. Barker, J.N., Alegre, V.A., and MacDonald, D.M.: J. Invest. Dermatol., *90*:117, 1988.
4. Bergstedt-Lindqvist, S. et al.: Eur. J. Immunol., *18*:1073, 1988.
5. Bernstein, I.L. et al.: Ann. Intern. Med., *94*:459, 1981.
6. Bernton, H.S., McMahon, T.F., and Brown, H.: Br. J. Dis. Chest, *66*:61, 1972.
7. Blumenthal, M.N. et al.: J. Allergy Clin. Immunol., *78*:962, 1986.
8. Bruynzeel-Koomen, C.A., and Bruynzeel, P.L.B.: Allergy (43 Suppl.), *5*:15, 1988.
9. Bruynzeel-Koomen, C.A. et al.: Br. J. Dermatol., *118*:229, 1988.
10. Buist, A.S.: Chest, *93*:449, 1988.
11. Burge, P.S.: Br. J. Dis. Chest, *81*:105, 1987.
12. Chan-Yeung, M., and Malo, J-L.: Chest, *91*:130S, 1987.
13. Chapman, M.D.: Allergy (43 Suppl.), *5*:7, 1988.
14. Chapman, M.D. et al.: Chest, *94*:185, 1988.
15. The Committee on Skin Test Standardization of the Netherlands Society of Allergology. Clin. Allergy, *18*:305, 1988.
16. Conner, B.L., and Georgitis, J.W.: Primary Care, *14*:457, 1987.
17. Coombs, R.R.A., and Gell, P.G.H.: *Clinical Aspects of Immunology.* Edited by P.G.H. Gell, R.R.A. Coombs, and P.J. Lachman. Oxford, Blackwell Scientific Publications, 1975.
18. DelPrete, G. et al.: Eur. J. Immunol., *16*:1509, 1986.
19. DelPrete, G. et al.: J. Immunol., *140*:4193, 1988.
20. Dorrington, K.J., and Bennich, H.: Immunol. Rev., *41*:3, 1978.
21. Dorsch, W.: Allergy (43 Suppl.), *5*:38, 1988.
22. Dreskin, S.C., and Metzger, H.: JAMA, *260*:1265, 1988.
23. Dreskin, S.C. et al.: J. Clin. Invest., *79*:1764, 1987.
24. Dykewicz, M.S.: Prim. Care, *14*:559, 1987.
25. Ewan, P.W.: J. R. Soc. Med., *78*:234, 1985.

26. Finkelman, F.D. et al.: J. Immunol., *140*:1022, 1988.

27. Fleekop, P.D. et al.: J. Allergy Clin. Immunol., *80*:140, 1987.

28. Frajman, M. et al.: Allergy, *42*:81, 1987.

29. Friedman, M.M., and Kaliner, M.A.: Am. Rev. Respir. Dis., *135*:1157, 1987.

30. Gaddy, J.N., and Busse, W.W.: Am. Rev. Respir. Dis., *134*:969, 1986.

31. Ganguly, N.K. et al.: J. Clin. Microbiol., *26*:739, 1988.

32. Geha, R.S., and Leung, D.Y.M.: Int. Arch. Allergy Appl. Immunol., *82*:389, 1987.

33. Geha, R.S., and Leung, D.Y.M.: J. Allergy Clin. Immunol., *78*:995, 1986.

34. Gleich, G.J. et al.: J. Allergy Clin. Immunol., *70*:261, 1982.

35. Gleich, G.J. et al.: J. Allergy Clin. Immunol., *80*:412, 1987.

36. Gontzes, P., and Bahna, S.L.: Prim. Care, *14*:547, 1987.

37. Gordon, J., and Guy, G.R.: Immunol. Today, *8*:339, 1987.

38. Gordon, J. et al.: Blood, *72*:367, 1988.

39. Grunbacher, F.J.: Arch. Oral Biol., *33*:121, 1988.

40. Haak-Frendscho, M., Dinarello, C., and Kaplan, A.P.: J. Allergy Clin. Immunol., *82*:218, 1988.

41. Haak-Frendscho, M. et al.: J. Clin. Invest., *82*:17, 1988.

42. Hatteuig, G., Kjellman, B., and Bjorksten, B.: Clin. Allergy, *17*:571, 1987.

43. Helm, B. et al.: Nature, *331*:180, 1988.

44. Holgate, S.T., Beasley, R., and Twentyman, O.P.: Clin. Sci., *73*:561, 1987.

45. Holgate, S.T., Robinson, C., and Church, M.K.: Allergy (43 Suppl.), *5*:22, 1988.

46. Ishizaka, K.: Annu. Rev. Immunol., *6*:513, 1988.

47. Ishizaka, K., Ishizaka, T., and Lee, E.H.: Immunochemistry, *7*:687, 1970.

48. Ishizaka, T., White, J.R., and Saito, H.: Int. Arch. Allergy Appl. Immunol., *82*:327, 1987.

49. Jouault, T. et al.: Eur. J. Immunol., *18*:237, 1988.

50. Kaliner, M.: Chest, *91*:171S, 1987.

51. Kane, P.M., Holowka, D., and Baird, B.: J. Cell. Biol., *107*:969, 1988.

52. Kemeny, D.M., and Richards, D.: J. Immunol. Methods, *108*:105, 1988.

53. Kershaw, C.R.: J. R. Soc. Med., *80*:683, 1987.

54. Kinet, J.P. et al.: Proc. Natl. Acad. Sci. U.S.A., *85*:6483, 1988.

55. Larsen, G.L.: Chest, *93*:1287, 1988.

56. Lichtenstein, L.M.: J. Allergy Clin. Immunol., *81*:814, 1988.

57. Lindberg, R.E., and Arroyave, C.: J. Allergy Clin. Immunol., *78*:614, 1986.

58. Liu, F.T., Albrandt, K., and Robertson, M.W.: Proc. Natl. Acad. Sci. U.S.A., *85*:5639, 1988.

59. Lomnitzer, R., Lanner, A., and Rabson, A.R.: Clin. Allergy, *18*:39, 1988.

60. MacDonald, S.M. et al.: J. Immunol., *139*:506, 1987.

61. MacGlashan, D., and Lichtenstein, L.M.: J. Immunol., *130*:2330, 1983.

62. MacGlashan, D.W., Jr. et al.: Fed. Proc., *42*:2504, 1983.

63. Maggi, E. et al.: Eur. J. Immunol., *18*:1045, 1988.

64. Marsh, D.G. et al.: Allergy, *43*:161, 1988.

65. McLean, D.C.: Prim. Care, *14*:513, 1987.

66. McRury, J. et al.: Clin. Exp. Immunol., *65*:631, 1986.

67. Metzger, H., Alcaraz, G., Kinet, J-P., and Quarto, R.: Biochem. Soc. Symp., *51*:59, 1986.

68. Morita, Y., Goto, M., and Miyamoto, T.: Allergy, *42*:104, 1987.

69. Morita, Y. et al.: Allergy, *43*:100, 1988.

70. Murlas, C.G.: Chest, *93*:1278, 1988.

71. Naclerio, R.M. et al.: N. Engl. J. Med., *313*:65, 1985.

72. Nagata, S., and Glovsky, M.M.: J. Allergy Clin. Immunol., *80*:24, 1987.

73. Nakajima, T., Sarfati, M., and Delespesse, G.: J. Immunol., *139*:848, 1987.

74. Novembre, E., deMartino, M., and Vierucci, A.: J. Allergy Clin. Immunol., *81*:1059, 1988.

75. O'Byrne, P.M.: Ann. N.Y. Acad. Sci., *524*:282, 1988.

76. O'Byrne, P.M., Dolovich, J., and Hargreave, F.E.: Am. Rev. Respir. Dis., *136*:740, 1987.

77. Olssen, P., Hammarlund, A., and Pipkorn, U.: J. Allergy Clin. Immunol., *82*:291, 1988.

78. Paller, A.S.: Prim. Care, *14*:491, 1987.

79. Peltonen, L., Havu, V.K., and Mattila, L.: Allergy, *43*:152, 1988.

80. Pène, J. et al.: Eur. J. Immunol., *18*:929, 1988.

81. Pène, J. et al.: J. Immunol., *141*:1218, 1988.

82. Pollart, S.M., Chapman, M.D., and Platts-Mills, T.A.: Prim. Care, *14*:591, 1987.

83. Pruzansky, J.J., and Patterson, R.: Immunology, *64*:307, 1988.

84. Reed, C.E.: Chest *94*:175, 1988.

85. Reilly, K.M. et al.: Int. Arch. Allergy Appl. Immunol., *84*:424, 1987.

86. Reisman, R.E., and Osur, S.L.: Ann. Allergy, *59*:429, 1987.

87. Ridel, P.R. et al.: J. Immunol., *141*:978, 1988.

88. Rodriguez, G.E., and Dyson, M.C.: Prim. Care, *14*:447, 1987.

89. Romagnani, S., DelPrete, G.F., and Maggi, E.: Allergy (43 Suppl.), *5*:32, 1988.

90. Sampson, H.A.: J. Allergy Clin. Immunol., *81*:495, 1988.

91. Savliwala, M.N., and Reisman, R.E.: J. Allergy Clin. Immunol., *80*:741, 1987.

92. Settipane, G.A.: Arch. Intern. Med., *141*:328, 1981.

93. Shalit, M. et al.: J. Immunol., *141*:821, 1988.

94. Sheffer, A.L. et al.: J. Allergy Clin. Immunol., *75*:479, 1985.

95. Sheller, J.R.: Am. J. Med. Sci., *293*:298, 1987.

96. Smith, T.F.: Prim. Care, *14*:421, 1987.

97. Snapper, C.M., Finkelman, F.D., and Paul, W.E.: J. Exp. Med., *167*:183, 1988.

98. Snapper, C.M., Finkelman, F.D., and Paul, W.E.: Immunol. Rev., *102*:51, 1988.

99. Soto-Aguilar, M.E., deShazo, R.D., and Waring, N.P.: Postgrad. Med., *82*:154, 1987.

100. Stankus, R.P., and Lehrer, S.B.: Postgrad. Med., *82*:213, 1987.

101. Stark, B.J., and Sullivan, T.J.: J. Allergy Clin. Immunol., *78*:76, 1986.

102. Stevenson, D.D., and Simon, R.A.: J. Allergy Clin. Immunol., *68*:26, 1981.

103. Subramanian, N., and Bray, M.A.: J. Immunol., *138*:271, 1987.

104. Suliaman, F., and Townley, R.G.: Prim. Care, *14*:475, 1987.

105. Tang, R.B. et al.: J. Asthma, *23*:245, 1986.

106. Tipton, W.R., Prim. Care, *14*:623, 1987.

107. Turner, K.J. et al.: Int. Arch. Allergy Appl. Immunol., *82*:398, 1987.

108. Valentine, M.D., and Lichtenstein, L.M.: JAMA, *258*:2881, 1987.

109. vanderZee, J.S. et al.: J. Allergy Clin. Immunol., *82*:270, 1988.

110. Wardlaw, A.J., and Kay, A.B.: Allergy, *42*:321, 1987.

111. Wasserman, S.I.: Ann. Allergy, *60*:477, 1988.

112. Weber, R.W.: Prim. Care, *14*:435, 1987.

113. Wedner, H.J.: Prim. Care, *14*:523, 1987.

114. Welch, M.J., and Kemp, J.P.: Prim. Care, *14*:575, 1989.

115. Withington, D.E. et al.: Anaesthesia, *42*:850, 1987.

116. Witkin, S.S., Jeremias, J., and Ledger, W.J.: Am. J. Obstet. Gynecol., *159*:32, 1988.

117. Youlten, L.J.: Practitioner, *231*:502, 1987.

IgE Quantitation by Enzyme Immunoassay[2]

PRINCIPLE. In the IgE enzyme immunoassay (EIA), beads coated with rabbit antihuman IgE are incubated with samples (standards, control and patient specimens). During this incubation, IgE present in the sample is bound to the solid phase anti-IgE. After aspiration of unbound material and washing, the beads are incubated with goat antihuman IgE conjugated with horseradish peroxidase (HRPO). The presence of the enzyme attached to the antibody-IgE complex on the bead surface is detected by incubating the washed bead with o-Phenylenediamine (OPD) substrate containing hydrogen peroxide. During incubation, a yellow-orange color develops in proportion to the amount of IgE bound to the antibody coated bead. The enzyme reaction is stopped by the addition of 1 N Sulfuric Acid. The assay absorbance values of the standards, control and patient specimens are obtained with a spectrophotometer set at a wavelength of 492 nm. A standard curve is obtained by plotting the absorbance value (Y-axis) against the corresponding concentration of the standards (X-axis). The IgE concentrations of the patient specimens and the control, which are run concurrently with the standards, can then be determined from the standard curve.

EQUIPMENT AND MATERIALS

1. IgE EIA Kit components-Abbott Laboratories:

a. Antibody to human IgE (rabbit) coated beads

b. One vial (20 mL) antibody to human IgE (Goat):Peroxidase (horseradish) conjugate. Minimum concentration: 0.05 μg/mL in saline with protein stabilizers and antimicrobial agents

c. Five vials (0.8 mL each) IgE (human) standards: 0, 10, 40, 75 and 200 IU/mL each in saline solution with protein stabilizers and antimicrobial agents

d. One vial (45 mL) specimen dilution buffer. Phosphate buffer

e. One bottle (10 tablets) OPD (o-Phenylenediamine · 2 HCl) tablets. OPD/tablet: 12.8 mg

f. One bottle (55 mL) diluent for OPD (o-Phenylenediamine · 2 HCl). A citrate-phosphate buffer containing 0.02% hydrogen peroxide

g. One vial (1 mL after reconstitution) IgE control. 30 to 120 IU IgE/mL (assay value on vial label). A human serum with anti-microbial agents

h. One vial (2 mL) reconstitution solution for IgE control

2. Reaction trays (20 or 60 wells per tray)

3. Cover seals

4. Assay tubes with identifying cartons and covers (for transfer of beads from reaction trays).

5. 1-N sulfuric acid

6. Precision pipettes, to deliver 200 μL, 300 μL, 1 mL and 5 mL

7. Precision pipette with disposable tips to deliver 50 μL

8. Precision pipette or similar equipment to deliver 450 μL

9. Disposable tips.

10. Device for delivery of rinse solution such as a Gorman-Rupp dispensing pump or equivalent

11. Test tubes and rack for predilution if required

12. An aspiration device for washing beads such as a Pentawash II with a vacuum source such as a Gast vacuum pump or equivalent and a trap for retaining the aspirate

13. Water bath capable of maintaining temperature at 37° C ± 2° C

14. Spectrophotometer capable of reading absorbance at 492 nm

15. Nonmetallic forceps

16. Single bead dispenser for dispensing one bead at a time from a 100 bead bottle

17. Membrane seal puncture tool for acid bottles

18. Vortex mixer or equivalent

19. Rectilinear graph paper (if quantum analyzer is not used)

20. 1 N sulfuric acid

PRECAUTIONS

For In Vitro Diagnostic Use:

1. Do not mix kit reagents from different master lots.

NOTE: Any OPD reagent lot or acid lot may be used with any Abbott IgE EIA Diagnostic Kit lot.

2. Do not use kit components beyond the expiration date.

3. Avoid microbial contamination of reagents when opening and removing aliquots from the primary vials.

4. After use, tightly recap reagents to avoid evaporation.

5. Use a dedicated pipette to deliver the conjugate in order to avoid any possible neutralization of the goat anti-human IgE: HRPO conjugate by contamination.

6. Store water for washing in clean containers to prevent contamination.

7. Avoid contact of OPD and sulfuric acid with skin and mucous membranes. If these reagents come into contact with skin, wash with water.

8. Do not expose OPD reagents to strong light during storage or incubation.

9. Avoid contact of the OPD Substrate Solution with any oxidizing agent. Do not allow Substrate Solution to come into contact with any metal parts. Rinse glassware used with OPD Solution thoroughly with 1 N acid (sulfuric or hydrochloric) using approximately 10% of the container volume followed by three washes of distilled water at the same volume prior to use.

10. If the desiccant obstructs the flow of beads, remove from bead bottle prior to dispensing beads. Replace desiccant in bottle and tightly cap bottle for storage. Do not store beads with bead dispenser attached to bottle.

REAGENT PREPARATION. Instructions for Reconstitution of IgE Control.

Prior to use, the control must be reconstituted with reconstitution solution for IgE control. Once reconstituted, the IgE control is stable for 3 months when stored at 2 to 8° C.

1. Using a clean pipette, transfer 1.0 mL of reconstitution solution to the vial of IgE control.

2. Mix gently to obtain a homogeneous solution.

STORAGE INSTRUCTIONS

1. Store kit reagents and reconstituted IgE Control at 2 to 8° C. OPD tablets and 1 N sulfuric acid may be stored at room temperature.

2. All reagents must be brought to room temperature (15 to 30° C) before use, but should be returned to storage conditions indicated above immediately after use.

CAUTION: Do not open OPD Tablet bottle until it is at room temperature.

3. Retain desiccant bags in OPD tablet bottle at all times during storage.

4. Reconstituted OPD solution MUST be held at room temperature and MUST be used within 60 minutes.

5. Indications of instability or deterioration of reagents:

a. The OPD substrate solution (OPD plus diluent for OPD) should be colorless to pale yellow. A yellow-orange color indicates that the reagent has been contaminated and must be discarded.

b. Precipitates in the reagent solutions and/or unexpected test results for IgE standards are generally considered indications of reagent instability or deterioration.

SPECIMEN COLLECTION AND PREPARATION. Serum or EDTA or heparinized plasma may be tested by Abbott IgE EIA. As in any quantitative assay, plasma collected in fluid anticoagulant should be avoided due to possible dilution of IgE levels. Remove serum or plasma from the clot or red cells as soon as possible to avoid hemolysis.

Clear nonhemolyzed specimens should be used. Specimens containing any particulate matter should be clarified before testing.

Specimens may be stored at 2 to 8° C for up to 7 days. For longer storage, the specimens should be frozen. Avoid repeated freezing and thawing.

Do not use heat-inactivated specimens.

PROCEDURE: PRELIMINARY COMMENTS

1. A specimen from a patient in which a level of over 200 IU/mL of IgE is expected may be diluted 1:10 (50 µL specimen + 450 µL specimen dilution buffer) prior to performing the assay.

2. Assay each standard, control, and specimen in duplicate. All standards MUST be included in each run of patient specimens. The IgE control must also be included in each run.

Ensure that all reaction trays containing Standards, Controls and/or patient specimens are subjected to the same processing and incubation times.

CAUTION: Use a separate disposable pipette tip for each transfer to avoid cross-contamination.

NOTE: Once the assay has been started, all subsequent steps should be completed without interruption.

3. Prior to beginning the assay procedure, bring all reagents to room temperature (15 to 30° C) and mix gently. Adjust water bath to 37° C ± 2° C.

4. Identify the reaction tubes and tray wells for each standard, control, and specimen in the run.

PROCEDURAL NOTES: FIRST AND SECOND INCUBATION

1. When pipetting standards, control, or specimens, be careful not to splash sample outside of well or high up on well rim, as it will not be removed in subsequent washings and may be transferred to the assay tubes, causing test interference.

2. When dispensing beads, remove cap from bead bottle, attach single bead dispenser and dispense beads into wells of the reaction tray as directed in the single bead dispenser insert.

3. Do not splash liquid while tapping trays.

4. When washing beads, follow the directions in *Wash Procedure Details* in the kit insert.

5. Do not splash enzyme conjugate reagent outside of well or high up on well rim, as it will not be removed in subsequent washings and may be transferred to the tubes causing test interference.

6. During the last 5 to 10 minutes of the second incubation, prepare OPD substrate solution as previously described.

7. After the second wash, remove all excess water from top of tray by aspiration or blotting.

COLOR DEVELOPMENT

1. When transferring beads from wells to assay tubes, align inverted rack of oriented tubes over the reaction tray. Press the tubes tightly over the wells and invert tray and tubes together so that beads fall into corresponding tubes. Blot excess water from top of tube rack.

2. Avoid strong light during color development.

3. Do not allow acid solution to contact metal.

PROCEDURE

1. Pipette 200 µL of specimen dilution buffer into each reaction well.

2. Add 50 µL of each standard, control, specimen, or diluted specimen to the appropriate reaction tray wells in duplicate as indicated on worksheet.

3. Add one bead to each well.

4. Apply cover seal. Tap tray gently to ensure bead is covered, sample is mixed, and any air bubbles are released.

5. Incubate 30 ± 2 minutes in water bath (37° C ± 2° C).

6. Discard cover seal. Wash each bead 3 times.

7. Add 200 µL of antibody to human IgE-peroxidase enzyme conjugate to each reaction well.

8. Apply new cover seal. Tap tray gently.

9. Incubate 30 ± 2 minutes in water bath (37° C ± 2° C).

10. During the last 5 to 10 minutes of the enzyme conjugate incubation, prepare OPD substrate solution.

11. Instructions for Preparation of OPD Substrate Solution:

The OPD (o-Phenylenediamine · 2 HCl) tablets must be dissolved in diluent for OPD immediately before use. The solution must not be stored longer than 60 minutes before use.

During the last 5 to 10 minutes of the second incubation period, prepare the OPD substrate solution as follows:

NOTE: 300 μL is required for each standard, control, or sample well and for two reagent blanks.

CAUTION: Use pipettes and containers known to be metal free; for example, use plastic ware or acid washed / distilled-water rinsed glassware.

a. Using a clean pipette or dispenser, transfer 5 mL of diluent for OPD for each tablet to be dissolved into a suitable container.

b. Transfer OPD tablet from bottle into container with diluent for OPD using a nonmetallic forceps or equivalent. Return desiccant to bottle immediately, if removed to obtain a tablet, and close bottle tightly. Allow tablet to dissolve. *DO NOT USE A TABLET THAT IS NOT INTACT.*

c. Just prior to dispensing for the final incubation of the assay, swirl gently to obtain a homogeneous solution.

12. Discard cover seal. Wash each bead 3 times.

13. Immediately transfer beads to EIA assay tubes.

14. Add 300 μL OPD substrate solution to each assay tube.

15. Cover and incubate 30 ± 2 minutes at room temperature (15 to 30° C).

16. Add 1.0 mL 1N sulfuric acid to each tube. Vortex to mix.

17. Select a wavelength of 492 nm on a spectrophotometer or use the Quantum II Analyzer.

18. Visually inspect both blanks and discard those that are contaminated (indicated by yellow-orange color). If both blanks are contaminated, the entire run must be repeated.

19. Blank the instrument by using one of the two substrate blank tubes. Read the standards followed by the control and the patient specimens.

20. If there is an interruption during the reading of samples, repeat the blank (using the second substrate blank tube if necessary). Continue reading specimens. All absorbence values should be determined within 2 hours after addition of acid.

CALCULATION

1. For the IgE EIA run to be valid, the following criteria must be met:

a. The mean absorbance assay value of the 200 IU / mL IgE Standard should be between 1.100 and 2.000.

b. The difference in absorbance values between the 10 and 0 IU / mL Standards should be between 0.150 and 0.500.

2. If any absorbance is less than 0.100, values for duplicates should be within 0.030 absorbance units of the mean of those values. For mean absorbance values of 0.200 or greater, duplicate values should be expected to lie within 15% of the mean absorbance. Duplicate values that differ from the mean by greater than 15% should be considered suspect.

3. The IgE concentration for the Abbott IgE Control should be within 20% of the label value.

4. If a photometer or spectrophotometer other than a Quantum Analyzer is used, calculate the IgE values as follows:

a. Using a rectilinear graph paper, construct a standard curve for each run by plotting the mean absorbance obtained for each IgE Standard on the vertical (Y-axis) versus the corresponding IgE concentration on the horizontal (X-axis).

b. Using the mean absorbance value for each patient specimen and control, determine the corresponding concentration of IgE in IU / mL obtained from the standard curve.

5. For all instruments: If the specimen requires additional dilution for its assay value to fall on the standard curve, the value from the standard curve must also be adjusted by the dilution factor.

REPORTING. Report patient IgE values in IU / ml, as determined from the standard curve.

INTERPRETATION OF RESULTS. Healthy, nonallergic adults have an expected IgE concentration of approximately 10 IU / mL to 180 IU / mL.[3] Children without allergic symptoms can be expected to have significantly less IgE, with a range that is approximately 10 to 20% of the adult value.[1]

LIMITATIONS OF THE PROCEDURE. Low levels of IgE do not necessarily indicate the absence of allergies; high levels do not necessarily confirm an allergic state.

IgE concentrations may vary as a result of diet, genetic background, geographical location, and other influences. Each laboratory should establish its own expected normal range for the population of interest.

REFERENCES

1. Kjellman, N-I.M., Johansson, S.G.O., and Roth, A.: Clin. Allergy, 6:51–59, 1976.
2. Package insert, IgE EIA Kit, Abbott Laboratories, North Chicago, Ill. 1985.
3. Wittig, H.J., Belloit, J., De Fillippi, I., and Royal, G.: J. Allergy Clin. Immunol., 66:305–313, 1980.

AUTOIMMUNITY

RHEUMATOID ARTHRITIS

Rheumatoid arthritis (RA) is a chronic, systemic inflammatory disease which primarily affects the joints. Of worldwide distribution, RA has a prevalence of approximately 1 to 2%, with females afflicted about three times more commonly than males.[32,50] Onset of the disease occurs most frequently between the ages of 35 and 50 but may occur at any age.[50] Criteria used in the diagnosis of RA were devised by the American Rheumatism Association (ARA) in 1956[78] and revised in 1958[79] and 1987.[7] Recommendations have also been proposed by the Third International Symposium of Population Studies of Rheumatic Disease (New York criteria).[9] By the ARA 1987 classification system, a diagnosis of RA is made if the patient satisfies at least four of seven clinical and laboratory criteria.[7]

Patients with RA often have initially nonspecific symptoms such as fatigue, anorexia, weight loss, and transient joint and muscle pain until arthritis becomes evident, with pain, swelling, and tenderness localized to specific joints.[32,39,50,58] Typically, the arthritis occurs in multiple joints in a symmetric fashion, although asymmetric involvement of joints is possible. Joint stiffness is frequently present, especially after periods of inactivity, e.g. upon waking up in the morning. Arthritis commonly appears in the small joints of the hands and feet in the early stages of disease. Progression of RA often leads to involvement of larger joints, such as those of the knees, hips, elbows, shoulders, and cervical spine, although these joints may be affected early in the course of the disease in some patients. Permanent joint deformities associated with severe loss of function, atrophy of skeletal muscle, and osteoporosis are common manifestations of the persistent inflammation and immobilization of the joints.

Approximately 20 to 30% of patients develop rheumatoid nodules.[32,39,50] These firm, subcutaneous or subperiosteal masses appear primarily over bony eminences but may also be present in other body sites, including the heart, lungs, and brain. Other extra-articular manifestations of RA, which tend to occur in patients with longstanding disease include vasculitis, neuropathy, pleuritis, pericarditis, and ocular disease.[10,39,50] An estimated 10 to 30% of patients may develop Sjogren's syndrome, characterized by the presence of keratoconjunctivitis sicca (dry eyes) and xerostomia (dry mouth).[32,39,50] Felty's syndrome, a triad of polyarthritis, splenomegaly, and neutropenia, occurs in less than 1% of RA patients, usually those with long-standing disease.[39,50] Juvenile rheumatoid arthritis, developing in persons under 16 years of age, may appear clinically as systemic illness (Still's disease), polyarthritis, or asymmetric involvement of one or two joints.[14,32]

The course of RA is highly variable, ranging from spontaneous remission (usually within 1 to 2 years after onset) to sustained, progressively active disease culminating in severe deformity and disability.[32] Most patients with RA experience daily or weekly fluctuations in disease activity, which usually assumes an overall course of gradual progression, or a polycyclic pattern characterized by periods of disease activity alternating with periods of improvement.[33,39,50] Joint deformity is variable in degree but is a significant contributor to disability and loss of productive working years.[33,39] Although RA is not usually a terminal disease, death may result in individuals with severe extraarticular manifestations or complications of drug therapy.[32,39,50] A wide variety of treatment protocols, aimed at relieving the symptoms of RA, are available. Pharmacologic therapy can be divided into three groups: (1) traditional agents such as aspirin or other nonsteroidal anti-inflammatory drugs, (2) disease-modifying drugs such as gold compounds, D-penicillamine, and hydroxychloroquine, and (3) corticosteroids and cytotoxic immunosuppressive therapy, generally reserved for patients with severe symptoms.[39,50,68] Physical and occupational therapy also play important roles in patient management, and reconstructive surgery may be performed on severely damaged joints.

Recognition of RA as an autoimmune disease began with the discovery of rheumatoid factors in the serum of patients with RA.[100] By definition, rheumatoid factors (RF) are antibodies directed against the Fc portion of IgG molecules. RF are classically 19S IgM antibodies, but may belong to any immunoglobulin class.[26] RF are found in the majority of patients with RA and have di-

agnostic usefulness for the disease.[7] However, they are not specific for RA, also being present in some normal individuals and patients with microbial infections, autoimmune diseases other than RA (e.g. Sjögren's syndrome, SLE, scleroderma), and B cell lymphoproliferative disorders with IgM paraproteins (e.g. Waldenström's macroglobulinemia, chronic lymphocytic leukemias, essential mixed cryoglobulinemias).[17,30,31] Genes coding for RF have been discovered in the normal human genome, suggesting that RF may serve a physiologic function, perhaps facilitating the clearance of immune complexes by amplifying weak antigen-antibody interactions, and that RF may become pathogenic only under abnormal conditions which lead to its overproduction and persistence.[17,30,31] Some RF have been found to react with the Fab region of IgG molecules, suggesting that they may serve as anti-idiotype antibodies participating in an immunoregulatory idiotype network.[17]

Autoantibodies other than RF also appear commonly in RA and include antinuclear antibodies, anticollagen antibodies, antibodies directed against cytoskeletal filamentous proteins, cold-reacting anti-lymphocyte antibodies, immunoconglutinins, and mixed cryoglobulins.[11,53,56,59,60,65,101,105]

Multiple complex mechanisms appear to contribute to the chronic inflammation and destruction of the joints seen in RA. The histologic appearance of the rheumatoid synovium varies considerably with the duration and state of disease activity.[29,41,53] Infiltrates of small lymphocytes are evident, particularly in the early stages of disease. Synovial biopsies from patients with long-standing RA reveal lymphoid follicles with germinal centers, close contact between lymphocytes and macrophages (seen via electron microscopy), and a large influx of immunoglobulin-producing plasma cells.

The abundance of immune complexes in synovial fluid, coupled with evidence of complement catabolism, has lead to speculation that immune complex mechanisms

(Gell and Coombs Type III hypersensitivity)[20] may play a role in the pathogenesis of RA.[107,108] Autoantibodies (e.g. RF, ANA, anti-collagen antibodies, cryoglobulins) are thought to react with antigen, activating the classical pathway of complement. Subsequent release of chemotaxins and anaphylatoxins then leads to an influx of leukocytes (see also Chaps. 1 and 6). Large numbers of polymorphonuclear cells (PMN) are evident in the synovial fluid during the acute phases of disease[41,52] and are thought to release their lysosomal enzymes upon cell death or after ingestion of immune complexes.[103] Among the numerous enzymes that may be released from the lysosomes[22] are collagenase, gelatinase, elastase, and cathepsin G, which are capable of destroying the cartilage matrix. In addition, a metabolic burst of oxidation in the PMN results in the release of reactive oxygen species (e.g. hydroxyl radical, superoxide anion, hypochlorous acid), which are capable of destroying matrix molecules such as hyaluronic acid.[52] Furthermore, stimulation of arachidonic acid metabolism results in the synthesis of prostaglandins, which may perpetuate the influx of PMN.[52] The release of the C5a component of complement via the action of lysosomal enzymes on C5 may also result in increased leukocyte chemotaxis.[103]

Cell-mediated immunity is also thought to play a role in the pathogenesis of RA. An increased number of CD4+ 4B4+ T lymphocytes (i.e. helper/inducer cells) are found in the subsynovium of patients with RA,[29,49,69] and are thought to provide help for the stimulation of B lymphocytes in immunoglobulin synthesis, as well as elaborate lymphokines inherent to immune and inflammatory processes (e.g. interleukin-2, interleukin-3, interferon gamma, migration inhibition factor).[2,29,53,91]

Proliferation of synovial lining cells, including fibroblasts, macrophages, mast cells, and stellate cells with long dendritic processes, results in the formation of a "pannus," an organized mass of proliferating cells that grows into the joint space, and invades the articular cartilage and subchondral bone.[41,52] Cells of the pannus secrete a number of factors that contribute to the destruction of the joints and bones, including collagenase, interleukin-1, and prostaglandins.[41,52]

The etiology of RA is unknown. A role for genetic factors is strongly suggested by the close association of RA with the HLA-DR4 haplotype;[42,90,106] approximately 70% of patients with seropositive RA (i.e. positive for RF) have this haplotype, as compared to only 30% of healthy control individuals.[57,66] However, a less than perfect correlation exists, and further studies are needed to provide more information on the genetics of disease susceptibility.

Classification of RA as an autoimmune disease implies a disturbance of normal immunoregulatory mechanisms. Increased levels of serum immunoglobulins are commonly seen in patients with RA,[93] and increased numbers of B cells spontaneously secreting immunoglobulin have been described in patients with active disease.[1,8] The number of peripheral blood B cells seen in RA patients is not significantly different from the number seen in healthy controls,[53,77] but an increased proportion of immature B cells capable of forming rosettes with mouse erythrocytes[53,77] or positive for the CD5 surface marker[53,70] have been detected in RA.

A number of T cell abnormalities have also been described. Increased numbers of activated T cells (Ia+)[5,13] and helper/inducer T cells (CD4+, 4B4+),[5,49,69] and decreased numbers of suppressor T cells (CD8+, Leu 15+) and suppressor inducer cells (CD8+, 2H4+)[35] have been described in the peripheral blood or synovial fluid of RA patients by some investigators. However, percentages and ratios of CD4+ and CD8+ T cells have been reported as normal, increased, or decreased by different investigators (reviewed in reference 5) and may vary with the disease activity of the patients studied.

Reported abnormalities in T cell function include increased in vitro helper activity,[47] decreased helper activity,[27] decreased interleukin-2 production,[3,19,46] and impaired Con A induced suppression.[16,83]

Of particular interest is the impaired ability of T lymphocytes from RA patients to inhibit the proliferation of Epstein Barr virus (EBV) infected B cells in vitro.[23,95] This observation coupled with the occurrence of increased antibody levels to EBV-induced antigens,[6,15,73] and the higher prevalence of EBV-transformed B cells in the peripheral blood of RA patients[96] suggests a possible role for EBV in the pathogenesis of RA. Some patients, however, have been described who lack antibodies to EBV,[24,28] and it remains to be determined whether this virus is a causative agent of disease or simply represents reactivation of a latent infection.[64] In those patients infected with the virus, EBV may act as a perpetuator of the disease by serving as a polyclonal stimulator of B cell activation.[64,99]

Two parvoviruses are also being considered as etiologic agents of RA:[18,88] B19, a virus identified as a cause of acute, and occasionally persistent arthropathy[71,104] and RA-1, which has been isolated from the synovial tissue of a patient with rheumatoid arthritis.[84] Other viruses under consideration include the rubella virus and hepatitis B virus.[97]

The diagnosis of RA is based on clinical manifestations, laboratory results, and radiographic findings.[7] One of the most useful laboratory assessments involves the measurement of rheumatoid factor, classically detected by agglutination methods. The Rose-Waaler test[80,100] was the first of these methods developed and involves agglutination of sheep red blood cells sensitized with rabbit IgG. Latex agglutination tests, first devised by Singer and Plotz,[86] and later modified,[72,85,87] are used most widely. Comparisons of the Rose-Waaler test and latex agglutination have generally found the former to be more specific, but the latter, more sensitive.[37,40,45,51,89,102] Agglutination tests us-

ing bentonite[12] or charcoal[36] have also been developed.

Despite their widespread routine use, agglutination tests have lacked standardization, and display considerable interlaboratory variation.[34,74,76] It must also be noted that all of the above tests, because they involve agglutination reactions, primarily detect IgM rheumatoid factors. Approximately 60 to 90% of all diagnosed RA cases are "seropositive," i.e. they exhibit positive RF agglutination tests.[17,26,43,44] The remaining patients may contain RF at a level lower than the sensitivity limit of the test used, RF of an immunoglobulin class other than IgM, or "hidden" RF (see below), or may truly be negative for RF.[26] Newer methods have been developed to detect RF[26] including nephelometry,[75] radioimmunoassay,[48] and enzyme linked immunosorbent assay;[94] these methods have improved sensitivity over the agglutination tests and the capability of determining immunoglobulin class-specific RF,[26] but their clinical value remains to be determined.[26,92]

"Hidden" IgM rheumatoid factors, undetectable by traditional methods because of strong complexing to patient IgG, can be detected in some cases of seronegative RA following gel filtration in an acid medium.[4,44] Hidden RF are especially common in patients with juvenile rheumatoid arthritis,[61] in whom they appear to correlate with disease activity.[62]

Other laboratory tests commonly performed in the assessment of RA include assays for markers of the acute phase response, e.g. erythrocyte sedimentation rate (ESR), C-reactive protein (CRP)), complement (C3, C4), and autoantibodies (antinuclear antibodies, cryoglobulins). CRP and the ESR are commonly elevated in RA, and levels of these parameters appear to correlate with disease activity.[21,25,54,55] Complement levels in the sera of RA patients are usually normal or elevated, indicating acute phase reactivity and probably a lack of catabolism.[55,63] Complement components are synthesized in increased quantities in the synovial membranes of RA as compared with degenerative or trauma-related arthritis.[82] However, synovial fluid from RA patients demonstrates decreases in classical pathway components of complement and in CH_{50},[50,81] indicative of complement activation and consumption, and more pronounced depressions are associated with more severe disease.[101] A number of autoantibodies can also be detected in the sera of RA patients (see above), including antinuclear antibodies (in approximately 25 to 60% of patients)[60] and mixed cryoglobulins (approximately 20% of patients).[101] Hematologic changes, such as a normochromic, normocytic anemia and thrombocytosis, are often present in active disease.[50]

Studies designed to investigate the association of clinical and laboratory parameters with prognosis of RA (reviewed in reference 98) have found the following to be indicators of a less favorable clinical outcome: presence of RF, especially of the IgA class, persistently increased CRP or ESR values, decreased hemoglobin, and the appearance of subcutaneous nodules. See also *Antinuclear Antibodies; Complement; C Reactive Protein; Cryoglobulins*.

REFERENCES

1. Al-Balaghi, S., Strom, H., and Moller, E.: Scand. J. Immunol., 16:69, 1982.
2. Al-Balaghi, S., Strom, H., and Moller, E.: Immunol. Rev., 78:7, 1984.
3. Alcocer-Varela, J., Laffon, A., and Alarcon-Segovia, D.: Rheumatol. Int., 4:39, 1984.
4. Allen, J.C., and Kunkel, H.G.: Arthritis Rheum., 9:758, 1966.
5. Alpert, S.D. et al.: Rheum. Dis. Clin. North Am., 13:431, 1987.
6. Alspaugh, M.A. et al.: J. Clin. Invest., 67:1134, 1981.
7. Arnett, F.C. et al.: Arthritis Rheum., 31:315, 1988.
8. Bell, D.A., and Pinto, J.: Clin. Immunol. Immunopathol., 31:272, 1984.
9. Bennett, P.H., and Burch, T.A.: Bull. Rheum. Dis., 17:453, 1967.
10. Bernhard, G.: In *Rheumatoid Arthritis*. Edited by P.D. Utsinger, N.J. Zvaifler, and G.E. Ehrlich. Philadelphia, J.B. Lippincott Co., 1985.
11. Bienenstock. J., and Bloch, K.J.: Arthritis Rheum., 10:187, 1967.
12. Bozecevich, J. et al.: Proc. Soc. Exp. Biol. Med., 97:180, 1958.
13. Burmester, G.R. et al.: Arthritis Rheum., 24:1370. 1981.
14. Butler, J.L.: In *Clinical Rheumatology*. Edited by G.V. Ball and W.J. Koopman. Philadelphia, W.B. Saunders Co., 1986.
15. Catalano. M.A. et al.: J. Clin. Invest., 65:1238, 1980.
16. Chattopadhyay. C. et al.: Scand. J. Immunol., 10:479, 1979.
17. Chen, P.P., Fong, S., and Carson, D.A.: Rheum. Dis. Clin. North Am., 13:545, 1987.
18. Cohen, B.J. et al.: Ann. Rheum. Dis., 45:832,1986.
19. Coombe, B. et al.: Clin. Exp. Immunol., 59:520, 1985.
20. Coombs, R.R.A., and Gell, P.G.H.: In *Clinical Aspects of Immunology*. Edited by P.G.H. Gell, R.R.A. Coombs, and P.J. Lachmann. Oxford, Blackwell Scientific Pub., 1975.
21. Dawes, P.T. et al.: Br. J. Rheumatol. 25:44, 1986.
22. deDuve, C.: Scand. J. Rheumatol., 5 (Suppl. 12):63, 1975.
23. Depper, J.M., Bluestein, H.G., and Zvaifler, N.J.: J. Immunol., 127:1899, 1981.
24. Depper, J.M., and Zvaifler, N.J.: Arthritis Rheum., 24:755, 1981.
25. Dixon, J.S. et al.: Scand. J. Rheumatol., 13:39, 1984.
*26. Dorner, R.W., Alexander, R.L., and Moore, T.L.: Clin. Chim. Acta, 167:1, 1987.
27. Egeland, T., Lea, T., and Mellbye, O.J.: Scand. J. Immunol., 18:355, 1983.
28. Ferrell, P.B., et al.: J. Clin. Invest., 67:681,1981.
29. Firestein, G.S., and Zvaifler, N.J.: Rheum. Dis. Clin. North Am., 13:447, 1987.
30. Fong, S. et al.: Pathol. Immunopathol. Res., 5:305, 1986.
31. Fong, S. et al.: Concepts Immunopathol., 5:168, 1988.
32. Fye, K.H., and Sack, K.E.: In *Basic and Clinical Immunology*. 6th ed. Edited by D.P. Stites, J.D. Stobo, and J.V. Wells. Norwalk, Appleton and Lange, 1987.
33. Gabriel, S.E., and Luthra, H.S.: Mayo Clin. Proc., 63:58, 1988.
34. Goddard, D.H., and Moore, M.E.: Arthritis Rheum., 31:432, 1988.
35. Goto, M. et al.: J. Rheumatol., 13:853, 1986.
36. Gottlieb, C.W., Lan, K.S., and Herbert, V.: Arthritis Rheum., 10:199, 1967.
37. Greenburg, C.L.: J. Clin. Pathol., 13:325, 1960.
38. Haraoui, B. et al.: J. Immunol., 133:697, 1984.
*39. Hardin, J.G.: In *Clinical Rheumatology*. Edited by G.V. Ball and W.J. Koopman. Philadelphia, W.B. Saunders Co., 1986.
40. Hedberg, H.: Acta Rheum. Scand., 7:43, 1961.
41. Hough, A.J., and Sokoloff, L.: In *Rheumatoid Arthritis*. Edited by P.D. Utsinger, N.J. Zvaifler, and G.E. Ehrlich. Philadelphia, J.B. Lippincott Co., 1985.
42. Husby, G., et al.: Lancet, 1:549, 1979.
43. Jacoby, R.K., Jayson, M.I.V., and Cash, J.A.: Br. Med. J., 2:96, 1973.
44. Johnson, P.M., and Faulk, W.P.: Clin. Immunol. Immunopathol., 6:414, 1976.

45. Julkunen, H. et al.: Acta Rheum. Scand., 7:48, 1961.

46. Kitas, G.D. et al.: Clin. Exp. Immunol., 73:242, 1988.

47. Kluin-Nelemans. et al.: J. Rheumatol., 11:272, 1984.

48. Koopman, W.J., Schrohenloher, R.E., and Solomon, A.: J. Immunol. Methods, 50:89, 1982.

49. Lasky, H.P., Bauer, K., and Pope, R.M.: Arthritis Rheum., 31:52, 1988.

50. Lipsky, P.E.: In Harrison's Principles of Internal Medicine. 11th ed. Edited by E. Braunwald et al. New York, McGraw-Hill Book Co., 1987.

51. MacSween, R.N.M. et al.: Scand. J. Rheumatol., 1:177, 1972.

52. Mainardi, C.L.: Rheum. Dis. Clin. North Am., 13:215, 1987.

53. Maini, R.N., Plater-Zyberk, C., and Andrew, E.: Rheum. Dis. Clin. North Am., 13:319, 1987.

54. Mallya, R.K. et al.: Clin. Exp. Immunol., 48:747, 1982.

55. Mallya, R.K. et al.: J. Rheumatol., 9:224, 1982.

56. Marcus, R.L., and Townes, A.S.: J. Clin. Invest., 50:282, 1971.

57. McCuster, C.T., and Singal, D.P.: J. Rheumatol., 15:1050, 1988.

58. McKenna, F., and Wright, V.: In Rheumatoid Arthritis. Edited by P.D. Utsinger, N.J. Zvaifler, and G.E. Ehrlich. Philadelphia, J.B. Lippincott Co., 1985.

59. Michaeli, D., and Fudenberg, H.H.: Clin. Immunol. Immunopathol., 2:153, 1974.

60. Molden, D.P.: Diagn. Med., June, 1985, p. 12.

61. Moore, T.L. et al.: Arthritis Rheum., 21:935, 1978.

62. Moore, T.L. et al.: J. Rheumatol., 9:599, 1982.

63. Moxley, G., and Ruddy, S.: Arthritis Rheum., 30:1097, 1987.

64. Musiani, M. et al.: Ann. Rheum. Dis., 46:837, 1987.

65. Nakamura, R.M., and Tan, E.M.: Clin. Lab. Med., 6:41, 1986.

66. Olsen, N.J., Stastny, P., and Jasin, H.E.: Arthritis Rheum., 30:841, 1987.

67. Osung, O.A., Chandra, M., and Holborow, E.J.: Ann. Rheum. Dis., 39:599, 1980.

68. Pinals, R.S.: Am. Fam. Physician, 37:145, 1988.

69. Pitzalis, C. et al.: Clin. Immunol. Immunopathol., 45:252, 1987.

70. Plater-Zyberk, C. et al.: Arthritis Rheum., 28:971, 1985.

71. Reid, D.M. et al.: Lancet, 1:422, 1985.

72. Rheins, M.S. et al.: J. Clin. Lab Med., 50:113, 1957.

73. Rhodes, G., et al.: J. Immunol., 134:211, 1985.

74. Rippey, J.H., and Biesecher, J.L.: Am. J. Clin. Pathol. (Suppl.), 80:599, 1983.

75. Roberts-Thomson, P.J. et al.: Ann. Rheum. Dis., 44:379, 1985.

76. Roberts-Thomson, P.J. et al.: Ann. Rheum. Dis., 46:417, 1987.

77. Room, G.R.W. et al.: Rheumatol. Int., 2:175, 1982.

78. Ropes, M.W. et al.: Bull. Rheum. Dis., 7:121, 1956.

79. Ropes, M.W. et al.: Bull. Rheum. Dis., 9:175, 1958.

80. Rose, H.M. et al.: Proc. Soc. Exp. Biol. Med., 68:1, 1948.

81. Ruddy, S., and Austen, K.F.: Arthritis Rheum., 13:713, 1970.

82. Ruddy, S., and Colton, H.R.: N. Engl. J. Med., 290:1284, 1974.

83. Sakane, T. et al.: J. Immunol., 129:1972, 1982.

84. Simpson, R.W. et al.: Science, 224:1425, 1984.

85. Singer, J.M.: Bull. Rheum. Dis., 26:868, 1975–76.

86. Singer, J.M., and Plotz, C.M.: Am. J. Med., 21:888, 1956.

87. Singer, J.M., and Plotz, C.M.: Arthritis Rheum., 1:142, 1958.

88. Smith, C.A., Woolf, A.D., and Lenci, M.: Rheum. Dis. Clin. North Am., 13:249, 1987.

89. Stage, D.E., and Mannik, M.: Bull. Rheum. Dis., 23:720, 1973.

90. Stastny, P.: N. Engl. J. Med., 298:869, 1978.

91. Stastny, P. et al.: Arthritis Rheum., 18:237, 1975.

92. Stone, R. et al.: J. Clin. Pathol., 40:107, 1987.

93. Synderman, R.: In Rheumatoid Arthritis. Edited by P.D. Utsinger, N.J. Zvaifler, and G.E. Ehrlich. Philadelphia, J.B. Lippincott Co., 1985.

94. Teitsson, I., and Valdimarsson, H.: J. Immunol. Methods, 71:149, 1984.

95. Tosato, G., Magrath, I.T., and Blaese, R.M.: J. Immunol., 128:575, 1982.

96. Tosato, G. et al.: J. Clin. Invest., 73:1789, 1984.

97. Utsinger, P.D., Zvaifler, N.J., and Weiner, S.B.: In Rheumatoid Arthritis. Edited by P.D. Utsinger, N.J. Zvaifler, and G.E. Ehrlich. Philadelphia, J.B. Lippincott Co., 1985.

98. van der Heijde, D.M.F.M., et al.: Semin. Arthritis Rheum., 17:284, 1988.

99. Vaughan, J.H.: Hosp. Pract., 19:101, 1984.

100. Waaler, E.: Acta Pathol. Microbiol. Scand., 17:172, 1940.

101. Wager, O.: Ann. Clin. Res., 7:168, 1975.

102. Waller, M.: Ann. N.Y. Acad. Sci., 168:5, 1969.

103. Wiesman, G.: N. Engl. J. Med., 286:141, 1972.

104. White, D.G. et al.: Lancet, 1:419, 1985.

105. Winchester, R.J. et al.: J. Clin. Invest., 541:1082, 1974.

106. Wooley, P.H., Panayi, G.S., and Batchelor, R.J.: Ann. Rheum. Dis., 38:188, 1979.

107. Zvaifler, N.J.: Adv. Immunol., 16:265, 1973.

108. Zvaifler, N.J.: Arthritis Rheum., 17:297, 1974.

Rheumatoid Factor Screening by Liposome Enhanced Latex Agglutination[1]

PRINCIPLE. RF Rheumatoid Factor Test Kits contain a suspension including both latex particles that have been coated with IgG, as well as liposomes coated with antiglobulin that act as enhancers. When serum containing rheumatoid factor is mixed with the Liposome-Latex Reagent, macroscopic agglutination of the latex particles will occur.

EQUIPMENT AND MATERIALS. The Leap RF Rheumatoid Factor Test Kit—Cooper Biomedical[1] consisting of:

1. Liposome-latex reagent, 5 ml—polystyrene latex particles coated with heat-aggregated human IgG and liposomes coated with antiglobulin prepared as a suspension in glycine saline buffer

2. Positive control, 2 ml—human serum containing a high titer of rheumatoid factor, prediluted in glycine saline buffer solution. This control can be utilized as supplied. The approximate RF value in international units (IU/ml) for each lot of this reagent appears on the vial label. This value has been established using a comparison of titers obtained with a standard that has been assayed against the National Reference Preparation obtained from the CDC. (The CDC preparation is comparable to the WHO International Reference Standard.)

3. Negative control, 2 ml—normal human serum, prediluted in glycine saline buffer

4. Low-level positive control, 2 ml—human serum containing a low titer of rheumatoid factor, prediluted in glycine saline buffer

5. Glycine saline buffer diluent, 100 ml, pH 8.1 ± 0.2.

Controls and glycine saline buffer diluent are ready to use as supplied. The liposome-latex reagent is a turbid reagent that should be mixed well prior to use. The positive, negative, and low-level positive controls, and glycine saline buffer diluent should not be used if turbid. All reagents should be handled carefully to avoid contamination by human serum, chemicals, or microorganisms. This product should not be used if the LEAP RF positive and negative controls do not react properly with the liposome-latex reagent. Leaking vials should not be used. Do not use beyond expiration date. Store at 2 to 8° C. *DO NOT FREEZE.* For in vitro diagnostic use only.

6. Nine-well glass slide with black background.

Materials not included in kit:

7. Serologic pipets

8. Test tubes and test tube rack

9. Transfer pipets

10. Wooden applicator sticks

11. Mechanical rotator (optional)

12. Stopwatch or timer

SPECIMEN COLLECTION AND PREPARATION. Collect the specimen into a tube without anticoagulant using an acceptable phlebotomy technique. Serum specimens may be tested immediately or held at 2 to 8° C for 24 hours. If a delay in testing is unavoidable, the serum should be frozen. Serum specimens to be shipped should be maintained continuously at 2 to 8° C.

PRECAUTION. Reagents contain sodium azide, which may react with lead or copper plumbing to form highly explosive azides. When disposing of reagents, flush with large volumes of water.

PROCEDURE
Rapid Slide Test Method:

1. Bring all reagents to room temperature prior to use.

2. Prepare a 1:20 dilution of the serum to be tested by pipeting 0.95 ml of the glycine saline buffer diluent and 0.05 ml of serum into a 12 × 75 mm test tube. Mix before using. Alternatively, approximate 1:20 dilution can be made by adding one drop ($\simeq 0.05$ ml) of serum to 1 ml of diluent.

3. Place one drop of diluted serum on one of the numbered sections of the clean glass slide.

4. Place one drop of the LEAP RF positive control serum on the appropriate section of the slide.

5. Place one drop of the LEAP RF negative control serum on the appropriate section of the slide.

6. Place one drop of the LEAP RF low-level positive control serum on the appropriate section of the slide.

7. Mix the LEAP RF liposome-latex reagent thoroughly. Add one drop of the reagent to each serum on the slide.

8. Mix the contents of each section with a separate wooden applicator stick or toothpick, and spread within the area of the oval.

9. Tilt the slide back and forth slowly or place on a mechanical rotator. Observe for agglutination for 2 minutes. Microscopic examination is not required.

NOTE: If a mechanical rotator is used, the rotation speed should not exceed 180 rpm.

10. It is recommended that the LEAP RF positive, negative and low-level positive control sera supplied be tested each time a test is performed. Satisfactory performance of the reagents is indicated by the following reactions:

Liposome-latex reagent + positive control serum: Strong agglutination of the latex suspension.

Liposome-latex reagent + low-level positive control serum: Weak agglutination of the latex suspension.

Liposome-latex reagent + negative control serum: No agglutination of the latex suspension.

If at any time throughout the shelf life of the product the controls do not perform as expected, the kit should not be used.

REPORTING. Results are reported as positive or negative for rheumatoid factor.

INTERPRETATION OF RESULTS. All results should be interpreted upon test completion as positive agglutination (visible clumping) of the latex particles by the serum under test, or negative, i.e., no agglutination of the latex particles by the serum under test. Approximately 80% of patients with a clinical diagnosis of rheumatoid arthritis produce positive tests.[2,3] Sera from 5% or less of the normal population produce a positive test. Titers below 20 are considered negative for rheumatoid factor. A titer value of 20 or above indicates the presence of rheumatoid factor.[2,3]

LIMITATIONS OF THE PROCEDURE

1. Falsely positive reactions may result because of drying if slide tests are observed for periods longer than 2 minutes.

2. Falsely positive results may occur in tests employing lipemic or contaminated serum or serum not diluted 1:20 prior to testing.

3. The liposome-latex reagent should be kept tightly capped when not in use to prevent evaporation, which may result in clumping of the latex particles.

REFERENCES

1. Leap, R.F.: Cooper Biomedical, Malvern, PA, 1985.

2. Singer, J.M.: Am. J. Med., *31*:766, 1961.

3. Waller, M., Toone, E.C., and Vaughan, E.: Arthritis Rheum., *7*:513, 1964.

Rheumatoid Factor Latex Tube Test

PRINCIPLE. Latex particles with adsorbed gamma globulin are reacted with serial dilutions of patient serum. The presence of IgM rheumatoid factor in the dilutions is indicated by latex agglutination.[1]

EQUIPMENT AND MATERIALS

1. 0.81 Latex Suspension (Difco): Store at 2 to 8° C. Do not freeze

2. RA Buffer (Difco): pH 8.2. Store at 15 to 30° C. Dissolve 17.5 g in 1 l of distilled water. Store reconstituted solution at 4° C. May be used indefinitely if solution remains clear

3. Gamma Globulin—Cohn Fraction II (Sigma): Store desiccated at 0 to 5° C. Add 200 mg to 20 ml of RA buffer. Mix well and allow to stand overnight in the refrigerator. Centrifuge and use supernate for testing. Store reconstituted at 2 to 8° C. Can be used up to 3 weeks after reconstitution. Each new lot must be tested with positive control serum and proper reactivity confirmed before use

4. Rheumatoid Factor Positive Control Serum (Difco): Rehydrate with 3 ml distilled water. Shake gently. Store at 2 to 8° C. Positive control serum should demonstrate the designated reactivity, and be discarded if greater than a twofold deviation is observed. Run a new control vial in parallel with the existing control before routine use. Discard any control not demonstrating proper reactivity

5. Patient Sample: Serum samples should be used fresh or may be frozen at −20° C prior to testing

6. 13 × 100 mm test tubes: 20 per patient and 10 per control

7. 0.1, 0.5, 1.0, and 5.0 ml pipets

8. Erlenmeyer flask

9. 56° C water bath

PROCEDURE

1. Prepare Cohn fraction II—latex suspension: For every 10 tubes (include positive control) to be tested, pipet 10 ml of RA buffer into an Erlenmeyer flask. Add 0.5 ml Cohn fraction

II and then 0.1 ml of latex. This suspension can be used only at the time prepared.

2. Place 20 test tubes in a rack for each specimen and 10 for the positive control.

3. Reconstitute the positive control if necessary (*Equipment and Materials #4*).

4. Add 1.9 ml RA buffer to the first tube and 1.0 ml to remainder of tubes for each specimen.

5. Add 0.1 ml of positive control serum to the first tube of an appropriately labeled row.

6. With a 1.0 ml pipet, mix and serially transfer 1.0 ml from tube 1 through tube 9 of the positive control row, discarding 1.0 ml from tube 9. Tube 10, which contains no serum, will be used as a negative control. The dilutions are 1:20, 1:40, 1:80, etc.

7. Pipet 0.1 ml of each patient specimen into the first tube of an appropriately labeled row. Mix and transfer 1.0 ml from tube 1 through tube 20, discarding 1.0 ml from tube 20.

8. Add 1.0 ml of the Cohn fraction II—latex suspension (from Procedure: Step 1) to each tube.

9. Shake to obtain a uniform suspension.

10. Incubate in a 56° C water bath for $1\frac{1}{2}$ hours.

11. Centrifuge at 2300 rpm for 3 minutes.

12. Agitate tubes and read for agglutination using transmitted light. The titer is recorded as the reciprocal of the last tube showing definite agglutination, as compared to the negative control (tube 10 of the positive control row).

13. The positive control must read ± one doubling dilution from the titer designated for that control.

REPORTING. Titers are reported as the reciprocal of the last serum dilution with definite agglutination, where "serum dilution" refers to the dilution prior to the addition of antigen.

LIMITATIONS OF THE PROCEDURE. A positive rheumatoid factor test cannot be considered diagnostic of rheumatoid arthritis, as it is commonly found in normals and in a variety of disease states.

A negative rheumatoid factor assay does not rule out the possibility of rheumatoid arthritis.

REFERENCE

1. Singer, J.M., and Plotz, C.M.: Am. J. Med., *21*:888, 1956.

SYSTEMIC LUPUS ERYTHEMATOSUS

Systemic lupus erythematosus (SLE) is a chronic inflammatory disease affecting multiple organs of the body. Although the disease may occur in either males or females and may develop at any age, 90% of cases occur in women, primarily those between 20 and 40 years of age.[38,47,118] In the United States, the prevalence of SLE has been estimated at 15 to 50 per 100,000,[47] with the disease affecting blacks more commonly than whites;[47,100] racial predilection, however, is questionable, as the incidence of SLE is apparently low in blacks residing in Africa.[118]

The clinical manifestations of SLE are diverse and virtually any organ system may be involved. Symptoms frequently overlap with a number of other disorders, and it is not unusual for establishment of a diagnosis to take 3 to 4 years.[33] In order to facilitate more accurate classification of the disease, preliminary criteria for SLE were published by the American Rheumatism Association in 1971[26] and revised in 1982.[114] In the revised classification system, an individual is diagnosed as having SLE if at least 4 of 11 criteria, consisting of common clinical manifestations and laboratory findings, are present simultaneously or serially.[114]

Vague, nonspecific symptoms, including fever, malaise, fatigue, and weight loss, are often present initially and may also occur at any time during the course of disease.[33] Involvement of one or more organ systems may be evident at initial presentation of the SLE patient. The most common clinical manifestation of SLE involves the musculoskeletal system, with polyarthralgias or arthritis occurring in approximately 95% of cases.[21,38,47] Mild symptoms are frequently evident at the onset of disease. Many patients develop frank arthritis, which is usually symmetric and involves the small joints of the hands, wrists, and knees, although any joint may be affected.[21,29,47] The arthritis is typically migratory and transient in nature, resolving within 1 to 2 days; severe joint deformities and bony erosions are uncommon.

Mucocutaneous involvement is also common in SLE, presenting in approximately 80% of cases.[21,47] Skin lesions are varied, and may be classified into acute, subacute, and chronic forms.[18,87] Acute cutaneous lupus is most commonly manifested as the classic malar ("butterfly") rash, appearing as an erythematous rash covering the cheeks and nose and occurring in approximately one-third of patients. The rash is acute in onset, exacerbated by exposure to sunlight, and heals without scarring. Acute lesions may also occur as photosensitivity dermatitis involving other areas of the body, generalized erythema, or bullous eruptions. Subacute cutaneous lupus is a widespread rash, consisting of annular or papulosquamous eruptions that are nonscarring and predominant in sun-exposed areas of the body. Chronic cutaneous lupus presents primarily as discoid lesions, appearing as erythematous raised patches with changes in pigmentation, scaling, and production of scars and telangiectasias. Other cutaneous manifestations of lupus include vasculitic lesions, mucosal ulcerations, and alopecia (loss of scalp hair).

Central nervous system involvement has been observed in 35 to 75% of cases[87] and is most commonly manifested as organic brain syndrome with or without psychosis, generalized seizures, cranial or peripheral neuropathies, cerebrovascular accidents, chorea, and/or transverse myelitis.[14]

Renal involvement occurs in nearly all SLE patients, as evidenced by renal biopsy, but produces clinical symptoms, or lupus nephritis, in only about one-half of patients.[47,87] Renal lesions vary in histologic morphology and clinical severity, and may be classified as (1) mesangial glomerulonephritis, (2) focal glomerulonephritis, (3) diffuse proliferative glomerulonephritis, or (4) membranous glomerulonephritis.[38,84] Prognosis of patients with the mesangial or membranous forms of glomerulonephritis is generally thought to be better than that of

patients with proliferative forms.[84,87] Lupus nephritis is commonly associated with proteinuria, hematuria, white blood cells in the urine, urinary casts, and elevated serum creatinine.[47,87]

Cardiopulmonary manifestations occur in approximately half of the patients with SLE and include pericarditis, myocarditis, endocarditis, pleurisy, and pneumonitis.[21,47,87] Gastrointestinal and liver involvement are seen in 30 to 40% of cases and most frequently produce nonspecific symptoms such as nausea and mild abdominal pain;[47,87] more serious consequences, including vasculitis of the intestine, acute pancreatitis, and chronic active hepatitis with elevated liver enzymes are less frequent. Ocular involvement occurs in about 20% of patients with SLE and most commonly includes conjunctivitis and episcleritis.[38,47,87] Less frequently, retinal vasculitis may occur, resulting in the degeneration of retinal nerve fibers and the formation of characteristic white fluffy exudates called cytoid bodies, with the potential of producing blindness. Vasculitis is common in SLE and affects primarily small to medium-sized arteries and veins.[21,38,47] Resulting symptoms include Raynaud's phenomenon, thrombosis, cutaneous ulceration, bowel infarction, and cerebrovascular accidents.

Hematologic abnormalities are frequent, occurring in approximately 80% of cases and including anemia, leukopenia, and thrombocytopenia.[21,47,87]

There is a great degree of variation in the pattern and prognosis of SLE: it may follow a relatively benign course or pursue a fulminant path leading to death in a few weeks or months. Treatment varies according to disease severity; those with mild symptoms may be managed successfully with nonsteroidal anti-inflammatory drugs (e.g. salicylates), antimalarial drugs, and local corticosteroid treatment, while those with more severe symptoms often require more intensive treatment involving systemic corticosteroids and/or cytotoxic drugs.[11,38,47,62,73] Prognosis has improved throughout the twentieth century, with the advent of mechanisms for earlier diagnosis, effective therapeutic agents (e.g. immunosuppressive drugs and antibiotics), and treatment modalities (e.g. hemodialysis and renal transplantation).[41,42] Most patients experience flare-ups of disease activity interspersed with long periods of remissions with relatively few symptoms. Death in SLE occurs most commonly from infection (as a result of aggressive immunosuppressive therapy or hemodialysis) or active organ disease, with active lupus nephritis most frequently responsible, followed by active central nervous system involvement.[41] The overall survival rate of SLE patients approaches 80% 10 years after the onset of multisystem disease.[41,48]

The etiology of SLE is unknown. The variable presentation of the disease suggests the involvement of multiple factors. Much evidence favors a role for genetic factors in predisposition to SLE. The incidence of SLE is greater in individuals who have a monozygotic twin affected with SLE than those with an affected dizygotic twin, and in persons who have a first degree relative affected with the disease than in those who do not.[5,13,73,108] An increased risk of developing SLE has been associated with the presence of HLA types DR2 or DR3 in Caucasian populations[43,73,108,125] (see also *HLA Antigens*), and the inbred strains of mice, New Zealand Black (NZB), NZB × NZW F1 hybrids, MRL-1pr/1pr, and BXSB exhibit a markedly high risk for developing murine lupus.[73,108,109,117]

Female sex hormones and environmental factors such as viral or bacterial infections have also been implicated in playing a role in the development of SLE.[24,73,111] Several drugs, most notably procainamide and hydralazine, are known to induce a lupus-like syndrome.[52,103] Fortunately, renal and central nervous system manifestations are rare in these instances and symptoms usually subside once the drug is withdrawn.

Abnormalities in regulation of the immune system are thought to be central to the pathophysiologic mechanisms of SLE. A markedly heterogeneous population of autoantibodies has been described in SLE,[38,47,51,85] including various antinuclear antibodies,[51,76,124] mixed cryoglobulins,[49,85,104] immunoconglutinins,[12] rheumatoid factors,[85] antilymphocyte antibodies,[77] anticardiolipin antibodies,[6] antierythrocyte antibodies,[38,47,85] antiplatelet antibodies,[38,47,85] and antineuronal antibodies[14,47,85] (See also *Anti-cardiolipin Antibodies; Anti-Nuclear Antibodies; Cryoglobulins; Rheumatoid Arthritis.*)

The plethora of autoantibodies produced is thought to result from polyclonal B cell hyperactivity,[73,93] which has been demonstrated by the increased number of immunoglobulin-secreting cells,[93,107] increased spontaneous immunoglobulin production in vitro,[17,61,93] increased in vitro proliferative capacity of peripheral blood B cells,[68,93] and hypergammaglobulinemia[73] seen in SLE patients, as compared to healthy individuals. Despite the spontaneous B cell hyperactivity observed, SLE patients have demonstrated decreased in vitro proliferative responses to lipopolysaccharide[1] and pokeweed mitogen[81] (suggesting prior stimulation of B cells), decreased antigen-specific in vitro antibody production,[81,83] and decreased in vivo antibody response to vaccination.[44,81] The B cell abnormalities in SLE may be due to a primary defect in the B lymphocytes and/or to defects in T lymphocytes and cytokines which exert an immunoregulatory role for B cell activity[56] (see also Chap. 1; Chap 7). Decreased numbers of CD8+ cells (T suppressor cells)[31,78] and decreased ability to generate T suppressor cell signals in vitro[15,66,92] have been described in SLE patients, and may contribute to the hyperproduction of autoantibodies associated with SLE. These defects, however, are variable, being seen primarily in periods of disease activity and becoming normal during remission.[15,23,92]

Data regarding T helper cells and lymphokine production in SLE are also conflicting.[23] Some patients exhibit a reduction in the absolute number of CD4+ T cells[10] and

CD4/CD8 subset ratio,[22,102] while others have reported normal or increased CD4/CD8 ratios.[78,102] Likewise, deficiencies in T helper cell function have been reported by some investigators for in vivo[1,44] and in vitro systems,[7,32] while normal T helper cell function has been demonstrated by others.[75,80,81] Anergy, as detected by skin testing, is common with SLE and fluctuates with disease activity.[89] Studies on production of lymphokines such as interleukin-2[4,70,99,120] and gamma interferon[55,99] have also produced variable results. The marked variation in research findings with regard to immune function in SLE may be due to heterogeneity of the SLE syndrome, status of disease activity at the time of testing, and differences in the experimental systems used.[23] Furthermore, some of the immune abnormalities reported may indeed contribute to the pathogenesis of SLE, while others are probably secondary manifestations occurring as a result of disease activity. Antilymphocyte antibodies are found in the vast majority of SLE sera,[69,74,106,116] and bind to both T and B cells, but are more often T cell specific.[69] These antibodies become lymphocytotoxic when complement is bound.[105] High titers of antilymphocyte antibodies have been found to correlate strongly with disease activity, lymphopenia, and reduction of specific lymphocyte subsets.[56,77] Further studies will be necessary to clarify the significance of the immunologic abnormalities in SLE.

Although cell-specific antibodies in lupus are thought to induce symptoms involving the appropriate cell type (e.g. antiplatelet antibodies are associated with thrombocytopenia, antineuronal antibodies with diffuse central nervous system symptoms),[47] the pathogenesis of SLE appears to be largely the result of deleterious effects caused by formation of soluble immune complexes, resulting in a chronic immune complex syndrome.[25] Normally, most immune complexes are cleared by the reticuloendothelial system. In immune-complex syndromes, however, the system may be overwhelmed by the chronic load of antigens and anti-

bodies,[95] or the ability to clear complexes may be rendered less efficient by other means. For example, the complement receptor type I (CR1), which is found on erythrocytes, monocytes, polymorphonuclear leukocytes, B lymphocytes, glomerular epithelial cells, and follicular dendritic cells, is capable of binding to the complement components C3b, iC3b, C3i, and C4b, and is thus thought to play a role in mediating the elimination of immune complexes through immune adherence and opsonization[119] (see also Chap. 6). Erythrocytes are thought to bind immune complexes via CR1 and transport them to the more fixed cells of the reticuloendothelial system. Decreased levels of CR1 have been observed on erythrocytes of SLE patients;[53,58,59] this in turn is thought to result in less binding of immune complexes and to reduce the efficiency of their clearance.[119] Decreases in the level of CR1 have also been found to correlate with disease activity.[58]

Immune complex syndromes involve the type III hypersensitivity reaction described by Gell and Coombs.[27,122] (See also Chap. 1.) This reaction is initiated and perpetuated by the formation of antigen- antibody complexes, either in the circulation, or in situ after binding of antigen to a target organ. Activation of complement, with subsequent accumulation of phagocytic cells, occurs at the sites of immune complex deposition, resulting in the release of lysosomal enzymes from these cells and damage to adjacent tissues.

The class of immunoglobulin, the nature of the antigen, and the physiochemical properties of the resultant immune complexes appear to influence their ability to cause pathogenesis.[16,72] Complement-fixing IgG antibodies with an acidic pH appear to be most pathogenic.[9] Deposition of immune complexes in the vessel walls is favored when complexes are greater than 19S in size, while intermediate sized complexes (9-15S) are preferentially deposited in the glomerular basement membrane.[95] The nature of the antigen and the tissue involved may favor deposition of immune complexes at particular sites in the body; for example, the affinity of the major autoantigen, DNA, for the glomerular basement membrane (GBM)[30] and the presence of C3 receptors on the GBM[35] enhance the likelihood of immune complex formation or deposition at this common site.[9,95] Antibodies to native DNA (nDNA) have been most closely associated with severe pathogenesis in SLE.[19,36,39,50,57,88,96,97,121] However, the role of immune complex hypersensitivity in the pathogenesis of this disease remains hypothetical, as circulating complexes of DNA-anti-DNA have been detected only infrequently in SLE patients.[9,95] On the other hand, this mode of pathogenesis is strongly supported by a multitude of other evidence, including detection of immunoglobulin, complement, and DNA in kidneys of SLE patients,[64,67,82] detection of immunoglobulin and complement in skin and other tissues or body fluids,[8,20,113] elution of antinuclear antibodies from renal lesions in lupus nephritis,[64,67] and elevated levels of uncharacterized immune complexes in the sera of clinically active lupus patients, as detected by numerous assays.[95]

Diagnosis and monitoring of the SLE patient involves a wide spectrum of laboratory assays, several of which are designed to detect autoantibodies or measure complement. One of the most prevalent features of SLE is the presence of antinuclear antibodies (ANA), which are found in 95 to 99% of SLE patients after screening with one of the available fluorescent antinuclear antibody tests.[76,124] Particular ANA's are associated with given fluorescent patterns (see *Antinuclear Antibodies*) and their specificity can be determined with greater certainty with the use of other assays. Antibodies to histones are present in approximately 70% of SLE patients[115] and can be detected by radioimmunoassay (RIA), enzyme-linked immunosorbent assay (ELISA), or Western blot.[37,90] Antibodies to deoxyribonucleoprotein (DNP), which is composed primarily of DNA-histone complexes, are also present

in approximately 70% of SLE patients[124] and are responsible for production of the LE cell phenomenon.[34] Antihistones and anti-DNP, however, are not specific for SLE and may be found in a variety of other diseases.[34,90,124]

On the other hand, antibodies to native DNA (nDNA), although present in fewer cases (approximately 40%),[115] are highly specific for SLE.[115,124] These are most commonly detected by RIA or a special immunofluorescence test using *Crithidia luciliae* as the substrate.[124] These tests are also used to monitor SLE patients, as elevated antibodies to nDNA are often associated with clinical exacerbations, especially involving the kidney.[51,110]

Antibody to the nonhistone nuclear antigen, Sm (Smith antigen), is also highly specific for SLE, but is detected in only about 30% of SLE patients,[115,124] most commonly by double immunodiffusion.[124] The presence of Sm antibody is associated with a higher incidence of renal disease, central nervous system complications, vasculitis, and a poor prognosis,[54,60] and rising titers frequently predict disease relapse.[60] Antibodies to two other nonhistone nuclear antigens, ribonucleoprotein (RNP) and SS-A/Ro are seen in approximately 35% of SLE patients,[115] and are measured most frequently by double immunodiffusion.[51,124] The former, when present in the absence of anti-Sm, is associated with a milder course of disease,[60] while the latter has been associated with heterogeneous clinical manifestations of lupus.[86] Antibodies to other nuclear antigens have a lower prevalence in SLE patients.[115]

Measurement of complement consumption is also performed frequently in the management of lupus patients. Serum levels of complement components are depressed at some time in most patients with SLE.[94,101] Patients with active lupus nephritis tend to have markedly low serum levels of C1q, C4, C2, C3, and Factor B, and decreased total hemolytic complement function (CH_{50}).[95] Indeed, lowered complement levels and demonstration of anti-DNA are the most consistent findings in active lupus nephritis.[46,94,95,96] Levels of C1q, C4, and CH_{50} tend to decline early in disease, whereas levels of C3 decline most notably later in disease, during the peak of illness. Patients with extensive cutaneous involvement, nonrenal exacerbations, or mild kidney disease may have mild to moderate reductions in complement.[65] Many studies have noted a correlation between depression of complement levels and active disease, with decreases often preceding exacerbations.[46,71,94,95,96] Other studies, however, have failed to demonstrate such an association,[3,19] possibly because single laboratory values represent only a static measurement of complement activity. Some investigators have found that complement activity is more accurately assessed through the performance of serial complement measurements, or better yet, through metabolic studies of complement;[71,95] however, tests for the latter measurement are not available for routine use. Examination of tissue biopsies for histologic changes or by immunofluorescence for deposition of immunoglobulins and complement may also be performed on kidney or other tissues. Kidney biopsies may be useful in classification and detection of renal disease.[63] Performance of the immunofluorescent lupus band test (LBT) on biopsies from normal-appearing skin of SLE patients reveals immune complex deposition at the dermal-epidermal junction in 40 to 60% of cases;[28,40,45,112,123] lesional skin usually reveals subepidermal deposits.[63]

VDRL tests frequently give false-positive results in patients with SLE[98] and are useful to include in the battery of tests performed in the diagnosis of SLE. High levels of cardiolipin antibody, as measured by ELISA or RIA, have been correlated with an increased incidence of thrombosis, thrombocytopenia, and fetal distress and loss[6] (see also *Anti-cardiolipin Antibodies*).

Tests for other autoantibodies have also been found to be positive in the following frequencies in SLE patients: anti-erythrocyte antibodies (found in 10 to 50% of cases), antiplatelet antibodies (<10%), antineuronal antibodies (40 to 60%), antilymphocyte antibodies (70%), and rheumatoid factor (30%).[47,51] Serum immunoglobulin levels are frequently elevated due to the spontaneous production of immunoglobulins in SLE patients and the multitude of autoantibodies produced.[73]

In addition to tests for antibodies and complement, a number of other nonspecific, adjunct tests are also useful, including evaluation of acute phase reactants, cryoglobulins, cbc, hematocrit, qualitative urine protein, and serum creatinine. The erythrocyte sedimentation rate (ESR) has been found to be a sensitive indicator of disease activity in SLE, but may also be elevated as a result of infection.[63] C-reactive protein (CRP) is not significantly elevated during SLE flareups, but becomes markedly increased during infections.[63] Proteinuria greater than 2+, severe azotemia (creatinine >3.0), and low hematocrit (<37%) have all been associated with a significant decrease in patient survival time.[41,42] Periodic performance of a variety of laboratory assays is thus necessary for successful diagnosis and evaluation of the heterogeneous disease, SLE. (See also *Anti-Cardiolipin Antibodies; Antinuclear Antibodies; Cryoglobulins; Rheumatoid Arthritis*.)

REFERENCES

1. Abe, T., and Homma, M.: Acta Rheumatol. Scand., 17:35, 1971.
2. Abe, T. et al.: Scand. J. Immunol., 15:475, 1982.
3. Abrass, C.K. et al.: Arthritis Rheum., 23:273, 1980.
4. Alcocer-Varela, J., and Alarcon-Segovia, D.: J. Clin. Invest., 69:1388, 1982.
5. Arnett, F.C., and Shulman, L.E.: Medicine, 55:313, 1976.
6. Asherson, R.A., and Harris, E.N.: Intern. Med., 8:73, 1987.
7. Ashman, R.F. et al.: J. Allergy Clin. Immunol., 70:465, 1982.
8. Atkins, C.J. et al.: Ann. Intern. Med., 76:65, 1972.
9. Bach, J.F. et al.: Ann. N.Y. Acad. Sci., 475:231, 1986.
10. Bakke, A.C. et al.: Arthritis Rheum., 26:745, 1983.
11. Ballou, S.P.: Postgrad. Med., 81:157, 1987.
12. Bienenstock, J., and Bloch, K.J.: Arthritis Rheum., 10:187, 1967.

13. Block, S.R. et al.: Am. J. Med., *59*:533, 1975.

14. Bluestein, H.G.: N. Engl. J. Med., *317*:309, 1987.

15. Bresnihan, B., and Jasin, H.E.: J. Clin. Invest., *59*:106, 1977.

16. Budd, J.J., Moore, T.L., and Osborn, T.G.: J. Rheumatol., *15*:247, 1988.

17. Budman, D.R. et al.: Arthritis Rheum., *20*:829, 1977.

18. Callen, J.P.: Rheum. Dis. Clin. North Am., *14*:79, 1988.

19. Cameron, J.S. et al.: Clin. Exp. Immunol., *25*:418, 1976.

20. Carr, R.I. et al.: J. Rheumatol., *2*:184, 1975.

21. Cassidy, J.T.: In *Clinical Medicine.* Vol. 4. Edited by R.G. Slavin and G.G. Hunder. Philadelphia, Harper and Row Publishers, 1986.

22. Chatenoud, L., and Bach, M.A.: Kidney Int., *20*:267, 1981.

23. Chiorazzi, N.: In *Systemic Lupus Erythematosus.* Edited by R.G. Lahita. New York, John Wiley and Sons, 1987.

24. Christian, C.L.: In *Systemic Lupus Erythematosus.* Edited by R.G. Lahita. New York, John Wiley and Sons, 1987.

25. Cochrane, C.G., and Koffler, D.: Adv. Immunol., *16*:185, 1973.

26. Cohen, A.S. et al.: Bull. Rheum. Dis., *21*:643, 1971.

27. Coombs, R.R.A., and Gell, P.G.H.: In *Clinical Aspects of Immunology.* Edited by P.G.H. Gell, R.R.A. Coombs, and P.J. Lachmann. Oxford, Blackwell Scientific Publications, 1975.

28. Cormane, R.H. et al.: Clin. Exp. Immunol., *1*:207, 1966.

29. Cronin, M.E.: Rheum. Dis. Clin. North Am., *14*:99, 1988.

30. Cukier, R., and Tron, F.: Clin. Exp. Immunol., *62*:143, 1985.

31. DeHoratius, R.: Arthritis Rheum., *25*:828, 1982.

32. Delfraissy, J.F. et al.: J. Clin. Invest., *66*:141, 1980.

33. Dubois, E.L., and Wallace, D.J.: In *Dubois Lupus Erythematosus,* 3rd ed. Edited by D.J. Wallace and E.L. Dubois. Philadelphia, Lea & Febiger, 1987.

34. Dubois, E.L., Strain, L.A., and Wallace, D.J.: In *Dubois Lupus Erythematosus.* 3rd ed. Edited by D.J. Wallace and E.L. Dubois. Philadelphia, Lea & Febiger, 1987.

35. Fearon, D.T., and Wong, W.W.: Ann. Rev. Immunol., *1*:243, 1983.

36. Friend, P.S., Kim, Y., and Michael, A.F.: Br. Med. J., *1*:25, 1977.

37. Fritzler, M.J.: In: *Manual of Clinical Laboratory Immunology.* 3rd. ed. Edited by N.R. Rose, H. Friedman, and J.L. Fahey. Washington, D.C., American Society for Microbiology, 1986.

38. Fye, K.H., and Sack, K.E.: In *Basic and Clinical Immunology.* 6th ed. Edited by D.P. Stites, J.D. Stobo, and J.V. Wells. Norwalk, Appleton and Lange, 1987.

39. Gershwin, M.E., and Steinberg, A.D.: Arthritis Rheum., *17*:947, 1974.

40. Gilliam, J.N. et al.: J. Clin. Invest., *53*:1434, 1974.

41. Ginzler, E., and Berg, A.: J. Rheumatol., *14*(Suppl. 13):218, 1987.

42. Ginzler, E.M., and Schorn, K.: Rheum. Dis. Clin. North Am., *14*:67, 1988.

43. Goldstein, R., and Arnett, F.C.: Rheum. Dis. Clin. North Am., *13*:487, 1987.

44. Gottlieb, A.B. et al.: J. Clin. Invest., *63*:885, 1979.

45. Grossman, J., Callerame, M.L., and Condemi, J.J.: Ann. Intern. Med., *80*:496, 1974.

46. Hadler, N.M. et al.: Arthritis Rheum., *16*:507, 1973.

47. Hahn, B.H.: In *Harrison's Principles of Internal Medicine.* 11th ed. Edited by E. Braunwald et al. New York, McGraw-Hill Book Co., 1987.

48. Halberg, P. et al.: Clin. Rheumatol., *6*:13, 1987.

49. Hanau, L.B., and Christian, C.L.: J. Clin. Invest., *46*:400, 1967.

50. Harbeck, R.J. et al.: J. Clin. Invest., *52*:789, 1973.

51. Harley, J.B., and Gaither, K.K.: Rheum. Dis. Clin. North Am., *14*:43, 1988.

52. Hess, E.: N. Engl. J. Med., *318*:1460, 1988.

53. Holme, E. et al.: Clin. Exp. Immunol., *63*:41, 1986.

54. Homma, M. et al.: J. Rheumatol., *14* (Suppl. 13):188, 1987.

55. Hooks, J.J. et al.: N. Engl. J. Med., *301*:5, 1979.

56. Horwitz, D.A.: In *Dubois Lupus Erythematosus.* 3rd ed. Edited by D.J. Wallace and E.L. Dubois. Philadelphia, Lea & Febiger, 1987.

57. Hughes, G.R.V., Cohen, S.A., and Christian, C.L.: Ann. Rheum. Dis., *30*:259, 1971.

58. Iida, K., Mornaghi, R., and Nussenzweig, V.: J. Exp. Med., *155*:1427, 1982.

59. Inada, Y. et al.: Clin. Exp. Immunol., *50*:189, 1982.

60. Insert, ENA I Test Kit: RNP and Sm Autoantibody Reagents, Calbiochem Behring, La Jolla, 1983.

61. Jasin, H.E., and Ziff, M.: Arthritis Rheum. *18*:219, 1975.

62. Kimberly, R.P.: Rheum. Dis. Clin. North Am., *14*:203, 1988.

63. Koffler, D.: In *Systemic Lupus Erythematosus.* Edited by R.G. Lahita. New York, John Wiley and Sons, 1987.

64. Koffler, D., Schur, P.H., and Kunkel, H.G.: J. Exp. Med., *126*:607, 1967.

65. Koffler, D. et al.: J. Exp. Med., *134*:169, (Suppl.), 1971.

66. Krakauer, R.S. et al.: Clin. Immunol. Immunopathol., *14*:327, 1979.

67. Krishnan, C., and Kaplan, M.H.: J. Clin. Invest., *46*:569, 1967.

68. Kumagai, S. et al.: J. Immunol., *128*:258, 1982.

69. Lies, R.B., Messner, R.P., and Williams, R.C.: Arthritis Rheum., *16*:369, 1973.

70. Linker-Israeli, M. et al.: J. Immunol., *130*:2651, 1983.

71. Lloyd. W., and Schur, P.H.: Medicine, *60*:208, 1981.

72. Mannik, M.: J. Rheumatol., *14*(Suppl. 13):35, 1987.

73. Manolios, N., and Schreiber, L.: Aust. N.Z. J. Med., *16*:729, 1986.

74. Messner, R.P., Kennedy, M.S., and Jelinek, J.G.: Arthritis Rheum., *18*:201, 1975.

75. Miller, K.B., and Salem, D.: Am. J. Med., *73*:487, 1982.

76. Molden, D.P.: Diagn. Med., p. 12, June, 1985.

77. Morimoto, C., and Schlossman, S.F.: Arthritis Rheum., *30*:225, 1987.

78. Morimoto, C. et al.: J. Clin. Invest., *66*:1171, 1980.

79. Nies, K.M., and Louie, J.S.: Arthritis Rheum., *21*:51, 1978.

80. Nies, K.M., Stevens, R.H., and Louie, J.S.: J. Clin. Lab. Immunol., *4*:69, 1980.

81. Nies, K. et al.: Arthritis Rheum., *23*:1343, 1980.

82. Paronetto, F., and Koffler, D.: J. Clin. Invest., *44*:1657, 1965.

83. Pelton, B.K., and Denman, A.M.: Clin. Exp. Immunol., *48*:513, 1982.

84. Pollak, V.E., and Kant, K.S.: In *Systemic Lupus Erythematosus.* Edited by R.G. Lahita. New York, John Wiley and Sons, 1987.

85. Quismorio, F.P.: In *Dubois Lupus Erythematosus.* 3rd ed. Edited by D.J. Wallace and E.L. Dubois. Philadelphia, Lea & Febiger, 1987.

86. Reichlin, M., and Harley, J.B.: J. Rheumatol., *14*(Suppl. 13):112, 1987.

87. Reeves, W.H., and Lahita, R.G.: In *Systemic Lupus Erythematosus.* Edited by R.G. Lahita. New York, John Wiley and Sons, 1987.

88. Robitalle, P., and Tan, E.M.: J. Clin. Invest., *52*:316, 1973.

89. Rosenthal, C.J., and Franklin, E.C.: Arthritis Rheum., *18*:207, 1975.

90. Rubin, R.L., and Waga, S.: J. Rheumatol., *14*(Suppl. 13):118, 1987.

91. Sakane, T., Steinberg, A.D., and Green, I.: Arthritis Rheum., *21*:657, 1978.

92. Sakane, T., Steinberg, A.D., and Green, I.: Arthritis Rheum., *23*:225, 1980.

93. Sakane, T. et al.: Arthritis Rheum., *31*:80, 1988.

94. Schur, P.H.: Adv. Nephrol., *6*:63, 1976.

95. Schur, P.H.: In *Dubois Lupus Erythematosus.* 3rd ed. Edited by D.J. Wallace and E.L. Dubois. Philadelphia, Lea & Febiger, 1987.

96. Schur, P.H., and Sandson, J.: N. Engl. J. Med., *278*:533, 1968.

97. Sharp, G.C. et al.: J. Clin. Invest., *50*:350, 1971.

98. Shulman, L.E.: In *Dubois Lupus Erythematosus.* 3rd ed. Edited by D.J. Wallace and E.L. Dubois. Philadelphia, Lea & Febiger, 1987.

99. Sibbitt, W.L. et al.: Clin. Immunol. Immunopathol., *32*:166, 1984.

100. Siegel, M., Holley, H.L., and Lee, S.L.: Arthritis Rheum., *13*:802, 1970.

101. Singsen, B.H. et al.: J. Pediatr., *89*:358, 1976.

102. Smolen, J.S. et al.: Am. J. Med., *72*:783, 1982.

103. Solinger, A.M.: Rheum. Dis. Clin. North Am., *14*:187, 1988.

104. Stastny, P., and Ziff, M.: N. Engl. J. Med., *280*:1376, 1960.

105. Stastny, P., and Ziff, M.: Arthritis Rheumatol., *14*:733, 1971.

106. Stastny, P., and Ziff, M.: Clin. Exp. Immunol., *8*:543, 1971.

107. Steinberg, A.D., et al.: Ann. Intern. Med., *91*:587, 1979.

108. Steinberg, A.D., and Klinman, D.M.: Rheum. Dis. Clin. North Am., *14*:25, 1988.

109. Steinberg, A.D. et al.: J. Rheumatol., *14*Suppl. 13):166, 1987.

110. Swaak, T., and Smeek, R.: Clin. Rheumatol., *6*(Suppl. 1):56, 1987.

111. Talal, N.: In *Dubois Lupus Erythematosus.* 3rd ed. Edited by D.J. Wallace and E.L. Dubois. Philadelphia, Lea & Febiger, 1987.

112. Tan, E.M.: J. Invest. Dermatol., *67*:360, 1976.

113. Tan, E.M., and Kunkel, H.G.: Arthritis Rheum., *9*:37, 1966.

114. Tan, E.M. et al.: Arthritis Rheum., *25*:1271, 1982.

115. Tan, E.M. et al.: Clin. Immunol. Immunopathol., *47*:121, 1988.

116. Terasaki, P.I., Mattironi, V.D., and Barnett, E.V.: N. Engl. J. Med., *283*:724, 1970.

117. Theofilopoulos, A.N., and Dixon, F.J.: In *Systemic Lupus Erythematosus.* Edited by R.G. Lahita. New York, John Wiley and Sons, 1987.

118. Wallace, D.J., and Dubois, E.L.: In *Dubois Lupus Erythematosus,* 3rd ed. Edited by D.J. Wallace and E.L. Dubois. Philadelphia, Lea & Febiger, 1987.

119. Walport, M.J., and Lachmann, P.J.: Arthritis Rheum., *31*:153, 1988.

120. Warrington, R.J.: J. Rheumatol., *15*:616, 1988.

121. Weitzman, R.J., and Walker, S.E.: Ann. Rheum. Dis., *36*:44, 1977.

122. Wells, J.V.: In *Basic and Clinical Immunology.* 5th ed. Edited by D.P. Stites, J.D. Stobo, H.H. Fudenberg, and J.V. Wells. Los Altos, Lange Medical Publications, 1984.

123. Wertheimer, D., and Barland, P.: Arthritis Rheum., *19*:1249, 1976.

124. Wilson, M.R.: In *Dubois Lupus Erythematosus.* 3rd ed. Edited by D.J. Wallace and E.L. Dubois. Philadelphia, Lea & Febiger, 1987.

125. Woodrow, J.C.: J. Rheumatol., *15*:197, 1988.

ANTINUCLEAR ANTIBODIES

Antinuclear antibodies, or ANAs, are autoantibodies which are directed against constituents of the nucleus. A markedly heterogeneous population of antibodies, ANAs can be formed against antigenic sites on DNA (single-stranded or double-stranded), RNA, or a number of nuclear proteins. ANAs have been described from all five immunoglobulin classes, but most are IgG or IgM.[6] While they are found in a small percentage of normal healthy individuals and individuals with disorders not classified as autoimmune (e.g. certain viral infections), they occur most commonly in patients with systemic rheumatic diseases.[38]

The first method devised for detecting an ANA was the LE cell phenomenon of Hargraves,[9] whereby antinuclear antibody (the LE factor) and complement induce opsonization and subsequent phagocytosis of nuclei by polymorphonuclear leukocytes.

Although a number of techniques have been developed to detect ANAs, screening for ANAs is most commonly performed using a fluorescent antinuclear antibody assay (ANA or FANA test), as this method has a high degree of sensitivity and is readily adaptable for use in the routine clinical laboratory.[7] Briefly, this is an indirect immunofluorescence technique involving incubation of patient serum with a cellular substrate (the source of nuclear antigens), which is fixed onto a microscope slide. The slides are then washed, incubated next with a fluoresceinated anti-human immunoglobulin, washed again, and observed under a fluorescent microscope. Presence of ANAs in test serum is indicated by apple-green fluorescence in the cell nuclei. Different patterns of fluorescence are characteristically produced in the presence of antibodies to particular nuclear antigens. The major fluorescent patterns visible by the ANA method are the following:

1. *Homogeneous pattern* (also known as the diffuse pattern)—This is the most common pattern seen and involves uniform fluorescence of the entire nucleus (Fig. 11–1A). This pattern is produced in the presence of antibodies which react with double-stranded DNA or with both single-stranded and double-stranded DNA, with histones, or with DNA-histone complexes known as deoxyribonucleoprotein (DNP).[7] The latter antibody is thought to be identical to the "LE factor" responsible for the LE cell phenomenon.[38]

2. *Peripheral pattern* (also known as the rim, outline, or shaggy pattern)—This pattern is characterized by fluorescence circling around the outer edge of the nucleus (Fig. 11–1B) and is produced primarily in the presence of antibodies to double-stranded, or native DNA (nDNA), but may also be produced in the presence of antibodies to histones or DNP.[7]

3. *Speckled pattern*—In this pattern, discrete fluorescent speckles are evident throughout the nucleus (Fig. 11–1C). Speckles may range in size from small to large, depending on the specificity of the ANAs, and are induced by antibodies to the nuclear constituents, Sm, RNP, and other extractable nuclear antigens[7] (see below).

4. *Nucleolar pattern*—This pattern is characterized by fluorescent staining of the nucleolus, seen as one or two large dots within each nucleus (Fig. 11–1D). It is produced most frequently in the presence of antibody to nucleolar RNA.[7]

Mixed patterns, in which more than one of the above is produced, may also be observed, as patients with rheumatic diseases may have antibodies to multiple nuclear antigens. Mixed patterns may be seen simultaneously at a given dilution, or they may become evident only as serum concentration is weakened by further dilution.

Standardization of ANA assays has been difficult, and considerable variation in results may be produced by different laboratories testing the same clinical specimens.[25,27,28,36] Problems with reproducibility may also be encountered in a single laboratory. Factors contributing to this variation include technical differences such as the type of substrate and method of substrate fixation used, the concentration, specificity, and fluorescein/protein ratios of the antibody conjugate, the microscope optics used, judgmental differences in interpretation of the results, and differences in the reference ranges established.[7,26,27]

Standardization of the ANA test can be improved with the use of ANA reference sera available through the Centers for Disease Control,[34] standard optical systems, and uniform assay conditions.[7,26,27] It is also recommended that laboratories establish their own reference ranges with patient populations containing a representative number of individuals both under and over the age of 40, because the incidence of

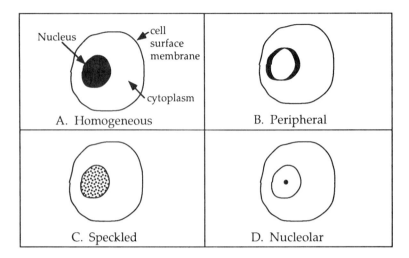

Fig. 11–1. Fluorescent patterns seen in the ANA test.

ANAs, although generally present in low titers, is increased in elderly individuals.[38] Our laboratory screens for ANAs using a 1:10 dilution of test serum, and has established a reference range of < 10.

The type of substrate used is particularly important. A large number of substrates are commercially available, but because each has inherent advantages and disadvantages, no single substrate is recommended for general use by all laboratories, and each laboratory must choose the substrate(s) best suited to its individual needs. Cryostat sections of rodent (mouse or rat) kidney or liver have been used for several years, and have the capability of detecting most nuclear antibodies and smooth muscle antibodies as well (see *Smooth Muscle Antibodies*); they are also free from interference from heterophile antibodies to blood group antigens, or from viral antibodies, which may cause false positive results with some cultured cell substrates.[7,38] Commercial kits containing human tissue culture cell substrates (e.g. human epithelial cells) have become more widely available. These cells have larger nuclei, which facilitate the reading of results, and are capable of detecting a wide variety of antinuclear antibodies, some of which are undetectable when the rodent cryostat sections are used (e.g. an-

tibodies to centromere, proliferating cell nuclear antigen (PCNA), and SS-A/Ro—see below).[4,7,14,38] Cell culture substrates, however, may contain passenger viruses which could cause false-positive results upon reaction with specific anti-viral antibodies, and unlike the cryostat sections, are unable to detect anti-smooth muscle antibodies, as they do not contain sections of smooth muscle layers.[7,38] Other substrates, including human amnion or mouse fibroblasts, have also been utilized for ANA testing.[18] A number of studies have been published which compare the sensitivities and specificities of various substrates.[2,4,8,18,21,22,24,26]

Despite the difficulties encountered in standardizing test results, the fluorescent ANA technique has proved to be a valuable method in screening for ANA. The sensitivity of the method is high, yielding positive results in 95 to 99% of SLE patients, depending on the type of substrate used.[25,38] Some laboratories find it beneficial to use more than one substrate, as this process detects a larger variety of ANAs, and reduces the number of false-negative ANA results obtained with lupus patients.[7,38]

ANA test results are generally reported as titer and pattern, as the latter gives some indication of the specificity of the ANA present (see above). Once a positive ANA screen has been obtained, however, additional tests are usually performed to determine the specificity of the ANA more precisely, as described below.

One group of ANA are those directed against histones, which consist of five major classes of basic proteins (H1, H2A, H2B, H3, and H4) that are complexed with DNA to form nucleosomes, the subunits of chromatin fibers. Antibodies to histones have been detected in approximately 50% of patients with SLE, 95% of patients with drug-induced lupus syndrome, 25% of patients with rheumatoid arthritis and in some patients with mixed connective tissue disease or progressive systemic sclerosis.[11,30,37] Antihistone antibodies usually produce a homogeneous pattern in the fluorescent ANA test, may less frequently produce a peripheral pattern, or may induce both.[7,37] Antibodies to the histone, H3, have also been associated with a pattern of variable large speckles.[7,27] Antibodies to histones may be more specifically characterized by immunofluorescence with specially prepared substrates, radioimmunoassay (RIA) or enzyme-linked immunosorbent assay (ELISA).[27,37]

Antibodies directed against complexes of DNA and histones known as deoxyribonucleoprotein (DNP) are also associated primarily with the homogeneous pattern of immunofluorescence in the ANA test, and are seen frequently in patients with SLE and drug-induced lupus.[11,37] Because anti-DNP is thought to be identical to the LE factor,[38] it may be demonstrated through the use of the LE cell prep.

Antibodies to DNA may react with antigenic determinants on double-stranded (ds) DNA, single-stranded (ss) DNA, or both.[27,37] Antibodies to denatured, or ss DNA are reactive with the nucleotide bases of the molecule, and are seen in SLE and a wide variety of other autoimmune diseases.[7,27] These antibodies are rarely detected using the immunofluorescent technique, since mammalian tissue sections contain negligible ss DNA, but they may be detected by a variety of other laboratory assays.[7]

Antibodies to ds, or native DNA (nDNA), on the other hand, are highly specific for SLE.[27,35] Although some investigators have reported anti-nDNA in association with other diseases, this observation is currently thought to be due to contamination of the DNA preparations used with ss DNA.[35] Antibodies to nDNA are thought to be reactive with the sugar-phosphate backbone or other conformational determinants of ds DNA[27,37] and may produce either a peripheral or homogeneous pattern (or both) in the immunofluorescent ANA test.[7] They may be detected more specifically by several different assays, the most common of which are immunofluorescence with *Crithidia luciliae,* and RIA utilizing the Farr technique; ELISA techniques are also becoming more available.[15,16] The *C. luciliae* assay is a special indirect immunofluorescence assay which was first introduced by Aarden et al.[1] in 1975 and uses the hemoflagellate organism, *C. luciliae,* as the cellular substrate. The presence of anti-nDNA is indicated by fluorescence in the kinetoplast, a circular organelle which is located near the flagellum of the organism and is composed primarily of ds DNA (Fig. 11–2).

In the RIA assay most frequently performed to detect anti-nDNA, patient serum is incubated with radiolabeled DNA. The Farr technique[5] is then utilized, whereby 50% ammonium sulfate is added, precipitating the antigen-antibody complexes, while leaving the soluble antigen DNA in solution.[39] While both assays have been useful, they also have a number of limitations: the RIA/Farr assay does not detect low affinity antibodies, which may become dissociated as a result of the ammonium sulfate precipitation step, does not distinguish between immunoglobulin and other substances in the test sample which may bind to DNA, and may detect antibodies to ss DNA, which may be present as a contaminant of the "ds DNA" preparations used.[16,37] The *C. luciliae* assay does not have

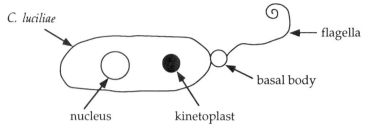

Fig. 11–2. *Crithidia luciliae* immunofluorescence test.

the quantitative capability of the RIA / Farr assay, and may also detect antibodies to histones, which may be present in the kinetoplast.[3] Test performance is highly dependent upon the growth medium, harvest time, and other conditions used in the preparation of *C. luciliae.*[17] Studies comparing the two assays as well as other assays have obtained different assessments of sensitivity, specificity, and patient results;[16,19] thus, each laboratory must decide which tests are most suited to their needs. Nevertheless, anti-nDNA assays are valuable in screening for antibodies to ds DNA, which, when detected, are specific for SLE.[35,38] These assays have also been helpful in monitoring SLE patients over time, as constant low titers are indicators of inactive disease with good prognosis, while a rapid rise in titer is a good predictor of disease exacerbation[10,32,37] (see also *Systemic Lupus Erythematosus*).

Another group of nuclear antigens to which autoantibodies may develop are the nonhistone proteins. Some of these have been referred to as *Extractable Nuclear Antigens (ENAs)*, so named because of their presence in saline solution extracts of certain nonhuman cells. The most common ENAs are Sm and RNP (see below). An expanding number of nonhistone proteins and corresponding autoantibodies have been identified.[35,37] Some of the more common antigens are described below.

1. *Sm*—The Sm antigen is a nuclear component toward which antibodies were first described in a patient named Smith.[33] The term Sm actually describes a family of small nuclear riboproteins consisting of at least eight different proteins in association

with five uridine-rich RNA species (U1, U2, U4, U5, or U6).[23,35] Sm antibodies are highly specific for SLE, and are found in approximately 30% of patients with the disease.[12,13,27,35] Anti-Sm produce a finely speckled pattern of nuclear fluorescence in the ANA screen.[7,14]

2. *RNP* (also referred to as Mo, nRNP, or U1 RNP)—RNP is a ribonucleoprotein containing the U1 species of small nuclear RNA in association with seven or eight nonhistone proteins.[23,35] Antibodies to RNP are found in high titer in most patients with a combination of overlapping rheumatologic symptoms known as mixed connective tissue disease, but are also found, usually in lower levels, in smaller percentages of patients with SLE and several other autoimmune rheumatic diseases, including scleroderma, dermatomyositis, Sjögren's syndrome, and rheumatoid arthritis.[13,25,27,37] Antibodies to RNP produce a finely speckled pattern in the fluorescent ANA screen.[7,14] RNP occurs in close association with Sm in multimolecular complexes, and antisera to the two antigens produce a line of partial identity when reacted in double immunodiffusion (Ouchterlony) tests.[13]

3. *SS-A / Ro.*—The SS-A / Ro antigen contains a 60,000 molecular weight protein in complex with 2 to 5 Y RNA species (Y = cytoplasmic) and has been detected primarily in the cytoplasm but also in the nucleus of cells.[23,35] Antibodies to SS-A / Ro are found in approximately 70% of patients with Sjögren's syndrome, 40 to 50% of patients with SLE, where they are frequently associated with subacute cutaneous lupus erythematosus, and in a lower prevalence

in patients with other connective tissue diseases.[10,25,27] Development of neonatal lupus, with photosensitive dermatitis and congenital heart block, is frequently associated with the presence of anti-SS-A/Ro antibodies in the mother and her newborn infant.[20,29,31] SS-A/Ro antigen is absent or present only in low concentrations in several mammalian tissues, causing many of the false-negative results for SLE patients tested in the fluorescent ANA screen using rodent substrates.[10,25,35] Most anti-SS-A/Ro antibodies are detectable using human epithelial cell line substrates, which give a finely speckled pattern of nuclear fluorescence.[25]

4. *SS-B/La.*—The SS-B/La antigen is a nuclear phosphoprotein with a molecular weight of approximately 45,000 daltons, which is found in complex with certain small RNAs, some of which appear to be of viral origin.[23,35] Anti-SS-B/La has been detected in approximately 40% of patients with Sjögren's syndrome and 15% of patients with SLE.[27,35] The SS-B/La and SS-A/Ro antigens have a physical affinity for one another and patients frequently have antibodies to both.[10] SS-B/La antibodies cause a fine speckled pattern of nuclear fluorescence in the fluorescent ANA screen.[7,14]

5. *Scl-70*—The Scl-70 antigen (formerly referred to as Scl-1), is a nuclear protein of molecular weight 70,000 daltons, which has been characterized as a degradation product of DNA topoisomerase I.[35,37] Antibodies to Scl-70 are seen in approximately 20% of patients with diffuse scleroderma, and are highly specific for this disease.[25,27] These antibodies produce a fine speckled pattern with or without nucleolar staining in the fluorescent ANA test.[7,25]

6. *Centromere*—Antibodies to proteins in the centromere region of the chromosome are often found in a subset of scleroderma known as the CREST syndrome (Calcinosis, Raynaud's phenomenon, Esophageal dysmotility, Sclerodactyly, and Telangiectasia).[25,27,35,37] Detection in the ANA screen requires the use of tissue culture cells as substrate; fluorescence appears in a discrete speckled pattern in interphase and metaphase cells.[7,14,37] Immunofluorescence using chromosomal spread preparations reveals the presence of two small dots, located at the kinetochores of the centromere.[37]

7. *PM-Scl* (also referred to as PM-1)— Antibodies to PM-Scl are directed against three proteins found in the nucleoplasm and nucleolus[35,37] and are present in the majority of patients with overlapping polymyositis-scleroderma, and in smaller percentages of patients with dermatomyositis or scleroderma alone.[27] These antibodies cause a nucleolar or speckled pattern in the ANA screen.[7,37]

8. *RANA*—Antibodies to rheumatoid arthritis-associated nuclear antigen (RANA) are directed against a nuclear antigen associated with Epstein Barr Virus (EBV) infection,[37] and are present in 90% of patients with rheumatoid arthritis.[27] These antibodies yield negative results on the ANA screen using traditional substrates, but produce a finely speckled pattern when immunofluorescence is performed on EBV-infected cell lines.[7,37]

A number of autoantibodies to nonhistone nuclear proteins other than those listed above have also been identified.[7,27,35,37,38] Although most antibodies to nonhistone proteins are detectable by the fluorescent ANA screen and produce a speckled pattern of immunofluorescence, this pattern is not specific for any one antibody. In addition, speckled patterns may sometimes not be evident on initial testing if other anti-nuclear antibodies are present which produce interfering patterns. Several procedures are available to characterize antibodies to nonhistone proteins more specifically. Most commonly used are immunodiffusion methods such as Ouchterlony double immunodiffusion and counterimmunoelectrophoresis; other methods, including ELISA, are also available.[7,15]

Nucleolar fluorescence in the ANA screen is most commonly caused by antibodies to 4-6S RNA in the nucleolus, present in a large percentage of patients with progressive systemic sclerosis, and in a smaller percentage of patients with SLE or other connective tissue disorders.[25] Nucleolar staining may also be caused by antibodies to other nucleolar RNA species, RNP, and PM-Scl.[7,14,27]

Thus, autoantibodies may be produced against a variety of nuclear antigens. Frequently, multiple ANAs are present in SLE and other connective tissue disorders. Although most ANAs are not specific for any one disease, some ANAs show a high degree of specificity, for example, anti-Sm and anti-nDNA are highly specific for SLE. Nevertheless, characteristic ANA profiles may be used to distinguish many of the autoimmune rheumatic diseases.[27,35] The fluorescent ANA assay has been a valuable screening test for antinuclear antibodies and may be used to monitor patients over time. A variety of other laboratory methods are available to characterize ANA more specifically.

REFERENCES

1. Aarden, L.A., deGroot, E.R., and Feltkamp, T.E.W.: Ann. N.Y. Acad. Sci., *254*:505, 1975.

2. Cleymaet, J.E., and Nakamura, R.M.: Am. J. Clin. Pathol., *58*:388, 1972.

3. Deng, J.-S. et al.: Arthritis Rheum., *28*:163, 1985.

4. Deng, J.-S. et al.: Diagn. Clin. Immunol., *5*:151, 1987.

5. Farr, R.S.: J. Infect. Dis., *103*:239, 1958.

6. Fernandez-Madrid, F., and Mattioli, M.: Semin. Arthritis Rheum., *6*:83, 1976.

7. Fritzler, M.J.: In *Manual of Clinical Laboratory Immunology*. 3rd ed. Edited by N.R. Rose, H. Friedman, and J.L. Fahey. Washington, D.C., American Society for Microbiology, 1986.

8. Hahon, N., Eckert, H.L., and Steward, J.: J. Clin. Microbiol., *2*:42, 1975.

9. Hargraves, M.M., Richmond, H., and Morton, R.: Proc. Mayo Clin., *23*:25, 1948.

10. Harley, J.B., and Gaither, K.K.: Rheum. Dis. Clin. North Am., *14*:43, 1988.

11. Hess, E.: N. Engl. J. Med., *318*:1460, 1988.

12. Homma, M. et al.: J. Rheumatol., *14* (Suppl 13):188, 1987.

13. Insert—ENA I Test Kit: RNP and Sm Autoantibody Reagents, Behring Diagnostics, Inc., Somerville, N.J., 1987.

14. Insert—AFT HEp System: HEp-2 Antinuclear Autoantibody Reagents, Behring Diagnostics, La Jolla, 1986.

15. Isenberg, D.A., and Maddison, P.J.: J. Clin. Pathol., *40*:1374, 1987.

16. Isenberg, D.A. et al.: Ann. Rheumatic Dis., *46*:448, 1987.

17. Jansen, E.M. et al.: Am. J. Clin. Pathol., *87*:461, 1987.

18. Kozin, F., Fowler, M., and Koethe, S.: Am. J. Clin. Pathol., *74*:785, 1980.

19. Lachman, P.J.: Ann. Rheum. Dis., *36*(suppl):67, 1977.

20. Lee, L.A. et al.: Am. J. Med., *83*:793, 1987.

21. Lipscomb, M.F. et al.: Diagn. Immunol., *2*:181, 1984.

22. McCarty, G.A., and Rice, J.R.: J. Rheumatol., *7*:339, 1980.

23. McNeilage, L.J., Whittingham, S., and MacKay, I.R.: J. Clin. Lab. Immunol., *15*:1, 1984.

24. Miller, M.H. et al.: J. Rheumatol., *12*:265, 1985.

25. Molden, D.P.: Diag. Med., p. 12, June, 1985.

26. Molden, D.P., Nakamura, R.M., and Tan, E.M.: Am. J. Clin. Pathol., *82*:57, 1984.

*27. Nakamura, R.M., and Tan, E.M.: Clin. Lab Med., *6*:41, 1986.

28. Nakamura, R.M., and Rippey, J.H.: Arch. Pathol. Lab. Med., *109*:109, 1985.

29. Reed, B.R. et al.: J. Pediatr., *103*:889, 1983.

30. Rubin, R.L., and Waga, S.: J. Rheumatol., *14*(suppl 13):118, 1987.

31. Scott, J.S. et al.: N. Engl. J. Med., *309*:209, 1983.

32. Swaak, T., and Smeek, R.: Clin. Rheumatol., *6*(suppl 1):56, 1987.

33. Tan, E.M., and Kunkel, H.G.: J. Immunol., *96*:464, 1966.

34. Tan, E.M. et al.: Arthritis Rheum., *25*:1003, 1982.

*35. Tan, E.M. et al.: Clin. Immunol. Immunopathol., *47*:121, 1988.

36. Taylor, R., Fulford, K., and Przybyszewski, V.A.: In *Antinuclear Antibodies*. Atlanta, U.S. Dept. of Health and Human Services, Centers for Disease Control, 1980.

*37. Wiik, A.: Allergy, *42*:241, 1987.

38. Wilson, M.R.: In *Dubois Lupus Erythematosus*. 3rd ed. Edited by D.J. Wallace and E.L. Dubois. Philadelphia, Lea & Febiger, 1987.

39. Wold, R.T. et al.: Science, *161*:806, 1968.

ANTIMITOCHONDRIAL ANTIBODIES

Testing for antimitochondrial antibodies (AMA) has been a valuable aid in the diagnosis of primary biliary cirrhosis, a progressive liver disease, probably of autoimmune origin, which is characterized by chronic inflammation and destruction of the intrahepatic bile ducts. AMA are considered a reliable indicator of the disease, as these antibodies have been detected in approximately 80 to 95% of cases of primary biliary cirrhosis, usually in high titer.[7,9,14,15] A much smaller percentage of patients with other liver diseases such as chronic active hepatitis and drug-induced hepatitis, and certain other disorders (e.g. collagen diseases) also have detectable AMA, but these are usually of lower titer.[7,10,14]

AMA are most commonly detected by indirect immunofluorescence; cryostat sections from various mammalian organs, or human epithelial cells may be used as substrate. The presence of AMA is indicated by fluorescence in the cytoplasm of the cells, corresponding to their mitochondrial distribution.[4] Recently, RIA, ELISA, fluorometric immunoassays, and immunoblotting methods using mitochondrial fractions as antigen have been used to study AMA.[6,11] On the basis of their reactivity in these tests as well as their staining patterns in immunofluorescence assays, AMA have been classified into nine categories (M1–M9).[1,8] Antibodies to the M2 antigen[2,5,13] and possibly the M4 and M8 antigen[3,16] appear to be specific for primary biliary cirrhosis, whereas antibodies to the other mitochondrial antigen groups are associated with other clinical disorders.[1,13] Further studies of these specificities by DNA cloning methods will more fully characterize these specificities and their clinical significance.[5]

Currently, detection of AMA via immunofluorescence, along with quantitation of IgM and liver enzymes, both of which tend to be elevated in primary biliary cirrhosis[12,14] constitute a reliable protocol for laboratory diagnosis of this disease.

REFERENCES

1. Baum, H., and Berg, P.A.: Semin. Liver Dis., 1:309, 1981.
2. Berg, P.A., Klein, R., and Lindenborn-Fotinos, J.J.: J. Hepatol., 2:123, 1986.
3. Berg, P.A. et al.: Lancet, 2:1329, 1980.
4. Bigazzi, P.E., Burek, C.L., and Rose, N.R.: In Manual of Clinical Laboratory Immunology. 3rd ed. Edited by N.R. Rose, H. Friedman, and J.L. Fahey. Washington, D.C., American Society for Microbiology, 1986.
5. Gershwin, M.E. et al.: J. Immunol., 138:3525, 1987.
6. Hussami, O.A. et al.: J. Clin. Lab. Immunol., 21:195, 1986.
7. Klatskin, G., and Kantor, F.S.: Ann. Intern Med., 77:533, 1972.
8. Klein, R. et al.: Clin. Exp. Immunol., 58:283, 1984.
9. Ladefoged, K., Andersen, P., and Jorgensen, J.: Acta Med. Scand. 205:103, 1979.
10. Ludwig, R.N.: Cleve. Clin. Q., 38:105, 1971.
11. Mendel-Hartvig, I., Frostell, A., and Totterman, T.H.: Int. Arch. Allergy Appl. Immunol., 83:265, 1987.
12. Taylor, K.B., and Thomas, H.C.: In Basic and Clinical Immunology. 6th ed. Edited by D.P. Stites, J.D. Stobo, and J.V. Wells. Norwalk, Appleton and Lange, 1987.
13. Triger, D.R.: In Clinical Immunology of the Liver and Gastrointestinal Tract. Edited by D.R. Triger. Bristol, John Wright and Sons, Ltd., 1986.
14. Ward, A.M., Ellis, G., and Goldberg, D.M.: Am. J. Clin. Pathol., 70:352, 1978.
15. Walker, J.G.: Ann. Clin. Biochem., 7:93, 1970.
16. Weber, P. et al.: Hepatology, 6:553, 1986.

ANTISMOOTH MUSCLE ANTIBODIES

The presence of antismooth muscle antibodies (ASMA) has been reported in a number of disorders, including autoimmune diseases of the liver, viral diseases such as infectious hepatitis, infectious mononucleosis, and cytomegalovirus infection, a variety of malignant diseases, and in a small percentage of healthy individuals.[1,12,14,16]

Most notable is the association of ASMA with chronic active hepatitis (CAH),[2,6,7,17] defined by most investigators as progressive inflammation of the liver persisting for at least 6 months.[13] Numerous reports in the literature have found the incidence of ASMA in CAH to range from 40 to 80%.[5,11,12,15,16] Although the clinical specificity of ASMA is low, high persistent titers tend to be associated with CAH, while ASMA in other diseases are usually transient and present in lower titers.[8,16] The ASMA in CAH are primarily of the IgG class.[16]

ASMA are detected in the laboratory by indirect immunofluorescence with cryostat sections of any of a number of organs containing smooth muscle as the substrate (e.g. thymus, liver, kidney, and stomach).[5,9,16] Our laboratory uses mouse kidney sections as substrate.[5] Through electron microscopy and immunofluorescence performed on rodent kidney substrates, ASMA have been found to be a heterogeneous group of antibodies reacting with microfilaments, microtubules, or intermediate filaments,[14] and staining vessels only (SMA-V), vessels and renal glomeruli only (SMA-G), or vessels, glomeruli, and intracellular fibrils (SMA-T).[1,14] The ASMA in CAH display the SMA-T pattern of staining[1,14] and are specifically directed against actin,[3,9] whereas ASMA in other disorders are thought to have different specificities which have not yet been fully characterized.[1,4,10,14]

Detection of ASMA by immunofluorescence is a useful aid in determining the presence of CAH and the subsequent need for therapy when used in conjunction with other laboratory tests such as those to evaluate liver enzymes, anti-nuclear antibodies, and IgG levels. All of these are elevated in the majority of patients with CAH.[15,16]

REFERENCES

1. Bottazzo, G.-F. et al.: J. Clin. Pathol., 29:403, 1976.
2. Doniach, D. et al.: Clin. Exp. Immunol., 1:237, 1966.
3. Gabbiani, G. et al.: Am. J. Pathol., 72:473, 1973.
4. Garbarz, D. et al.: Clin. Exp. Immunol., 43:87, 1981.
5. Insert—AFT System I, Behring Diagnostics, La Jolla, CA., 1986.
6. Ironside, P.N., Deboer, W.R.G.M., and Nairn, R.C.: Lancet, 1:1210, 1966.
7. Johnson, G.D., Holborow, E.J., and Glynn, L.E.: Lancet, 2:878, 1965.
8. Jorde, R., Skogen, B., and Rekvig, O.P.: Acta Med. Scand., 222:471, 1987.
9. Kurki, P. et al.: Gut, 21:878, 1980.
10. Kurki, P., and Virtanen, I.: J. Immunol. Methods, 76:329, 1985.
11. Ladefoged, K., Andersen, P., and Jorgensen, J.: Acta Med. Scand., 205:103, 1979.
12. Ludwig, R.N., Deodhar, S.D., and Brown, C.H.: Cleve. Clin. Q., 38:105, 1971.
13. Taylor, K.B., and Thomas, H.C.: In Basic and Clinical Immunology, 6th ed. Edited by D.P. Stites, J.D. Stobo, and J.V. Wells. Norwalk, Appleton and Lange, 1987.
*14. Toh, B.H.: Clin. Exp. Immunol., 38:621, 1979.
15. Walker, J.G.: Ann. Clin. Biochem., 7:93, 1970.
*16 Ward, A.M., Ellis, G., and Goldberg, D.M.: Am. J. Clin. Pathol., 70:352, 1978.
17. Whittingham, S. et al.: Gastroenterology, 51:499, 1966.

Autoantibody Tests[1]:
Antinuclear Antibody Test (ANA)
Antimitochondrial Antibody Test (AMA)
Antismooth Muscle Antibody Test (ASMA)

PRINCIPLE. This procedure is used for the detection and quantitative estimation of antinuclear (ANA), antimitochondrial (AMA), and antismooth muscle (ASMA) antibodies in human serum by the indirect fluorescent antibody technique. Frozen sections of mouse kidney containing vessels with smooth muscle lining in renal tubules and mitochondria as well as nuclei are used as the antigen substrate. When this substrate is overlaid with the patient's serum, antinuclear (ANA), antimitochondrial (AMA) and antismooth muscle (ASMA) antibodies, if present, will bind to their specific antigen sites in the substrate. The excess serum is then removed by washing and fluorescein-labeled anti-human IgG is added which will bind to the human antibody. The slide is washed to remove excess fluorescein-labeled conjugate and observed under the fluorescence microscope. The presence of ANA, AMA or ASMA in the serum sample is demonstrated by a yellowish-green (apple green) fluorescence when observed under a fluorescence microscope. The type of autoantibody bound by the substrate is determined by noting the specific pattern of this fluorescence. The titer of the autoantibody is measured by determining the highest dilution of serum sample producing a positive reaction.

EQUIPMENT AND MATERIALS

1. AFT System I, Autoantibody test reagents, (Calbiochem-Behring Corp.):

a. Anti-human IgG, H & L Chain (Goat), Fluorescein Isothiocyanate Labeled, F/P ratio 1.5, 0.1% Sodium azide. Store between 2 and 8°C

b. Buffered Diluent, pH 7.1, 0.1% Sodium azide. Use only the buffered diluent supplied with the kit for dilution of test specimens. Use of other reagents may cause nonspecific fluorescence in the test system. Store buffered diluent between 2 and 8° C

c. Substrate slides (mouse kidney) 8 wells per slide

d. Phosphate buffered saline

e. Antimitochondrial Antibody (AMA) Positive Control (Calbiochem-Behring Corp. Cat. No. 879016)

f. Antismooth Muscle Antibody (ASMA) Positive Control (Calbiochem-Behring Corp. Cat. No. 879017)

2. Additional materials required:

a. Distilled or deionized water

b. Moist chamber

c. Coplin jar

d. Pasteur pipets and bulbs or 25 μl pipets with disposable tips

e. Mounting fluid

f. Cover slips

g. ANA positive control: Use undiluted patient serum that is known to be positive

h. ANA negative control: Use undiluted patient serum that is known to be negative

SPECIMEN COLLECTION AND PREPARATION. This procedure should be performed with a serum specimen.

Turbidity, hemolysis, visible bacterial growth, or drugs capable of fluorescing in the test specimen may interfere with the performance and accuracy of the test. Do not use hemolyzed or lipemic serum specimens.

Serum specimens may be stored at 2 to 8° C for up to 5 days. If longer storage is desired, store at −20° C.

PROCEDURE: SCREENING TESTS:

ANA procedure: Dilute serum 1:10 with buffered diluent supplied (0.1 ml serum in 0.9 ml buffer).

ANA positive control: Dilute 1:10, 1:50, 1:250, and 1:1250 in buffered diluent supplied.

ASMA and AMA procedure: Dilute patient serum 1:10 with buffered diluent supplied.

Do not dilute ASMA and AMA positive controls, or negative control. These controls are supplied in the proper dilution.

1. Remove substrate slide from refrigerator and allow to warm to room temperature. Cut end of foil bag with scissors and carefully remove slide to avoid damaging mouse kidney tissue. Caution: If moisture of condensation deposits on slide (because of inadequate warming before cutting foil bag), allow slide to dry completely before proceeding with test. Failure to do so may cause loss of sections from slide.

2. Label slide in space provided and record specimens to be tested on a worksheet.

3. Place substrate slide in moist chamber.

4. For the antinuclear antibody (ANA) test, place approximately 25 μl of ANA positive control dilutions into rings 1, 2, 3, and 4 and approximately 25 μl of autoantibody negative control into ring 5.

For the antimitochondrial antibody (AMA) test, place approximately 25 μl of buffered diluent and AMA negative control into rings 1 and 2, and approximately 25 μl of autoantibody positive control into ring 3.

For the antismooth muscle antibody (ASMA) test, place approximately 25 μl of buffered diluent and ASMA negative control into rings 1 and 2, and approximately 25 μl of autoantibody positive control into ring 3.

5. Place approximately 25 μl of properly diluted patient specimen into each of the remaining rings, as recorded on worksheet.

Do not disturb specimen or allow it to run over the ring once placed on the slide.

6. Place lid on moist chamber and incubate slide for 30 minutes at room temperature. Remove slide from chamber and rinse gently with 5 to 10 ml of phosphate buffered saline solution (PBS) using a Pasteur or serologic pipet. Use a direct stream of PBS to midline of slide to minimize cross-contamination between wells.

7. Tap edge of slide on paper towel to remove excess phosphate buffered saline. Replace slide in moist chamber and immediately cover slide with antihuman IgG, fluorescein labeled. *DO NOT ALLOW SLIDE TO DRY.*

The conjugate dilution has been adjusted to allow for dilution by residual phosphate buffered saline that may remain on the slide. Thus, the presence of phosphate buffered saline will not interfere with this step of the reaction.

8. Replace lid on moist chamber and incubate slide with anti-human IgG, fluorescein labeled, for 30 minutes at room temperature.

9. Remove lid from chamber, remove slide and rinse with PBS. Place in Coplin jar containing phosphate buffered saline for 10 minutes.

10. Remove slide from the Coplin jar and tap side of slide on paper towel to remove excess moisture. Place two drops of mounting medium on each slide and cover with a coverslip. Read slide within 60 minutes. If slide cannot be read within 60 minutes, it may be stored between 2

and 8° C in the dark for up to 24 hours before reading.

11. Examine slide under the fluorescence microscope at both low and high dry magnification. Do not expose slide to long periods of excitation light from the fluorescence microscope, as this will cause fading of fluorescence.

The ANA positive control should yield a positive reaction, while the autoantibody negative control should show no pattern of fluorescence. Occasional background fluorescence may be observed, and is usually due to improper washing techniques. The background fluorescence of the conjugate may be determined by comparison to buffered diluent; no nonspecific background staining should be observed with the buffered diluent.

Production of unexpected results by the control sera may be due to several factors:

a. Improper storage of sera (look for signs of contamination, and if found, discard control sera).

b. Improper use of optical system.

c. Improper reading (compare carefully with negative control).

d. Improper dilution techniques (repeat test following directions given under "Screening Test").

e. Partial drying of sera and/or conjugate (this can lead to false negative reactions).

If a repeat test fails to yield the expected results, then the controls and/or conjugate should be discarded and new reagents used. Care should be taken to ensure that the slide is not moved once samples have been applied. In addition, no more than 25 μl of sample should be applied per well. If by accident the samples should spill into each other, then the slide should be discarded and the test repeated.

TITRATION OF POSITIVE SPECIMENS. All specimens giving a positive test reaction should be titrated. Determine the highest dilution producing a positive reaction. It is important that both the titer and the pattern of the positive response be determined.

1. Prepare fivefold serial dilutions of all specimens yielding a positive ANA, AMA, or ASMA reaction in the screening test as follows:

For each specimen to be titered, place 0.9 ml buffered diluent in the first of four test tubes. Place 0.4 ml buffered diluent in the remaining three test tubes. Pipet 0.1 ml of serum to be titered into the first tube. This is a 1:10 dilution. Pipet 0.1 ml of 1:10 dilution into the second tube. Continue mixing and transferring 0.1 ml through the fourth tube. The dilutions prepared are 1:10, 1:50, 1:250, and 1:1250.

2. Repeat assay procedure given in steps 1 through 11 under "Screening Test." For autoantibody titration, use appropriate positive control (ANA, AMA, ASMA), autoantibody negative control, and the 1:10, 1:50, 1:250, and 1:1250 dilutions of specimen(s) to be titered.

3. Determine the highest dilution producing a positive reaction.

READING OF SLIDES. Examine several fields, reading those parts of the tissue sections with well-defined cells for evaluation of ANA or AMA, or with blood vessels for evaluation of ASMA. Several fields of a single well might have to be scanned in order to locate blood vessels required for the detection of ASMA. Initial examination under low magnification ($100-200\times$) may aid in locating the vessels. Not all cells will appear optimal because of possible disruption during sectioning. Identify any fluorescent staining observed on the sections as nuclear, nucleolar, mitochondrial or smooth muscle. Observed fluorescent staining should be compared to the appropriate positive and negative controls.

REPORTING. Results are reported as positive or negative for ANA, AMA, or ASMA. Titers for positive specimens are determined and reported. For ANA, the type of fluorescent pattern observed is also reported (see below).

INTERPRETATION OF RESULTS

Positive Reactions for Antinuclear Antibodies (ANA):

Fluorescent staining of the nucleus with diffuse homogeneous, peripheral, speckled, or nucleolar patterns is considered specific for antinuclear antibodies. Fluorescent staining of the nucleus may be classified by pattern as follows[1] (see package insert for illustrations of fluorescent patterns):

1. A diffuse homogeneous pattern is defined as a uniform, solid fluorescent stain throughout the nucleus.

2. A peripheral pattern has a characteristic fluorescent staining of the rim or edge of the nucleus.

3. A nucleolar pattern refers to fluorescent staining of the nucleolus.

4. A speckled pattern has numerous, discrete specks of fluorescent staining throughout the nucleus.

Positive Reaction for Antimitochondrial Antibodies (AMA):

Fluorescent staining of the mitochondria is considered specific for antimitochondrial antibodies.

The AMA autoantibodies that react with the proximal and the distal tubules of the mouse kidney need to be distinguished by their morphology from the less common antimicrosomal antibodies that react with the proximal tubules only and from antibodies that give only diffuse immunofluorescence staining patterns.[1]

Positive Reactions for Antismooth Muscle Antibodies (ASMA):

Fluorescent staining of the smooth muscle of blood vessels is considered specific for antismooth muscle antibodies. A positive sample should produce fluorescence on the inner and outer lining of the vessel.[1]

Negative Reaction:

The absence of specific fluorescent staining of the nucleus, nucleolus, mitochondria, or smooth muscle is considered negative for ANA, AMA, and ASMA.[1]

Unusual patterns that may be observed include the staining of the brush borders of the kidney tubules, the tubular basement membrane, the glomeruli (with an appearance of glomerular basement membrane staining), or of the connective tissue (with a pattern of reticulin antibodies).[1] These patterns have not been found to have any clinical or diagnostic significance. At least some of them are caused by unusual heterophile antibodies. These patterns are sometimes mistaken for AMA antibodies.

LIMITATIONS OF THE PROCEDURE. The fluorescein-labeled antihuman IgG is prepared from an anti-human IgG, H & L chain (GOAT). This conjugate, while primarily reacting with autoantibodies of the IgG class, will cross-react through the light chain with autoantibodies of other classes such as IgM or IgD.

The results of this test may not correlate with systemic lupus erythematosus if the patient has been treated with corticosteroids or immunosuppressive drugs. The analyst should be aware of the possibility of prozone, nonspecific patterns and interference phenomena in reading slides.[2,3]

Prozone may be observed when a significant excess of autoantibody occurs for antigen available, such as in the case of high serum titers of ANA run at low dilutions. The result is a doubtful positive or even negative reaction given by a serum which usually yields a strongly positive result at a high dilution. In order to avoid misreading clinically important immunofluorescent reactions as false negatives, suspect sera (doubtful positives) should be titrated.

Interference phenomena may be present when there are two or more autoantibodies in a serum specimen which gives a positive immunofluorescence reaction. When this occurs, one of the antibodies present (usually the stronger one) predominates and suppresses the reaction of the other(s). Titrations of such sera may reveal first one and then another antibody. Repeat titrations often yield divergent titers. When this phenomenon occurs, the presence of all discernible autoantibodies and their apparent titers should be reported.

It should also be noted that the actual titer of the weaker autoantibody may have been suppressed due to the interference phenomenon.

Different clinical populations may warrant a change in the initial screening for ASMA to dilutions higher than 1:10.

It is advantageous to have alternate substrates available such as the human epithelial cell line, HEp-2. HEp-2 cells are large in size, making ANA patterns easily discernible. HEp-2 is also the recommended substrate for detecting centromere antibodies and appears to be highly selective for the CREST variant of progressive systemic sclerosis.

REFERENCES

1. Insert, AFT System I Autoantibody Reagents, Behring Diagnostics, La Jolla, CA, 1987.
2. Ladefogel, K., Anderson, P., and Jorgensen, J.: Acta Med. Scand., *205*:103, 1979.
3. Nakamura, R.M., Chisari, F.V., and Edgington, T.S.: *Progress in Clinical Pathology*. Edited by M. Stefanini. New York, Grune & Stratton, 1975.

Anti-dsDNA Test: Farr Technique[1]

PRINCIPLE. Complexes composed of radiolabeled dsDNA and anti-DNA from patient sera are precipitated with the use of ammonium sulfate. Radio-labeled dsDNA not bound by the reaction is left in solution. The radioactivity of the precipitates is measured using a gamma counter. A graph is prepared, plotting concentration of each standard against its radioactive count, and patient results are read from this graph.

EQUIPMENT AND MATERIALS

1. Anti-dsDNA Kit (Amersham Corporation), containing: (50 and 100 test packs available)

a. Anti-DNA Standards (6): Freeze-dried vials of buffered human serum, each with a different anti-DNA binding activity, assigned arbitrarily, but in accordance with a standard prepared and kept by Amersham Corporation. Assigned values are stated on the label

b. ^{125}I Labeled dsDNA: DNA ^{125}I in solution with not more than 2 μCi ^{125}I, in buffer. This is supplied ready for use

c. Ammonium sulfate: Contains at least 55 ml of 93% saturated ammonium sulfate solution. This is supplied ready for use. Keep at 2 to 8° C prior to use

d. Tube rack

e. Polystyrene assay tubes (50)

f. Graph paper

2. Anti-DNA Controls (Amersham):

a. Control 6 is freeze-dried 10% (v/v) human serum and 0.9% bovine serum albumin

b. Control 7 is freeze-dried 10% (v/v) human serum and 0.9% bovine serum albumin

Upon reconstitution, each vial contains 200 μl of 10% (v/v) human serum. The expected anti-DNA values for the constituents are given under the "Expected Values" section of the control package insert. Controls are to be reconstituted with 200 μl of distilled water and do not need any further diluting prior to testing. Store the controls at 2 to 4° C before reconstitution. Controls should be used immediately after reconstitution and not stored for use in subsequent assays.

3. Precision micropipets for dispensing 25 μl, 200 μl, and 1000 μl, with disposable tips.

4. Vortex mixer

5. Water baths maintained at 37° C $\pm$ 0.5° C

6. Thermometer

7. Refrigerator at 2 to 4° C

8. Centrifuge

9. Aspirator

10. Gamma scintillation counter, calibrated for ^{125}I

11. Distilled water

PREPARATION OF REAGENTS. Standards: To reconstitute the freeze-dried standards, tap the vials to dislodge any large particles from the stoppers. For each vial remove the closure and stopper, taking care not to lose any small particles of freeze-dried material adhering to the stopper. Add 2000 μl freshly distilled water to the zero standard vial and 200 μl freshly distilled water to each of the other serum standard vials. Replace the stoppers and leave the contents of the vials to dissolve at room temperature for 10 minutes. The contents of the vials should then be further mixed by gentle inversion and swirling until complete solution is obtained. Vigorous agitation and foaming should be avoided.

STORAGE INSTRUCTIONS

1. Store unreconstituted standards and other components at 2 to 8° C; do not freeze.

2. Reconstituted standards should be used at once and then stored at $-20°$ C for future use. Avoid repeated freezing and re-thawing. Do not thaw more than twice.

3. Expiration date is stated on the package label.

SPECIMEN COLLECTION AND PREPARATION. Patient sample: Serum samples can be fresh, frozen or quick frozen (1 week at $2°$ C, up to 8 weeks at $-20°$ C, unknown length of time at $-70°$ C). Repeated freezing and thawing should be avoided.

PROCEDURE

PERFORM STEPS IN AN AREA DESIGNATED FOR RADIOACTIVITY.

The order of the steps should be followed exactly:

1. Label and arrange the assay tubes as required. Run each standard, control, and specimen in duplicate.

2. Pipette 25 μl of standards, controls and specimens into the appropriate tubes.

3. Dispense 200 μl ^{125}I-labeled dsDNA solution (red) into each tube using a precision pipette or repeating dispenser.

4. Vortex to mix all the tubes thoroughly. Cover the tubes (e.g. with plastic film) and incubate at $37°$ C for 1 hour $\pm$ 10 minutes.

5. Remove the ammonium sulfate solution from the refrigerator and add 1000 μl to the appropriate tubes. Vortex to mix all tubes thoroughly.

6. Centrifuge all tubes together for 15 minutes at 1500 g at room temperature (18 to $28°$ C) or at 2 to $8°$ C.

7. Immediately after centrifugation invert the tubes to pour off the supernatant liquids, and place the inverted tubes on a pad of absorbent tissues to drain for 10 to 15 minutes.

8. Firmly blot the rims of the tube on the tissue pad to remove any last drops of liquid and turn upright. Do not re-invert the tubes once they have been turned upright.

9. Count all the tubes in a suitable gamma counter for the time required to accumulate at least 1,000 counts in the zero standards tubes.

10. Plot ^{125}I counts per minute (cpm) obtained against the anti-DNA binding activity of the six standards. Draw the best curve (using a french curve) through the mean of the duplicate samples, rejecting grossly aberrant counts.

11. Read the counts for the control duplicates from the standard curve and calculate the mean values. The controls must be $\pm$ 2 standard de-viations from the means established for the run to be acceptable.

12. Read count for each patient sample duplicate from the standard curve and calculate the mean value for that sample.

13. If the sample result is greater than the highest standard, the sample should be further diluted and retested.

NOTE: Radioactive materials should be disposed of in accordance with institutional policies.

REPORTING. The mean value of each sample is reported in units/ml.

INTERPRETATION OF RESULTS

<15 U/ml = negative

$15-25$ U/ml = intermediate

>25 U/ml = positive

LIMITATIONS OF THE PROCEDURE

1. Differences in avidities between individual sera are not accounted for using this procedure. The anti-DNA activity levels detected are a function of both the concentration of anti-DNA antibodies and their avidity.

2. The method of preparation of the radioactive DNA ensures that it is essentially, although not entirely, double stranded DNA.

REFERENCE

1. Package insert, Anti-dsDNA Kit, Immunoradioassay for DNA binding activity in serum, Amersham Corporation, Arlington Heights, IL, 1989.

Extractable Nuclear Antigens (ENA): RNP and SM Autoantibody[1]

PRINCIPLE. Extractable nuclear antigens (ENA) are a mixture of RNP, Sm, and other soluble nuclear antigens found in saline extracts of mammalian tissue (in this kit, calf thymus). In this Ouchterlony double-immunodiffusion procedure, a solution containing ENA is placed in the central well of an agarose plate, while patient samples and controls are placed in surrounding wells. Antigens and patient antibodies diffuse through the agarose and form a visible precipitate in the zone of equivalence if the sample contains antibodies to any of the extractable nuclear antigens present. No precipitate forms in the absence of specific antibodies. Precipitin lines from patient samples are compared to control antisera results and are identified as Sm, RNP or "other" based on whether the lines formed are of identity, partial identity or non-identity relative to the controls.

EQUIPMENT AND MATERIALS

ENA test kit, Behring Diagnostics, consisting of:

1. Agarose Plates. Eight seven-well agarose plates (one central well surrounded by six peripheral wells) (0.1% sodium azide)

2. ENA (extractable nuclear antigen) from calf thymus, 2×0.45 ml, lyophilized from buffer containing 0.1% sodium azide

3. RNP Positive Control, human, 0.7 ml in buffer containing 0.1% sodium azide

4. Sm positive control, human, 0.7 ml in buffer containing 0.1% sodium azide

5. Eight protocol sheets

6. Four image film packages

Not Included in Kit:

1. Test tubes

2. Normal saline (Dissolve 0.9 g sodium chloride in sufficient distilled water to make 100 mL of solution)

3. Serologic pipets

4. Capillary pipets

5. Small spotlight (or viewing chamber)

6. Magnifying glass

7. Distilled water

NOTE: In order to use the image film included with the kit, the following materials are also needed:

8. Bulb (GE EBV2 photolamp)

9. Plastic box with lid (or moist chamber)

10. Ammonium hydroxide (30%)

11. Filter paper

12. Ruler

13. Timer

PRECAUTIONS. Sodium azide may react with copper or lead plumbing to form highly explosive metal azides. Upon disposal, flush with large amounts of water to prevent azide buildup.

PREPARATION OF REAGENTS

1. ENA (Extractable Nuclear Antigen): Remove cap and stopper from vial. (Vent carefully since vial contents may be vacuum

sealed.) Pipet 0.45 ml of distilled water into vial. Replace stopper and rotate gently until dissolved. Write reconstitution date on label.

2. Control sera: Ready for use as supplied.

STORAGE INSTRUCTIONS. Store at 2 to 8° C. Reconstituted ENA solution is stable for 14 days at 2 to 8° C. Do not use the controls if turbidity or a precipitate is observed. Reconstituted antigen may be stored frozen in aliquots, but should not be frozen and thawed more than once.

SPECIMEN COLLECTION AND PREPARATION. This procedure should be performed with a serum specimen.

Turbidity, hemolysis or visible bacterial growth may interfere with the performance and accuracy of the test.

Serum specimens may be stored at 2 to 8° C for up to 5 days. If longer storage is desired, store at $-20°$ C.

PROCEDURE

Use one of the enclosed protocol sheets for recording data.

1. Reconstitute a vial of ENA with 0.45 ml distilled water.

2. Prepare a 1:4 dilution of the sera to be tested with normal saline solution (e.g., 0.1 ml serum $+$ 0.3 mL saline solution). Do not dilute the control sera. They are supplied in the proper concentration for use.

3. Remove the lid from one agarose plate. Using a calibrated pipet or pasteur pipet, fill the peripheral wells with controls and patient samples (undiluted and 1:4 dilutions) as shown in Figure 11–3. Use a clean pipet for each specimen. Fill wells until the fluid is level with the agarose surface. Approximate fill volume for sample well is 65 μl.

NOTE: A small plate orientation mark appears next to one of the peripheral wells. This is well 1; peripheral wells 2 through 6 proceed clockwise (Fig. 11–3).

4. Fill the central well (well 7) with reconstituted ENA solution. Approximate fill volume is 90 μl.

CAUTION:

1. Reasonable care in filling the wells is important. The wells will hold approximately 90 μl of antigen, and 65 μl of samples and controls. Under- or overfilling the wells, or damaging the agarose during filling, may produce irregular diffusion.

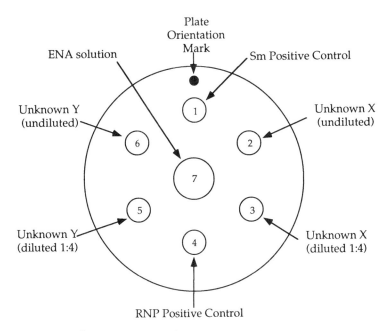

Plate
Orientation
Mark

ENA solution

Sm Positive Control

Unknown Y
(undiluted)

Unknown X
(undiluted)

Unknown Y
(diluted 1:4)

Unknown X
(diluted 1:4)

RNP Positive Control

Fig. 11–3. ENA agarose plate assay protocol.

2. The format depicted in Figure 11–3 must be followed exactly. A maximum of two patient samples (undiluted and 1:4 dilution) can be tested per plate.

5. Cover the plate immediately after all wells have been filled.

6. Incubate plate at room temperature on a level, vibration-free surface for 24 hours.

7. Remove plate lid, and examine against a dark background for presence or absence of precipitin lines. Use a magnifying glass and a small spotlight or pen light if necessary. Optimal results may be obtained by using commercially available viewers with an indirect light source. Plates should be rechecked at 48 hours for the appearance of any newly formed precipitin lines. Record results on protocol sheet.

8. A permanent record of ENA precipitation reactions can be made using the Image Film included in the kit. To produce a better image, rinse the developed plate in normal saline solution, then fill all the wells to the top with normal saline solution. Remove a sheet of photosensitive paper from the foil pouch and place it (glossy side up) under the plate. Expose paper and plate (lid removed) to light from an EBV-2 GE photolamp* for approximately 8 minutes. The bulb

*The GE EBV-2 photolamp is 500 watts, and the bulb heat may melt the lamp socket if the lamp is not rated for 500 watts. Use a lamp rated for 500 watts, without a shade or reflector.

should be approximately 14 inches from the paper and directly above the plate. Prepare a developing chamber by placing a piece of filter paper in a small plastic box somewhat larger than the sheet of Image Film. Saturate the filter paper with a 30% solution of ammonium hydroxide. Place the exposed image film in the developing chamber, using two pencils to keep the film from touching the wet filter paper. *DO NOT* place the film directly on top of the wet filter paper. The image will develop within 3 to 5 minutes, and can be attached to the protocol sheet for a permanent record.

The plate can also be stained and photographed using techniques developed for preparing permanent records of IEP plates.

QUALITY CONTROL. The RNP and Sm positive controls must be assayed on each agarose plate. A line of precipitation must be observed between each positive control well and the antigen well in order for results on unknown samples to be considered valid.

REPORTING. Results are reported as positive or negative for either RNP or Sm. Titer results may be generated depending on physician's request.

INTERPRETATION OF RESULTS. Examine the area between patient sample and central well for lines of identity, partial identity or non-identity with the precipitin line of the positive control sera (Fig. 11–4, A, B, C).

Examples of patterns of immunoprecipitin lines which may be encountered during ENA testing are given in Figures 11–5, 11–6, 11–7. Figure 11–5 depicts a patient serum positive for Sm antibody. Figure 11–6 depicts a patient serum containing antibodies reactive against ENA other than Sm or RNP (non-Sm, non-RNP). Figure 11–7 depicts the precipitin reaction of a patient serum containing both Sm and RNP antibodies.

Patient sera that fail to produce precipitin reactions are negative for ENA antibodies.

LIMITATIONS OF THE PROCEDURE. Prozone phenomenon is observed when a significant excess of antibody exists relative to available antigen. Doubtful samples should be retested at 1:8 and 1:16 dilutions. If a serum sample exhibits multiple precipitin reactions, it may be difficult to determine if lines of identity, nonidentity or partial identity occur with the positive control. In such a case, retesting the sample at several dilutions may permit evaluation of results.

REFERENCE

1. Insert, ENA I Test Kit, Behring Diagnostics, Inc., Somerville, NJ, 1987.

ANTICARDIOLIPIN ANTIBODIES

Cardiolipin is an acidic phospholipid present in the inner mitochondrial membrane, where it plays a role in the activity of cytochrome c oxidase and cytochrome P-450.[31,39] Its concentration varies in different tissues, and is particularly high in the heart.[31]

Antibodies to cardiolipin and other negatively charged phospholipids are present most commonly in patients with systemic lupus erythematosus (SLE) or SLE-like disorders, but may also be seen in patients with other autoimmune diseases (e.g. rheumatoid arthritis, Sjögren's syndrome, mixed connective tissue disease, ulcerative colitis) and a variety of other disorders such as malignancies, acute infections, multiple cerebral infarctions, and recurrent deep venous thrombosis).[3,12,22,28,32,38]

Anticardiolipin antibodies (ACA), the lupus anticoagulant (LAC), and antibodies responsible for the biologic false-positive test for syphilis are thought to be closely related members of a family of autoantibodies directed against phospholipids.[20] The lupus anticoagulant, first described by Conley and Hartmann in 1952,[12] defines a heterogeneous group of autoantibodies of the IgG or IgM class, thought to be present in approximately 5 to 10% of SLE patients,[7] but not specific for SLE.[5,40] Through their interactions with phospholipids, LAC inhibit the generation of the prothrombin activator complex in the clotting pathways, resulting in prolongation of phospholipid-dependent coagulation tests such as the activated partial thromboplastin time (APTT). Cardiolipin has been found to block the effects of LAC on the APTT,[17] and approximately 50

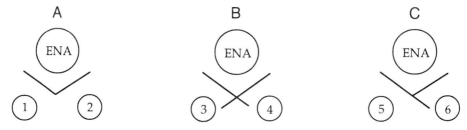

Fig. 11–4. A. Line of identity. The antibodies in wells 1 and 2 recognize the same antigenic determinants.
B. Line of non-identity. The antibodies in wells 3 and 4 recognize different antigenic determinants.
C. Line of partial identity. The antibodies in wells 5 and 6 react with some common antigenic determinants. Moreover, antibodies in well 5 react with antigenic determinants not recognized by the antibodies in well 6.

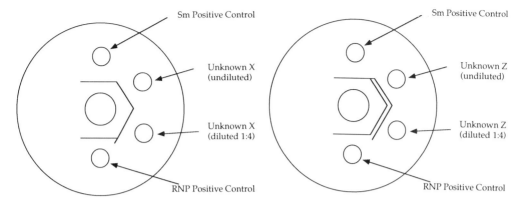

Fig. 11–5. Unknown X forms a line of identity with the Sm positive control, indicating that the serum contains Sm antibodies. At the same time serum X forms a line of partial identity (or spur) with the RNP positive control. This occurs because RNP antigen is always complexed with Sm. The RNP line is inhibited from crossing the Sm line. Free Sm molecules can penetrate the precipitin line to react with Sm antibodies, producing the spur.

to 70% of patients with antibodies to cardiolipin have detectable LAC.[22,24] In addition, approximately 30% of patients with LAC or ACA demonstrate a biologic false positive result in tests which employ a mixture of cardiolipin, lecithin, and cholesterol as antigen (e.g. VDRL, RPR).[23]

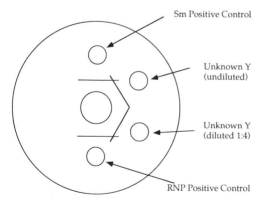

Fig. 11–6. Patient sample Y contains neither Sm nor RNP antibodies, indicated by the lines of nonidentity of serum Y with the precipitin lines of both the Sm and the RNP Positive Controls.

Fig. 11–7. Patient sample Z contains antibodies to both Sm and RNP, indicated by two precipitin lines, one forming a line of identity with the Sm positive control (outer line) and the other forming a line of identity with the RNP positive control (inner line). Moreover, as expected, the inner precipitin line forms a line of partial identity with the Sm positive control.

The presence of LAC and elevated titers of ACA have been correlated with an increased incidence of thrombosis, thrombocytopenia, and fetal loss in patients with SLE or SLE-like autoimmune disease.[2,4,22,24,28] These symptoms are collectively known as the antiphospholipid syndrome or the anticardiolipin syndrome.[3,29]

The most frequent clinical manifestation seen in patients with antiphospholipid antibodies is recurrent thrombosis, which occurs most commonly in the deep veins of the leg.[2,3] The pulmonary veins and cerebral arteries are also frequently affected, often resulting in pulmonary embolism and transient ischemic attacks or stroke, respectively.[2,12,32] Other sites that may be affected include renal veins, hepatic veins, retinal veins, and axillary veins.[2]

Several pathogenic mechanisms have been hypothesized to describe involvement of LAC and ACA in thrombotic events (reviewed in references 2, 3, 33, and 44). ACA and LAC may facilitate thrombosis by cross-reacting with phospholipid antigens present on endothelial cell membranes, thereby preventing the release of arachidonic acid, subsequently reducing prostacycline production, and promoting platelet aggregation.[1,9] Other proposed mechanisms involving antiphospholipid antibodies include inhibition of prekallikrein or plasminogen activator and subsequent reduction in fibrin clearance.[1,7,16,42] ACA and LAC may also interfere with feedback inhibition of coagulation by inhibiting thrombomodulin and the activation of protein C.[8,11]

Although thrombocytopenia is common in patients with antiphospholipid antibodies, hemorrhagic tendency is not usually seen unless the decrease in platelet count is severe or accompanied by another clotting defect.[2] Thrombocytopenia may result from cross-reaction of ACA and LAC with platelet phospholipids, promoting increased platelet destruction by the reticuloendothelial system.[23] The resulting increase in platelet adhesiveness could also contribute to thrombosis.[16]

Increased incidence of fetal distress and death is also frequently associated with the presence of LAC and high titers of ACA in pregnant women with SLE and women who have antinuclear antibodies but do not meet all the diagnostic criteria for SLE.[6,14,18,34] It has been proposed that ACA may play a role in this clinical outcome via the induction of decidual vasculopathy and placental infarction, or by reaction of the antibodies with a phospholipid antigen on the placenta, resulting in inhibition of placental growth and nutrient transport to the fetus.[6,15,34]

Measurement of ACA has been recommended for all pregnant women with SLE and patients with a history of recurrent fetal death.[3] Lockshin et al.[35] found detection of ACA by enzyme linked immunosorbent assay (ELISA) to be a better predictor of fetal death than the APTT. Measurement of ACA may thus be a valuable aid in monitoring pregnant women at increased risk for fetal death and assessing the need for therapies which may increase fetal salvage.[3,6,37] Some studies have indicated that thrombosis and fetal loss may occur more frequently in individuals with moderate to high titers of ACA, as compared to those with low ACA concentrations,[25,34] while other studies have not documented these correlations.[19,38,43] These findings underscore the need for an accurate, reliable method to measure ACA.

In 1983, Harris et al.[22] developed a radioimmunoassay to detect ACA. Since that time, a number of modifications to the assay have been introduced,[10,21] and ELISA methods have also been developed.[34,36,41] Because of the number of variables in methodology, there is a need for standardization in ACA testing, and an international workshop was held in 1986 to evaluate methods for detecting ACA.[26] This workshop, which included participants from 30 laboratories, found that diluents containing 10% fetal calf serum or 10% adult bovine serum were preferable in the assay, and that invalid results were obtained if phosphate buffered saline solution (PBS) alone, PBS-Tween, or 0.3% gelatin were used as diluent. The study also concluded that comparison of results from different laboratories would be facilitated if results were reported as "high," "medium," or "low" positive based on binding activity of the test samples as compared to that of the standards, rather than defining a specific cutoff point for positivity. When this method was used, the participating laboratories with valid assays were in agreement in their identification of high and medium positive samples; however, determination of borderline low values, or the distinction between "abnormal" and "normal" results, was more difficult. Accuracy and reproducibility may be improved with the use of standard samples covering a wide range of ACA concentrations; such samples are now available to investigators.[27] With improved standardization and identification of positive results, the clinical significance of anticardiolipin antibodies will likely become clearer in future years.

REFERENCES

1. Angles-Cano, E., Sultan, Y., and Clauvel, J.-P.: J. Clin. Lab. Med., *94*:312, 1979.

*2. Asherson, R.A., and Harris, E.N.: Postgrad. Med. J., 62:1081, 1986.

*3. Asherson, R.A., and Harris, E.N.: Intern. Med., 8:73, 1987.

4. Boey, M.L., et al.: Br. Med. J., 287:1021, 1983.

5. Boxer, M., Ellman, K., and Carvalho, A.: Arthritis Rheum., 19:1244, 1976.

6. Branch, D.W. et al.: N. Engl. J. Med., 313:1322, 1985.

7. Byron, M.A.: Clin. Rheum. Dis., 8:137, 1982.

8. Cariou, R. et al.: N. Engl. J. Med., 314:1193, 1986 (letter).

9. Carreras, L.O. et al.: Lancet, 1:244, 1981.

10. Colaco, C.B., and Male, D.K.: Clin. Exp. Immunol., 59:449, 1985.

11. Comp, P.C. et al.: Blood, 62 (Suppl. 1): 299, 1983.

12. Conley, C.L., and Hartmann, R.C.: J. Clin. Invest., 31:621, 1952 (abstr).

13. Coull, B.M. et al.: Stroke, 18:1107, 1987.

14. Derue, G.J. et al.: J. Obstet. Gynaecol., 5:207, 1985.

15. DeWolf, F. et al.: Am. J. Obstet. Gynecol., 142:829, 1982.

16. Elias, M., and Eldor, A.: Arch. Intern. Med., 144:510, 1984.

17. Exner, T. et al.: Pathology, 7:319, 1975.

18. Feinstein, D.I.: N. Engl. J. Med., 313:1348, 1985.

19. Fort, J.G. et al.: Arthritis Rheum., 30:752, 1987.

20. Getahun, B., and Hurtubise, P.E.: ASCP Check Sample Immunopathology No. IP 86-6. American Society of Clinical Pathologists, Chicago, 1986.

21. Gharavi, A.E. et al.: Ann. Rheum. Dis., 46:1, 1987.

22. Harris, E.N. et al.: Lancet, 2:1211, 1983.

23. Harris, E.N. et al.: Br. J. Haematol., 59:227, 1985.

24. Harris, E.N., Gharavi, A.E., and Hughes, G.R.V.: Clin. Rheum. Dis., 11:591, 1985.

25. Harris, E.N. et al.: Arch. Intern. Med., 146:2153, 1986.

26. Harris, E.N. et al.: Clin. Exp. Immunol., 68:215, 1987.

27. Harris, E.N., Gharavi, A.E., and Hughes, G.R.V.: Arthritis Rheum., 30:835, 1987, (letter).

28. Hughes, G.R.V.: Br Med. J., 287:1088, 1983.

29. Hughes, G.R.V.: Clin. Exp. Rheumatol., 3:285, 1985.

30. Hughes, G.R.V., Harris, E.N., and Gharavi, A.E.: J. Rheumatol., 13:486, 1986.

31. Lehninger, A.L.: Biochemistry, 2nd ed. New York, Worth Publishers, Inc., 1975.

32. Levine, S.R. et al.: Stroke, 18:1101, 1987.

33. Levine, S.R., and Welch, K.M.A.: Arch. Neurol., 44:876, 1987.

34. Lockshin, M.D. et al.: N. Engl. J. Med., 313:152, 1985.

35. Lockshin, M.D. et al.: J. Rheumatol., 14:259, 1987.

36. Loizou, S. et al.: Clin. Exp. Immunol., 62:738, 1985.

37. Lubbe, W.F. et al.: Br. J. Obstet. Gynaecol., 91:357, 1984.

38. Manoussakis, M.N. et al.: Clin. Immunol. Immunopathol., 44:297, 1987.

39. Ming, C.H.: Am. J. Obstet. Gynecol., 158:441, 1988.

40. Mueh, J.R., Herbst, K.D., and Rapaport, S.I.: Ann. Intern. Med., 92:156, 1980.

41. Petri, M. et al.: Ann. Intern. Med., 106:524, 1987.

42. Sanfelippo, M.J., and Drayna, C.J.: Am. J. Clin. Pathol., 77:275, 1982.

43. Sturfelt, G. et al.: Arthritis Rheum., 30:382, 1987.

44. Sukenik, S., El-Roeiy, A., and Shoenfeld, Y.: Acta Haemat., 76:86, 1986.

Anticardiolipin Antibodies by ELISA

PRINCIPLE. This enzyme-linked immunosorbent assay (ELISA) for the detection of anti-cardiolipin antibodies (ACA) uses commercially prepared microtiter plates coated with cardiolipin. Nonspecific binding is eliminated by blocking the plates with 10% fetal calf serum in phosphate buffered saline solution. Patient sera are diluted and added to the wells. Cardiolipin antibody antigen complexes are then detected by the addition of antihuman immunoglobulin conjugated to peroxidase, which acts on azino-benzthiazoline sulfonate to form a green reaction.

EQUIPMENT AND MATERIALS:

1. MALAKIT (SciMedx) anti-cardiolipin kit containing:

a. 1 microtiter plate coated with bovine cardiolipin. 12 strips of 8 wells each

b. Diluent, 10× concentration (20 ml)

c. Wash buffer, 10× concentration (50 ml)

d. Low positive control, lyophilized serum pool, (200 µl). Can be stored for 2 weeks at 4° C or longer at −20° C

e. Negative control, lyophilized serum pool, (200 µl). Can be stored for 2 weeks at 4° C or longer at −20° C.

f. Conjugate, antitotal immunoglobulin linked to peroxidase, 100× concentration, (300 µl). Working dilution should be prepared just before use

g. Substrate, azino-benzthiazoline sulfonate (12 ml). If crystallized, the precipitate should be redissolved in 37° C water bath

h. Fixator solution (3 ml)

2. 10 μl, 100 μl and 1 ml pipettes

3. Distilled water

4. Absorbent paper

5. Moisture chamber

6. 37° C incubator

7. Microtiter plate washer

8. Microtiter plate spectrophotometer with 405 nm filter

SPECIMEN COLLECTION AND PREPARATION. Fresh or frozen serum or plasma may be used; no significant differences have been noted between the two.

The samples must be completely free of all platelet debris. Fixation of anticardiolipin antibodies to the platelet surface could diminish final values.

Inactivation of serum complement does not affect assay performance.

PROCEDURE

1. Make a 1:10 working dilution of diluent using 9 ml of distilled water.

2. Make a 1:10 working dilution of wash buffer using 36 ml of distilled water.

3. Reconstitute positive and negative controls with 200 μl of distilled water.

4. Dilute controls and patient sera by adding 10 μl of sample to 1 ml of diluent buffer.

5. For each run, include a reagent blank well, negative control well and positive control well.

6. Fill each well with 100 μl of control or sample.

7. Fill the reagent blank well with 100 μl of diluent buffer.

8. Incubate the wells at 37° C in a moist chamber for 1 hour.

9. Empty wells and wash three times with wash buffer using 200 μl per well.

10. Blot on absorbent paper.

11. Make an approximate 1:100 working dilution of conjugate by adding 10 μl to 1 ml of dilution buffer.

12. Fill each well with 100 μl of working dilution conjugate.

13. Incubate at 37° C in a moist chamber for 1 hour.

14. Repeat steps 9 and 10.

15. Fill each well with 100 μl of substrate as supplied by the manufacturer.

16. Incubate at 37° C in a moist chamber for 30 minutes.

17. Stop the reaction by the addition of 20 μl of fixator to each well.

18. Blank the instrument using the reagent blank well.

19. Read the plate on a microtiter plate spectrophotometer, set at 405 nm.

REPORTING. Patient and control results are reported as negative, low positive or high positive for cardiolipin antibodies.

INTERPRETATION OF RESULTS

Negative control: O.D. (as stated on bottle) corresponding to value for pool of normal patients.

Positive control: O.D. (as stated on bottle) corresponding to value for pool of patients with low level of anti-cardiolipin antibody.

Patient values: An O.D. equal to or less than the negative control indicates normal amounts of anti-cardiolipin antibody present. An O.D. between the negative and the low positive control indicates a LOW anticardiolipin antibody level. An O.D. greater than the low positive control indicates HIGH level of anti-cardiolipin antibody.

REFERENCE

1. Package insert, MALAKIT cardiolipin, Sci-Medx, Denville, NJ, 1988.

COLD AGGLUTININS

By definition, cold agglutinins are cold-reacting, autoimmune antibodies that are directed against antigens found on the membrane of red blood cells. Cold agglutinating antibodies attach to antigenic sites when temperatures are decreased, and can be eluted, or returned to solution, by warming. Like other antibodies, they are synthesized by B lymphocytes. Cold agglutinins are referred to as polyclonal if produced by a heterogeneous population of B cells; monoclonal if produced by a homogeneous or monoclonal B cell line.

Classification of cold agglutinins may be based on immunoglobulin class or by the antigen with which they react. The majority of cold agglutinating autoantibodies are composed of Mu heavy chains and kappa light chains,[9,12,14,56] and are thus designated IgMκ. IgM molecules with lambda light chains (IgMλ) are common within polyclonal cold agglutinins, albeit not as common as might be expected.[55] Monoclonal IgMλ occur,[20,23,24,30] but are usually atypical in their antigenic determinants,[30] physical properties[20,23] and/or the severity of associated disease (see below).[20] Homogeneous IgA cold agglutinins occur,[1,31] but are rare. Mixed cold agglutination activity has been described, consisting of both IgM and IgG antibody.[2,10]

Most cold agglutinins react with the I/i blood group antigens found on erythrocytes, lymphocytes, polymorphonuclear leukocytes (PMNs), mononuclear phagocytes, and platelets.[26] The I/i antigens are glycolipid molecules if produced by erythrocytes, or glycoprotein if secreted by cells into body fluids and adsorbed onto the red cell surface.[26] Erythrocytes in newborns are rich in i antigen. From birth, conversion to I antigen on the cell progresses until adult levels with predominately I antigen are reached at about 18 months of age.[31] Although both I and i are demonstrable on newborn and adult cells, the relative concentrations are vastly different. I/i antigens are complex and have multiple antigenic determinants, as defined by anti-I/anti-i antibodies.[8,26]

In combination with complement from non-human sources, cold agglutinins with anti-I or anti-i specificity are toxic to lymphocytes[28,45] and to polymophonuclear and mononuclear phagocytes.[26,29] Interaction of cold agglutinins, particularly anti-I, with antigen or erythrocytes and complement also induces complement activation. The thermal amplitude, or the highest temperature at which the antibody reacts with its antigen, is an important factor in the interaction of antibody, complement, and red cells in vivo.[26,42] As the majority of cold agglutinins are IgM, they are effective complement activators once attached to antigen, but the hemolytic action of complement depends on the existing plasma complement levels, the number of activation sites available on the cells, the temperatures, and the

competitive adherence of C3b-coated cells to phagocytes in the liver and spleen.[7] Coated cells may be phagocytized, or may be freed by the breakdown of C_3b, releasing cells coated with the C_3d fragment into circulation. C_3d-coated red cells are resistant to cold agglutinin/complement mediated hemolysis, as well as to phagocytosis.[7]

Rarely, cold agglutinating autoantibodies are described with specificities other than anti-I/anti-i; examples are anti-P;[5,53] anti-BI,[4] anti-A_1,[30,40] anti-M,[15] anti-1H,[41,51] and others.[33]

In 1979, Roelcke et al.[36] described two IgM autoantibodies that agglutinated red blood cells in cold temperatures only after the cells were pretreated with proteolytic enzymes. This was the first of many "cryptic membranous antigens"[25] to be reported; a new type of cold agglutinin. Cryptic antigens may be unveiled by treatment of erythrocytes with proteases (e.g. papain) or with neuraminidase (NANA). The effects of such pretreatment on the red cells results in altered I/i antigens (I_{cr}, i_{cr}), as well as other apparently distinct antigens, designated Pr[38] (Pr_1, Pr_2, Pr_3, Pr_a),[32,33,35,39] Gd,[48] and others.[37,49] Antibodies to cryptic antigens comprise a small proportion of reportable cold agglutinins,[27,48] and appear capable of causing clinical disease,[27,36] albeit rarely.[6] In addition to detection of antibody by agglutination of treated cells, anti-cryptic antibodies may be demonstrated by immunofluorescence.[55]

Because of the method used to define cryptic antigens, differentiation from T antigens is necessary. Called "human carcinoma-associated precursor antigens,"[47] T antigens, with Tn, are immediate precursors of the M and N antigens of the MNSsU blood group system.[18] First described as the Thomson-Friedenreich phenomenon, T antigens can be exposed by bacterial, as well as experimental, neuraminidase,[11] inducing panagglutination of red cells by the anti-T found as an isoagglutinin in all human sera.[47] Greater than 90% of anti-T is IgM,[18] and thermodependent (i.e. cold agglutinating) activity is often present.[18,27] Anti-T occurs in low titers in normals. Polyclonal titers may increase in atypical pneumonia and liver cirrhosis.[18] Anti-T has not been described as a monoclonal protein.

Anti-T can be definitely differentiated from antibodies to cryptic antigens;[27,34] however, such differentiation is not usually performed in clinical situations.

Cold agglutinins may occur in asymptomatic individuals, or may induce hemolytic anemia and/or obstruction of microcirculation due to in vivo interaction with antigen and complement. A role for the antibody in thrombocytopenia and leukopenia has also been speculated.[2]

Polyclonal, or heterogeneous cold agglutinins are transient, arising in conjunction with certain infectious and autoimmune disorders,[26,27] most notably *Mycoplasma pneumoniae* infection (anti-I)[46] and infectious mononucleosis (anti-i).[17,22] Polyclonal cold agglutinins exhibit broad-banded electrophoretic patterns on total protein electrophoresis, indicating heterogeneous populations of IgM and occasionally IgG.[2,50] Titers characteristically rise during the second or third week of illness and may reach 8000 before dropping rapidly to normal levels. Clinical symptoms are temperature-dependent, and usually restricted to pallor or cyanosis of peripheral body parts. Occasionally, hemolytic episodes are observed.

Persistent polyclonal cold-agglutinating antibodies have been described in persons infected with human immunodeficiency virus (HIV).[25]

Homogeneous persistent cold agglutinins are detected primarily in that small percentage[19,41] of lymphoproliferative disorders wherein the proliferating cell represents a mature, antibody-producing B or plasma cell which happens to be producing an autoantibody with cold agglutinating activity.[44] Thus, in diseases such as Waldenström's macroglobulinemia, reticulosarcoma, B cell lymphomas, B cell chronic lymphocytic leukemia (CLL), lymphosarcoma, Hodgkin's disease, plasmacytoma,

and Kaposi's sarcoma, symptoms and pathology of the primary disease may be complicated by the presence of cold agglutinating antibody. Reticulosarcoma, more often than others, is associated with atypical cold agglutinins as determined by immunoglobulin class or by antigenic determinant.[23,24] If the antibody produced in any of the above disorders is an IgMλ, rather than the typical IgMκ, a more aggressive primary disease is usually observed.[20,23]

Three classic disease entities have primary symptoms that arise directly from the presence of cold-reacting antibodies. *Chronic cold agglutinin disease* (CCAD),[16] also known as *chronic hemagglutinin disease* (CHAD), is characterized by high titers of cold agglutinins which do not vary with time. Cold intolerance and chronic and/or acute onset hemolytic anemia are usual symptoms. Although titers of 1×10^6 are common,[21] low titer cold agglutinins have also been implicated in disease.[42,50] Cold intolerance usually manifests as Raynaud's phenomenon,[13] although acrocyanosis secondary to intravascular agglutination may also be present.[7] The hemolytic anemia associated with CCAD is most often chronic, occurring independent of significant cold exposure. In addition to detectable cold agglutinins, laboratory findings include anemia of varying degree, polychromasia with variable numbers of spherocytes, positive direct Coomb's tests, and, often, decreased complement levels. The monoclonal cold agglutinin often appears as an abnormal peak on total protein electrophoresis.[3,43] A small percentage[24] of patients with CCAD also have cryoprecipitate,[19,20,24] and Bence-Jones protein is present, although in low concentrations, in most.[19]

A second disease where cold-reacting antibody relates directly to primary symptoms is the form of autoimmune hemolytic anemia known as *cold antibody hemolytic anemia* (AIHA:CAHA).[31] IgM antibodies, usually with anti-I activity, are most commonly found.[52]

Paroxysmal cold hemoglobinuria is caused by a biphasic antibody known as the Donath-Landsteiner antibody. The antibody reacts with P antigen in cold temperatures, initiating complement activation, which induces cell lysis as the temperature rises.[5]

REFERENCES

1. Angevine, C.D., Anderson, B.R., and Barnett, E.V.: J. Immunol., *96*:578, 1966.
2. Capra, J.D., Dowling, P., Cook, S., and Kunkel, H.C.: Vox Sang., *16*:10, 1969.
3. Christensen, W.N., Dacie, J.V., Croucher, B.E.E., and Charlwood, P.A.: Br. J. Haematol., *3*:262, 1957.
4. Dodds, A.J., Klarkowski, D., Cooper, D.A., and Isbister, J.P.: Am. J. Clin. Pathol., *71*:473, 1979.
5. Donath, J., and Lansteiner, K.: Munch. Med. Wochenschr., *51*:1590, 1904.
6. Dybkjaer, E., and Kissmeyer-Nielson, F.: Vox Sang., *12*:429, 1967.
7. Evans, R.S., Turner, E., Bingham, M., and Woods, R.: J. Clin. Invest., *47*:691, 1968.
8. Feizi, T.: Immunol. Commun., *10*:127, 1981.
9. Feizi, T.: Science, *156*:1111, 1967.
10. Goldberg, L.S., and Barnett, E.V.: J. Immunol., *99*:803, 1967.
11. Gray, J.M., Beck, M.L., and Oberman, H.A.: Vox Sang., *22*:379, 1972.
12. Harboe, M., and Lind, K.: Scand. J. Haematol., *3*:269, 1966.
13. Harboe, M., and Torsvik, H.: Scand. J. Haematol., *6*:416, 1969.
14. Harboe, M. et al.: Scand. J. Haematol., *2*:259, 1965.
15. Hysell, J.K., Beck, M.L., and Gray, J.M.: Transfusion, *13*:146, 1973.
16. Iwai, S., and Mei-Sai, N.: Jpn. Med. World, *5*:119, 1925.
17. Jenkins, W.J., Koster, H.G., Marsh, W.L., and Carter, R.L.: Br. J. Haematol., *11*:480, 1965.
18. Kim, Y.D., Prakash, U., Weber, G.T., and Hargie, M.: Immunol. Com., *8*:397, 1979.
19. Krajny, M., and Pruzanski, W.: Can. Med. Assoc. J., *114*:899, 1976.
20. Kuenn, J.W., Weber, R., Teague, P.O., and Keitt, A.S.: Cancer, *42*:1826, 1978.
21. Macris, N. et al.: Am. J. Med., *48*:524, 1970.
22. Marsh, W.L., and Jenkins, W.J.: Nature, *188*:753, 1960.
23. Pascali, E., Pezzoli, A., Melato, M., and Falconieri, G.: Acta Haematol., *64*:94, 1980.
24. Pruzanski, W., Cowan, D.H., and Parr, D.: Clin. Immunol. Immunopathol., *2*:234, 1974.
25. Pruzanski, W., Roelcke, D., Donnelly, E., and Lui, L.C.: Acta Haematol. (Basel), *75*:171, 1986.
26. Pruzanski, W., and Shumak, K.: N. Engl. J. Med., *297*:538, 1977.
27. Pruzanski, W. et al.: Am. J. Hematol., *26*:167, 1987.
28. Pruzanski, W. et al.: Clin. Immunol. Immunopathol., *4*:248, 1975.
29. Pruzanski, W., Farid, N., Keystone, E., and Armstrong, M.: Clin. Immunol. Immunopathol., *4*:277, 1975.
30. Rochant, H. et al.: Vox Sang., *22*:45, 1972.
31. Roelcke, D.: Clin. Immunol. Immunopathol., *2*:266, 1974.
32. Roelcke, D.: Eur. J. Immunol., *3*:206, 1973.
33. Roelcke, D., Dahr, W., and Kalden, J.R.: Vox Sang., *51*:207, 1986.
34. Roelcke, D., Ebert, W., and Anstee, D.J.: Vox Sang., *27*:429, 1974.
35. Roelcke, D., Ebert, W., and Geisen, H.P.: Vox Sang., *30*:122, 1976.
36. Roelcke, D., Meiser, R.J., and Brucher, H.: Blut, *39*:217, 1979.
37. Roelcke, D., Riesen, W., Geisen, H.P., and Ebert, W.: Vox Sang., *33*:304, 1977.
38. Roelcke, D., and Uhlenbruck, G.: Vox Sang., *18*:478, 1970.
39. Roelcke, D. et al.: Vox. Sang., *20*:218, 1971.
40. Rochant, H. et al.: Vox. Sang., *1*:45, 1972.
41. Sandhaus, L.M., Raska, K., Jr., and Wu, H.V.: Am. J. Clin. Pathol., *86*:120, 1986.
42. Schreiber, A.D., Herskovitz, B.S., and Goldwein, M.: N. Engl. J. Med., *296*:1490, 1977.
43. Schubothe, H.: Schweiz. Med. Wochenschr., *84*:1109, 1954.
44. Seligmann, M., and Brouet, J.C.: Semin. Hematol., *10*:163, 1973.
45. Shumak, K.H., Rachkewich, R.A., Crookston, M.C., and Crookston, J.H.: Nature, *231*:148, 1971.
46. Spigam, C.L., and Jones, J.P.: Arch. Intern. Med., *76*:75, 1945.
47. Springer, G.F. et al.: Prog. Allergy, *26*:42, 1979.
48. Staub, C.A.: Transfusion, *25*:414, 1985.
49. Suzuki, S.: Nippon Ketsueki Gakkai Zasshi, *48*:1074, 1985.
50. Szymanski, I.O., Teno, R., and Rybak, M.E.: Vox. Sang., *51*:112, 1986.
51. Uchikawa, M., and Tohyama, H.: Transfusion, *26*:240, 1986.
52. VanLoghem, J.J. et al.: Vox. Sang., *7*:214, 1962.
53. Vondem Borne, A.E.G. et al.: Br. J. Haematol., *50*:345, 1982.
54. Weiner, A.S., Unger, L.J., Cohen, L., and Feldman, J.: Ann. Intern. Mcd., *44*:221, 1956.
55. Winchester, R.J., Fu, S.M., Winfield, J.B., and Kunkel, H.G.: J. Immunol., *114*:410, 1975.
56. Worlledge, S.M., and Blajchman, M.A.: Br. J. Haematol., *23*(Suppl.):61, 1972.

Cold Agglutinins Test

PRINCIPLE. Dilutions of patient serum are reacted with human type O red blood cells at refrigerator temperatures. Cold agglutinins, if present, react with antigens found on adult human red blood cells, and agglutinate the cells.

EQUIPMENT AND MATERIALS

1. Refrigerator at 4° C
2. 37° C water bath

3. 13 × 100 mm test tubes

4. 2 ml and 0.5 ml serologic pipets

5. 0.9% (w/v) sodium chloride

6. Erythrocytes: Human type O blood in versene or other suitable anticoagulant. Day-old blood is used to prepare erythrocyte suspension, which can be kept at 4° C for 2 days after preparation. Erythrocytes from certain group O donors may agglutinate more readily than others, so pooled O cells are desirable and/or care should be taken that control titers do not vary more than a twofold dilution from day-to-day

7. Serum: All serum or plasma should be free of hemolysis and need not be inactivated. Serum separated from the clot may be stored frozen (−20° C) until use. Avoid repeated freezing and thawing

8. Control Serum: Pooled sera of known titer may be prepared by adding a known serum containing high cold agglutinating antibody levels to a pool of 'normal' serum, with the resulting pool assayed and adjusted to a titer of 128 to 256. Test to ensure the pool is HBsAg and HIV negative. Freeze in 0.5 ml aliquots at −70° C. May be used as long as proper reactivity is maintained. Run in parallel with the old control for at least 10 runs before placing in routine use

SPECIMEN COLLECTION AND PREPARATION. *Blood must be at least as warm as room temperature before separating serum or plasma from cells.* Refrigerated blood can be eluted by placing in 37° C waterbath until completely warmed; up to 1 hour for 7 ml clot tubes, shorter for smaller amounts.

PROCEDURE

1. Wash human type O cells at least three times in saline solution. Add 0.2 ml of packed cells to saline solution in a 100 ml volumetric flask and qs to 100 ml with saline solution to make a 0.2% suspension. (Different volumes may be prepared as long as the suspension is 0.2% O cells.)

2. Set up one row of eight 13 × 100 mm tubes for each serum and control to be tested.

3. Add 0.6 ml of saline solution to tube 1 and 0.4 ml to tubes 2 to 8.

4. Add 0.2 ml of positive control to the first tube of Row 1. Mix and transfer 0.4 ml through tube 7. Discard 0.4 ml from tube 7.

5. Tube 8 serves as a negative control. For the patient(s), add 0.2 ml of serum or plasma to the first tube of the appropriate row. Mix and transfer 0.4 ml through tube 8. Remove 0.4 ml from tube 8 and discard it.

6. Add 0.4 ml of "O" cell suspension to each tube. The final dilutions are 1:8, 1:16, 1:32, etc.

7. Incubate in refrigerator overnight.

8. Read *immediately* after taking from refrigerator, as any warming may cause a decrease in titer of a cold agglutinin. The titer is the reciprocal of the last dilution showing definite agglutination. The positive control must read ± one tube from the assayed titer and the negative control must be negative for the run to be accepted. Record and initial control results.

9. Any agglutination observed must be warmed in a 37° C waterbath and allowed to elute before being reported as a cold agglutinating antibody (a few seconds is usually sufficient for elution to occur). Any sera which cause agglutination that does *not* elute at 37° C are referred to the blood bank for further testing.

REPORTING. The titer is reported as the reciprocal of the last tube with agglutination which is reversible upon warming. Titers in which no agglutination is observed are reported as negative.

INTERPRETATION OF RESULTS. A titer of less than 64 may be seen in normal healthy people. Higher titers may be indicative of a variety of disease states.[3]

In diagnosing *M. pneumoniae,* the most significant finding is a fourfold rise or fall in titer associated with clinical symptoms. Paired specimens should be taken 1 to 2 weeks apart and, wherever possible, run simultaneously using the same red blood cells. Cold agglutinins exceed a titer of 64 on initial testing of approximately 61% of patients with *M. pneumoniae* infection.[3]

REFERENCES

1. Adinolfi, M.: Immunology, *9*:43, 1965.
2. Department of the Army Technical Manual: Laboratory Procedures in Clinical Serology. Washington, D.C., U.S. Government Printing Office, 1960.
3. Felber, N.: Postgrad. Med., *60*:89, 1976.
4. Spigam, C.L., and Jones, J.P.: Arch. Intern. Med., *76*:75, 1945.

CRYOGLOBULINS

Cryoglobulins, as the term implies, are immunoglobulins that precipitate reversibly at lowered temperatures. First described by Wintrobe and Buell in a patient with multiple myeloma,[24] cryoglobulins usually appear in cooled serum as dense flocculates, but may be crystalline or gelatinous in nature. Although most authors describe these proteins quantitatively, in grams per deciliter (g/dl), clinical laboratories are likely to express them as percent of total volume, as determined by the observation of precipitate in refrigerated serum in Wintrobe tubes (cryocrit method).[8] The temperature at which precipitation occurs varies; however, in general, the presence of higher protein concentrations in a sample increases the temperature at which cryoglobulin insolubility occurs.[16,22]

Separation of cryoglobulins from other precipitating plasma proteins,[8,16,22] e.g. fibrinogen, is accomplished by the use of serum rather than plasma for testing.

The term *cryoglobulinemia* refers to those pathologic conditions invoked by the presence of circulating cryoglobulins. Large amounts of cryoglobulin can be present without related symptoms in some individuals,[8,16] while relatively small concentrations in others may induce disease.[8] Cryoglobulins have been described in an ever increasing list of diseases,[5,7,22] most notably lymphoproliferative or autoimmune disorders; however, idiopathic cryoglobulins account for approximately 30% of cases.[5]

Cryoglobulins are classified[5] into three types on the basis of their composition. Up to one-third of cases described[5,8] are *Type I* or *monoclonal cryoglobulins,* comprised of a single homogeneous protein. Although many of these are associated with lymphoproliferative disorders such as multiple myeloma or Waldenström's macroglobulinemia, idiopathic, nonmalignant monoclonal cryoglobulinemia (NCG) accounts for a small number of cases.[20]

Types II and III are classified as mixed cryoproteins. *Type II,* or *mixed cryoglobulins,* are composed of a monoclonal component, usually IgM, which exhibits rheumatoid factor antibody activity toward, and is present in

association with, a polyclonal IgG component. Although often seen in collagen-vascular diseases, about 50%[15] of Type II cryoglobulins are idiopathic, designated *essential mixed cryoglobulinema* (EMC). *Type III,* or *polyclonal cryoglobulins,* include all mixed cryoglobulins which lack a monoclonal component, and thus are polyclonal and heterogeneous in nature.

Monoclonal cryoglobulins, whether idiopathic or associated with hematopoietic disease, are usually IgM or IgG, rarely IgA, and on occasion, may be Bence-Jones protein.[3,8] Roughly 5% of myeloma proteins and 7% of paraproteins associated with Waldenström's macroglobulinemia are cryoglobulins.[16] Self-association and polymerization of the molecules occur on cold exposure, and may induce partial or complete occlusion of small blood vessels, with or without accompanying vasculitis.[20] Symptoms are variable, but may include hyperviscosity, cold urticaria, Raynaud's phenomenon, purpura, cutaneous vasculitis with or without ulceration, or retinal hemorrhage.[8,16] Monoclonal cryoglobulins have unique structural and serologic properties which distinguish them from normal or myelomatous immunoglobulin.[1,3,5] Data show that build up of circulating cryoglobulin is probably because of increased synthesis rather than lack of ability to catabolize.[2]

Idiopathic, nonmalignant monoclonal cryoglobulinemia may be related to a c-myc protooncogene rearrangement,[20] which may, in turn, relate to the clonal expansion and high rate of synthesis of cryoglobulin in nonmalignant B cells.

Type II mixed cryoglobulins[19] may appear without symptoms, but more often induce purpura, weakness, and arthralgia. Hepato- and splenomegaly are quite common, and liver function abnormalities are frequently noted.[8] Approximately half of cases exhibit nephritis which may be mild and reversible, but is often progressive.[8] The monoclonal component characteristic of Type II cryoglobulins is usually IgM with kappa light chains.[7,8,13,23] Some authors argue that its appearance is a result of an otherwise undetected lymphoproliferative disorder;[7] others see it as a highly restricted immune response to as yet undefined antigens.[7,8,15] IgG or IgA monoclonal components have also been described.[5]

Antibody activity against polyclonal IgG (i.e. rheumatoid factor activity) is characteristic of virtually all of the monoclonal constituents of Type II cryoglobulins described. Occasionally, antibody activity toward another antigen has been demonstrated within cryoprecipitate,[7,8,10,14] presumably a result of the specificity of captured IgG.

Early complement components, e.g. C_2, are severely depleted in mixed cryoglobulinemia,[6,7,21,22] and patients may appear deficient in C_1 esterase inhibitor.[6,22] Later components such as C_6 and C_9 are most often normal or slightly increased. Moderate hypergammaglobulinemia may be present, but monoclonal spikes are usually absent on serum protein electrophoresis.[6]

Essential mixed cryoglobulinemia, or EMC, is slightly more common in females than males,[7,22] with onset generally during the third or fourth decade of life. The incidence of severe disease varies with geographic area, occurring more frequently in the latin countries of southern Europe.[7] The clinical picture of EMC[15] is typical for mixed cryoglobulins, with recurrent palpable purpura, polyarthralgias, and renal disease. Hepatic dysfunction, ranging from minimal involvement to chronic active hepatitis or cirrhosis, is seen in most patients.

Renal and dermal involvement in cryoglobulinemia appears to be the result of immune complex formation.[7,9,10,15,22] In one study, complexes were demonstrable in normal appearing skin of most EMC patients,[9] and subendothelial deposits of immunoglobulin and complement are usually detectable in the kidney.[10,15,22] The high concentration of protein in glomerular capillaries, induced by the natural filtration process, may enhance localized precipitation,[7,22] leading to interluminal thrombi.[22]

Cryoprecipitation in the area triggers the accumulation of massive numbers of activated macrophages which may act as scavengers and also mediate local damage via liberation of certain monokines.[7] The presence of monocytes and/or their products may contribute to the glomerular cell proliferation, which is almost always present in this disease.[22] Symptomatic glomerulonephritis may take two forms:[7] (1) recurrent, time-limited episodes of cryoprecipitation in the glomeruli may induce acute nephrotic syndrome and/or mesangial sclerosis and (2) progressive impairment of renal function may result from chronic deposition of cryoglobulin on glomerular basement membrane. Survival rates for EMC are best if the kidneys are not involved; however, prognosis, even for patients experiencing acute renal failure or acute nephrotic syndrome is not always dire.[22]

Treatment for EMC has involved plasma exchange, steroids, and the use of cytotoxic drugs, with early and rapid symptomatic relief in some cases,[18] and measured success in others.[7] Clinical trials with alpha interferon have also been attempted.[4]

Association of EMC with hepatitis B virus (HBV) has been debated,[11,12,17,22] and, more recently, EMC has been linked to Epstein-Barr virus.[7]

Polyclonal mixed cryoglobulins (Type III) account for many of the cryoglobulins detected;[5] however, many of these are found in low concentrations, and/or are associated with infections which, when resolved, are reflected in disappearance of the precipitating protein.[25]

REFERENCES

1. Abraham, G.N., Podell, D.N., Welch, E.H., and Johnston, S.L.: Immunology, 48:315, 1983.
2. Abraham, G.N., Waterhouse, C., and Condemi, J.J.: Clin. Exp. Immunol., 35:89, 1979.
3. Abraham, G.N. et al.: Clin. Exp. Immunol., 36:63, 1979.
4. Bonomo, L., Casato, M., and Afeltra, A.: Am. J. Med., 83:726, 1987.
5. Brouet, J.C. et al.: Am. J. Med., 57:775, 1974.
6. Casali, P. et al.: Acta Hematol., 59:277, 1978.

7. D'Amico, G. et al.: Adv. Nephrol., *17*:219, 1988.

8. Franklin, E.C.: J. Allergy Clin. Immunol., *66*:269, 1980.

9. Gabrielli, A. et al.: Arthritis Rheum., *30*:884, 1987.

10. Gamble, C.N., Kimchi, A., Depner, T.A., and Christensen, D.: Am. J. Clin. Pathol., *77*:347, 1982.

11. Garcia-Bragado, F., and Ercilla, G.: Arthritis Rheum., *30*:1440, 1987.

12. Garcia-Bragado, F. et al.: N. Engl. J. Med., *312*:187, 1985.

13. Geltner, D., Franklin, E.C., and Frangione, B.: J. Immunol., *125*:1530, 1980.

14. Goldman, M. et al.: Arthritis Rheum., *30*:1318, 1987.

15. Gorevic, P.D. et al.: Am. J. Med., *69*:287, 1980.

16. Grey, H.H., and Kohler, P.F.: Semin. Hematol., *10*:87, 1973.

17. Levo, Y. et al.: N. Engl. J. Med., *296*:1501, 1977.

18. Lockwood, C.M. et al.: Lancet, *1*:63, 1977.

19. Meltzer, M., and Franklin, E.C.: Am. J. Med., *40*:828, 1966.

20. Perl, A. et al.: J. Immunol., *139*:3512, 1987.

21. Reithmuller, G., Meltzer, M., Franklin, E.C., and Miescher, P.A.: Clin. Exp. Immunol., *1*:337, 1966.

22. Tarantino, A. et al.: Q. J. Med., *50*:1, 1981.

23. Williams, J.M., Gorenic, P.D., and Looney, R.J.: Immunology, *62*:529, 1987.

24. Wintrobe, M.M., and Buell, M.V.: Bull. Johns Hopkins Hosp., *52*:156, 1933.

25. Yrivarren, J.L., and Lopez, L.R.: J. Clin. Immunol., *7*:471, 1987.

Cryoglobulin Determination

PRINCIPLE. Sera suspected of containing cryoglobulins are incubated at refrigerator temperatures. Precipitated cryoglobulins are quantitated in percent of total volume, and, if applicable, assayed to determine their composition.

EQUIPMENT AND MATERIALS

1. Wintrobe hematocrit tubes—two per patient

2. 9" pasteur pipets

3. Refrigerator

4. Refrigerated centrifuge

5. 37° C water bath

6. Patient Serum: *Blood is collected and allowed to clot at 37° C. Blood for cryoglobulin determinations must not be refrigerated before testing.* Serum should be used immediately.

SPECIMEN COLLECTION AND PREPARATION. Blood is collected by routine venipuncture and put into a tube containing no anticoagulants. The tube should be kept warm (at least 37° C) and transported to the laboratory as soon as possible. If the sample has been refrigerated, it is not suitable for testing, as cryoglobulins in refrigerated whole blood may precipitate prior to serum separation.

PROCEDURE

NOTE: There is no control run with this procedure.

1. Allow blood to clot for at least 1 hour at room temperature, preferably at 37° C.

2. Centrifuge at room temperature.

3. Remove serum with a 9" pasteur pipet and fill two Wintrobe tubes to the 10 mark, taking care to avoid all cells and fibrin. Filling Wintrobe tubes from the bottom prevents air bubbles, which must be avoided. Label carrier tubes with the patient's name, the date, and the time of refrigeration.

4. Refrigerate and observe every 24 hours for at least 3 days; or until precipitate is noted. Precipitates observed at 24 hours should be allowed to incubate an additional day to ensure complete precipitation.

5. If precipitate is observed, centrifuge at 4° C for 30 minutes at 2000 rpm. Observe percent of cryoglobulin (v/v). Record cryoglobulins of ≤1% as "trace" on the computer sheets. If >1%, perform the following:

   a. Warm one of the tubes at 37° C for at least 30 minutes to dissolve precipitate.

    (1) If precipitate does not dissolve, report estimated percentage.

    (2) If precipitate does dissolve, proceed with the following:

     (a) Remove other tube from refrigerator.

     (b) Centrifuge at 4° C, 2000 rpm for 30 minutes.

     (c) Remove supernatant and discard. Wash the precipitate three times in cold saline solution.

     (d) Resuspend precipitate in 1 ml warm saline solution. Warm in 37° C water bath if necessary, to completely resuspend.

     (e) Run protein electrophoresis on half of the cryoglobulin suspension.

     (f) Run immunofixation electrophoresis on the remainder of the precipitate suspension. (See *Immunofixation Electrophoresis (IFE)*).

6. If no precipitate is observed after 3 days, record as negative for cryoglobulins.

RESULTS. Results are reported as negative, trace, or % present. Immunofixation electrophoresis results are reported as to protein composition.

INTERPRETATION OF RESULTS. Cryoglobulins of greater than 1% occur in a variety of disease states, including monoclonal malignant disorders such as Waldenström's macroglobulinemia and in the rheumatic diseases such as rheumatoid arthritis. Cryoglobulins of less than 1% may be considered normal.

LIMITATIONS OF THE PROCEDURE

1. Excessive fibrin will appear as strands throughout the Wintrobe tube and could interfere with the reading or be incorrectly interpreted as positive.

2. Testing on refrigerated whole blood can give false-negative results.

AUTOIMMUNE THYROIDITIS

The thyroid gland is located in the anterior region of the neck, where it is bound firmly to the trachea, covering the second, third, and fourth tracheal rings. The fundamental functional and structural unit of the thyroid, the follicle, is a spherical entity lined by cuboidal epithelial cells and surrounded by a rich capillary and lymphatic network.

Within each follicle is found the substance known as colloid, whose primary constituent, thyroglobulin (Tg), is comprised of the thyroid hormones triiodothyronine (T_3) and thyroxine (T_4).

Secretion of the thyroid hormones is initiated by the hypothalamus gland production of thyrotropin-releasing hormone (TRH), which acts on the pituitary, inducing the release of thyroid-stimulating hormone (TSH, thyrotropin). TSH, in turn, bind to receptors (TSH receptors) on the cell membrane of the thyroid gland, causing the breakdown of thyroglobulin into secretable hormones.

TRH ———————→ TSH
(Hypothalamus)   (Pituitary)
                         |
                         ↓
                    Thyroid hormones (Thyroid)

Autoimmune thyroid diseases (autoimmune thyroiditis) are examples of both organ-specific autoimmunity and autoimmune endocrinopathy.[54] As such, they are diseases of the thyroid that exhibit evidence of humoral and/or cell mediated immune responsiveness to constituents of the organ. Among the many disorders of the thyroid are two that are considered autoimmune: *Graves' disease* (also known as diffuse toxic goiter, hyperthyroidism, and thyrotoxicosis), and *Hashimoto's thyroiditis* (also known as chronic lymphocytic thyroiditis). A third disease, *primary adult myxedema* (also known as autoimmune atrophic thyroiditis or primary hypothyroidism) may also be autoimmune in nature.[53] In general, the generation of autoimmune disease can be divided into two stages: (1) an initiation stage where development of autoantibodies and autoreactive cells takes place and (2), development of tissue damage as a result of immune reactions.[12] Many of the defects described below are seen in patients with normal thyroid ("euthyroid") or with thyroid diseases not considered to be autoimmune. In some cases, the presence of autoreactivity may herald the initiation of autoimmune disease;[23] in others, no such progression is observable.

Autoimmune thyroid diseases have some immune abnormalities in common. Lymphocytes from the majority of these patients can be induced to undergo blastogenesis by the addition of thyroglobulin to cell culture.[6] It appears that helper T cells[16,37] are the responsive cells to this stimulus. Suppressor T cell abnormalities,[20,36,51] perhaps confined to their specific response to thyroid antigens,[24] have been described and may be related to autoantibody hyperproduction and/or to the cell-mediated pathogenesis of these diseases[15,20] Hyperproduction of a spectrum of autoantibodies[21] (see below) may have pathogenic significance; in fact, the functional and morphologic status of the gland at any time may be the result of the balance established among them.[21] There is also evidence to support a specific B-cell defect in autoimmune thyroid diseases.[62] And, in certain syndromes, lymphoid and monocytic infiltrate of the thyroid is extensive.[10]

An observation important to understanding of autoimmune thyroid disease relates to major histocompatibility complex (MHC) gene products which, in man, are known as human leukocyte antigens (HLA). HLA antigens are polymorphic membrane glycoproteins that play a major regulatory role in cell interactions (see also Chap 13). MHC, Class I-coded antigens, also known as HLA A, B and C, are expressed on all nucleated cells of the body and are recognized by certain T lymphocytes.[37] MHC, Class II-coded antigens, or HLA-DR, DP, and DQ, are normally found on immune cells, e.g. B cells, activated T cells, and cells of the mononuclear phagocytic system. MHC, Class III genes are represented by components of the complement system. Normally, thyroid cells have Class I antigen, but Class II antigen found in the thyroid is confined to the dendritic cells of monocytic lineage. Under certain conditions, notably in autoimmune thyroid disease or in other situations where focal thyroiditis with lymphocytic infiltrate occurs,[29] aberrant HLA-DR antigens are expressed on the surface of thyroid epithelial cells (thymocytes).[23,26,29] Increased incidence of HLA-DR + T lymphocytes in the thyroid is also observed, as well as a higher concentration of MHC Class I (HLA-A, B, C) antigens.[23,29] Speculation that intrathyroid T lymphocyte production of lymphokines (e.g. gamma interferon) induces expression of the HLA-DR antigens on thymocytes, perhaps in response to a viral infection,[12,37] has come from several authors.[12,29,37,55,56] HLA-DR antigens, in combination with the antigens normally found on thyroid cells (e.g. thyroglobulin), might allow the T helper cells to recognize those antigens, initiating an immune response against them[12,29,37,55,56] in both humoral (i.e. autoantibodies) and cell-mediated (i.e. autoreactive lymphocytes) systems. Whether or not autoimmune disease actually develops may depend on co-existing T suppressor abnormalities.[12] Regardless of the validity of these suppositions in the initiation of autoimmune thyroid manifestations, it seems likely that the interactions described serve to perpetuate autoimmune activity, once initiated.[32]

Circulating autoantibodies[21] are the hallmark of autoimmune thyroid disease. Produced in apparently healthy[58] as well as diseased thyroid glands, these antibodies may have significance in diagnosis and/or they may be implicated in the pathogenesis of the disease. Autoantibodies found in autoimmune thyroid diseases[21] are listed here, with references:

Antithyroglobulin Antibody (ATgAb)[43]
Antimicrosomal Antibody (AMcAb)[4]
Thyroid Stimulating Hormone (TSA) Receptor Antibodies, (TRAb)[27]
    Long-Acting Thyroid Stimulator (LATS)[2]
    Long-Acting Thyroid Stimulator Protector (LATS-P)[1]
    Thyroid Stimulating Immunoglobulin (TSIg)[41]
    Thyrotropin-Binding-Inhibiting Immunoglobulin (TBII)[50]
    Anti-Post Receptor Effect Antibody[58]
    Thyroid Growth-Stimulating Immunoglobulin (TGI)[18]
    Thyroid Growth-Inhibiting Immunoglobulin (TGII)[19]
Thyroid Hormone Autoantibodies[42,46]

Autoantibodies to thyroglobulin (ATgAbs) were among the first of these antibodies to be described,[43] and are still used clinically in the diagnosis of autoimmune thyroid disease.[5,47] Relatively low titers may be detected in healthy individuals[58] or in persons with apparently unrelated autoimmune disorders,[46] while high titers are common in chronic lymphocytic thyroiditis (Hashimoto's disease) and moderate titers, in Graves' disease and primary adult myxedema. The antibodies may be detected by passive hemagglutination, precipitation, or complement fixation;[5,63] however, a negative result, particularly with hemagglutination, does not mean thyroglobulin antibodies are absent,[63] and precipitating antibodies may be restricted to sera from patients with Hashimoto's disease.[5] Although ATgAbs are usually IgM or IgG, IgA antibodies have also been described for these and for microsomal antibodies.[61] IgG cytophilic ATgAbs,[14,48,60] adherent to macrophages[52] and lymphocytes,[14] have been implicated in antibody-dependent cellular cytotoxicity (ADCC) of thyroglobulin-coated cells in in vitro studies,[14,33] suggesting a role for the antibody in pathogenesis.

Another antithyroid antibody of diagnostic value[5,47] is known as antimicrosomal antibody (AMcAb).[4] Unlike antithyroglobulin, AMcAb is almost invariably associated with autoimmune thyroid disease or focal thyroiditis,[47] being present in the vast majority of cases of Hashimoto's and Graves' diseases.[21] Assay results with hemagglutination and precipitating test systems[5,63] are similar to those described for ATgAbs. Antimicrosomal antibodies may mediate antibody-dependent cellular cytotoxicity by macrophages in patients with Hashimoto's disease.[11] Recently, experimental evidence has suggested that thyroid peroxidase and the microsomal antigen are identical.[31,34,35,44]

Antibodies that interact with the TSH receptor (TRAbs) may cause thyroid stimulation via activation of the receptor, or they may decrease the secretion of thyroid hormones by blocking receptor activation by TSH. Autoantibodies with stimulatory effect include long-acting thyroid stimulator (LATS), long-acting stimulator protector (LATS-P), and thyroid-stimulating immunoglobulin (TSIg). Inhibitory effects are mediated by thyrotropin-binding inhibiting immunoglobulin (TBII), by the antipostreceptor effect antibody, as well as by thyroid growth-inhibiting immunoglobulin (TGII). In practical terms, the balance between stimulatory and blocking antibodies in a given patient may determine, at any given time, the functional state of the gland.[21]

Normally, thyroid hormones circulate in blood bound to serum proteins; for example, most circulating thyroxine (T_4) is bound to thyroxine-binding globulin, to thyroxine-binding prealbumin, or to albumin. Autoantibodies reactive with thyroid hormones[22,38,39,42] are found in varying percentages of patients with autoimmune thyroid disease, as well as in many other disease states.[46] Almost always, antibodies to thyroid hormones are discovered because of discrepancies between clinical observations and thyroid hormone levels as detected by radioimmunoassay.[55] Reports vary on the actual effect of these antibodies on hormone metabolism,[46] and, as yet, no role in pathogenesis has been defined. Hormone autoantibodies are detectable by electrophoresis, immunoelectrophoresis, column chromatography, radioimmunoassay, or by polyethylene glycol (PEG) treatment of serum.[3,45]

Graves' Disease

Graves' disease is the most common cause of hyperthyroidism, or overproduction of thyroid hormone, in man. Also known as diffuse toxic goiter, symptoms of the disease form a triad of hyperthyroidism, infiltrative ophthalmopathy, and infiltrative dermopathy.

Exophthalmos, a large-eyed, staring expression, is usually present. Hyperthyroid hormone production increases the body's metabolic rate, inducing such symptoms as heat intolerance, restlessness, palpitations of the heart, and weight loss. Onset is usually insidious, developing slowly, and may go undiagnosed early in the disease. Along with other autoimmune disorders, Graves' disease has been linked to HLA DR3, where the relative risk is approximately 3%. Associations with other HLA antigens (e.g. B8, B35) have been reported.[37]

Diagnosis of overt Graves' disease may be made on the basis of clinical observations and TSH, T_3, and T_4 levels.[27] Autoantibodies to thyroglobulin are present in about half of cases; antimicrosomal antigens are virtually always found.[21] Probably the most significant of autoantibodies are the thyroid stimulating hormone receptor antibodies (TRAbs) described above. Sera from Graves' disease patients may exhibit several of these antibodies; however, pathogenesis may be linked to those factors, e.g. thyroid stimulating immunoglobulin (TSIg), chronically able to stimulate the receptor to induce thyroglobulin dissociation into thyroid hormones. Goiters, when present in Graves' disease, may result from thyroid growth-stimulating immunoglobulin (TGI).[18] As noted in the general discussion on autoimmune thyroid disease, patients with Graves' disease exhibit suppressor T cell defects[25,57] and T subset imbalances may be present.[20] The thyroid gland is often infiltrated with lymphocytes, and antibody dependent cellular cytotoxicity (ADCC) may occur.[8]

Hashimoto's Thyroiditis

As the name implies, Hashimoto's thyroiditis is characterized by a progressive, chronic inflammation of the thyroid gland, accompanied by a lymphocytic infiltrate and the presence of antithyroid autoantibodies. Many individuals with the disease are initially euthyroid; clinical symptoms usually appear later in the disease as thyroid hormone secretion decreases (hypothyroidism). Metabolic rates may slow, with fatigue, anorexia, and dry skin and hair may occur. Goiter may or may not be present. That Hashimoto's disease is genetically influenced is supported by family aggregation studies and by evidence of association with the inheritance of certain MHC-coded antigens, e.g. DR5.[37]

Autoreactive behavior of the immune system is characteristic of Hashimoto's thyroiditis. Antithyroglobulin antibodies, often with high titers, are present in approximately 60% of patients. Antibodies to microsomal antigen appear in virtually all patients. A small number of individuals demonstrate TRAbs,[50] mimicking those seen in Graves' disease. Blocking type antibodies, e.g. TBII, may play a role in inhibiting

TSH receptor activity; hence, contributing to diminished hormone levels,[7] and thyroid growth immunoglobulin (TGI) may induce goiter formation.[18] A small number of Hashimoto's cases have been shown to convert to Graves' disease while undergoing treatment for Hashimoto's.[49]

Imbalances of T lymphocyte subsets[9,15] and thyroid-specific defects in suppressor T cell activity[59] have also been described in Hashimoto's disease. T and B lymphocytes in the thyroid gland have demonstrable specificity for thyroid antigens,[17] and cytotoxic lymphocytes[13,28,30] and antibody-dependent cellular cytotoxicity[14] are present. Complement in sera from these patients can cause thyroid cell destruction in culture.[40] And, histologic studies of the thyroid gland in patients with clinical Hashimoto's disease reveal patterns similar to that of a lymph node, with its predominately lymphoid cell constituency.

Primary Adult Myxedema

Primary adult myxedema is characterized by progressive atrophy of the thyroid gland, apparently as a result of autoimmune processes.[53] Symptoms in common with hypothyroidism include cold, dry skin, coarse hair, cold intolerance, and lethargy.

REFERENCES

1. Adams, D.D., and Kennedy, T.H.: J. Clin. Endocrinol. Metab., 27:173, 1967.
2. Adams, D.L., and Purves, H.D.: Proc. Univ. Otago Med. School, 40:6, 1956.
3. Allen, D.J., Murphy, F., and Needham, C.A.: Lancet, 2:824, 1982.
4. Anderson, J.R., Goudie, R.B., and Gray, K.G.: Scott. Med. J., 4:64, 1959.
5. Anderson, J.W. et al.: J. Clin. Endocrinol. Metab., 27:937, 1967.
6. Aoki, N., and DeGroot, J.: Clin. Exp. Immunol., 38:523, 1979.
7. Arikawa, K. et al.: J. Clin. Endocrinol. Metab., 60:953, 1985.
8. Bagner, U., Wall, J.R., and Schleusener, H.: Acta. Endocrinol. (Suppl.), 281:133, 1987.
9. Benveniste, P., Row, V.V., and Volpe, R.: Clin. Exp. Immunol., 61:274, 1985.
10. Biörklund, A., and Sönderström, N.: Acta Otolaryngol., 82:204, 1976.
11. Bogner, U., Schleusener, H., and Wall, J.R.: J. Clin. Endocrinol. Metab., 59:734, 1984.

12. Bottazzo, G.F., Pujol-Borrell, R., and Hanafusa, T.: Lancet, 2:1115, 1983.

13. Calder, E.A., Penhale, W.J., Barnes, E.W., and Irvine, W.J.: Clin. Exp. Immunol., 14:19, 1973.

14. Calder, E.A. et al.: Clin. Exp. Immunol., 14:153, 1973.

15. Canonica, G.W. et al.: Clin. Immunol. Immunopathol., 23:616, 1982.

16. Canonica, G.W. et al.: Clin. Immunol. Immunopathol., 32:132, 1984.

17. DelPrete, G.F. et al.: Acta. Endocrinol. (Suppl.), 281:111, 1987.

18. Drexhage, H.A. et al.: Lancet, 2:287, 1980.

19. Drexhage, H.A. et al.: Lancet, 1:594, 1981.

20. Eguchi, K. et al.: Clin. Exp. Immunol., 70:403, 1987.

21. Frey, H.: Acta. Med. Scand., 222:289, 1987.

22. Ginsberg, J., Segal, D., Ehrlich, R.M., and Walfish, P.G.: Clin. Endocrinol., 8:133, 1978.

23. Hanafusa, T. et al.: Lancet, 2:1111, 1983.

24. Hara, Y., Sridama, V., Mori, H., and DeGroot, L.J.: Endocrinol. Jpn., 34:203, 1987.

25. Ishikawa, N. et al.: J. Clin. Endocrinol. Metab., 64:17, 1987.

26. Jansson, R., Karlssen, A., and Forsum, U.: Clin. Exp. Immunol., 58:264, 1984.

27. Larsen, P.R. et al.: Arch. Pathol. Lab. Med., 111:1141, 1987.

28. Laryea, E., Row, V.V., and Volpe, R.: Clin. Endocrinol., 2:23, 1973.

29. Lucas-Martin, A. et al.: J. Clin. Endocrinol. Metab., 66:367, 1987.

30. McLachlan, S.M. et al.: Acta. Endocrinol. (Suppl.), 281:125, 1987.

31. Mariotti, S. et al.: J. Clin. Endocrinol. Metab., 65:987, 1987.

32. Matsunaga, M. et al.: J. Clin. Endocrinol. Metab., 62:723, 1986.

33. Mitsunaga, M.: Acta. Med. Okayama, 41:205, 1987.

34. Nakajima, Y. et al.: Mol. Cell. Endocrinol., 53:15, 1987.

35. Nilsson, M., Mölne, J., Karlsson, F.A., and Ericson, L.T.: Mol. Cell. Endocrinol., 53:177, 1987.

36. Okita, N., Row, V.V., and Volpe, R.: J. Clin. Endocrinol. Metab., 52:528, 1981.

37. Piccinini, L.A., Roman, S.H., and Davies, T.F.: Clin. Endocrinol., 26:253, 1987.

38. Premachandra, B.N., and Blumenthal, H.T.: J. Clin. Endocrinol. Metab., 27:931, 1967.

39. Pryds, O., Hadberg, A., and Kastrup, K.W.: Acta. Paediatr. Scand., 76:685, 1987.

40. Pulvertaft, R.V., Doniach, D., Roitt, I.M., and Hudson, R.V.: Br. J. Exp. Pathol., 42:496, 1961.

41. Rees Smith, B., and Hall, R.: Lancet, 2:427, 1974.

42. Robbins, J., Rall, J.E., and Rawson, R.W.: J. Clin. Endocrinol. Metab., 16:573, 1956.

43. Roitt, I.M. et al.: Lancet, 2:820, 1956.

44. Ruf, J. et al.: Acta. Endocrinol. (Suppl.), 281:49, 1987.

45. Sakata, S., Komaki, T., and Nakamura, S.: Clin. Chem., 31:1252, 1985.

46. Sakata, S., Nakamura, S., and Miura, K.: Ann. Intern. Med., 103:579, 1985.

47. Scherbaum, W.A.: Acta. Endocrinol. (Suppl.), 281:325, 1987.

48. Shishiba, Y.: J. Clin. Endocrinol. Metab., 28:1389, 1968.

49. Skare, S., Frey, H.M.M., and Konow-Thorsen, R.: Acta Endocrinol. (Copenh), 105:179, 1985.

50. Smith, B.R., and Hall, R.: Lancet, 2:427, 1974.

51. Sridama, V., Pacini, F., and DeGroot, L.: J. Clin. Endocrinol. Metab., 54:316, 1982.

52. Suzuki, S. et al.: J. Clin. Endocrinol. Metab., 51:446, 1980.

53. Takasu, N., Naka, M., Mori, T., and Yamada, T.: Clin. Endocrinol. 21:345, 1984.

54. Theofilopoulos, A.N.: In Basic and Clinical Immunology. 6th ed. Edited by D.P. Stites, J.D. Stobo, and J.V. Wells. Norwalk, Conn., Appleton and Lange, 1987.

55. Todd, I., Pujol-Borrell, R., Belfiore, A., and Bottazzo, G.F.: Acta Endocrinol. (Suppl.), 281:27, 1987.

56. Todd, I., Pujol-Borrell, R., Hammond, L.J., and Bottazzo, G.F.: Clin. Exp. Immunol., 61:265, 1985.

57. Ueki, Y. et al.: J. Clin. Endocrinol. Metab., 65:922, 1987.

58. Villalpando, S., Cisneros, I., and Garcia-Bulnes, G.: Acta. Endocrinol., 99:500, 1982.

59. Volpe, R., and Row, V.V.: In Autoimmunity and the Thyroid. Edited by P.G. Walfish, J.K. Wall, and R. Volpe. New York, Academic Press, 1985.

60. Wasserman, J., vonStedingk, L.V., Perlmann, P., and Jonsson, J.: Int. Arch. Allergy, 47:473, 1974.

61. Weetman, A.P.: Int. Arch. Allergy Appl. Immunol., 83:432, 1987.

62. Weiss, I., DeBernardo, E., and Davies, T.F.: Clin. Immunol. Immunopathol., 23:50, 1982.

63. Wilkin, T.J. et al.: Clin. Endocrinol., 10:507, 1979.

Thyroglobulin Hemagglutination: Thyroid Antibody[1]

PRINCIPLE. Thyroglobulin is bound to the surface of sensitized, tanned erythrocytes. The coated cells are agglutinated by thyroglobulin antibodies in test serum, yielding an even carpet of cells at the bottom of a microtiter well.

EQUIPMENT AND MATERIALS

1. Thymune-T Hemagglutination Kit (Wellcome Diagnostics) containing:

a. Thyroglobulin sensitized test cell suspension: A freeze-dried, aldehyde treated, tanned turkey red blood cell suspension, coated with human thyroglobulin, in phosphate buffered saline solution, pH 7.2, containing 5% sucrose, 1.5% normal rabbit serum, and 0.1% sodium azide. Store at 4° C. Expiration date is noted on the label. Reconstitute with distilled water to the volume indicated on the bottle label. After reconstitution, cells should be stored at $-20°$ C.

b. Control cell suspension: A freeze-dried, aldehyde treated 1% tanned turkey red blood cell suspension preserved exactly as the above. Store at 4° C. Expiration date is noted on the label. Reconstitute with distilled water to the volume stated on the label. After reconstitution, store cells at $-20°$ C.

c. Diluent: Contains optimal concentrations of normal human and turkey serum in sterile, isotonic saline solution; 0.1% sodium azide is added as a preservative. Store at 4° C. May be used until expiration date noted on label. *NOTE: DO NOT MIX REAGENTS BETWEEN KITS.*

d. Positive control serum: A positive control serum of established thyroglobulin antibody titer is provided with the kit. Store at 4° C. May be used until the expiration date noted on the label.

e. Negative control serum: A negative control sample that does not agglutinate the red cells is provided with the kit and stored as described for the positive control serum.

2. Microtiter plates with u-shaped wells

3. 0.025 ml microdiluters

4. Go-no-go blotters (Dynatech Laboratories, Inc.)

5. 0.025 ml pipette and tips

6. Disposable 0.025 ml droppers or micropipettes

7. Bunsen burner

8. Beaker of distilled water

9. Microtiter viewing mirror

SPECIMEN COLLECTION AND PREPARATION. Serum samples are used fresh, or frozen to $-20°$ C until use. Avoid repeated freezing and thawing. Samples must be heat-inactivated before use. Plasma samples are not suitable for testing.

PROCEDURE

1. Inactivate all samples at 56° C for 30 minutes.

2. Prepare sufficient thyroglobulin sensitized cells (0.025 ml per sample/control) and control cells (0.025 ml per sample/control) for the run.

3. Wipe the back of a u-shaped microtiter plate with a wet paper towel to dispel static electricity. Label one row for each specimen/control to be tested.

4. Using a 0.025 ml dropper, place four drops of diluent into well 1 and one drop into each remaining well of all rows to be used.

5. Flame microtiter diluters. Cool, and check volume by touching surface of distilled water in a beaker and blotting on go-no-go blotter.

6. For each serum/control, pick up 0.025 ml of serum. Add to well 1 of the appropriate row. Mix and transfer 0.025 ml to well 2—this is the serum control well. Discard 0.025 ml from well 2.

7. With a clean micropipette tip or microdiluter, transfer 0.025 ml of absorbed serum from well 1 of each row to well 3. Mix and serially transfer 0.025 ml through to well 12. Discard 0.025 ml from well 12.

8. Using a disposable 0.025 ml dropper, add 0.025 ml of thyroglobulin sensitized cells to wells 3 to 11 of all rows.

9. Using a disposable 0.025 ml dropper, add 0.025 ml of control cells to well 2 of each row. Mix contents by tapping the plate thoroughly on all four sides. *CAUTION:* Failure to mix properly will result in erratic settling patterns and lower sensitivity.

10. Cover and incubate at room temperature 30 to 60 minutes.

11. Read for agglutination by placing plate on the microtiter viewing mirror.

12. In the event that a serum agglutinates the control cells (step #9), absorb 0.1 ml of serum with packed cells obtained by centrifugation of 0.5 ml of the control cell suspension. Shake and incubate for 10 minutes at room temperature. Serofuge at high speed 4 to 5 minutes and separate absorbed serum. Repeat the test using absorbed serum.

13. If complete agglutination is still present at the final dilution of 1:5120, prepare a 1:100 dilution of the serum in the diluent supplied, titrate as a normal sample and repeat the test. If an endpoint is still not obtained, repeat the titration starting with a higher dilution, e.g. 1:1000. Or, titer the patient serum out for two or more rows instead of one.

REPORTING. Strong agglutination (4+) is evidenced by a diffuse carpet of cells; negative reactions appear as a button of cells. The control well (well 2) of each row must be negative before test results can be reported. Agglutination in well 2 indicates antibody reactant with control cells and the test samples must be absorbed as described above. The positive and negative control must perform to the established criteria before any results are reported. Record control results as required. Weakly positive reactions may result in intermediate patterns. The endpoint should be read as the highest dilution of the sample giving approximately 50% agglutination of the test cells (i.e. 2+ agglutination). A prozone (one or more wells showing unexpectedly weak agglutination) is sometimes seen at low dilutions of some strongly positive sera, and care should be taken not to misinterpret such results.

The dilutions in wells 3 to 12 are twofold and range from 1:10 to 1:5120. If all controls, including the serum control well, exhibit the proper reactivity, the patient serum is reported as the reciprocal of the last dilution with at least 2+ reactivity. Negative samples are reported as "negative."

INTERPRETATION OF RESULTS. The normal range for antithyroglobulin, established in this laboratory, is <20.

LIMITATIONS OF THE PROCEDURE. Plasma and bacterially contaminated serum samples are unsuitable for testing.

REFERENCE

1. Insert, Thymune-T, Wellcome Diagnostics, Dartford, England, 1987.

Microsomal Hemagglutination: Thyroid Antibody[1]

PRINCIPLE. Microsomal antigen is bound to the surface of sensitized, tanned erythrocytes. The coated cells are agglutinated by microsomal antibodies in the test serum, yielding an even carpet of cells at the bottom of a microtiter well.

EQUIPMENT AND MATERIALS

1. Thymune-M Hemagglutination Kit (Wellcome Diagnostics) containing:

a. Microsomal antigen sensitized test cell suspension: A freeze-dried 1% suspension of aldehyde-treated, tanned turkey red blood cells, coated with microsomal antigen; in PBS, pH 7.2 with 5% sucrose, 1.5% normal rabbit serum and 0.1% sodium azide. Store at 4° C. Expi-

ration date is noted on the label. Reconstitute with distilled water to the volume stated on the label. Reconstituted cells may be used up to 5 days at 4° C or up to a month if stored at −20° C.

b. Control cell suspension: An aldehyde-treated tanned turkey red blood cell suspension, suspended and preserved as above. Store at 4° C. Expiration date is noted on the label. Reconstitute with the amount of distilled water noted on the label. Reconstituted cells may be used up to 5 days, if stored at 4° C, or may be stored at −20° C for up to 18 months.

c. Diluent: A sterile, isotonic saline solution containing normal human serum, normal turkey serum, 0.1% sodium azide, and 100 mg/l human thyroglobulin. Store at 4° C. May be used until expiration date noted on the label. NOTE: DO NOT MIX REAGENTS BETWEEN KITS.

d. Positive control serum: A positive control serum of established microsomal antibody titer is provided with the Wellcome kit. Store at 4° C. May be used until the expiration date noted on the label.

e. Negative control serum: A sample that does not agglutinate the red cells in this test is provided with the kit. Store as described above.

2. Microtiter plate: "U" bottom wells

3. 0.025-ml droppers

4. 0.025-ml microdiluters or micropipettes

5. Go-no-go blotters (Dynatech Laboratories, Inc.)

6. 0.025-ml pipette and tips

7. Bunsen burner

8. Beaker filled with distilled water

9. Microtiter viewing mirror

SPECIMEN COLLECTION AND PREPARATION. Serum samples are used fresh, or frozen to −20° C until used. Avoid repeated freezing and thawing. Sera must be heat-inactivated before testing. Plasma samples are not suitable for testing.

PROCEDURE

1. Thaw and inactivate sera to be tested.

2. Wipe the back of a u-shaped microtiter plate with a wet paper towel to dispel static electricity. Label a row for each specimen/control to be tested.

3. Flame microtiter diluters, touch to surface of distilled water in beaker, and test by blotting on go-no-go blotter.

4. Using a standard 0.025-ml dropper, add four drops of diluent to wells 1 and 2, and three drops to wells 3 to 12. Do this for each row to be used.

5. Pipette 0.025 ml of serum into well 1. Using a micropipette or microdiluter mix and transfer 0.025 ml to well 2.

6. With a clean micropipette tip or microdiluter, transfer 0.025 ml from well 2 to well 3— this is the serum control well. Discard 0.025 ml from well 3.

7. With a clean micropipette tip or microdiluter, transfer 0.025 ml from well 2 to well 4; mix and transfer 0.025 ml to well 5. Continue fourfold dilutions to well 12. Discard 0.025 ml from well 12.

8. Immediately add 0.025 ml of control cells to well 3 and 0.025 ml of test cells to wells 4 to 12.

9. Mix contents by tapping the plate thoroughly on all four sides.

CAUTION: Failure to mix properly will result in erratic settling patterns and lower sensitivity.

10. Incubate plate at room temperature out of direct sunlight and free from any vibration for 1 hour.

11. Place the microtiter plate on the viewing mirror and observe for agglutination.

12. Should agglutination be evident in the control well (3) of any test serum row, the serum should be adsorbed by mixing the packed cells obtained by centrifugation of 0.5 ml of the control cell suspension with 0.1 ml inactivated serum. Following a 10-minute incubation at room temperature, centrifuge and collect the adsorbed serum. Repeat the test using adsorbed serum.

REPORTING. Strong agglutination (4+) is evidenced by a diffuse carpet of cells; negative reactions appear as a compact button of cells. Any serum dilution causing 2+ (50% agglutination) or greater agglutination is considered positive; therefore, the end point is taken as the last well with at least 2+ agglutination. The control well (3) of each row must be negative and the positive and negative control sera must demonstrate proper reactivity before results can be reported. Positive control should be 2+ at the titer indicated in the package insert (± one serum dilution); negative control should be negative. Record control results as required. Weakly positive reactions may result in intermediate patterns. The end point should be read as the highest dilution of the sample giving approximately 2+ agglutination of the test cells. A prozone (one or more wells showing unexpectedly weak agglutination) is sometimes seen at low dilutions of some strongly positive sera and care should be taken not to misinterpret such results.

The dilutions in wells 4 to 12 are fourfold and range from 1:100 to 1:6,553,600.

Serum samples which agglutinate the test cell suspension are reported as positive, with the reciprocal of the last dilution exhibiting at least 2+ agglutination as the titer, e.g. positive, titer 1600.

Negative samples are recorded as "negative."

INTERPRETATION OF RESULTS. Titers of ≤ 100 are considered normal in this laboratory.

LIMITATIONS OF THE PROCEDURE. A high proportion of strongly positive sera give prozones in the test and for this reason a full titration must be carried out on every test serum.

Plasma and bacterially contaminated serum samples are unsuitable for testing.

REFERENCE

1. Insert, Thymune-M, Wellcome Diagnostics, Dartford, England, 1983.

Chapter | 12

TUMOR MARKERS

Tumor markers can be defined as products of tumor cells or nonmalignant tissues whose synthesis is associated with the presence of a tumor.[3] These markers may be present in cell-bound form in cancerous tissues, or may be circulating in elevated levels in body fluids of patients with neoplastic disease.

Tumor markers are varied in nature and may be classified into the following major categories: (1) *Oncofetal antigens,* which are found on both neoplastic tissues in the adult and normal tissues in the fetus, (2) *Hormones,* produced in excessive amounts, or produced ectopically by tissues not normally producing that hormone, (3) *Enzymes,* produced in excess, or ectopically, and (4) *Antigens defined by monoclonal antibodies.* Table 12–1 lists some of the more commonly employed tumor antigens, their classification, and the malignant diseases for which their measurement is useful.

Recently, there has been renewed interest in tumor markers, leading to their increased use in clinical evaluations and to the discovery of new markers. When used in conjunction with other tests, tumor markers have provided useful information to the clinician regarding diagnosis, prognosis, and treatment of patients with tumors. Analysis of cell-associated tumor markers in histo-logic sections has been helpful in the classification and staging of tumors. Measurement of circulating tumor markers has been beneficial in assessing the extent of malignancy in newly diagnosed patients, and in monitoring patients for tumor recurrence following therapy.

Tumor markers have not been useful as a screening tool for early detection of cancer in the general population because they lack the necessary sensitivity and specificity. To date, no tumor marker has been found that is unique to a particular malignant disease; all markers described thus far are also produced by normal cells,[1-3] and markers may be present in elevated concentrations in noncancerous disease states as well. Although inappropriate as a general screening tool, detection of tumor markers in patients suspected of malignancy or being treated for malignancy has been useful in establishing diagnosis and predicting prognosis, when used together with other laboratory and clinical findings. (See also *Alpha-feto Protein, Carcinoembryonic Antigen, Human Chorionic Gonadotropin, Lysozyme.*)

REFERENCES

1. Cohn, S.L., Lincoln, S.T., and Roseen, S.T.: Cancer Invest., *4*:305, 1986.
2. Garrett, P.E., and Kurtz, S.R.: Med. Clin. North Am., *70*:1295, 1986.
3. McLellan Guy, J.: Lab. Med., *16*:273, 1985.

Table 12–1. Tumor Markers[1,3]

Marker	Associated Malignancy
Oncofetal	
Alpha-fetoprotein (AFP)	Nonseminomatous testicular; Hepatocellular
Carcinoembryonic antigen (CEA)	Colorectal; Breast; Lung
Hormones	
Calcitonin	Medullary thyroid
Human chorionic gonadotropin (hCG)	Testicular
Enzymes	
Lysozyme	Monocytic leukemias; Acute and chronic mye-lomonocytic leukemias
Neuron-specific enolase (NSE)	Small cell carcinoma of lung
Prostatic acid phosphatase (PAP)	Prostrate
Terminal deoxynucleotidal transferase (TdT)	Acute lymphocytic leukemia (Common, Pre-B, Null); Chronic myelogenous leuke-mia (Lymphoid or mixed; Blastic phase)
Defined by Monoclonal Antibodies	
CA 19-9	Pancreatic; Gastrointestinal
CA 125	Ovarian

ALPHA-FETOPROTEIN

Alpha-fetoprotein (AFP) is a glycoprotein that is synthesized primarily in fetal liver and yolk sac, and to a lesser extent, in the gastrointestinal tract of the fetus.[6,7,10,11,15] First isolated in 1956,[3] AFP has a molecular weight of approximately 70,000 daltons with a carbohydrate content of approximately 3 to 4%, and migrates with the alpha globulins on electrophoresis of cord serum.[6,7,10,11,15] It shares many physicochemical properties with albumin, and comparison of the two proteins in humans shows a 39% amino acid sequence homology.[11] Although the function of AFP is unknown, it has been speculated that the glycoprotein may play multiple roles in the fetus by (1) acting as a fetal albumin, (2) permitting hepatocyte proliferation by blocking VLDL synthesis, which has been shown to inhibit the growth of liver cells, and (3) providing immunoregulatory protection to the fetus, as it has been shown to suppress immune responses in laboratory animals and in vitro.[11,14]

Synthesis of AFP by the human embryo peaks at 12 to 14 weeks of gestation, when fetal serum concentrations of about 3 mg/mL are evident.[11] Thereafter, production decreases as gestation progresses to term, at which time it virtually ceases. Serum levels drop with the half-life of the protein (approximately 3.5 days),[6] until adult concentrations of less than 20 ng/mL are reached by about 6 to 12 months of age.[6,11] Elevated AFP levels reappear subsequently in adult serum during pregnancy or in the presence of tumors of endodermal origin.

AFP was first recognized as an oncofetal tumor marker in 1963 by Abelev et al.,[1] who detected the marker in the sera of mice and rats with chemically-induced hepatomas, and shortly thereafter, by Tatarinov, who observed AFP in the sera of human patients in association with hepatocellular carcinoma (HCC).[17] The use of AFP as a tumor marker has been most beneficial in the evaluation of patients with primary HCC or nonseminomatous testicular tumors, although elevations of AFP are also evident in the sera of a smaller percentage of patients with other endodermally derived tumors, including carcinomas of the gastrointestinal tract.[6,7]

As 70 to 80% of patients with primary HCC have elevated concentrations of serum AFP,[6,10,15] measurement of the tumor marker has been useful in confirming this diagnosis. Some studies have shown that monitoring AFP levels in individuals with chronic Hepatitis B infections may be helpful in detecting progression to HCC, often at a stage when the tumor is resectable.[8,15] However, more than 30% of patients with small tumors have AFP levels within the reference range,[15] but measurement of AFP may be beneficial when combined with other laboratory results in detection of early HCC.[12,18]

AFP levels have been observed to correlate with prognosis in some populations of HCC patients; higher values are associated with decreased survival.[9,13] Except for early HCC, monitoring AFP values in individual patients also correlates with response to therapy, with increases in AFP often preceding detection of recurrent tumor growth by several months;[6,20] but, as chemotherapy is relatively ineffective in treating HCC, AFP testing appears to be more valuable as a diagnostic tool in this type of malignancy.[15]

Another major use of AFP as a tumor marker has been in the evaluation of nonseminiferous germ cell tumors of the testes. Measurement of AFP should be performed simultaneously with measurement of the tumor marker hCG (see *Human Chorionic Gonadotropin*) in order to provide optimal information in the clinical evaluation of this malignancy, as fluctuations in the levels of these two markers often do not parallel each other.[19] Studies have shown that one or both of these markers are elevated in 50 to 90% of patients with nonseminomatous testicular tumors, and that the increasing frequency of elevated markers prior to surgery correlates with a more advanced stage of the tumor.[7,19] In addition, measurement of both markers is helpful in typing the testicular tumor; continual elevations of AFP alone indicate a nonseminomatous testicular tumor, while elevations of hCG only may be indicative of a pure seminomatous tumor, a mixed testicular tumor, or a nonseminomatous tumor.[19] Monitoring AFP and hCG levels following therapy is also an important part of the clinical evaluation of patients with testicular tumors, as failure of elevated markers to decline to normal levels indicates the presence of residual tumor cells, while

a decline in markers followed by an elevation is indicative of tumor recurrence. AFP values obtained too soon after surgery, however, may appear elevated due to residual AFP in the serum, which has not yet declined to normal as a result of the half-life of AFP, hence, the importance of obtaining serial measurements.[19]

Although AFP testing plays an important role in the diagnosis and management of patients with hepatocellular carcinomas and nonseminomatous testicular tumors, it is not appropriate for use as a screening tool for malignancy in the general population. Elevations of AFP are also evident in noncancerous disease states, including ataxia telangiectasia, hereditary tyrosinemia, and nonmalignant liver diseases in which hepatic regeneration is occurring.[6,10] Although AFP elevations in most patients with HCC are usually greater than 500 ng/mL, and AFP elevations associated with benign liver diseases are usually less than 100 ng/mL, the point at which AFP levels are considered diagnostic for HCC varies in different laboratories.[20] Recently, a variant form of AFP has been discovered, in which the carbohydrate portion is fucosylated.[2] Elevations of fucosylated AFP are evident in many patients with HCC, and may be valuable in distinguishing malignant from benign liver disease.[20]

In addition to its use as a tumor marker, AFP testing is commonly used as a screening tool for fetal neural tube defects (NTD) during pregnancy. The most common of these are anencephaly, a lethal condition associated with absence of the cranial vault and cerebral hemispheres, and spina bifida, a condition varying widely in severity and characterized by exposure of the neural tissue because of failure of the bony spinal canal to close during fetal development.

In a normal pregnancy, AFP is excreted from the fetal urine into the amniotic fluid, where its concentration peaks at about 50 mg/mL at 13 to 17 weeks of gestation, then steadily declines until term.[4,10,11] AFP in the amniotic fluid diffuses across the placenta into the maternal serum, where it rises throughout pregnancy from the normal adult concentration (less than 20 ng/mL) before 6 weeks' gestation, to about 250 ng/mL at 32 weeks' gestation.[10] In open NTD, AFP levels in amniotic fluid and maternal serum are elevated above these expected concentrations because of leakage of AFP from fetal serum and cerebrospinal fluid directly into the amniotic fluid and subsequent diffusion into the maternal serum. AFP elevations in pregnancy, however, are not specific to NTD. Other conditions, including other open fetal malformations, such as omphalocele or gastroschisis, intestinal atresias leading to decreased swallowing and digestion of AFP by the fetus, congenital nephrosis leading to increased excretion of AFP in fetal urine, errors in estimating gestational age, multiple pregnancies, and fetal demise also result in abnormal increases in AFP.[4,10,11] Thus, elevated results obtained by AFP screening of maternal serum must be accompanied by confirmatory procedures in the detection of NTD; these include testing for AFP in amniotic fluid, diagnostic ultrasound or amniography, and amniotic fluid acetylcholinesterase testing, the latter giving a positive result in NTD due to leakage of the enzyme from the exposed central nervous system into the amniotic fluid.[4,10,11] Conversely, abnormally low levels of AFP have been associated with molar pregnancy, missed abortion, pseudocyesis, overestimated gestational age, and Down syndrome;[4,10,11] diagnosis must subsequently be confirmed by ultrasound and amniocentesis.

Methods of choice for AFP measurement are radioimmunoassay and ELISA.[4,7,10,11] The development of monoclonal antibody reagents may allow for greater specificity of test results, but procedures using these reagents appear to require modifications in order to achieve an acceptable level of sensitivity.[5,16]

REFERENCES

1. Abelev, G.I. et al.: Transplantation, *1*:174, 1963.

2. Aoyagi, Y. et al.: Biochim. Biophys. Acta, *830*:217, 1985.

3. Bergstrand, C.G., and Czar, B.: Scand. J. Clin. Lab. Invest., *8*:174, 1956.

*4. Burton, B.K.: Adv. Pediatr., *33*:181, 1986.

5. Chan, D.W. et al.: Clin. Chem., *32*:1318, 1986.

*6. Cohn, S.L., Lincoln, S.T., and Rosen, S.T.: Cancer Invest., *4*:305, 1986.

7. Garrett, P.E., and Kurtz, S.R.: Med. Clin. North Am., *70*:1295, 1986.

8. Heyward, W.L. et al.: JAMA, *254*:3052, 1985.

9. Johnson, P.J. et al.: Br. J. Cancer, *44*:502, 1981.

10. Insert—AFP-EIA Kit, Abbott Laboratories, North Chicago, IL, 1985.

*11. Knight, J.A., and Wu, J.T.: Lab. Med., *19*:219, 1988.

12. Liaw, Y.F. et al.: Liver, *6*:133, 1986.

13. Matsumoto, Y. et al.: Cancer, *49*:354, 1982.

14. Murgita, R.A. et al.: Nature, *267*:257, 1977.

15. Rustin, G.J.S.: In *Tumor Markers in Clinical Practice.* Edited by A.S. Daar. Oxford, Blackwell Scientific Publications, 1987.

16. Shahangian, S., Fritsche, H.A., and Hughes, J.I.: Clin. Chem., *33*:583, 1987.

17. Tatarinov, Y.S.: Vopr. Med. Khim., *10*:90, 1964.

18. Tatsuta, M. et al.: Oncology, *43*:306, 1986.

19. Vessella, R.L., and Lange, P.H.: Lab. Med., *16*:298, 1985.

20. Warnes, T.W., and Smith, A.: Baillieres Clin. Gastroenterol., *1*:63, 1987.

Alpha-Fetoprotein by EIA[1]

PRINCIPLE. The Abbott AFP-EIA system is a solid phase enzyme immunoassay based on the "sandwich" principle. Beads coated with goat anti-AFP are incubated with specimens or the appropriate standards and controls. During this incubation, AFP present in the specimens, standards, and controls is bound to the solid phase. Unbound materials present in the specimens, standards, and controls are removed by aspiration of fluid and washing of the beads. Goat anti-AFP conjugated with horseradish peroxidase is incubated with the beads and, if AFP is present in the specimen, the anti-AFP:horseradish peroxidase conjugate is bound to the AFP on the beads. Unbound conjugate is removed by aspiration and the beads are washed. The beads are next incubated with enzyme substrate solution (hydrogen peroxide and ortho-phenylenediamine ·2HCl) to develop a color, which is a measure of the amount of bound anti-AFP:horseradish peroxidase conjugate. The enzyme reaction is stopped by the addition of 1N sulfuric acid, and the intensity of color developed is read using a spectrophotometer set at 492 nm. The intensity of the color formed by the enzyme reaction is proportional to the concentration of AFP in the specimen within the working range of the assay. A standard curve is obtained by plotting the AFP concentration of the standards vs. the absorbance. The AFP concentration of the specimens and of the controls run concurrently with the standards can be determined from the curve.

EQUIPMENT AND MATERIALS

Kit reagents:

1. Anti-AFP (goat) coated beads in phosphate buffer. Preservative: Thimerosal

2. Anti-AFP (goat):peroxidase (horseradish) conjugate in tris buffer with protein stabilizer. Minimum concentration of antibody: 0.01 μg/mL

3. AFP (human) standards: 0, 2, 5, 10, 20, 40 and 60 ng/mL in phosphate buffer with protein stabilizer. Preservative: Thimerosal

4. OPD (o-phenylenediamine·2HCl) tablets. OPD/tablet: 12.8 mg

5. Diluent for OPD (o-phenylenediamine·2HCl). Citrate-phosphate buffer containing hydrogen peroxide. Preservative: Thimerosal

6. AFP (human) Control I: 10 to 30 ng AFP (human)/mL calf serum (assay value on vial label). Preservative: Thimerosal

7. AFP (human) Control II: 150 to 300 ng AFP (human)/mL calf serum (assay value on vial label). Preservative: Thimerosal

Materials not included in kit:

8. Reaction trays

9. Cover seals (tear along perforation for use)

10. Reaction tubes with identifying cartons (for transfer of beads from reaction trays)

11. 1N sulfuric acid

12. Precision pipettes to deliver 25 μL, 175 μL, 200 μL and 10 mL

13. EIA pipetting package to deliver 200 μL, 300 μL and 1 mL or equivalent for dispensing antibody conjugate and/or OPD substrate solution

14. Device for delivery of rinse solution such as a Gorman-Rupp Pump, or equivalent

15. An aspiration device for washing coated beads such as a Pentawash II with a vacuum source and two traps for retaining the aspirate

16. Vacuum pump or equivalent for use with a Pentawash II

17. Water bath capable of maintaining temperature at 45°C $\pm$ 1°C

18. Rectilinear graph paper

19. Nonmetallic forceps

20. Spectrophotometer capable of reading absorbance at 492 nm (Quantum I, Quantum II or equivalent)

PRECAUTIONS

1. For in vitro diagnostic use only.

2. Do not mix reagents from different master lots. EXCEPTION: Any sulfuric acid lot may be used with any AFP-EIA kit lot.

3. Do not use kit components beyond the expiration date.

4. Do not expose OPD reagents to strong light during storage or incubation.

5. Avoid microbial contamination of reagents when opening and removing aliquots from the vials.

6. Use pipette with disposable tips for pipetting standards and specimens.

7. Avoid contact of the OPD substrate solution with any oxidizing agent. Do not allow substrate solution or 1N sulfuric acid to come into contact with any metal parts. Rinse glassware used for the diluent for OPD or 1N sulfuric acid thoroughly with 1N sulfuric acid. Use approximately 10% of the container volume followed by three washes of distilled water at the same volume prior to use. NOTE: Each 110 mL bottle of 1N sulfuric acid supplied as an accessory to the kit contains a sufficient volume for only 100 tests. Additional reagent grade acid should be prepared for washing glassware as required.

8. The standards and controls of this kit contain human blood components. They

have been tested and found nonreactive for hepatitis B surface antigen and HIV Ab by a test which meets the requirements of the United States Food and Drug Administration for third generation sensitivity. No known test method can offer complete assurance that products derived from human blood will not transmit hepatitis and other viral infections. Therefore, all blood derivatives should be considered potentially infectious.

9. Do not pipette by mouth.

10. Do not smoke, eat, or drink in areas in which specimens or kit reagents are being handled.

11. Wear gloves during and wash hands thoroughly after handling of kit reagents.

12. Handle OPD tablets, solution containing OPD and 1N sulfuric acid with care, as they may cause irritation to the skin.

REAGENT PREPARATION. The OPD (o-phenylenediamine·2HCl) tablet must be dissolved in diluent for OPD immediately before use. The solution must not be stored longer than 60 minutes before use and should not be exposed to strong light.

During the last 10 to 15 minutes of the second incubation period, prepare the OPD substrate solution as follows:

NOTE: 300 μL is required for each test well.

1. Using a clean pipette or dispenser, transfer into a suitable container, 5 mL of diluent for OPD for each tablet to be dissolved. Caution: use pipettes and containers known to be metal free. For example, use disposable plastic ware or acid-washed and distilled water-rinsed glassware.

2. Transfer tablet(s) from bottle into diluent for OPD using a nonmetallic forceps or equivalent. Return desiccant to bottle immediately if removed to obtain tablet(s) and close bottle tightly. Allow tablet(s) to dissolve.

3. Just prior to dispensing for the final incubation of the assay, swirl gently to obtain a homogeneous solution.

REAGENT STORAGE

1. Store AFP-EIA kit reagents at 2 to 8° C. OPD tablets and 1N sulfuric acid may be stored at 2 to 30° C.

2. Bring all reagents to room temperature (15 to 30° C) for use and return to storage conditions indicated above. Caution: Do not open OPD tablet bottle until it is a room temperature.

3. Avoid unnecessary exposure to light.

4. Retain desiccant bags in OPD tablet bottle at all times during storage.

5. Reconstituted OPD solution MUST be stored at room temperature and MUST be used within 60 minutes.

Indications of Instability or Deterioration of Reagents:

The substrate solution (OPD plus diluent for OPD) should be colorless to pale yellow. A yellow-orange color indicates that the reagent has been contaminated and must be discarded.

SPECIMEN COLLECTION AND PREPARATION. Only serum specimens can be tested by the Abbott AFP-EIA procedure. Specimens should be collected in such a way as to avoid hemolysis. If the test is to be run within 24 hours after collection, the specimen should be stored in the refrigerator at 2 to 8° C. If testing will be delayed more than 24 hours, the specimen should be frozen.

PROCEDURE

CAUTION: Bring serum specimens and reagents to room temperature and mix well before use. Use a clean pipette or disposable tip for each transfer to avoid cross-contamination.

NOTE: Each standard, control, and specimen should be assayed in duplicate each time the test is performed.

NOTE: Careful control of the timing of all steps is critical when more than one reaction tray is used. Add the beads to the first tray and start the incubation for this tray. It is recommended that beads be added to each additional tray at 5-minute intervals and the incubations begun immediately after bead addition. This time interval should be maintained between trays throughout the assay, including the steps of the enzyme reaction. The procedure ensures sufficient time to complete all manipulations for a given tray or reaction carton, and allows for identical timing for all samples.

1. Adjust temperature of water bath to 45°C ± 1° C.

2. Identify reaction tray wells with data sheet for testing the standards, controls, and specimens.

3. Using precision pipettes, add 200 μL of standards to their assigned wells.

4. Pipette 25 μL of each specimen or AFP control into its assigned well. Then add 175 μL of 0 ng/mL standard to each well containing a specimen or control. Gently tap tray to mix specimens or controls in wells. Alternatively, the specimen or control may be diluted in a test tube by adding 100 μL of the specimen or control and 700 μL of the 0 ng/mL standard. Mix well and pipette 200 μL of the diluted specimen or control into its assigned well. This is an eightfold dilution of each specimen and control.

NOTE: For increased sensitivity the specimen and controls may be run at a 1:2 dilution, using 100 μL test sample and 100 μL 0 ng/ml standard. The Quantum II's data base must be edited to reflect this change.

5. Using a clean forceps, raise the basket holding the beads out of its bottle, allowing excess liquid from the basket to drain back into the bottle. Place the basket in the inverted cap of the bead bottle. Use forceps to dispense one bead into each well containing a test sample. As an alternative, attach a plastic pipette tip with a small orifice to an aspirator. Using the suction of the aspirator, transfer the bead to the well. Release the bead into the well by breaking the vacuum. Using forceps, immediately replace the bead basket in its bottle and cap the bottle. Do not handle the bead basket with bare hands.

6. Apply cover seal to each tray. Gently tap trays to ensure that each bead is covered with the sample and that any air bubbles are released. Be careful not to splash liquid onto cover.

7. Incubate the trays in the 45° C ± 1° C water bath for 2 hours ± 5 minutes.

8. At the end of the 2-hour incubation period, remove the trays from the water bath. Carefully remove and discard the cover seals. Aspirate the liquid and wash each bead two times with 4 to 5 mL of distilled or deionized water for a total wash volume of 8 to 10 mL (see Wash Procedure Details in the kit insert).

NOTE: Excessive drying of beads is detrimental to assay results. Release beads from Pentawash II or equivalent immediately after aspiration of wash water.

9. Add 200 μL of Anti-AFP (goat):peroxidase (horseradish) conjugate to each well containing a bead.

10. Apply a new cover seal to each tray. Make sure that beads are completely covered with liq-

uid by tapping the trays to release any air bubbles that may be trapped in the solution.

11. Incubate the trays for 2 hours ± 5 minutes in the 45° C ± 1° C water bath.

12. During the last 10 to 15 minutes of the 2-hour incubation, prepare OPD substrate solution as described under Reagent Preparation.

13. At the end of the 2-hour incubation, remove the trays from the water bath. Remove and discard the cover seals. Aspirate the liquid and wash each bead two times with 4 to 5 mL of distilled or deionized water for a total wash volume of 8 to 10 mL. Remove all excess liquid from tray by aspiration or blotting. NOTE: Excessive drying of beads is detrimental to assay results. Release beads from Pentawash II or equivalent immediately after aspiration of wash water.

14. Immediately transfer beads from wells to properly identified reaction tubes. Align inverted rack of oriented tubes over the tray, press tubes tightly over wells, then invert tray and tubes together so that beads fall into corresponding tubes.

15. Pipette 300 μL of the freshly prepared OPD substrate solution into each tube containing a bead. The incubation period begins when OPD solution is added to the first tube. NOTE: Substrate solution should be clear to pale yellow. Do not allow substrate to come into contact with metal.

16. Incubate tubes at 15 to 30° C for 30 ± 1 minutes. To prevent foreign material from contaminating the mixture and excessive light from affecting color development, cover the box until incubation is complete.

17. Stop the enzyme reaction by adding 1.0 mL of 1N sulfuric acid to each tube at 30 ± 1 minutes after the addition of OPD substrate solution to that tube. Add the acid at the same rate and in the same sequence as followed in the addition of OPD substrate solution in step 15.

18. Mix (vortex or equivalent) each tube. Do not allow acid solution to come into contact with metal. Air bubbles should be removed prior to reading absorbance. All absorbance values should be determined within 2 hours after addition of 1N sulfuric acid.

19. Set Quantum II in appropriate mode. Refer to the Instruction Manual for operating procedures.

Blank the Quantum II using a reaction tube containing distilled or deionized water. Read AFP standards, controls and specimens.

If the Quantum II is not used, set the photometer or spectrophotometer at 492 nm and zero the instrument using distilled or deionized water. Determine the absorbance of the standards, controls and specimens. Be sure that the cuvette is free of color residue from previous specimens.

Procedure for assay of specimens with greater than 480 ng AFP/mL:

If in an initial assay, a specimen is found to contain greater than 480 ng AFP/mL, dilute the specimen with an appropriate amount of 0 ng/mL AFP standard. It is desirable to perform the dilution so that the diluted specimen reads above 3 ng/mL on the standard curve. Assay specimen according to assay procedure and perform calculations using dilution factor as described in Results.

Example: A tenfold dilution is prepared by adding 100 μL of the specimen to 900 μL of 0 ng/mL AFP standard. Mix thoroughly before assaying.

RESULTS. *NOTE:* The mean absorbance value of the 60 ng/mL AFP standard should be above 0.8. If the 60 ng/mL standard absorbance value is below 0.8, specimen values derived from the standard curve may be suspect.

1. If the Quantum II is used, AFP values will be automatically calculated and recorded on the printout.

2. If a photometer or spectrophotometer other than a Quantum is used, calculate the AFP values as follows:

a. Construct the standard curve by plotting the mean absorbance obtained for each AFP standard on the vertical (Y) axis versus the corresponding AFP concentration on the horizontal (X) axis, using rectilinear graph paper.

Values for duplicates should be within 0.02 absorbance units of the mean absorbance value if the mean value is less than 0.2. For mean absorbance values of 0.2 or greater, duplicate values generally should be expected to lie within 10% of the mean absorbance.

b. Using the mean absorbance value for each specimen, determine the corresponding concentration of AFP in ng/mL obtained from the standard curve. Multiply the value read on the X-axis by 8 since the specimen was diluted eightfold in the assay.

3. If the specimen required additional dilution for its assay value to fall on the standard curve, the value from the standard curve must also be adjusted by the dilution factor. For the example given above, the specimen was diluted tenfold before assaying; therefore the value determined from the X-axis should be multiplied by 80.

LIMITATIONS OF THE PROCEDURE. Abbott AFP-EIA is to be used as an aid in the management of nonseminomatous testicular cancer patients in conjunction with information available from the clinical evaluation and other diagnostic procedures. Increased serum AFP concentrations have also been observed in ataxia telangiectasia, hereditary tyrosinemia, primary hepatocellular carcinoma, gastrointestinal tract cancers with and without liver metastases, and in benign hepatic conditions such as acute viral hepatitis, chronic active hepatitis and cirrhosis.

AFP testing is not recommended as a screening procedure to detect cancer in the general population.

AFP testing for prenatal screening should be performed only if appropriate background data are available. Data should include AFP ranges for each week of gestational age. These ranges must be based on regional populations.

Additional support should be readily available to the patient including ultrasound, amniocentesis, cytogenetics, and counseling.

REPORTING. When reporting results, it is important to add the comment *"NOT FOR PERINATAL SCREENING"*—unless laboratory is licensed for perinatal testing.

SPECIFICITY. Lipemic, icteric, and hemolyzed specimens and serum proteins such as alpha-globulins, gamma-globulins, ceruloplasmin, transferrin or alpha-1-antitrypsin do not interfere with the AFP-EIA.

SENSITIVITY. The sensitivity of the AFP-EIA system is better than 0.6 ng/mL which, after taking into account the eightfold dilution of the specimen in the assay, is equivalent to a concentration of 4.8 ng AFP/mL of patient specimen. The sensitivity was calculated as the concentration which is two standard deviations above the zero standard.

REFERENCE

1. Package Insert—AFP-EIA, Abbott Laboratories, North Chicago, IL, 1987.

CARCINOEMBRYONIC ANTIGEN

Carcinoembryonic antigen (CEA)[4,10] is a glycoprotein that has a molecular weight of approximately 200,000 daltons and migrates to the beta globulin region during serum electrophoresis. It is heterogeneous in nature, with protein-carbohydrate ratios varying from 1:5 to 1:1 in tumors derived from different sources.[4]

An oncofetal protein, CEA was originally isolated by Gold and Freedman in 1965 from human fetal intestine and adult colon carcinomas.[11] It is also present on fetal liver and pancreas, and in small amounts, in normal adult colon tissue.[4,10]

CEA has become the most widely used tumor marker.[10] Its greatest value is in the clinical evaluation of colorectal carcinomas; several studies have shown that 50 to 90% of patients with these carcinomas demonstrate elevated serum CEA levels prior to treatment.[10] Initially, it was hoped that CEA would be a specific marker for the presence of colorectal carcinoma. However, subsequent studies have shown that CEA assays are inappropriate for diagnostic screening of the general population, since CEA levels may also be elevated in the sera of a small percentage of healthy nonsmokers, and in some cigarette smokers,[1,4] as well as in a significant number of patients with a variety of nonmalignant conditions, including collagen vascular disease, cirrhosis of the liver, nonspecific colitis, diabetes mellitus, arteriosclerosis, and functional bowel disease.[4,5] Patients with these conditions, however, generally do not demonstrate extreme elevations of CEA, with levels only rarely exceeding 10 ng/mL.[4]

More appropriately, CEA assays have served as a prognostic tool in monitoring patients who are being treated for colorectal carcinomas. A clinical response to treatment is generally accompanied by a decline in serum CEA.[10] Conversely, a steady, progressive increase in CEA levels in patients who have undergone surgical resection of a colorectal tumor strongly suggests tumor recurrence. Monitoring CEA levels postoperatively has been shown to identify tumor recurrence with a sensitivity of approximately 80%.[8]

The sensitivity of CEA monitoring appears to be best in the detection of metastatic recurrence, as opposed to local recurrence; the usefulness of this marker as a guide to second-look surgery in patient follow-up is therefore controversial,[8,9,13] but may be most appropriate for a select group of patients. This was suggested by one study of over 400 patients with colorectal carcinoma, which indicated that detection of resectable, recurrent tumors was most successful in patients with CEA levels less than 11 ng/mL, in whom other tests had been performed to rule out the possibility of unresectable metastases.[13]

Although CEA levels are also elevated in some patients with other types of carcinomas, including carcinomas of the breast, lung, and pancreas, CEA measurement has had a more limited role in the clinical evaluation of these diseases. With these carcinomas, CEA assays have been most useful in assessing prognosis of disease, as highly elevated levels are present most consistently in patients with advanced disease involving bone or visceral metastases, and are associated with a poor prognosis.[3,6,15]

CEA may also play a role in histologic classification of tumors, although it is controversial whether CEA measurement provides information above that obtained through staging.[8,12] Even so, presence of CEA in histologic sections of lung carcinoma has been found to be strongly predictive of a poor prognosis.[3] In addition, elevated levels of CEA in effusions from patients with an unknown primary tumor are reportedly diagnostic of a metastatic carcinoma of breast, lung, or gastrointestinal origin.[14]

Measurement of CEA in the laboratory is performed by RIA or ELISA. Normal ranges vary with the method used, and the laboratory performing the method, but are generally considered to be less than 5 ng/mL.[10,12] Clinically significant differences have been found when comparing the available methods, and may be due partly to the heterogeneity of the CEA molecules in patient specimens.[7,8] Because of these variations, serial measurements on specimens from the same patient should be performed using one assay, and results from different laboratories should be cautiously interpreted.[7,8] One study showed that between-laboratory variation may be decreased considerably by conversion of the results to international units on the basis of the international reference CEA standard.[16] In the future, the use of monoclonal antibodies may also decrease variability in CEA measurement, by allowing for specific detection of CEA epitopes.

REFERENCES

1. Alexander, J.C., Silverman, N.A., and Chretien, P.B.: JAMA, 235:1975, 1976.
2. Beard, D.B., and Haskell, C.M.: Am. J. Med., 80:241, 1986.
3. Bishopric, G.A., and Ordonez, N.G.: Cancer, 58:1316, 1986.
*4. Cohn, S.L., Lincoln, S.T., and Rosen, S.T.: Cancer Invest., 4:305, 1986.
5. Costanza, M.E. et al.: Cancer, 33:583, 1974.
6. Del Favero, G.: Cancer, 57:1576, 1986.
7. Fleisher, M. et al.: Clin. Chem., 30:200, 1984.
*8. Fletcher, R.H.: Ann. Intern. Med., 104:66, 1986.
9. Fucini, C. et al.: Tumori, 69:359, 1983.
*10. Garrett, P.E., and Kurtz, S.R.: Med. Clin. North Am., 70:1295, 1986.
11. Gold, P., and Freedman, S.O.: J. Exp. Med., 121:439, 1965.
12. Holyoke, E.D.: Lab. Med., 16:295, 1985.
13. Minton, J.P. et al.: Cancer, 55:1284, 1985.
14. Pinto, M.M. et al.: Acta Cytol. 31:113, 1987.
15. Waalkes, T.P., and Shaper, J.H.: Lab. Med., 16:279, 1985.
16. Zucchelli, G.C. et al.: Clin. Chem., 32:1942, 1986.

HUMAN CHORIONIC GONADOTROPIN

Human chorionic gonadotropin (hCG)[5,8,11,13] is a member of the human gly-coprotein hormone family, which also includes the pituitary hormones, luteinizing hormone (LH), follicle-stimulating hormone (FSH), and thyroid stimulating hormone (TSH). Each of these hormones consists of two noncovalently linked subunits: alpha and beta. The alpha subunit is virtually identical in all four hormones, and has a molecular weight of approximately 14,900, while the beta subunit confers hormonal specificity, and is therefore unique to each glycoprotein. A significant amount of homology does exist among the beta subunits of the four hormones, though, and is especially evident between hCG and LH, which exhibit about an 80% homology in their N-terminal sequence of 115 amino acids. The beta subunit of hCG contains a unique carboxy terminal region consisting of 24 additional amino acids, and has a molecular weight of approximately 23,000. Modern assays to detect hCG take advantage of this fact and are specific for the beta subunit.

Synthesized by the syncytiotrophoblast cells of the placenta, hCG functions to maintain the corpus luteum and stimulate the production of progesterone during the first 6 to 8 weeks of gestation.[11,13] As such, hCG has long been utilized as the major laboratory marker for early detection of pregnancy, detectable in maternal plasma by 8 to 13 days after ovulation by most assays,[8] and reaching its peak levels (24 to 70 IU/mL, equivalent to approximately 5 to 14 µg/mL) at 8 to 10 weeks in a normal pregnancy and declining thereafter.[3,8,13] Routine screening for pregnancy is performed qualitatively, by detection of hCG in maternal urine, because urinary hCG values generally parallel serum values, and are detectable approximately 1 day after serum hCG is evident.[7] Detection of hCG is also being used with increased frequency in determining the success of implantation following in vitro fertilization and embryo transfer.[11]

Quantitative measurement of hCG has been useful in evaluating complications of pregnancy. For a given gestational age, patients with ectopic pregnancy or threatened or subclinical abortion have lower hCG serum concentrations than those found in normal pregnancy, while women with multiple pregnancies have higher hCG concentrations than those with single-infant pregnancies.[8]

As a tumor marker, hCG is particularly valuable in the evaluation of trophoblastic disease and testicular tumors. In contrast to a normal pregnancy, in which hCG levels decline after 8 to 10 weeks gestation, patients with fetal chorion tumors, such as hydatiform mole, invasive mole, and choriocarcinoma, demonstrate consistent production of the hormone.[3,8] Correct identification of patients with trophoblastic tumors has been significantly enhanced when ultrasonography (to detect fetal heart movement) is supplemented with serial hCG measurements, which fail to decline after the first trimester of pregnancy in the presence of such tumors.[8,12] Patients diagnosed with hydatiform mole are further monitored by serial measurements of hCG after molar evacuation in order to detect residual tumor or progression to invasive mole or choriocarcinoma. Regression curves generated from patients after successful evacuation of a molar pregnancy show an initial rapid decline in serum hCG level followed by a more variable decline (with a half-life of 1 to 3 days[8]), in which hCG may remain detectable for as long as 12 to 15 weeks after evacuation.[3,8] The presence of residual tumor and treatment with chemotherapy are indicated in patients with detectable levels of hCG after this time, while complete remission is reliably indicated by persistence of undetectable hCG levels for 1 year following evacuation.[3,8]

Serial measurement of hCG has also been important in monitoring patients with invasive mole or choriocarcinoma for effectiveness of chemotherapy, with remission indicated by maintenance of undetectable hCG levels for at least 3 consecutive weeks.[8] In addition, quantitative hCG levels are im-

portant in staging patients with these trophoblastic tumors, and are directly related to fatality rate.[1,3,8] Another prognostic indicator may be the detection of unique hCG variants by isoelectric focusing (IEF). While sera from normal pregnant women contain seven isoelectric variants of hCG with pIs ranging from 3.9 to 7.0, and patients with hydatiform mole or invasive mole demonstrate similar IEF patterns, sera from patients with advanced choriocarcinoma contain unique additional variants, whose presence is associated with a poor survival rate.[8,16] Finally, cerebrospinal fluid (CSF) values of hCG have been used to establish the presence of brain metastases, which are indicated by a serum hCG:CSF hCG ratio of less than 60:1.[8,13]

As a marker for testicular tumors, hCG should be measured in conjunction with alpha-fetoprotein (AFP) in order to obtain maximal information for clinical evaluation of the patient (see also *Alpha Feto Protein*). In normal, nonpregnant adults, serum hCG levels are less than 1 ng/mL.[14] Elevated levels of hCG and/or AFP are found in 50 to 90% of patients with nonseminomatous testicular tumors, and elevated hCG alone is seen in 10 to 30% of patients with pure seminomas.[5,9,15] Quantitative measurement of hCG has been helpful in classifying, staging, and clinically monitoring patients with these tumors. For patient monitoring, serial measurements demonstrating rising levels of hCG are seen as unequivocal evidence of persistent tumor, while declining levels frequently indicate a decrease in tumor burden, although not definitively, as residual tumor cells which do not produce hCG (or AFP) may remain after therapy.[3,5,15]

Although hCG is produced ectopically by a wide range of tumors other than those of trophoblastic or testicular origin, its clinical utility in these diseases is limited, as serum values are generally low.[8,13] The free beta subunit of hCG, however, may be a promising new marker of nontrophoblastic gynecologic malignancies. In recent studies in which assays specific for the free beta subunit were utilized, 50 to 74% of women with these malignancies exhibited detectable urinary levels, significantly higher than the percentage of patients exhibiting intact hCG.[4,10] Detection of the free hCG beta subunit will need to be evaluated further to establish its role in clinical evaluation of patients with gynecologic tumors.

A large number of hCG laboratory tests are available commercially. These assays commonly use antisera to the hCG beta subunit, but may detect intact hCG only, free hCG beta subunit only, or both. Qualitative hCG tests are used to screen for early pregnancy, and have been performed by a number of different methods, including direct hemagglutination, latex agglutination, latex agglutination inhibition, and enzyme immunoassay. The newest methods, enzyme immunoassays with monoclonal antibody reagents, have a sensitivity level of approximately 25 to 50 mIU/mL (5 to 10 ng/mL), and can detect pregnancy as soon as 23 to 25 days after the last menstrual period.[2,6] The use of monoclonal antibodies has circumvented the problem of cross-reactivity with LH, and has reduced interference caused by proteinuria.[2,6] As a tumor marker or indicator of pregnancy complications, hCG is measured quantitatively by radioimmunoassays that are capable of detecting as little as 0.2 ng/mL hCG.[5]

REFERENCES

1. Bagshawe, K.D.: Cancer, 38:1373, 1976.
2. Bandi, Z.L., Schoen, I., and DeLara, M.: Am. J. Clin. Pathol., 87:236, 1987.
3. Cohn, S.L., Lincoln, S.T., and Rosen, S.T.: Cancer Invest., 4:305, 1986.
4. Cole, I.A. et al.: Cancer Res., 48:1356, 1988.
5. Garrett, P.E., and Kurtz, S.R.: Med. Clin. North Am., 70:1295, 1986.
6. Gelletlie, R., and Nielson, J.B.: Clin. Chem., 32:2166, 1986.
7. Hay, D.L. et al.: Aust. N.Z.J. Obstet. Gynaecol., 24:206, 1984.
*8. Hussa, R.O.: The Clinical Marker hCG. New York, Praeger Publications, 1987.
9. Javadpour, N.: Cancer, 45:1755, 1980.
10. O'Connor, J.F. et al.: Cancer Res., 48:1361, 1988.
11. Puett, D.: Bioassays, 4:70, 1986.
12. Romero, R. et al.: Obstet. Gynecol., 66:553, 1985.
13. Rustin, G.J.S.: In Tumor Markers in Clinical Practice. Edited by A.S. Daar. Oxford, Blackwell Scientific Publications, 1987.
14. Vaitukaitis, J.L., Braunstein, G.D. and Ross, G.T.: Am. J. Obstet. Gynecol., 113:751, 1972.
15. Vessella, R.L., and Lange, P.H.: Lab. Med., 16:298, 1985.
16. Yazaki, K., Armstrong, E.G., and Koide, S.S.: Cancer, 59:795, 1987.

Human Chorionic Gonadotropin (Beta Subunit) Quantitative Test[1]

PRINCIPLE. Tandem-R HCG (Total β-HCG) kit is a solid phase, two-site immunoradiometric assay to measure both the intact HCG molecule and free β-subunit of the HCG molecule. Patient samples are reacted with a plastic bead (solid phase) coated with two monoclonal antibodies, one directed to the intact HCG molecule and one to the free β-subunit of the HCG molecule. A monoclonal anti-HCG labelled with ^{125}I is added. After the formation of the solid phase/antigen/labeled antibody sandwich, the bead is washed to remove unbound labeled antibody. The radioactivity bound to the solid phase is measured with a gamma counter. The level of radioactivity is directly proportional to the concentration of the intact HCG molecule and free β-subunit of HCG present in the test sample.

EQUIPMENT AND MATERIALS

Kit includes:

Tandem-R HCG (Total β-HCG) kit— Hybritech Inc.

1. Tracer Antibody. Monoclonal mouse IgG (against HCG) labeled with ^{125}I in a protein matrix containing less than 10 μCi per vial, a blue dye, and 0.1% sodium azide

2. Beads. Monoclonal mouse IgG against intact HCG and a monoclonal mouse IgG against the free β-unit of HCG coated on plastic beads in buffer containing 0.1% sodium azide

3. Negative Control (0 mIU/mL calibrator). Human serum containing no detectable concentration of HCG and 0.1% sodium azide

4. Positive Reference (25 mIU/mL calibrator). Human serum containing 25 mIU HCG/mL and 0.1% sodium azide

5. Positive Control (100 mIU/mL calibrator). Human serum containing 100 mIU HCG/mL and 0.1% sodium azide

6. Wash concentrate. Buffer containing 0.3% sodium azide

Provided separately: Tandem-HCG Quantitative set—Hybritech Inc.

7. Zero Diluent. Human serum containing no detectable concentration of HCG and 0.1% sodium azide

8. Calibrators. Human serum containing 5, 10, 25, 100, 200, and 400 mIU HCG/mL and 0.1% sodium azide

9. Wash concentrate. Buffer containing 0.3% sodium azide

Not Provided:

10. 12 × 75 mm plastic test tubes

11. Test tube rack

12. Gamma counter

13. Repeating precision pipettor: 100 μL

14. Repeating pipettor: 2 mL

15. Disposable tip precision pipettor: 50 μL

16. Aspiration device

17. 37° C waterbath

18. Parafilm or equivalent for covering tubes

19. Millipore water

20. Forceps

21. Container for storage of wash solution

22. Small decant rack

STORAGE. Tandem-R HCG reagents are to be stored at 2 to 8° C until expiration date of kit.

Calibrators are supplied ready-to-use and are stable until the expiration date when stored at 2 to 8° C.

Wash solution is stable at 2 to 8° C until expiration date.

Follow appropriate radioactive material storage protocols.

SPECIMEN COLLECTION. Serum—100 μL. Plasma samples should not be used. Specimens may be stored for 7 days at 2 to 8° C prior to assaying. Specimens held for longer times should be frozen only once at −20° C.

WARNINGS AND PRECAUTIONS

1. Follow universal blood and body fluid precautions.

2. Follow proper radioactive materials handling and storage protocols.

PROCEDURE

1. Bring all liquid reagents to room temperature and thoroughly mix all liquid reagents by gentle agitation or swirling.

2. To prepare the wash solution, add the contents from one vial of the wash concentrate to 500 mL of distilled water and mix.

3. Three levels of control should be run with each assay.

4. Label 12 × 75 mm plastic tubes for standards, controls, and specimens.

5. Introduce 1 bead into each tube after blotting the residual droplet on the bead upon removal from its container. DO NOT permit the bead to dry.

6. Pipette 50 μL of calibrators, controls, and specimens into respective tubes.

7. Pipette 100 μL of tracer antibody into each tube.

8. Shake the test tube rack to ensure mixing and cover the tubes.

9. Incubate the tubes at 37° C for 1 hour.

10. Wash the beads three times (twice with buffer and once with Millipore water). Use decanting rack.

   a. Pipette 2 mL of wash solution into each tube.

   b. Decant the liquid from each tube. Shake rack and blot tubes.

   c. Repeat a and b.

   d. Pipette 2 mL Millipore water into each tube.

   e. Decant liquid. Shake rack and blot.

11. Count each tube in a gamma counter for 10,000 cpm and record the counts per minute.

12. Calculate results as described in the Calculations section.

CALCULATIONS

1. Automated: Use the cpm from the Packard Auto-Gamma 5650. Enter into calculator for final results.

Use the Hybritech Data Station:

   a. Turn power on.

   Prints "Hybritech Data Station"
       "Immunoassay Data Reduction System"

   Display reads: "Select Function"

   (1) Run protocol

   Pressing the scroll buttons (↑↓) allows you to scroll through the functions 1 to 7.

b. Select option (1) run protocol, press E (enter)

Display reads: "Select Protocol"

(1) TAN E-IgE

(2) etc etc

(13) TAN R-HCG

Press ↓ arrow to go from 1 to 13)

Select 13, TAN R-HCG—press E (enter)

Display reads: "List parameters"

Press 0 = No

or

Press 1 = Yes

c. Answer questions:

Data entry type

Select option (2) Manual—press enter

Data processing

Select option (1) real time—press enter

d. Enter the cpm of the standards

NOTE: If a wrong number is pushed, press "C" for clear and re-enter the correct number. If a wrong cpm is entered, edit the curve at the end of the standards cpm entry.

e. After last standard cpm is entered, display reads "Please wait—curve fitting."

f. Answer questions that appear on digital display

"Edit data?" 0 = No

1 = Yes

(1) If no—enter cpm of unknowns

(2) If yes—go through and change the incorrect cpm.

(3) Press EDIT. Select option 4—recalculate curve.

(4) Enter cpm of unknowns.

2. Manual: Using graph paper supplied by Hybritech, plot the cpm of the standards on the Y axis, and the standard concentrations on the X axis. Interpolate unknown cpm and read concentration.

RESULTS

Linearity 3 to 400 mIU/mL

Values greater than the highest standard should be diluted with zero standard and re-assayed. Multiply final result by dilution factor.

Reference Interval: <3.0 mIU/mL

INTERPRETATION OF RESULTS. HCG is not normally detected in the serum of healthy men and healthy nonpregnant women.

Pregnant women normally attain serum HCG concentrations up to 50 mIU/mL in the week following conception or in the third week after the last menstrual period. A maximum is reached by the second to third month, followed by a decrease to as low as 4,000 mIU/mL by the third trimester (6 to 9 months).

During the first 6 weeks of pregnancy, serum HCG concentrations have a doubling time of 1.5 to 3 days. Following delivery, HCG concentrations rapidly decrease and usually return to normal within several days postpartum.

Elevated serum HCG concentrations have been reported in patients diagnosed as having choriocarcinoma, hydatidiform mole, and some nontrophoblastic malignancies, including testicular tumors, prostatic cancer, breast cancer and lung cancer.

REFERENCE

1. Package Insert—Tandem-R HCG, Hybritech Incorporated, San Diego, Ca., 1987.

LYSOZYME (MURAMIDASE)

Originally described by Fleming in 1922 as a "remarkable bacteriolytic element found in tissues and secretions,"[6] lysozyme is a cationic enzyme, with a molecular weight of 14,000 daltons, which is capable of cleaving the beta (1,4) glycosidic bond between N-acetylmuramic acid and N-acetylglucosamine in the peptidoglycan of bacterial cell walls.[13,18] A ubiquitous enzyme, lysozyme has been isolated from humans, other vertebrates, invertebrates, plants, fungi, bacteria, and phages.[18] As such, it is believed to function primarily as a bacteriolytic constituent of nonspecific, primitive defense systems.[18] Other biologic roles for the enzyme have also been proposed, including modulation of the inflammatory response,[8] enhancement of bacteriolysis by antibody and complement,[7,34,36] and stimulation of phagocytosis.[18]

In humans, lysozyme is found in a variety of tissues[19,21] and body fluids.[12,15,31] Serum concentrations of lysozyme range from 4.0 to 13.0 μg/mL in normal individuals, with similar levels in umbilical cord serum, amniotic fluid, saliva, and seminal fluid.[12,15,31] The highest amount of lysozyme is present in tears, which contain 120 times the concentration found in serum, while gastric juice and breast milk contain 8 times normal serum levels.[12,15] Urine, bile, and cerebrospinal fluid, conversely, normally have negligible concentrations of lysozyme.[12,15,31]

The major source of lysozyme in the human body is thought to be the phagocyte: polymorphonuclear leukocytes (PMN), monocytes, macrophages, and their precursors. These are the only known hematopoietic sources.[13] In PMN, lysozyme synthesis occurs during the promyelocyte/myelocyte precursor stages of development and halts as the cells mature, at which time constant levels are maintained in the granules.[10,13] By contrast, synthesis by monocytes is continual, and may become enhanced by as much as 140 to 250% during cellular activation.[9]

Lysozyme is found in the body wherever phagocytes are congregated. Serum levels of the enzyme in normal individuals and in patients with myeloproliferative disorders are thought to reflect primarily the liberation of lysozyme by dying PMN (i.e. the rate of granulocyte turnover), since, in comparison to monocytes, PMN are present in greater numbers, contain a higher concentration of lysozyme, and have a shorter lifespan.[13,21] Serum levels in patients with granulomatous diseases or monocytic or myelomonocytic leukemias, on the other hand, are thought to result chiefly from secretion of lysozyme by stimulated monocytes and macrophages.[13,21] Lysozyme production also occurs normally by cartilage[10,13] and by glandular cells,[13,21] the latter of which are thought to be the primary contributors of the lysozyme found in tears, saliva, and other body secretions.[21] The contribution of these tissues to serum lysozyme is unknown, but is thought to be minor.[21]

The major use of lysozyme determination has been as a hematologic marker for granulocytes, monocytes, and their precursors in various malignant disorders. Marked increases in serum and urine lysozyme concentrations have been found in patients with monocytic leukemias and most acute and chronic myelomonocytic leuke-

mias.[2,23,31] Increased concentrations have also been observed in granulocytic leukemias,[14,27] in some cases of myelogenous leukemia,[35] and in a few cases of multiple myeloma.[31] Lysozyme levels in patients with lymphocytic or myeloblastic leukemias are normal, or may be decreased as a result of relative agranulocytopenia.[31,32,35]

Some disagreement exists among investigators as to the prognostic usefulness of serial lysozyme tests on persons with these disorders. Wiernik and Serpick[35] found it to be useful as a bone marrow aspirate, and Catovsky et al.[2] document some prognostic value, while Seligman et al.[32] deny any correlation with disease activity.

Increased levels of serum lysozyme have also been associated with benign monocyte hyperproliferation, as seen in tuberculosis[29] and sarcoidosis,[25] where levels appear to reflect the total mass of biologically active granulomas.[33] In addition, increased serum lysozyme activity has been found in patients with megaloblastic anemias (presumably as a result of increased granulocyte turnover),[28] ulcerative colitis,[22] and Crohn's disease.[5]

Laboratory measurement of lysozyme has also been applied to body fluids other than serum. Lysozyme determination in the urine, for example, has been a useful indicator of renal tubular damage. Lysomuria, or increased lysozyme in the urine, has been observed in a variety of conditions involving renal damage,[15] including renal allograft rejection,[4] urinary tract infections,[23] and glomerulonephritis.[30]

Increased lysozyme concentrations have been found in the cerebrospinal fluid of patients with inflammatory neoplastic diseases of the central nervous system,[3] and in the synovial fluid of patients with rheumatoid arthritis,[10,27] while decreased levels have been measured in the tears of patients with keratoconjunctivitis sicca.[16]

Various methods for determining lysozyme concentrations have been described. The technique used most commonly by clinical laboratories is the "lysoplate" method, originally developed by Osserman and Lawlor[23] since it is simple to perform and has a sensitivity of approximately 0.09 μg/mL.[15] In this method, lysozyme is determined by its ability to lyse the cell walls of the bacterium, *Micrococcus lysodeikticus* suspended in an agarose medium, thereby forming zones of clearance. Determination of lysozyme by lysis of *M. lysodeikticus* may also be measured by using turbidimetric assays.[20,24] Attempts to compare the lysoplate method to turbidimetric methods have shown variable degrees of correlation, which may be due to differences in factors influencing the lysoplate method, including quality of the agar diffusion medium, pH, ionic strength, temperature, and the possible presence of unidentified interfering substances in biologic specimens.[11,17,26] Immunochemical methods for measurement of lysozyme, including rocket electrophoresis, nephelometry, radioimmunoassay, and enzyme immunoassay, have also been developed.[1]

REFERENCES

1. Brouwer, J., Leeuuen-Herberts, T., and Otting-van de Ruit, M.: Clin. Chim. Acta, *142*:21, 1984.
2. Catovsky, D., Galton, D.A.G., and Griffin, C.: Br. J. Haematol., *21*:565, 1971.
3. DiLorenzo, N., Palma, L., Ferrante, L.: Neurochirurgia, *20*:19, 1977.
4. Ellis, L., McSwiney, R.R., and Tucker, S.M.: Ann. Clin. Biochem., *15*:253, 1978.
5. Falchuk, K.R., Perrotto, J.L., and Isselbacher, K.L.: N. Engl. J. Med., *292*:395, 1975.
6. Fleming, A.: Proc. R. Soc. Lond., *93*:306, 1922.
7. Glynn, A.A.: Immunology, *16*:463, 1969.
8. Gordon, L.I. et al.: J. Clin. Invest., *64*:226, 1979.
9. Gordon, S., Todd, J., and Cohn, Z.A.: J. Exp. Med., *139*:1228, 1974.
10. Greenwald, R.A.: Semin. Arth. Rheum., *6*:35, 1976.
11. Gupta, D.K., vonFigura, K., and Hasilik, A.: Clin. Chim. Acta, *165*:73, 1987.
12. Hankiewicz, Y., and Swierczek, E.: Clin. Chim. Acta, *57*:205, 1974.
*13. Hansen, N.E.: Ser. Haematol., *7*:7, 1974.
14. Hansen, N.E. et al.: Acta Neurol. Scand., *55*:418, 1977.
15. Insert—Quantiplate lysozyme test kit, Kallestad Laboratories, Inc., 1977.
16. Janssen, P.T., and van Bijsterveld, O.P.: Clin. Chim. Acta, *121*:251, 1982.
17. Jenzano, J.W., Hogan, S.L., and Lundblad, R.L.: J. Clin. Microbiol., *24*:963, 1986.
*18. Jolles, P., and Jolles, J.: Mol. Cell. Biochem., *63*:165, 1984.
19. Klockars, M., and Reitamo, S.: J. Histochem. Cytochem., *23*:932, 1975.
20. Litwack, G.: Proc. Soc. Exp. Biol. Med., *89*:401, 1955.
21. Mason, D.Y., and Taylor, C.R.: J. Clin. Pathol., *28*:124, 1975.
22. Meyer, K., et al.: Am. J. Med., *5*:496, 1948.
*23. Osserman, E.F., and Lawlor, D.P.: J. Exp. Med., *124*:921, 1966.
24. Parry, R.M., Chandan, R.C., and Shahani, K.M.: Proc. Soc. Exp. Biol. Med., *119*:384, 1965.
25. Pascual, R.S., Gee, J.B.L., and Finch, S.C.: N. Engl. J. Med., *289*:1074, 1973.
26. Peeters, T.L., and Vantrappen, G.R.: Clin. Chim. Acta, *74*:217, 1977.
27. Perellie, P.E., and Finch, S.C.: N. Engl. J. Med., *283*:456, 1970.
28. Perellie, P.E., Kaplan, S.S., and Finch, S.C.: N. Engl. J. Med., *277*:10, 1967.
29. Perellie, P.E., Khan, K., and Finch, S.C.: Am. J. Med. Sci., *265*:297, 1973.
30. Prockup, D.J., and Davidson, W.D.: N. Engl. J. Med., *270*:269, 1964.
*31. Pruzanski, W., and Saito, S.G.: Am. J. Med. Sci., *258*:405, 1969.
32. Seligman, B.R. et al.: Am. J. Med. Sci., *264*:69, 1972.
33. Selroos, O., and Klockars, M.: Scand. J. Respir. Dis., *58*:110, 1977.
34. Wardlaw, A.: J. Exp. Med., *115*:1231, 1962.
35. Wiernik, P.H., and Serpick, A.A.: Am. J. Med., *46*:330, 1969.
36. Wilson, L.A., and Spitznagel, J.K.: J. Bacteriol., *96*:1339, 1968.

Lysozyme (Muramidase) Test

PRINCIPLE. Patient sample, placed in a circular well cut into a gel containing a suspension of *Micrococcus lysodeikticus*, is compared to three known standard solutions with respect to its ability to lyse that bacterium.

EQUIPMENT AND MATERIALS

1. Quantiplates (Kallestad): Contain 2.4 ± 0.1 mL of a pH 8.6 buffered agarose-*Micrococcus lysodeikticus* mixture. 0.1% sodium azide added as a preservative. Store at 2 to 8° C in a Ziplock bag. Do not freeze. May be used until the expiration date noted on the package or until visual aberrancies (e.g., drying, clearing) occur

2. Standard solutions (Kallestad): Lyophilized, pooled human urine with known concentrations of lysozyme; standardized against company reference sera. Each vial contains 0.1% sodium azide as a preserva-

tive. Store at 2 to 8° C. Expiration dates and concentrations are noted on the labels. Reconstitute with 0.5 mL distilled water. Cap and mix gently by inversion. The rehydrated standards may be used up to 60 days, if stored at 2 to 8° C, unless visible contamination occurs

3. Patient sample: serum, urine, or tear samples may be used with this test. Icteric, lipemic or hemolyzed sera will give elevated values and are not acceptable. Random or 24-hour urine samples (collected without preservative) are equally suited for testing. Specimens may be stored up to 5 days at 2 to 8° C, or at −20° C for longer periods. Repeated freezing and thawing may cause enzyme deterioration. Tears should be diluted 1:100 in saline solution before testing

4. Positive control: A patient sample (or pooled samples, if available) is aliquoted and frozen to −70° C for use as a control on between run variations. New controls are run in parallel with existing controls for at least two runs before being placed in routine use. Two standard deviations from the mean of these is accepted for each run

5. Volumetric pipet, calibrated to deliver 5 μL, with tips

6. Two-cycle semi-logarithmic graph paper

7. Kallestad viewer or ruler

PROCEDURE

1. Bring all reagents, samples, and positive control to room temperature (23° C ± 2° C). If tear samples are to be run, dilute 1:100 in saline solution.

2. Remove the quantiplate from its Ziplock bag, open, and observe for moisture. If excess moisture is evident, allow the plate to sit, uncovered, until it evaporates.

3. Reconstitute standard solutions (see *Equipment and Materials* #2).

4. Obtain two-cycle semilog paper and record the solutions to be placed in each well on the reverse side (e.g. standard solutions #1–3 in wells 1–3; control in well 4; patients in 5 and 6).

NOTE: If more than one plate is to be used, all standards and the control should be included on each plate.

5. Using a 5 μL volumetric pipet, place 5 μL of standard solutions and 5 μL of the control and patient samples into the designated wells.

6. Cover the plate, return it to its plastic bag, and reseal the bag. A moisture chamber may be used for incubation instead of the plastic bag.

7. Incubate at room temperature (23° C ± 2° C) for 18 ± ½ hours, or at 37° C for 6 hours.

8. Using Kallestad viewer or ruler, measure the diameter of the cleared area around each well to the nearest 0.1 mm. All wells should be read in the same order in which they were filled, and using the same length of time, as fluctuations in time may adversely affect the results.

9. Plot the concentration (y-axis) vs. the zone diameter (x-axis) of the three standard solutions on the graph paper. Draw the best straight line between the points.

10. Determine the concentration of the control and patient samples by plotting the zone diameter on the standard curve and reading the intersecting concentration. Check to ensure that control results are within acceptable range.

11. If a sample zone diameter measures larger than that of the highest standard, the procedure (steps 1 to 10) should be repeated following dilution of the sample in saline solution. Multiply the result obtained by the dilution factor.

REPORTING. Serum, urine, and tear samples are reported in μg/mL of lysozyme as determined by plotting on the standard curve.

NOTE: Samples with zone diameters smaller than that of the lowest standard are reported as less than the value assigned to that standard.

INTERPRETATION OF RESULTS. The normal range for serum is 4.8 to 13.0 μg/mL. The normal range for urine ranges from 0 to 2.0 μg/mL.

The coefficient of variation using the lysoplate method[3] ranges up to 10%.[4] Kallestad[2] reports up to 8.2% variation.

The accuracy of the lysoplate method appears related to agarose concentration, pH, ionic strength, temperature, and the concentration of buffer salts and proteins.[4] Greenwald and May[1] caution those using commercial lysoplates, after observing considerable lot-to-lot variability; however, Kallestad was not among those tested.

REFERENCES

1. Greenwald, R.A., and May, W.W., Clin. Chim. Acta, 73:299, 1976.

2. Insert Quantiplate, Lysozyme Test Kit, Kallestad Laboratories, 1977.

3. Osserman, E.F., and Lawlor, D.P., J. Exp. Med., 124:921, 1966.

4. Peeters, T.L., and Vantrappen, G.R., Clin. Chim. Acta, 74:217, 1977.

Chapter 13

HLA ANTIGENS

A cluster of genes known as the *major histocompatibility complex* (MHC) codes for molecules that regulate immune responses to the plethora of antigens in our environment. The products of these genes are called *major histocompatibility antigens* because of their ability to evoke a strong rejection response when present on tissue transplanted into a genetically disparate individual.

The MHC has been studied most extensively in the mouse and in humans. The murine MHC, present on chromosome 17, is referred to as the *H-2 complex*.[57,76,77,91] The MHC in humans is located on the short arm of chromosome 6, comprises approximately 1/1000 of the human genome, and is called the *HLA* (Human Leukocyte Antigen or Histocompatibility Locus Antigen) *complex* because of the initial discovery of human MHC antigens on leukocytes.[10,23,43,102,138,144]

Some minor histocompatibility antigens, which induce a weaker rejection response, have been identified in the mouse[69,77,87] and are also thought to be present in humans and other species, but for the most part, are not well characterized.

A simplified schematic diagram of the genes in the HLA complex is illustrated in Figure 13–1. The gene loci of the MHC and their encoded products are categorized into two major classes based on the structure, function, and location of the expressed antigens[10] (see below). HLA-A, HLA-B, and HLA-C are defined as *Class I* HLA loci, while the HLA-D region, located closest to the centromere, is the *Class II* HLA locus. The HLA-D region has been divided further into five subregions, designated as DP (formerly known as SB), DN (formerly, DZα or DOα), DO (formerly, DOβ), DQ (formerly, DC, MB, DS, or LB-E), and DR.[6,21,46,67] Each HLA-D subregion contains one or more A and/or B genes (formerly designated α and β, respectively)[46,67] (Fig. 13–1).

An additional Class I gene, designated HLA-E, has recently been identified between the HLA-C and HLA-A loci.[79] Genes coding for the complement components, C2, Factor B, and C4 (see Chap 6) and for the enzyme, 21-hydroxylase, are located between the HLA-D and HLA-B regions, and have been referred to by some investigators as Class III genes;[80,144] the significance of their linkage to the HLA complex is not known.

The HLA system continues to be under intensive investigation, and will inevitably undergo further nomenclature changes as new genes are discovered.

The antigens coded for by the Class I and Class II MHC genes bear a remarkable de-

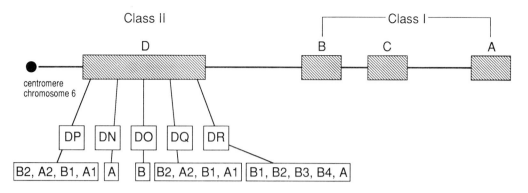

Fig. 13-1. HLA: The Major Histocompatibility Complex of Man.

gree of structural similarity to each other, to immunoglobulins, and to the T cell receptor, suggesting a common evolutionary origin of these molecules.[89,142,144] The molecules contain similar amino acid sequences, and distinct domains joined by disulfide bonds.

The HLA-A, B, and C antigens are comprised of a polymorphic glycoprotein chain (termed alpha, molecular weight 45,000), which is encoded by the MHC and noncovalently associated with beta-2-microglobulin, a 12-kilodalton protein encoded outside of the MHC (chromosome 15).[23,124,144] It was originally thought that these antigens were expressed by virtually all nucleated human cells, but subsequent studies have found that these determinants are not detectable on certain tissues, including sperm and trophoblast, and only weakly expressed by some other tissues.[28,41] Functionally, Class I antigens serve as recognition molecules for cytotoxic T lymphocytes[8,10] (see also Chap 1). The cellular expression of these antigens is increased in the presence of α, β, or γ interferon.[40,52,65]

The Class II antigens (the HLA-D or Ia molecules) are heterodimers consisting of an alpha chain (molecular weight 29 to 34 kilodaltons) noncovalently bound to a beta chain (molecular weight 25 to 28 kilodaltons).[10,124,144] The DP, DQ, and DR α/β heterodimers are coded for by a combination of one of the A genes, which codes for the

α polypeptide, and one of the B genes, which codes for the β portion of the molecule, in the respective D subregion[10,96] (Fig. 13-1). No protein product has been discovered for the DN or DO subregions, which contain only one A or one B gene, respectively.[10,96] The Class II antigens are more restricted in their tissue distribution as compared to the Class I antigens, but are not as limited as originally believed. HLA-D molecules have been known to be present on B lymphocytes, various cells of the macrophage lineage, and activated T lymphocytes, but more recent studies with monoclonal antibodies indicate that they are also widely (although not universally) distributed on endothelial cells throughout the body and on epithelial cells in a number of organs as well.[23,28,42,95,97] Gamma interferon has been shown to increase cell surface expression of the Class II antigens.[40,135] Functionally, Class II MHC antigens play a role in the presentation of antigen to T helper lymphocytes, which recognize antigen only when complexed with self Ia molecules[89,144] (see also Chap 1). The importance of both Class I and Class II molecules in immune responses is underscored by the severe immunologic impairment seen in the rare deficiency, Bare Lymphocyte syndrome,[35] which is characterized by the lack of expression of one or both types of MHC molecules.

The HLA system exhibits the most extensive polymorphism of any known human gene system.[10,144] Recognition of different specificities within this system has been made possible through the use of serologic and cellular typing reagents (see below) and most recently, molecular probes, and has been greatly aided by cooperation among investigators in a series of international collaborative workshops. At the 10th International Histocompatibility Testing Workshop, held in 1987, the number of allelles recognized for each HLA locus were as follows: HLA-A (24), HLA-B (52), HLA-C (11), HLA-D (26), HLA-DR (20), HLA-DQ (9), and HLA-DP (6).[46,67] By convention, antigens are assigned HLA A, B, C, or D numbers (e.g. HLA-A1, HLA-B5) when a consensus among international workers is reached on the definition of that antigen. Newly described antigens are given a provisional status, designated by a "w" (for workshop) before the allele number, until consensus is reached. Table 13–1 provides a complete listing of the HLA specificities recognized at the 1987 workshop.

Each individual possesses two chromosomes containing the MHC, and therefore, two alleles for each HLA locus, unless that individual is homozygous at any given locus. The mode of inheritance of these alleles is described in more detail below (see *Paternity Testing*).

HLA AND ORGAN TRANSPLANTATION

The importance of HLA antigens in clinical organ transplantation was recognized shortly after the discovery of the HLA system. Graft tissue containing MHC antigens different from those present in the transplant recipient can induce the generation of cytotoxic T lymphocytes and the formation of antibodies which mediate rejection of that graft[34,55,121] (see also Chap 1). These observations prompted the development of HLA typing techniques (see below) to match transplant recipients with HLA compatible donors. Individuals are routinely typed for HLA-A, B, C, and DR antigens by serological methods (see *Microcytotoxicity Test for HLA Antigens*, below). HLA-D types

can be determined, if desired, by performing a mixed lymphocyte culture (see below). Ideally, the donor and recipient would have the same MHC composition, but the extreme polymorphism characteristic of the MHC makes this a rare situation, except in the case of identical siblings.[15,56,94,103] Studies have thus been ongoing to determine the best possible protocol for matching despite inevitable HLA differences, and to reevaluate the significance of HLA testing in light of current immunosuppressive therapies.

Because the effects of HLA matching have been studied most extensively in renal transplantation, the following discussion will concentrate primarily in that area. Although initial studies reported a beneficial effect of HLA matching in kidney transplantation,[92,101] the results of more recent studies have not been as clear;[94,134] several investigators have reported a beneficial effect of HLA matching on graft survival,[3,56,98,103,115,140] but other investigators have observed little or no benefit in certain patient groups.[29,48,60,78,134] Results of these studies appear to be complicated by several other factors influencing graft survival, including age, sex, blood type and HLA phenotype of the recipient, pregraft blood transfusions, and type of immunosuppressive therapy received (reviewed in reference 134). With the recent success of cyclosporin therapy, some investigators have suggested that HLA matching is no longer necessary since high survival rates were achieved in their studies regardless of the degree of HLA match;[61,78,128] however, other investigators have reported that HLA matching positively influences the graft survival rate, even in cyclosporin-treated patients.[31,38,93,98] Overall the majority of multi- and single- center analyses suggest that matching for HLA-DR antigens produces the most pronounced beneficial effect on kidney graft survival, followed by matching for HLA-B antigens, and then HLA-A antigens;[94,134] maximum benefit appears to result from matching at both the DR and B loci.[94,134]

Table 13–1. Complete Listing of HLA specificities (1988)[a,b,c]

HLA-A	HLA-B	HLA-C	HLA-D	HLA-DR	HLA-DQ	HLA-DP
A1	B5	Cw1	Dw1	DR1	DQw1	DPw1
A2	B7	Cw2	Dw2	DR2	DQw2	DPw2
A3	B8	Cw3	Dw3	DR3	DQw3	DPw3
A9	B12	Cw4	Dw4	DR4	DQw4	DPw4
A10	B13	Cw5	Dw5	DR5	DQw5(w1)	DPw5
A11	B14	Cw6	Dw6	DRw6	DQw6(w1)	DPw6
Aw19	B15	Cw7	Dw7	DR7	DQw7(w3)	
A23(9)	B16	Cw8	Dw8	DRw8	DQw8(w3)	
A24(9)	B17	Cw9(w3)	Dw9	DR9	DQw9(w3)	
A25(10)	B18	Cw10(w3)	Dw10	DRw10		
A26(10)	B21	Cw11	Dw11(w7)	DRw11(5)		
A28	Bw22		Dw12	DRw12(5)		
A29(w19)	B27		Dw13	DRw13(w6)		
A30(w19)	B35		Dw14	DRw14(w6)		
A31(w19)	B37		Dw15	DRw15(2)		
A32(w19)	B38(16)		Dw16	DRw16(2)		
Aw33(w19)	B39(16)		Dw17(w7)	DRw17(3)		
Aw34(10)	B40		Dw18(w6)	DRw18(3)		
Aw36	Bw41		Dw19(w6)	DRw52		
Aw43	Bw42		Dw20	DRw53		
Aw66(10)	B44(12)		Dw21			
Aw68(28)	B45(12)		Dw22			
Aw69(28)	Bw46		Dw23			
Aw74(w19)	Bw47		Dw24			
	Bw48		Dw25			
	B49(21)		Dw26			
	Bw50(21)					
	B51(5)					
	Bw52(5)					
	Bw53					
	Bw54(w22)					
	Bw55(w22)					
	Bw56(w22)					
	Bw57(17)					
	Bw58(17)					
	Bw59					
	Bw60(40)					
	Bw61(40)					
	Bw62(15)					
	Bw63(15)					
	Bw64(14)					
	Bw65(14)					
	Bw67					
	Bw70					
	Bw71(w70)					
	Bw72(w70)					
	Bw73					
	Bw75(15)					
	Bw76(15)					
	Bw77(15)					
	Bw4					
	Bw6					

[a] From references 46 and 67

[b] Numbers in parentheses indicate broad specificities under which some of the HLA antigens are included; e.g. HLA-A23 is included under the HLA-A9 specificity

[c] The HLA-Bw4, Bw6, DRw52, and DRw53 antigens include multiple specificities, which are indicated in references 46 and 67

Problems of obtaining HLA-A and HLA-B matches may be alleviated by typing for public specificities (i.e. determinants that are common to more than one HLA antigen, and cross-react with typing antisera) rather than for private antigens, as suggested by some investigators who found that testing for public antigens resulted in better matched grafts.[115] Continued evaluation of factors such as these will likely improve graft survival and encourage the use of cost efficient approaches in renal transplantation. Ongoing studies should also provide a better understanding of the effects of HLA matching for transplantation of other tissues.

Transplantation of bone marrow may involve an additional problem. In this situation, the grafted tissue contains immunocompetent lymphocytes which may destroy host organs, resulting in graft-vs-host disease (GVH). Classically characterized by a skin rash, severe diarrhea and jaundice, GVH commonly occurs when an immunosuppressed individual receives immunocompetent cells, and has the potential of causing death.[55]

To avoid this problem, in addition to serologic typing for HLA antigens, a one-way mixed lymphocyte culture should be performed whereby the potential donor's lymphocytes are stimulated with lymphocytes from the recipient (see below); a low response is essential in order to avoid the occurrence of fatal GVH.[112] Recently, bone marrow transplantation using donors other than HLA-identical siblings has been made possible by depletion of immunocompetent T cells from the donor marrow using soybean lectin agglutination/rosette techniques or treatment with monoclonal antibodies and complement prior to transplantation.[14,55,108,109] However, transplantation of bone marrow so treated may result in a more limited engraftment associated with an increased incidence of infections.[55,99]

Preformed antibodies to donor HLA antigens, if present in a transplant recipient, can cause a rapid destruction of the graft tissue, a phenomenon known as hyperacute rejection.[55,121] Such antibodies are screened for by using the cross-match test (see below). A positive cross-match is a contraindication to transplantation.

PATERNITY TESTING

The application of HLA typing to paternity testing requires an understanding of the mode of inheritance of the HLA antigens, which follows the principles of simple Mendelian genetics. An individual contains two alleles for each of the HLA loci (HLA-A, B, C, and D (including D subregions)), because one chromosome containing the MHC is inherited from each parent. The alleles are codominantly expressed. Because they are closely linked, HLA-A, B, C, and D alleles are usually inherited as a single unit, known as a haplotype. An example illustrating the inheritance of HLA haplotypes is shown in Figure 13–2. In approximately 1% of cases,[121] recombination of chromosomes may occur during the formation of ova or sperm, resulting in the generation of a new haplotype which can be passed on to the child (e.g. a recombination of the maternal chromosomes in the example in Figure 13–2 might lead to the generation of the recombinant haplotype, A2, B12, Cw5, Dw7). Since the HLA loci are located in close proximity to each other, this is a rare occurrence.

The mode of inheritance described above makes HLA typing procedures useful in cases of disputed paternity, when used in conjunction with determinations of other inherited markers such as erythrocyte antigens (e.g. ABO, Rh, MNS), erythrocyte enzymes (e.g. adenosine deaminase, glucose-6-phosphate dehydrogenase), hemoglobin, and serum proteins (e.g. haptoglobin, Gm allotypes of IgG).[17] An accused male can be definitively excluded as a child's father if that child contains an HLA allele not present in either parent and/or if the child does not possess either of the two alleles for a given locus present in the al-

MOTHER

A2	B12	Cw5	Dw4
A23	B13	Cw8	Dw7

X

FATHER

A3	B7	Cw1	Dw2
A10	B21	Cw6	Dw15

Possible HLA Types of Children

1				2				3				4			
A2	B12	Cw5	Dw4	A2	B12	Cw5	Dw4	A23	B13	Cw8	Dw7	A23	B13	Cw8	Dw7
A3	B7	Cw1	Dw2	A10	B21	Cw6	Dw15	A3	B7	Cw1	Dw2	A10	B21	Cw6	Dw15

Fig. 13–2. Inheritance of HLA haplotypes: An example.

A *haplotype* is defined as a combination of alleles present on a single chromosome. In the illustration above, A2 is an example of an allele, while A2, B12, Cw5, and Dw4 is an example of a haplotype. The HLA alleles are inherited by simple Mendelian genetics, with each child receiving one maternal haplotype and one paternal haplotype. In the absence of chromosomal recombination, four different combinations of haplotypes are possible in the offspring. Thus, there is a 25% chance that two siblings will be HLA identical, a 25% chance that they will have nonidentical HLA types, and a 50% chance that they will be partially identical (i.e. share one haplotype).

leged father.[17] The case for exclusion is strengthened by repeat testing with different reagents on a fresh blood specimen, if possible, and by the finding of additional exclusionary genetic markers.[17]

If, however, the accused male possesses all of the HLA alleles present in the child that are not found in the mother, he will be included as a possible candidate for the child's true father. Such a finding is not definitive proof of paternity, however, because other males may also fit that description. Therefore, laboratory determinations of HLA alleles and other genetic markers are used to calculate the probability of paternity. These calculations are based on Mendel's First Law, the Hardy-Weinberg equilibrium principle, and probability theory, and consider the following factors: (a) the phenotypes of the mother, alleged father, and child, (b) the frequencies of the paternally-derived genes of the child in the population at large, and (c) estimates of the prior probability, based on the number of potential fathers and the frequency of encounters of each with the mother during the possible period of conception.[17,25] The estimated probability is most commonly ex-pressed in terms of the paternity index, defined as X/Y, where $X =$ the probability that the accused paternity is true, and $Y =$ the probability that the accused paternity is false.[17,25] Additional factors which need to be considered in special situations include linkage disequilibrium of compound loci such as HLA (see *HLA and Disease* below), consanguinity, and racial mixtures.[17,25]

HLA AND DISEASE

Through population and family studies, statistically significant associations between particular diseases and specific histocompatibility types have become apparent. The first association to be demonstrated was the linkage between susceptibility to virally-induced leukemias and specific H-2 types in mice.[85,86] This finding prompted a search for similar disease associations in man. The strongest association observed in humans is that between ankylosing spondilitis and HLA-B27:[27,119] approximately 90% of Caucasian patients with this disease possess the HLA-B27 antigen.[113,144] While other disease associations have not been as pronounced, over 50 diseases, the majority of which are autoimmune in nature, have been reported to possess statistically significant associations with particular HLA types.[90,144] A listing of some of the more well known disease associations can be found in Table 13–2.

HLA disease associations are commonly expressed in terms of a quantitative value known as the relative risk. *Relative risk* (RR) is defined as the number of times a disease occurs in individuals who possess a particular HLA antigen as compared to those who lack that antigen[104,126] and can be calculated by the following formula:[104,120]

$$RR = \frac{p^+ \times c^-}{p^- \times c^+}$$

where:

p^+ = number of patients with a given disease who have a specific HLA antigen

p^- = number of patients with a given disease who lack the HLA antigen

c^+ = number of controls without a given disease who have a particular HLA antigen

c^- = number of controls without a given disease who lack the HLA antigen

When performing the calculations, it is important to compare patients and controls of the same race, because the frequency of individual HLA antigens may vary significantly between different racial groups.[120] A relative risk equal to 1.0 indicates that the likelihood of developing a particular disease is the same in individuals with a particular HLA antigen as in individuals without that antigen.[104,120,126] An RR value greater than one indicates that individuals with a particular HLA antigen have a greater chance of developing a certain disease than individuals without that antigen; for example, an RR equal to 8.0 means that an individual with the pertinent HLA antigen is 8 times more likely to have the disease being evaluated than a person without that antigen. Estimated RR values for particular disease associations are given in Table 13–2.

Several hypotheses have been proposed to explain the mechanisms underlying HLA disease associations.[13,24,104,144] One hypothesis is that of molecular mimicry, or cross-reactivity between an infectious organism and an HLA antigen, resulting in inability of the host to respond to that pathogen. In support of this hypothesis is the reported cross-reactivity between the HLA-B27 an-

Table 13–2. HLA Associations with Disease[a]

HLA Antigen	Disease	Estimated Relative Risk
HLA-A3	Hemochromatosis	8
HLA-B27	Ankylosing spondylitis	87
	Reiter's disease	37
	Juvenile rheumatoid arthritis	3
	Anterior uveitis	10
HLA-Cw6	Psoriasis	13
HLA-DR2	Multiple sclerosis	4
	Narcolepsy	?
HLA-DR3	Systemic lupus erythematosus	6
	Graves' disease	4
	Myasthenia gravis	3
	Sicca syndrome	10
	Insulin-dependent diabetes[b]	8
HLA-DR4	Rheumatoid arthritis	5
HLA-DR5	Hashimoto's thyroiditis	3
	Pernicious anemia	5

[a] A partial list determined from studies on Caucasian populations; adopted from references 126 and 127. Note: variances will be seen in RR values obtained from different studies
[b] Associated with DR3, DR4, or both

tigen and *Klebsiella pneumoniae, Yersinia enterolitica,* and *Shigella flexneri.*[49,136] Alternatively, some HLA antigens may act as receptors for pathogenic organisms and thus play a key role in the establishment of infection. Another explanation for the association of HLA with disease states that structural modification of HLA antigens may occur as a result of their interaction with foreign agents, inducing an immune response against the modified antigens and subsequent development of disease. Yet another hypothesis states that HLA type determines which epitope(s) on an antigen will be recognized, and that individuals with particular diseases may bear HLA antigens which are unable to recognize a critical determinant of a pathogen, resulting in immunologic unresponsiveness and establishment of disease.[75] HLA Class II antigens may also be inappropriately expressed on target organs in patients with autoimmune diseases, stimulating an immune response to that organ.[13] Other hypotheses to explain the associations between HLA and disease have also been proposed,[13,75] and different mechanisms may be involved in different disease situations.[144]

Although HLA-disease associations appear to be a real phenomenon, they are not absolute: only a small percentage of individuals with a given HLA antigen actually develop a particular disease, and conversely, not all individuals with a particular disease possess the associated HLA antigen.[32,118] Possible factors which contribute to this lack of absolute association include the following:[118] association of a disease with a particular subtype of an HLA antigen, the heterogeneity of certain diseases, presence of a predisposing epitope on more than one HLA antigen, and the possible role of as yet undiscovered HLA antigens. In addition, combinations of two or more HLA antigens may be necessary to produce disease susceptibility.[118] Some haplotypes, e.g. B8, DR3, occur much more frequently in populations than expected from random association, a phenomenon known as *linkage dis-* equilibrium.[4,32,117] In some cases, the haplotype, rather than individual HLA alleles, may be responsible for the immune response produced against a given antigen; for example, certain haplotypes have been associated with unresponsiveness of some people to the hepatitis B vaccine.[39] Alternately, unidentified non-MHC genes linked to HLA genes may play a role in immune responsiveness.[104,118] Further studies will clearly be required to more completely elucidate the intriguing relationship between HLA and disease.

HLA TYPING

Microcytotoxicity Test for HLA Antigens

The microlymphocytotoxicity test is the standard method used for the typing of HLA A, B, C, and DR antigens.[5,44,70,129] The method involves incubation of live lymphocytes from the patient with a panel of antibodies known to be directed against particular HLA antigens (e.g. anti-A1, anti-B8). The addition of complement causes cytolysis when the cells are incubated in the presence of antibody of the appropriate specificity (e.g. when cells positive for HLA-A1 are incubated with anti-HLA-A1). Cytolysis is most commonly determined by dye exclusion: viability dyes such as eosin Y or trypan blue are excluded from live, intact cells, but enter through the damaged cell membranes of killed cells, which then appear stained under phase contrast microscopy. A high percentage of the cells tested will thus be stained in the presence of a typing serum specific for the antigens expressed by the cells.

The lymphocytotoxicity test is routinely performed as a micromethod, which was first introduced by Terasaki and McClelland in 1964,[130] and allows for the usage of small volumes of typing sera and patient cells. The HLA antisera are obtained primarily from multiparous women and transfusion or transplant patients, but may also be derived from volunteers after deliberate immunization.[44,70] After extensive testing, the antisera are placed in small wells of commercially available microtest trays, which can be stored frozen prior to use. It is desirable to use several antisera for the detection of each specificity, because of the cross-reactivity between some antigens and the limited availability of monospecific sera.[70] Several monoclonal HLA antibodies have been developed,[22,28,37,51,63] but many are unable to bind complement or have too limited a specificity for widespread use as typing reagents.[1,28] Monoclonal antibodies, however, have been invaluable tools in the biochemical characterization of new HLA antigens.[1,28,63]

Successful performance of the test also depends on the quality of the lymphocyte preparation: the mononuclear cell suspension obtained (fresh or stored frozen at −70° C) should have a high viability and be free from contamination with polymorphonuclear cells and platelets.[5,44,70] Typing for DR antigens requires the use of mononuclear cells enriched for B lymphocytes (e.g. by adherence to a nylon wool column and rosetting out of T lymphocytes), because T lymphocytes are mostly negative for this marker.[44]

Altered expression of HLA antigens on patient cells due to disease or drug therapy has been reported to have an effect on the test results.[70] In addition, cells homozygous for individual HLA antigens may exhibit stronger cross-reactions than heterozygous cells.[70]

Optimal cytotoxicity is best achieved by the use of rabbit serum as the source of complement.[44,70,107] The reading of cytotoxicity is most commonly performed by the use of vital dyes, as described above, but may also be accomplished by [51]chromium release, fluorochromasia, or electron microscopy.[44,107]

Although several minor modifications in the microcytotoxicity test have been implemented since its development in 1964, the basic test has remained the same. Details of these modifications and technical problems that may arise are described elsewhere.[44,70,107] (See also *Lymphocyte Microcytotoxicity Test*.) The success of this method is reflected in the results from the ASHI/CAP Histocompatibility Testing Program, which showed a greater than 90% consistency in the identification of most recognized HLA antigens among over 200 laboratories surveyed between 1981 and 1986.[47]

Mixed Lymphocyte Culture and Primed Lymphocyte Test

In 1964, Bain and co-workers observed that in vitro culture of leukocytes from two unrelated individuals resulted in the formation of blast cells undergoing mitosis and DNA synthesis.[12] This proliferative reaction was shown to be due to genetic differences between the leukocyte donors,[9,12] and served as a basis for the modern mixed lymphocyte culture (MLC).

In the MLC method,[44,45,107] lymphocytes (most commonly peripheral blood mononuclear cells) from two individuals are cultured in round bottomed microtiter plates[62] under sterile conditions for a period of 6 to 7 days. Reactivity of one donor's lymphocytes to alloantigens on cells from the other donor is selectively detected by a one-way MLC:[11,71] lymphocytes from one of the individuals are treated with sublethal irradiation or mitomycin-C prior to culture in order to block DNA synthesis, and therefore, proliferation of that cell population. The one-way MLC is set up as follows:

Lymphocytes from Individual A + (Responder cells)	Lymphocytes from Individual B (X-irradiated or Mitomycin-C treated) (Stimulator cells)

The untreated cells that are stimulated to proliferate are called responder cells; these have been characterized as T lymphocytes[30,50,64,108] and require the accessory function provided by cells of the monocyte/macrophage lineage[19] (see Chap 8). The proliferative response is stimulated primarily by differences in the HLA-D antigens of the lymphocyte donors,[7,9,30] although significant proliferation has been observed in some cultures of lymphocytes from HLA-D- identical individuals, suggesting that other antigens are involved in stimulation as well.[26] The X-irradiation or mitomycin-C—treated cells capable of providing this stimulation are called stimulator cells, and include B lymphocytes, monocytes, and activated T lymphocytes;[111,137] epithelial cells,[81] endothelial cells,[66] sperm cells,[84] and cells from certain tissues[114] may also provide stimulation.

Proliferation is most commonly measured by detecting the incorporation of radiolabeled (^{3}H) thymidine by the cultured cells: cultures are labeled with tritiated thymidine on approximately day 5 and incubated for an additional 12 to 18 hours. The cells are then harvested onto glass fiber discs using a cell harvester. The radioactivity retained by the glass fiber discs is determined by liquid scintillation counting and is proportional to the amount of cell proliferation. The results are expressed in terms of the *Stimulation Index* (SI) or *Relative Response* (RR) as follows:[45]

$$SI = \frac{\text{cpm from test culture}}{\text{cpm from autologous culture}}$$

$$RR = \frac{\text{cpm from test culture} - \text{cpm from autologous culture}}{\text{cpm from control culture} - \text{cpm from autologous culture}}$$

where: cpm = counts per minute

test culture = responder cells incubated with stimulator cells from a different individual

autologous culture = responder cells incubated with stimulator cells from the same individual

control culture = responder cells incubated with stimulator cells from an unrelated control individual or a pool of unrelated control individuals, all previously HLA typed

(See also *Mixed Lymphocyte Culture* below)

Traditionally, the test has been used to define new HLA-D alleles and to determine the HLA-D type of an individual by the use of homozygous typing cells (HTC)[132] as stimulator cells. HTC contain two identical HLA-D alleles (e.g. HLA-Dw1, Dw1). A low amount of proliferation indicates that the responder cells tested contain the same HLA-D antigens as the HTC; a high degree of proliferation indicates that the responder cells possess HLA-D antigens different than those of the HTC. Because HTC are obtained primarily from offspring of first cousin marriages or offspring of parents with HLA identical haplotypes,[44,45] they are precious reagents and are not used on a routine basis.

As an alternative to HTC, the primed lymphocyte typing test (PLT) may be used.[44,63] In this procedure, lymphocytes primed to certain HLA antigens are generated by culture for 9 to 10 days in a MLC with stimulator cells which differ from the responder cells by one HLA haplotype. The responder cells are then collected and cryopreserved for use at a later date; upon subsequent incubation with stimulator cells that possess HLA antigens contained on the original stimulator cells, the primed cells undergo accelerated proliferation, allowing results to be obtained within 1 to 3 days. This response has been shown to be stimulated primarily by differences in HLA-D, DR, and DP antigens,[53,63] although HLA-A and B antigens may also provide some stimulation.[125,146] Cells responding to one HLA determinant may be produced by cloning the primed cells.[63]

Because the MLC and PLT are labor intensive procedures with a long result turn around time, they are not often performed in routine laboratories to type HLA-D antigens. Instead, many laboratories type HLA-DR antigens by the microcytotoxicity method (see above), since a high correlation has been discovered between HLA-D and DR types (e.g. an individual who is HLA-DR3 positive will also be HLA-Dw3 positive).[2,16,100,106,139,141] However, as more has been discovered about the HLA system, disparities between HLA-DR typing and MLC reactivity have been revealed, particularly among non-Caucasoid populations.[53,96,122] For example, individuals typed as HLA-DR4 may be either HLA-Dw4, Dw10, Dw13, or Dw15 as defined by MLC.[67,96] A complete listing of currently defined HLA-D and DR relationships can be found in reference 67.

The MLC has also been useful in organ transplantation, especially in the testing of living related donors. The recipient's lymphocytes may be incubated with stimulator cells from potential donors in order to assess donor compatibility. Conversely, incubation of the donor's lymphocytes with stimulator cells from the recipient can be used to predict graft-vs-host disease in bone marrow transplantation. Several studies have noted increased survival of renal grafts when MLC reactivity was low.[59,82,105] The value of the MLC in predicting graft survival continues to be evaluated in light of new immunosuppressive therapies such as cyclosporin.[58]

Cross-Match Test: Screening for HLA Antibodies

Performance of the lymphocyte cross match test is essential to detect the presence of preformed HLA antibodies in future transplant recipients. Such antibodies, induced by prior exposure through situations such as multiparity or previous transfusions or transplants, are capable of causing accelerated or "hyperacute" graft rejection upon reaction with the appropriate HLA antigens on graft tissue.[55,74,121,143]

The routine procedure for the cross-match test is similar to the complement-mediated microcytotoxicity test for HLA antigens (see above), except that screening for HLA antibodies is performed by incubating the patient's serum with a panel of lymphocytes of known HLA types. The test results may be influenced by a number of factors, including incubation time, wash steps, handling or preparation of cells, source of complement, and use of an antiglobulin reagent to increase sensitivity.[116] More sensitive methods of detecting HLA antibodies, such as flow cytometry,[33,54,83,131] ^{51}Cr-release,[72,88] or antibody-dependent cell-mediated cytotoxicity,[73] have also been developed, but their clinical usefulness needs to be more completely evaluated.[116]

Presence of cytotoxicity in the cross-match test is a contraindication to transplantation of donor tissue containing HLA antigens to which the patient's antibodies are directed. Patients should be monitored regularly (e.g. monthly) while waiting for a transplant, since HLA antibody status may fluctuate with time.[145]

Differentiation between alloantibodies and autoantibodies may be accomplished by testing binding activities of the sera over a range of temperatures and by testing sera adsorbed with autologous and donor cells.[58]

The cross-match test can also be used to identify sera containing HLA antibodies for use as typing reagents.[107,145]

See also *Cytotoxic Antibody Screening.*

Future Trends: Restriction Fragment Length Polymorphisms (RFLP)

Identification of HLA types by nucleic acid hybridization is an area currently being investigated.[20,36,68] In this method, DNA is extracted, cleaved with restriction endonuclease enzymes, and identified by hybridization to DNA or RNA probes from a particular gene by Southern blotting.[18,123] The resulting patterns of restriction endonuclease fragments (polymorphisms) are analyzed, and may someday be characterized extensively enough for use in defining specific HLA genotypes and phenotypes in the routine typing laboratory.[67,120]

REFERENCES

1. Albrecht, J., and Muller, H.A.G.: Clin. Chem., 33:1619, 1987.

2. Albrechtsen, D., Solheim, B.G., and Thorsby, E.: Scand. J. Immunol., 6:419, 1977.

3. Albrechtsen, D. et al.: Transpl. Proc., 13:924, 1981.

4. Alper, C.A., Awdeh, Z., and Yunis, E.J.: Hum. Immunol., 15:366, 1986.

5. American Association of Blood Banks: *Technical Manual.* 9th ed. Arlington, American Association of Blood Banks, 1985.

6. Bach, F.H.: Immunol. Today, 6:89, 1985.

7. Bach, F.H., and Amos, D.B.: Science, 156:1506, 1967.

8. Bach, F.H., Bach, M.L., and Sondel, P.M.: Nature, 259:273, 1976.

9. Bach, F., and Hirschorn, K.: Science, 143:813, 1964.

*10. Bach, F.H., and Sachs, D.H.: N. Engl. J. Med., 317:489, 1987.

11. Bach, F., and Voynow, N.K.: Science, 153:545, 1966.

12. Bain, B., Vas, M.R., and Lowenstein, L.: Blood, 23:108, 1964.

13. Batchelor, J.R., and McMichael, A.J.: Brit. Med. Bull., 43:156, 1987.

14. Beatty, P.G. et al.: N. Engl. J. Med., 313:765, 1985.

15. Beatty, P.G. et al.: Transplantation, 45:714, 1988.

16. Berg, B., and Ringden, O.: Transplantation, 33:291, 1982.

17. Bias, W.B., and Zachary, A.A.: In *Manual of Clinical Laboratory Immunology.* 3rd ed. Edited by N.R. Rose, H. Friedman, and J.L. Fahey. Washington D.C., American Society for Microbiology, 1986.

18. Biro, P.A., and Glass, D.: In *Manual of Clinical Laboratory Immunology,* 3rd ed. Edited by N.R. Rose, H. Friedman, and J.L. Fahey. Washington D.C., American Society for Microbiology, 1986.

19. Blomgren, H.: Scand. J. Immunol., 6:857, 1977.

20. Bodmer, J. et al.: Proc. Natl. Acad. Sci., 84:4596, 1987.

21. Bodmer, J., and Bodmer, W.: Immunol. Today, 5:251, 1984.

22. Bodmer, J.G. et al.: In *Histocompatibility Testing.* Edited by E.D. Albert et al. New York, Springer Verlag, 1984.

*23. Bodmer, W.F.: J. Clin. Pathol., 40:948, 1987.

24. Bodmer, W.F., and Bodmer, J.G.: Br. Med. Bull., 34:309, 1978.

25. Borowsky, R.: Am. J. Hum. Genet., 42:132, 1988.

26. Bradley, B.A., and Festenstein, H.: Br. Med. Bull., 34:223, 1978.

27. Brewerton, D.A. et al.: Lancet, 1:904, 1973.

28. Brodsky, F.M. et al.: Immunol. Rev., 47:3, 1979.

29. Busson, M. et al.: Transplantation, 38:227, 1984.

30. Cantor, H., and Boyse, E.A.: J. Exp. Med., 141:1376, 1975.

31. Cats, S. et al.: N. Engl. J. Med., 311:675, 1984.

32. Chaplin, D.D., and Kemp, M.E.: Year in Immunol., 3:179, 1988.

33. Chapman, J.R. et al.: Transpl. Proc., 17:2480, 1985.

34. Cheung, K. W.-K., and Boral, L.I.: Lab. Management, p. 61, March, 1986.

35. Clement, L.T. et al.: J. Clin. Invest., 81:669, 1988.

36. Cohen, D. et al.: Proc. Natl. Acad. Sci. U.S.A., 81:7870, 1984.

37. Colombani, J. and Lepage, V.: Tissue Antigens, 24:209, 1984.

38. Cook, D.J., and Terasaki, P.I.: Transplant Proc. 20 (Suppl. 3):244, 1988.

39. Craven, D.E. et al.: Ann. Intern. Med., 105:356, 1986.

40. Cresswell, P.: Br. Med. Bull., 43:66, 1987.

41. Daar, A.S. et al.: Transplantation, 38:287, 1984.

42. Daar, A.S. et al.: Transplantation, 38:293, 1984.

43. Dausset, J.: Acta Haematol., 20:156, 1958.

*44. Dick, H.M., and Kissmeyer-Nielsen, F.K.: *Histocompatibility Techniques,* Amsterdam, Elsevier/North Holland Biomedical Press, 1979.

45. Dubey, D.P., Yunis, I., and Yunis, E.J.: In *Manual of Clinical Laboratory Immunology,* 3rd ed. Edited by N.R. Rose, H. Friedman, and J.L. Fahey. Washington D.C., American Society for Microbiology, 1986.

46. Dupont, B., ed.: *Histocompatibility Testing,* New York, Springer Verlag, 1988.

47. Duquesnoy, R.J., Marrari, M., and Walker, R.H.: Arch. Pathol. Lab. Med., 111:1101, 1987.

48. Dyer, P.A. et al.: Transpl. Proc., 15:137, 1983.

49. Ebringer, A., Baines, M., and Ptaszynska, T.: Immunol. Rev., 86:101, 1985.

50. Engleman, E.G. et al.: J. Exp. Med. 153:193, 1981.

51. Fauchet, R. et al.: In *Histocompatibility Testing.* Edited by E.D. Albert et al. Heidelberg, Germany, Springer Verlag, 1984.

52. Fellous, M. et al.: Eur. J. Immunol., 9:446, 1979.

53. Festenstein, H., and Ollier, B.: Br. Med. Bull., 43:122, 1987.

54. Garovoy, M.R. et al.: Transplant Proc., 15:1939, 1983.

55. Garovoy, M.R. et al.: In *Basic and Clinical Immunology.* 6th ed. Edited by D.P. Stites, J.D. Stobo, and J.V. Wells. Norwalk, Appleton and Lange, 1987.

56. Gilks, W.R. et al.: Transplantation, 43:669, 1987.

57. Gorer, P.A., Lyman, S., and Snell, G.D.: Proc. R. Soc. Lond., *135*:499, 1948.

58. Hansen, J.A. et al.: In *Manual of Clinical Laboratory Immunology*. 3rd ed. Edited by N.R. Rose, H. Friedman, and J.L. Fahey. Washington D.C., American Society for Microbiology, 1986.

59. Harmon, W.E. et al.: J. Immunol., *129*:1573, 1982.

60. Harris, K.R. et al.: Lancet, *2*:802, 1985.

61. Harris, K.R. et al.: Transplant. Proc., *17*:42, 1985.

62. Hartzman, R.J. et al.: Transplantation, *11*:268, 1971.

63. Hartzman, R.J., and Sheehy, M.J.: In *Manual of Clinical Laboratory Immunology*. 3rd ed. Edited by N.R. Rose, H. Friedman, and J.L. Fahey. Washington D.C., American Society for Microbiology, 1986.

64. Hayry, P. et al.: Transplant. Rev., *12*:91, 1972.

65. Heron, I., Hokland, M., and Berg, K.: Proc. Natl. Acad. Sci. U.S.A., *75*:6215, 1978.

66. Hirschberg, H. et al.: Transplantation, *19*:191, 1975.

*67. HLA Nomenclature Committee: Tissue Antigens, *32*:177, 1988.

68. Hyldig-Nielsen, J.J. et al.: Proc. Natl. Acad. Sci. U.S.A., *84*:1644, 1987.

69. Johnson, L.L., Bailey, D.W., and Mobraaten, L.E.: Immunogenetics, *14*:63, 1981.

70. Joysey, V.C., and Wolf, E.: Br. Med. Bull., *34*:217, 1978.

71. Kasakura, S., and Lowenstein, L.: J. Immunol., *101*:12, 1968.

72. Kerman, R., et al.: Transplant. Proc., *16*:1430, 1984.

73. Kirchoff, C., et al.: Transplant. Proc., *13*:1565, 1981.

74. Kissmeyer-Nielsen, et al.: Lancet, *2*:662, 1966.

75. Klein, J.: Adv. Exp. Biol. Med., *225*:1, 1987.

76. Klein, J.: J. Pediatr., *111*:996, 1987.

77. Klein, J., Figuerosa, F., and David, C.S.: Immunogenetics, *17*:553, 1983.

78. Klintmalm, G. et al.: Transplant Proc., *17*:1026, 1985.

79. Koller, B.H. et al.: J. Immunol., *141*:897, 1988.

80. Lachmann, P.J., and Hobart, M.J.: Br. Med. Bull., *34*:247, 1978.

81. Lane, J.T.L., Jackson, L., and Ling, N.R.: Transplantation, *19*:250, 1975.

82. Langhoff, E. et al.: Transplantation, *39*:18, 1985.

83. Lazda, V.A.: Transplantation, *45*:562, 1988.

84. Levis, W.R., Whalen, J.J., and Sherins, R.J.: Science, *191*:302, 1976.

85. Lilly, F.: Genetics, *53*:529, 1966.

86. Lilly, F.: J. Exp. Med., *127*:465, 1968.

87. Loveland, B., and Simpson, E.: Immunol. Today, *7*:223, 1986.

88. Lucas, Z.J. et al.: Transplantation, *10*:522, 1970.

89. Marrack, P., and Kappler, J.: Sci. Am., p. 36, February, 1986.

90. McDevitt, H.O.: Hosp. Pract. p. 57, July 15, 1985.

91. Melief, C.: Immunol. Today, *4*:58, 1983.

92. Morris, P.J. et al.: Lancet, *2*:803, 1968.

93. Morris, P.J. et al.: Lancet, *1*:98, 1984.

*94. Morris, P.J. et al.: Br. Med. Bull., *43*:184, 1987.

95. Natali, P.G. et al.: Transplantation, *31*:75, 1981.

96. Nepom, G.T.: Concepts Immunopathol., *5*:80, 1988.

97. Nixon, D.F., Pan-Yun Ting, J., and Frelinger, J.: Immunol. Today, *3*:339, 1982.

98. Opelz, G.: Transplantation, *40*:240, 1985.

99. O'Reilly, R.J. et al.: Vox Sang, *51* (suppl 2):81, 1986.

100. Park, M.S. et al.: Scand. J. Immunol., *6*:413, 1977.

101. Patel, R., Mickey, M.R., and Terasaki, P.I.: N. Engl. J. Med., *279*:501, 1968.

102. Payne, R., et al.: Cold Spring Harb. Symp. Quant. Biol., *29*:285, 1964.

103. Persijn, G.G. et al.: N. Engl. J. Med., *307*:905, 1982.

104. Peter, J.B., and Hawkins, B.R.: Diagnostic Med., p. 1, Jan/Feb, 1981.

105. Pineda, A.A. et al.: Transplantation, *29*:97, 1980.

106. Radvany, R.M., and Vaisruts, N.: Transplantation, *38*:347, 1984.

107. Ray, J.G., et al. (eds): *NIAID Manual of Tissue Typing Techniques*. Bethesda, National Institute of Allergy and Infectious Diseases, National Institutes of Health, 1976.

108. Reinherz, E.L. et al.: Proc. Natl. Acad. Sci. U.S.A., *76*:4061, 1979.

109. Reisner, Y. et al.: Lancet, *2*:1320, 1980.

110. Reisner, Y. et al.: Lancet, *2*:327, 1981.

111. Rode, H.N., and Gordon, J.: Cell. Immunol., *13*:87, 1974.

112. Rodey, G.E. et al.: Transplantation, *17*:84, 1974.

113. Sachs, J.A., and Brewerton, D.A.: Br. Med. Bull., *34*:275, 1978.

114. Sakai, A. et al.: Transplant. Proc., *9*:629, 1977.

115. Sanfilippo, F. et al.: N. Engl. J. Med., *311*:358, 1984.

116. Sanfilippo, F.P. et al.: Am. J. Clin. Pathol., *87*:258, 1987.

117. Schaller, J.G., and Hansen, J.A.: Hosp. Pract., p. 41, May, 1981.

118. Schiffenbauer, J., and Schwartz, B.D.: Rheum. Dis. Clin. North Am., *13*:463, 1987.

119. Schlosstein, L. et al.: N. Engl. J. Med., *288*:704, 1973.

120. Schwartz, B.D.: In *Basic and Clinical Immunology*, 6th ed. Edited by D.P. Stites, J.D. Stobo, and J.V. Wells. Norwalk, Appleton and Lange, 1987.

121. Sell, S.: *Immunology Immunopathology and Immunity*. 4th ed. New York, Elsevier Science Publishing Co., Inc., 1987.

122. Smith, R.A., and Belcher, R.: Ann. Clin. Lab. Sci., *17*:318, 1987.

123. Southern, E.M.: J. Mol. Biol., *98*:503, 1975.

124. Strominger, J.L.: Br. Med. Bull., *43*:81, 1987.

125. Suciu-Foca, N., and Rubinstein, P.: Transplant. Proc., *9*:385, 1977.

126. Svejgaard, A.: In *Manual of Clinical Laboratory Immunology*, 3rd ed. Edited by N.R. Rose, H. Friedman,

and J.L. Fahey. Washington D.C., American Society for Microbiology, 1986.

127. Svejgaard, A., Platz, P., and Ryder, L.P.: Immunol. Rev., *70*:193, 1983.

128. Taylor, R.J. et al.: Transplantation, *38*:616, 1984.

129. Terasaki, P.I. et al.: Am. J. Clin. Pathol., *69*:103, 1978.

130. Terasaki, P.I., and McClelland, J.D.: Nature, *204*:998, 1964.

131. Thistlewaite, J.R. et al.: Transplant Proc., *18*:676, 1986.

132. Thorsby, E., and Piazza, A.: In *Histocompatibility Testing.* Edited by F. Kissmeyer-Nielson. Copenhagen, Munksgaard, 1975.

133. Thorsby, E. et al.: Transplant Proc., *9*:393, 1977.

*134. Ting, A., and Morris, P.J.: Tissue Antigens, *25*:225, 1985.

135. Trinchieri, G., and Perussia, B.: Immunol. Today, *6*:131, 1985.

136. van Bohemen, C.H.G., Grumet, F.C., and Zanen, H.C.: Immunology, *52*:607, 1984.

137. van Oers, M.H.J., and Zeijlemaker, W.P.: Cell. Immunol., *31*:205, 1977.

138. van Rood, J.J., and van Leeuwen, A.: J. Clin. Invest., *42*:1382, 1963.

139. van Rood, J.J. et al.: Scand. J. Immunol., *6*:373, 1977.

140. van Rood, J.J. et al.: Transplant. Proc., *17*:681, 1985.

141. Walford, R.L. et al.: Scand. J. Immunol., *6*:393, 1977.

142. Williams, A.F.: Immunol. Today, *8*:298, 1987.

143. Williams, G.M. et al.: N. Engl. J. Med., *279*:611, 1968.

*144. Yunis, E.J.: Am. J. Clin. Pathol., *89*:268, 1988.

145. Zachary, A.A.: In *Manual of Clinical Laboratory Immunology.* 3rd ed. Edited by N.R. Rose, H. Friedman, and J.L. Fahey. Washington D.C., American Society for Microbiology, 1986.

146. Zier, K.S., Braunsteiner, H., and Albert, E.D.: Tissue Antigens, *10*:163, 1977.

HLA Antigen Typing: Microcytotoxicity Test Procedure[1-5]

PRINCIPLE. To screen for the presence of HLA-A,B,C antigens, patient lymphocytes are reacted with a panel of specific HLA antisera in Terasaki trays. Complement is added, producing changes in the membrane permeability of those cells possessing HLA antigens to which the antisera is directed. After incubation, a supravital dye is added. Cells which have the appropriate antigen react with the antisera and will take up the dye, appearing as "dead" cells microscopically. Negative cells will not take up the dye and appear refractile and unstained under the microscope.

HLA-DR antigens are present on the B lymphocyte population. In order to detect these antigens, peripheral blood lymphocyte suspensions must be enriched for B lymphocytes. This can be accomplished by adhering B lymphocytes to nylon wool columns and subsequent elution. Resulting B lymphocyte suspensions are tested in a similar manner as above.

EQUIPMENT AND MATERIALS

1. Repeating dispensers (Hamilton) with 1 μl syringe, 2 μl syringe, 5 μl syringe

2. Rabbit complement ($-70°$ C freezer). There are different lots of complement for HLA-A,B,C and HLA-DR typing

3. 5% eosin dye (5 g per 100 ml of Hanks Balanced Salt Solution. Should be filtered before use.)

4. Buffered formalin (37% formaldehyde. Buffered to a pH of 7.4 with 10% NaOH or HCL. Must be filtered before using.)

5. 75 $\times$ 50 mm glass slides

6. 72 well Terasaki trays (Robbins Scientific), with 2 μl of mineral oil dispensed into each well

7. Nylon-wool-pretreated (Associated Biomedic Systems)

8. Plastic drinking straws (approximately 0.5 inches in diameter)

9. 50 ml tubes (Falcon)

10. DR typing trays (Gen-Trak Inc.)

11. 16 $\times$ 150 mm tube

12. Inverted phase contrast microscope with a 10$\times$ objective

13. Positive control sera - the positive control is made up of pooled antisera

14. Negative control sera - pooled human sera tested to be free of detectable cytotoxic antibody

15. HLA antisera panel (see *Preparation of Reagents*)

SPECIMEN COLLECTION AND PREPARATION. Specimen requirement is generally 5 to 10 ml of heparinized blood. Minimum volume is dependent on patient's lymphocyte count. Other types of anticoagulant may be used;

however, Ca^{++} and Mg^{++} free Hanks' Balanced Salt Solution must be substituted to prevent clotting. Blood must be kept at room temperature and used within 4 hours of collection.

PREPARATION OF REAGENTS. Preparation of trays - Dispense 2 μl of light weight mineral oil into each well of a Terasaki microtiter plate. With each plate perform appropriate positive and negative controls by placing 1 μl positive control antisera in well 1A and 1 μl negative control antisera in well 1B. Dispense 1 μl of each antiserum from the HLA panel into the appropriate well of the tray. Separate typing trays are prepared for DR antigen testing. Trays prepared in this fashion may be stored at $-70°$ C. HLA antisera panel used is determined independently by each laboratory. In our laboratory we utilize a 70 HLA antisera panel along with positive and negative controls.

PREPARATION OF NYLON WOOL COLUMNS

1. Approximately 0.1 g of nylon wool is soaked in Hank's balanced salt solution (HBSS) with 5% fetal calf serum (FCS) in a 50-ml tube.

2. One end of the plastic straw is sealed with a warm flat iron. (Sealing the flex of the straw is easiest.)

3. Pack nylon wool into the straw to a length of approximately 4 cm. Do not pack nylon wool too tightly.

4. Add approximately 1 to 2 ml of HBSS with 5% FCS to the end of the column to keep it moist.

5. Straws may be stored frozen at $-20°$ C until they are used.

6. Thaw and prewarm column by incubating at $37°$ C for 30 minutes just prior to adding cells.

PROCEDURE

HLA-A,B,C Typing

1. Remove and thaw HLA antisera tray just prior to use.

2. Prepare mononuclear cells (see *Ficoll Hypaque Separation of Mononuclear Cells from Peripheral Blood*) from patient's whole peripheral blood. Adjust lymphocyte suspension to a concentration of 2×10^6 cells/ml in Hank's Balanced Salt Solution.

3. Thoroughly mix the lymphocyte suspension and with a 1-μl Hamilton syringe, add 1 μl of cell suspension to each well, being careful not to touch antisera with needle. Be sure antisera drop and cell drop are thoroughly mixed. Gently tap plate to mix.

4. Incubate the tray at room temperature for 30 minutes covered.

5. With a 5-μl Hamilton syringe, add 5 μl of rabbit complement to each well. Be sure all wells are mixed.

6. Cover and incubate at room temperature for 60 minutes.

7. With a 2-μl Hamilton syringe, add 2 μl of 5% eosin to each well.

8. After 2 minutes, gently add 5 μl of formalin to each well with a 5-μl Hamilton syringe.

9. Lower a clean 50 $\times$ 75 mm microscope slide onto the wells to flatten the tops of the droplets. There will be some running over of the fluid in the wells to the spaces on the plate between the wells.

10. Read plates with an inverted phase contrast microscope with a 10$\times$ objective. Living lymphocytes are small and refractile, whereas "dead" lymphocytes are larger, non-refractile, and appear darker in color. The background will appear orange. Cells tend to settle out to the periphery of the wells.

11. Observe the percentage of viable cells in the control wells and read the other wells according to whether a similar percentage of cells are killed. Score the percentage of dead cells.

DR Typing

1. Cut a small notch in the sealed end of straw so that it drips at the rate of about 2 to 5 ml/minute.

2. Holding column vertically add cells (suspended in 0.5 ml of HBSS with 5% FCS from step 2 of HLA-A,B,C typing) to the top of the column and allow to run into the nylon wool.

3. When cell-containing fluid has just completely run into the nylon wool, immediately turn the column horizontally.

4. Add approximately 1 ml of HBSS with 5% FCS to the end of the column to keep it moist.

5. Incubate at $37°$ C for 30 minutes in a horizontal position.

6. Place the column vertically over a 50-ml centrifuge tube and collect the non-adherent cells by allowing 20 ml of HBSS with 5% FCS to drip through the column. These cells may be centrifuged and resuspended in HBSS (1 ml HBSS with 5% FCS).

7. In a 16 $\times$ 150 mm tube, recover the B lymphocyte rich adherent cells by adding 3 to 5 ml of HBSS with 5% FCS to the column and

squeezing the straw vigorously in the area of the nylon wool while the media is running through.

8. Centrifuge the tube containing adherent cells at 200 × g for 10 minutes. Decant and resuspend cell button in 1.0 ml of HBSS with 5% FCS.

9. Perform cell count. Adjust cell count to 1.5 × 10⁶ cells/ml (1500 cells per mm³) for DR typing.

10. Continue as in step 3 of HLA-A,B,C with the following modifications: Step 4 - incubate at 37° C for 60 minutes, and Step 6 - incubate at room temperature for 120 minutes.

REPORTING. Score percentage of dead cells as follows:

1 = negative reaction in which the viability is the same as the negative control. Approximately 0 to 10% of the cells are dead.

2 = doubtful negative reaction with a detectable change in viability over the negative control. Approximately 10 to 20% more positive than the negative control.

4 = doubtful positive reaction with a detectable change. Approximately 50% of the cells are dead.

6 = positive reaction clearly different from the controls. 60 to 80% of the cells are dead.

8 = strong positive reaction with essentially all cells killed similar to positive control. Greater than 80% of the cells are dead.

0 = if no reading of the well can be made. Report positive antigen reactions for each patient.

INTERPRETATION OF RESULTS. HLA phenotype determination is based on the reaction of cells with the antisera for a given antigen. The reactions for the HLA-A,B,C specificities on the patient's cells are graded. Each HLA-A,B,C and HLA-DR antigen should be defined either by three antisera or by two monospecific antisera and their splits.

Cross-reactivity of antisera is common, therefore sufficient antisera combinations should be included to determine true reactivity versus cross-reactivity. Usually the reaction of an antiserum is strongest with

its homologous antigen and less so with cross-reacting antigens.

The positive control should demonstrate a 6 or 8 reaction. The negative control serum should demonstrate a 1 or 2 reaction. If the controls do not read as above, the typing must be repeated.

LIMITATIONS OF THE PROCEDURE

1. The accuracy of the procedure depends on the purity of the lymphocyte suspension used. If there is any degree of granulocyte contamination, this may lead to false-positive results.

2. Too large an amount of platelet contamination will lead to false-negative reactions. Platelets have HLA antigens and may neutralize the antisera within a well.

3. If the lymphocyte count of the cell suspension used is too high, false-negative reactions may occur.

4. Accurate readings cannot be obtained when the background positive reactions are too high. Any cell suspension that has more than 20% non-viable cells should not be used for screening.

5. Any typing which is inconclusive should be repeated with an alternate source of antisera.

6. Because even weak positive reactions may be significant in HLA-DR typing, the B lymphocyte suspension must have a viability as close to 100% as possible. Prompt handling of all specimens for HLA-DR typing ensures maximum viability.

7. In HLA-DR typing any reaction greater than a grade 2 reaction should be considered a positive reaction.

8. Because some lots of complement may be cytotoxic to B lymphocytes, complement should be pre-tested against known B lymphocyte suspensions using known HLA-DR antisera.

9. Nylon wool must be packed loosely enough in the straw so fluid drips rather quickly through it.

10. The many steps involved in the HLA-DR separation procedure provide an easy opportunity for bacterial contamination of the resulting B cell suspension. Hence these

cells should be tested immediately and not stored overnight.

11. The HLA-DR procedure may be stopped overnight at the step immediately following elution of the column. Be sure to leave cells in *dilute* suspension for overnight storage at room temperature. Storage in media with antibiotics (i.e. RPMI 1640) is preferred.

12. HLA-DR plates should be read immediately and again 12 to 24 hours later for correct interpretation.

REFERENCES

1. Danilous, J. et al.: Eighth International Histocompatibility Workshop Newsletter #6, December, 1978.

2. Mittal, K.K., Mickey, M.R., Singal, D.P., and Terasaki, P.I.: Transplantation, *6*:913, 1968.

3. Ray, J.G. (Ed.): DHEW Publication No. (NIH) 78-545, p. 22, 1976.

4. Terasaki, P.I., and McClelland, J.D.: Nature, *204*:998, 1964.

5. Winchester, R.J. et al.: J. Exp. Med., *14*:74, 1975.

Mixed Lymphocyte Culture (MLC) Procedure[1,2]

PRINCIPLE. Lymphocytes from two allogenic individuals, when cultured together for a period of 6 days, will undergo blastogenic changes proportional to the degree of genetic difference between the two individuals. This stimulation may or may not reflect differences at the HLA-D locus. The degree of stimulation is measured by the incorporation of a radioisotope (tritiated thymidine) by the cells between the sixth and seventh days of culture. One-way stimulation is measured by irradiating the stimulating cell population, which allows this population of lymphocytes to act as viable stimulating cells while at the same time, rendering them incapable of responding to the foreign antigens of the other cell population.

EQUIPMENT AND MATERIALS

1. Normal human serum [NHS] (North American Biologicals), heat inactivated, and stored in aliquots of 2 ml in $-20°$ C freezer

2. Isopaque-Ficoll gradient (LSM) (Bionetics)

3. RPMI 1640 tissue culture media with glutamine (M.A. Bioproducts)

4. Penicillin-streptomycin mixture (5000 units per ml) 20-ml bottles stored frozen (M.A. Bioproducts)

5. Hepes Buffer (N-2 hydroxyethylpiperazine-N-2-ethanesulfonic acid)

6. 96 well microtiter plates (Costar Plastics), round bottom with covers

7. 100-μl, 50-μl, and 25-μl pipettor with sterile disposable tips

8. Sterile, disposable pasteur pipettes

9. Sterile, disposable serologic pipettes, (1 ml, 5 ml, and 10 ml)

10. Sterile, disposable 50-ml centrifuge tubes, plastic

11. Sterile, disposable 16 × 125 mm plastic screw top tubes

12. Pressure sensitive film (Falcon Plastics)

13. Gamma cell 1000 irradiator (Isomedix, Inc., with a cesium - 137 chloride source

14. Incubator set at 37°C, 5% CO_2

15. Tritiated thymidine (Amersham) 1 μCi/ml. The tritiated thymidine is diluted 1:25 in RPMI 1640 when it is received. It is then aliquoted into small tubes and stored frozen at $-80°$ C in the freezer

16. Multiple automated sample harvester (MASH)

17. Glass fiber strips

18. Liquid scintillation counter

19. Scintillation vials

20. BetaFluor liquid scintillation fluid

21. Pool 4 - a pool of lymphocytes from four selected unrelated donors is prepared, irradiated and frozen in aliquots in the vapor phase of liquid nitrogen. These cells are used as a stimulation control in the mixed lymphocyte culture test. They should produce "maximum" proliferation of the responder cells.

SPECIMEN COLLECTION AND PREPARATION. Twenty ml of heparinized blood from each person is required. If several individuals from the same family are to be tested against one another, more samples may be necessary from each person to allow for all possible combinations. Also 20 ml of heparinized blood is required from a control individual mismatched at the HLA-DR locus.

PREPARATION OF REAGENTS

NOTE: All work should be done in the biologic safety cabinet to ensure the sterility of the culture.

Hepes Buffer:

a. 23.8 g of Hepes Buffer are added to 50 ml of distilled water in a 100-ml flask.

b. pH to 8.1 with 3N or 4N NAOH. This usually requires about 20 to 25 ml

c. Q.S. to 100 ml in a 100-ml graduated cylinder.

d. Filter sterilize with a millipore filter.

e. Store in a sterile bottle at 4° C. Outdate is 6 months.

Culture Media:

a. To a 500-ml bottle of RPMI 1640 with glutamine, add 10 ml of penicillin-streptomycin solution.

b. Add 15 ml of Hepes Buffer.

c. Store at 4° C. Shelf life is 2 months when processed using sterile technique.

PROCEDURE

1. It is essential to maintain the sterility of solutions and cell suspensions throughout. Only sterile tubes, pipettes, and glassware should be used. Work in the biologic safety cabinet.

2. Mononuclear cells are separated by the following:

Blood is overlayered on approximately 10 ml of Isopaque — Ficoll gradient in a 50-ml centrifuge tube for each patient to be tested. The tubes are centrifuged at 400 × g (1500 rpm) for 30 minutes. (See also *Ficoll-Hypaque Separation of Mononuclear Cells from Peripheral Blood*)

3. Cells at the interface are transferred to a new 50-ml centrifuge tube.

4. Cells are washed twice with approximately 20 ml of culture media (200 g, 1000 rpm, 10 minutes).

5. Cells are resuspended in 2 ml of culture media.

6. Perform a cell count on the lymphocyte suspensions and adjust cell count to 4×10^6 cells/ml, (4000×10^3 cells/mm^3) for each suspension using culture media as diluent.

7. Perform a cell viability on each cell suspension including the unrelated control. Record the results.

8. Divide each cell suspension into two 16 × 125 mm tubes, labeling one R and one R_x, one D and one D_x, or one C and one C_x for each cell suspension. The R corresponds to the recipient, the D to the donor, and the C to the control. The tubes labeled with only the letter are the untreated cells and the tubes labeled with "x" are the cell suspensions which are to be irradiated.

9. The tubes labeled R_x, D_x, and C_x are irradiated with 5000 rads in the Gammacell irradiator. The time necessary to achieve 5000 rads is dependent on the age of the irradiation source. Use appropriate table to find the correct time to irradiate the specimens.

10. Set up microtiter plate in the following manner:

a. Thaw the appropriate number of tubes of normal human serum (NHS) for the size of the culture to be set up (one tube is required for three microtiter rows).

b. Dilute the NHS with the appropriate amount of culture media. This will vary for each lot of NHS, and is pretested by the manufacturer for correct dilution.

c. Add 100 μl of diluted NHS to each well of the microtiter plate to be used.

d. Cell suspensions are added to the microtiter plate according to the following pattern. Fifty μl of untreated cells and 100 μl of irradiated cells are added to each designated well.

Column (wells):	1,2,3	4,5,6	7,8,9
Row A	$\overline{RR_x}$	$\overline{DR_x}$	$\overline{CR_x}$
B	RD_x	DD_x	CD_x
C	RC_x	DC_x	CC_x
D	RP_x	P_x	

P = pool 4

If cells from more than one donor are to be tested, label them D_1, D_2, etc. and add the appropriate combinations to the above chart.

11. Cover the microtiter plate with a piece of pressure sensitive film being sure that each filled well is covered and sealed.

12. Incubate the culture at 37° C, 5% CO_2, for 5 days. The day the culture is set up is counted as day 0.

13. The culture is "pulsed" on day 5. Twenty-five μl (0.025 ml) of tritiated thymidine is added to each well of the microtiter plate. Thaw one or more tubes of diluted thymidine to pulse culture. Remaining thawed thymidine may be stored at 4° C for 1 or 2 days, then discarded. Be sure to discard all radioactive materials following appropriate radioactivity disposal protocols.

14. Recover the microtiter plate with a new piece of pressure sensitive film and reincubate the culture at 37° C, 5% CO_2, for 16 to 24 hours. Cultures should be pulsed in the afternoon of the fifth day and harvested in the morning of the sixth day.

15. Harvest culture on day 6 using a MLC harvester. Transfer glass fiber filter strips to scintillation vials containing 3 ml BetaFluor liquid scintillation fluid.

16. Read vials on liquid scintillation counter, for 1 to 2 minutes.

17. An unrelated third party control and the pool 4 control are always run with each MLC. Stimulation of the control (C) by R_x and D_x and stimulation of R and D by C_x must be sufficiently high (greater than 20,000 CPM) or the MLC should be repeated. The mean count of the triplicate wells is determined for each combination.

From this, a relative response value is calculated by the following formula:

$$RR = \frac{(R + D_x) - (R + R_x)}{(R + C_x) - (R + R_x)} \times 100$$

using the mean value for each combination.

18. Also, calculate a relative response value using the pool control value:

$$RR = \frac{(R + D_x) - (R + R_x)}{(R + P_x) - (R + R_x)} \times 100$$

REPORTING. Patients results are reported as relative response when compared to allogenic control.

INTERPRETATION OF RESULTS. Individuals who are HLA-D region compatible will show low values for the relative response (e.g. 0.05). Individuals who have higher relative response values (e.g. 0.7) are probably mismatched for some HLA-D locus antigens even if they are serologically HLA-DR identical.

LIMITATIONS OF THE PROCEDURE

1. This is a biologic assay and hence is subject to the variation seen in individuals when measured on subsequent days. The assay should be reproducible in terms of showing stimulation or nonstimulation between two people; however, relative response values may be somewhat different if the assay is repeated.

2. Sterility is essential. Contamination of the culture with bacteria will result in failure of cell growth, resulting in failure of positive control combinations to show stimulation.

3. Normal human serum source is critical. Some lots of NHS are cytotoxic to lymphocytes. Other lots do not support cell growth adequately. Some lots of NHS will result in high background values, as the sera itself will stimulate a small population of cells. Each lot of NHS should be tested before use.

4. Caution should be observed in interpreting results from cultures on leukemic patients with a high blast count. This may result in significantly high autologous combinations—e.g. $\geq 20,000$ CPM—making it impossible to interpret donor-recipient combinations.

5. Controls - autologous controls and positive stimulation controls (C and P) are necessary to ensure that the culture conditions were appropriate and that non-stimulation combinations of donor-recipient reflect true compatibility.

6. Unexpected results that do not coincide with HLA typing results should be confirmed by repeat testing of the mixed lymphocyte culture.

REFERENCES

1. Bach, F.H., and Hirschorn, K.: Science, *145*:1315, 1964.

2. Bain, B., Vas, M.R., and Lowenstein, L.: Blood, *23*:108, 1964.

Cytotoxic Antibody Screening Procedure[1,2]

PRINCIPLE. To screen for the presence of HLA antibodies, patient serum is reacted with a panel of mononuclear cells of known HLA types in Terasaki trays. Complement is added, producing changes in the membrane permeability of the cells possessing those HLA antigens to which the patient's antibodies are directed. After incubation, a supravital dye is added. Cells which have sustained membrane damage will take up the dye and appear as "dead" cells microscopically. Undamaged cells will not take up the dye and will appear refractile and unstained under the microscope.

EQUIPMENT AND MATERIALS
Reagents:

1. Repeating dispensers (Hamilton) with 1-μl syringe, 2-μl syringe, 5-μl syringe

2. Rabbit complement (−70° C freezer). There are different lots of complement for anti-HLA-A,B,C and anti-HLA-DR typing

3. 5% eosin dye (5 g per 100 ml of Hanks Balanced Salt Solution). (Should be filtered before use)

4. Buffered formalin (37% formaldehyde. Buffered to a pH of 7.4 with 10% NaOH or HCL. Must be filtered before using)

5. 75 × 50 mm glass slides

6. 72-well Terasaki trays (Robbins Scientific), with 2 μl of mineral oil dispensed into each well

7. Inverted phase contrast microscope with a 10× objective

8. Positive control sera—pooled human sera positive for HLA antibodies

9. Negative control sera—pooled human sera negative for HLA antibodies

10. Panel of mononuclear cells prepared from at least 20 individuals with known HLA types. Can be fresh or stored frozen

SPECIMEN COLLECTION AND PREPARATION

1. Clotted tubes are spun and serum is transferred to a 12 × 75 mm plastic tube labeled with the patient's name and the date (including the year). Specimen should be stored at −20° C.

2. Specimens to be tested for cytotoxic antibody should be *heat inactivated* at 56° C for 30 minutes prior to testing.

PREPARATION OF REAGENTS.

Preparation of trays—Dispense 2 μl of lightweight mineral oil into each well of a Terasaki microtiter plate. With each plate perform appropriate positive and negative controls by placing 1 μl positive control sera in well 1A and 1 μl negative control sera in well 1B. Dispense 1 μl of serum from each patient to be tested into one well of the tray. Trays prepared in this fashion may be stored at −70° C. It may also be desirable to test sera at a 1:2 dilution. Each tray contains serum from multiple patients. One mononuclear cell type from the panel is added to each tray.

PROCEDURE

1. Remove and thaw patient sera trays just prior to use.

2. Prepare mononuclear cells (See *Ficoll Hypaque Separation of Mononuclear Cells from Peripheral Blood*) from a lymphocyte panel of known HLA types, generally a panel of cells from at least 20 individuals are used (healthy, control individuals). Adjust lymphocyte suspension to a concentration of 2 × 10⁶ cells/ml in Hank's Balanced Salt Solution.

3. Thoroughly mix the lymphocyte suspension and with a 1-μl Hamilton syringe, add 1 μl of cell suspension to each well, being careful not to touch antisera with needle. Be sure antisera drop and cell drop are thoroughly mixed by gently tapping plate.

4. Incubate the tray at room temperature for 30 minutes covered.

5. With a 5-μl Hamilton syringe, add 5 μl of the appropriate rabbit complement to each well (see Equipment and Materials). Be sure all wells are mixed.

6. Cover and incubate at room temperature for 60 minutes.

7. With a 2-μl Hamilton syringe, add 2 μl of 5% eosin to each well.

8. After 2 minutes, gently add 5 μl of formalin to each well with a 5 μl Hamilton syringe.

9. Lower a clean 50 × 75 mm microscope slide onto the wells to flatten the tops of the droplets. There will be some running over of the fluid in the wells to the spaces on the plate between the wells.

10. Read plates with an inverted phase contrast microscope with a 10× objective. The cells tend to settle out to the periphery of the wells. Living lymphocytes are small and refractile, whereas "dead" lymphocytes are larger, nonrefractile, and appear darker in color against an orange background.

11. Observe the percentage of viable cells in the control wells and read the other wells according to whether a similar percentage of cells are killed. Score the percentage of dead cells.

REPORTING

Score percentage of dead cells as follows:

1 = negative reaction in which the viability is the same as the negative control. Approximately 0 to 10% of the cells are dead.

2 = doubtful negative reactions with a detectable change in viability over the negative control. Approximately 10 to 20% more positive than the negative control.

4 = doubtful positive reaction with a detectable change. Approximately 50% of the cells are dead.

6 = positive reaction clearly different from the controls. Sixty to 80% of the cells are dead.

8 = strong positive reaction with essentially all cells killed similar to positive control. Greater than 80% of the cells are dead.

0 = if no reading of the well can be made.

Report positive antibodies for each patient.

INTERPRETATION OF RESULTS. A positive reaction against a lymphocyte population indicates cytotoxic effect. Patients are determined to have cytotoxic antibodies if greater than 5% of the normal lymphocyte panel is positive. Cytotoxic effect is most likely due to HLA antibodies but other cytotoxic antibodies cannot be ruled out utilizing this procedure.

The positive control serum should demonstrate a 6 or 8 reaction. The negative control serum should demonstrate a 1 or 2 reaction. If the controls do not read as above, the typing must be repeated.

LIMITATIONS OF THE PROCEDURE

1. The accuracy of the procedure depends on the purity of the lymphocyte suspension used. If there is any degree of granulocyte contamination, this may lead to false-positive results.

2. Too large an amount of platelet contamination will lead to false-negative reactions. Platelets have HLA antigens and may neutralize the antisera within a well.

3. If the lymphocyte count of the cell suspension used is too high, false-negative reactions may occur.

4. False-negative reactions may occur when sera are tested undiluted. It is common practice to test patient's sera both undiluted and at a 1:2 dilution.

5. Accurate readings cannot be obtained when the background positive reactions are too high. Any cell suspension that has more than 20% non-viable cells should not be used for screening.

REFERENCES

1. Ray, John G. (Ed.): *Manual of Tissue Typing Techniques.* DHEW Publication No. (NIH) 78-545, p. 22, 1976.

2. Zachary, A.A., and Braun, W.E. (Eds.): New York, *The American Association for Clinical Histocompatibility Testing,* 1981.

Page numbers in *italics* indicate figures; numbers followed by "t" indicate tables.